GPC	glycophorin C	ITP	idiopathic thrombocytopenic purpura
GPD	glycophorin D	IV	intravenous
GTP	good tissue practice	IVP	intravenous push
GVHD	graft-vs-host disease	LAL	limulus amebocyte lysate
Gy	Gray	LDH	lactate dehydrogenase
HAV	hepatitis A virus	Lin⁻	lineage negative
HAZMAT	hazardous material	LT-CIC	long-term culture-initiating cells
Hb	hemoglobin	MAC	membrane attack complex
HBc	hepatitis B core antigen	MHC	major histocompatibility complex
HBIG	hepatitis B immunoglobulin	MLC	mixed lymphocyte (leukocyte) culture
HBsAg	hepatitis B surface antigen	MLR	mixed lymphocyte (leukocyte) reaction
HBV	hepatitis B virus	mmol	millimole [one thousandth (10^{-3}) of a mole]
Hct	hematocrit		
HCT/Ps	human cells, tissues, and cellular and tissue-based products	MNC	mononuclear cell
		MoAb	monoclonal antibody
HCV	hepatitis C virus	mOsm	milliosmole(s)
HES	hydroxyethyl starch	mRNA	messenger ribonucleic acid
HEV	hepatitis E virus	MSDS	material safety data sheet
HIV	human immunodeficiency virus	NAT	nucleic acid testing
HLA	human leukocyte antigen	NC	nucleated cell
HPC	hematopoietic progenitor cell	NIH	National Institutes of Health
HPC-A	HPCs from apheresis	NK	natural killer
HPC-C	HPCs from cord blood	NMDP	National Marrow Donor Program
HPC-M	HPCs from marrow	NRC	Nuclear Regulatory Commission
HSCT	hematopoietic stem cell transplantation	NS	normal saline
HTLV-I	human T-cell lymphotropic virus, type I	NT	not tested
HTR	hemolytic transfusion reaction	OQ	operational qualification
HVAC	heating, ventilation, and air conditioning	OSHA	Occupational Safety and Health Administration
i-ATP	intracellular ATP		
IBW	ideal body weight	Osm	osmole(s)
iCa	Ionized calcium	p	probability
IDE	investigational device exemption	PBS	phosphate-buffered saline
Ig	immunoglobulin	PBPC	peripheral blood progenitor cell
IVIG	Intravenous immunoglobulin	PBSC	peripheral blood stem cell
IL-1α	interleukin 1 alpha	PCR	polymerase chain reaction
IL-1β	interleukin 1 beta	PEG	polyethylene glycol
IL-2	interleukin 2	PHA	phytohemagglutinin
IND	investigational new drug	PHS	Public Health Service (Act)
INR	international normalized ratio	PMA	premarket approval
IQ	installation qualification	PNA	p-nitroanaline
ISBT	International Society of Blood Transfusion	PO	per os (Latin: by mouth)
		PPE	personal protective equipment
ISCT	International Society for Cellular Therapy	PPLO	pleuropneumonia-like organism
		PQ	performance qualification

PRN	pro re nata (Latin: for the existing occasion; as needed)	SCF	stem cell factor
		SG	specific gravity
PT	proficiency test; prothrombin time test	SOP	standard operating procedure
PulseOx	pulse oximetry	SPA	staphylococcal protein A
PVC	polyvinyl chloride	SQ	subcutaneous
QA	quality assessment or quality assurance	SSO	single-strand or sequence-specific oligonucleotide
QC	quality control	SSP	sequence-specific primer
QSE	quality system essential	STS	serologic test for syphilis
RBCs	Red Blood Cells (blood donor unit)	T	temperature
RFLP	restriction fragment length polymorphism	TBV	total blood volume
		TCR	T-cell receptor
Rh	Rhesus factor	TNCs	Total nucleated cells
RLU	relative luminescence units	TNF-α	tumor necrosis factor alpha
RNA	ribonucleic acid	tRNA	transfer ribonucleic acid
RPM	revolutions per minute	UCB	umbilical cord blood
RR	repeatedly reactive or relative risk	UNOS	United Network for Organ Sharing
RT	room temperature or reverse transcriptase	μM	micromolar
SBT	sequence-based technology	WHO	World Health Organization

Cellular Therapy:

Principles, Methods, and Regulations

♦ ♦ ♦

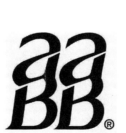

Other related publications available from the AABB:

Hematopoietic Stem Cell Transplantation: A Handbook for Clinicians
Edited by John R. Wingard, MD; Dennis A. Gastineau, MD; Helen L. Leather, B Pharm; Edward Snyder, MD, FCAP; and Zbigniew M. Szczepiorkowski, MD, PhD, FCAP

Standards for Cellular Therapy Product Services

Core Principles in Cellular Therapy
Edited by John D. Roback, MD, PhD

Circular of Information for the Use of Cellular Therapy Products

Cord Blood: Biology, Immunology, Banking, and Clinical Transplantation
Edited by Hal E. Broxmeyer, PhD

To purchase books or to inquire about other book services, including chapter reprints and large-quantity sales, please contact our sales department:
- 866.222.2498 (within the United States)
- +1 301.215.6499 (outside the United States)
- +1 301.951.7150 (fax)
- www.aabb.org>Bookstore

AABB customer service representatives are available by telephone from 8:30 am to 5:00 pm ET, Monday through Friday, excluding holidays.

Cellular Therapy:
Principles, Methods, and Regulations

Editor in Chief

Ellen M. Areman, MS, SBB(ASCP)
Biologics Consulting Group, Inc
Alexandria, Virginia

Associate Editor

Kathy Loper, MHS, MT(ASCP)
AABB
Bethesda, Maryland

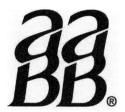

Mention of specific products or equipment by contributors to this AABB publication does not represent an endorsement of such products by AABB nor does it necessarily indicate a preference for those products over other similar competitive products.

AABB authors are requested to comply with a conflict of interest policy that includes disclosure of relationships with commercial firms. A copy of the policy is located at http://www.aabb.org.

Efforts are made to have publications of the AABB consistent with regard to acceptable practices. However, for several reasons, they may not be. First, as new developments in the practice of cellular therapy occur, changes may be recommended to the *Standards for Cellular Therapy Product Services*. It is not possible, however, to revise each publication at the time such a change is adopted. Thus, it is essential that the most recent edition of the CT Standards be consulted as a reference in regard to current acceptable practices. Second, the views expressed in this publication represent the opinions of the authors. The publication of this book does not constitute an endorsement by AABB of any view expressed herein, and the AABB expressly disclaims any liability arising from any inaccuracy or misstatement.

AABB
8101 Glenbrook Road
Bethesda, Maryland 20814-2749

ISBN 978-1-56395-296-8
Printed in the United States

Library of Congress Cataloging-in-Publication Data

Cellular therapy : principles, methods, and regulations / editors, Ellen M. Areman, Kathy Loper.
    p. ; cm.
Includes bibliographical references and index.
ISBN 978-1-56395-296-8
1. Cellular therapy. I. Areman, Ellen M., 1943- II. Loper, Kathy. III. AABB.
[DNLM: 1. Biological Therapy—standards—United States. 2. Biological Therapy—United States. 3. Biological Therapy—methods—United States. WB 365 C393 2009]

RM287.C386 2009
615.8'45—dc22

2009033309

Contributors

Brenda Alder, MS, MT(ASCP)SBB
Northside Hospital
Atlanta, Georgia

Julie G. Allickson, PhD, MS, MT(ASCP)
Cryo-Cell International, Inc
Oldsmar, Florida

Ellen Areman, MS, SBB(ASCP)
Biologics Consulting Group, Inc
Alexandria, Virginia

Karen Bieback, PhD
Institute for Transfusion Medicine and Immunology
University of Heidelberg
Mannheim, Germany

Eda Bloom, PhD
US Food and Drug Administration
Rockville, Maryland

Paula L. Brown, MT(ASCP), JD
University of Arkansas for Medical Sciences
Little Rock, Arkansas

Peter Bugert, PhD
Institute of Transfusion Medicine and Immunology
University of Heidelberg
Mannheim, Germany

Lizabeth Cardwell, MT(ASCP), MBA, RAC
Compliance Consulting
Seattle, Washington

Emer Clarke, PhD
ReachBio, LLC
Seattle, Washington

Philip H. Coelho, BSME
PHC Medical, Inc
Sacramento, California

Michele Cottler-Fox, MD
University of Arkansas for Medical Sciences
Little Rock, Arkansas

Melissa Croskell, MT(ASCP)
The Children's Hospital-Aurora
Aurora, Colorado

Herbert M. Cullis, MT
American Fluoroseal Corp
Gaithersburg, Maryland

Mary Dadone, PhD
Consultant
Annapolis, Maryland

Janice M. Davis-Sproul, MAS, MT(ASCP)SBB
Sidney Kimmel Comprehensive Cancer Center at Johns Hopkins
Baltimore, Maryland

Florinna Estioco Dekovic, MT(ASCP)BB, CQA(ASQ)
University of California-San Francisco
San Francisco, California

Meghan Delaney, DO
Puget Sound Blood Center
Seattle, Washington

Gary C. du Moulin, PhD, MPH
Genzyme Biosurgery
Cambridge, Massachusetts

Karen Edward, BS, MT(ASCP)
Advanced Cell and Gene Therapy, LLC
New York, New York

Julie Edwards, BS, MT(ASCP)
Sidney Kimmel Comprehensive Cancer Center
at Johns Hopkins
Baltimore, Maryland

Hermann Eichler, MD
Institute for Clinical Hematology and Transfusion Medicine
Saarland University Hospital
Homburg/Saar, Germany

Cynthia Elliott, MT, HP(ASCP), CQA(ASQ)
CT Auditing and Compliance Services, LLC
Sugar Hill, Georgia

Vicki Fellowes, MT(ASCP)
National Institutes of Health
Bethesda, Maryland

John Finkbohner, PhD
MedImmune, LLC
Gaithersburg, Maryland

Daniel H. Fowler, MD
National Institutes of Health
Bethesda, Maryland

Joyce L. Frey-Vasconcells, PhD
Pharmanet Consulting
Washington, District of Columbia

Nina K. Garlie, PhD
Aurora St Luke's Medical Center
Milwaukee, Wisconsin

John R. Godshalk, MSE, MBA
Biologics Consulting Group, Inc
Alexandria, Virginia

Nicholas Greco, PhD
Case Western Reserve University
Cleveland Cord Blood Center
Cleveland, Ohio

N. Rebecca Haley, MD
Duke Translational Medicine Institute
Durham, North Carolina

Karen M. Hall, MT(ASCP)
HemoGenix, Inc
Colorado Springs, Colorado

Liana Harvath, PhD
Liana Harvath, PhD, LLC
Rockville, Maryland

Terry O. Harville, MD, PhD
University of Arkansas for Medical Sciences
Little Rock, Arkansas

Richard L. Haspel, MD, PhD
Beth Israel Deaconess Medical Center
Boston, Massachusetts

Allison Hubel, PhD
University of Minnesota
Minneapolis, Minnesota

Betsy W. Jett, MT(ASCP), CQA, CQM/OE(ASQ)
National Institutes of Health
Bethesda, Maryland

Diane Kadidlo, MT(ASCP)SBB
University of Minnesota
St Paul, Minnesota

Grace S. Kao, MD
Dana-Farber Cancer Center
Harvard Medical School
Boston, Massachusetts

Safa Karandish, MT(ASCP)
Pall Life Sciences
Houston, Texas

Michael Keeney, FIMLS, FCSMLS(D)
London Health Sciences Centre
London, Ontario, Canada

Carolyn A. Keever-Taylor, PhD
Medical College of Wisconsin
Milwaukee, Wisconsin

Sarah Kennett, PhD
US Food and Drug Administration
Rockville, Maryland

Aisha Khan, MS, MBA
University of Miami Miller School of Medicine
Miami, Florida

Hanh Khuu, MD
National Institutes of Health
Bethesda, Maryland

Dave Krugh, MT(ASCP)SBB, CLS, CLCP(NCA)
OSU James Cancer Hospital and Solove Research Institute
Columbus, Ohio

Victoria A. Lake, BSc, BA, RAC
Fred Hutchinson Cancer Research Center
Seattle, Washington

Michael L. Linenberger, MD, FACP
Seattle Cancer Care Alliance
University of Washington
Fred Hutchinson Cancer Research Center
Seattle, Washington

Elina Linetsky, MSc, MT
University of Miami Miller School of Medicine
Miami, Florida

Kathy Loper, MHS, MT(ASCP)
AABB
Bethesda, Maryland

Amy McDaniel, PhD
Wyeth Biotech
Andover, Massachusetts

David H. McKenna, Jr, MD
University of Minnesota
St Paul, Minnesota

John D. McMannis, PhD
The University of Texas M.D. Anderson Cancer Center
Houston, Texas

Jeffrey S. Miller, MD
University of Minnesota Masonic Cancer Research Center
Minneapolis, Minnesota

Lynn O'Donnell, PhD
OSU James Cancer Hospital and Solove Research Institute
Columbus, Ohio

Daniel P. Offringa
The Biologics Consulting Group, Inc
Alexandria, Virginia

Jennifer L. Olson, PhD
Wake Forest University School of Medicine
Winston-Salem, North Carolina

Angela Ondo, MT(ASCP)
Sidney Kimmel Cancer Center at Johns Hopkins
Baltimore, Maryland

Douglas Padley, MT(ASCP)
Mayo Clinic
Rochester, Minnesota

Cynthia Porter, PhD
US Food and Drug Administration
Rockville, Maryland

Robert A. Preti, PhD
Progenitor Cell Therapy, LLC
Hackensack, New Jersey

Jo Lynn Procter, MEd, MT(ASCP)SBB
National Institutes of Health Clinical Center
Bethesda, Maryland

Donna Regan, MT(ASCP)
SSM Cardinal Glennon Children's Medical Center
St Louis, Missouri

Ivan N. Rich, PhD
HemoGenix, Inc
Colorado Springs, Colorado

Camillo Ricordi, MD
University of Miami Miller School of Medicine
Miami, Florida

Jerome Ritz, MD
Harvard Medical School
Dana-Farber Cancer Institute
Boston, Massachusetts

Tara Sadeghi, BS
MD Anderson Cancer Center
Houston, Texas

Elizabeth Smith
Dendreon Corporation
Seattle, Washington

Edward Snyder, MD, FACP
Yale University School of Medicine
Yale-New Haven Hospital
New Haven, Connecticut

Thomas R. Spitzer, MD
Massachusetts General Hospital
Boston, Massachusetts

Olive J. Sturtevant, MHP, MT(ASCP) SBB/SLS
Dana-Farber Cancer Institute
Boston, Massachusetts

Michele W. Sugrue, MS, MT(ASCP)SBB
University of Florida and Shands Hospital
Gainesville, Florida

D. Robert Sutherland, MSc
University of Toronto
University Health Network/Toronto General Hospital
Toronto, Ontario, Canada

Marcia Swearingen, MS, MT(ASCP)SBB
San Diego Blood Bank
San Diego, California

Zbigniew M. Szczepiorkowski, MD, PhD, FCAP
Dartmouth-Hitchcock Medical Center
Lebanon, New Hampshire

Bryan Tillman, MD, PhD
Wake Forest University School of Medicine
Winston-Salem, North Carolina

Sharon E. Tindle, MS
St. Vincent's Comprehensive Cancer Center
New York, New York

Darin J. Weber, PhD
The Biologics Consulting Group, Inc
Seattle, Washington

Theresa L. Whiteside, PhD
Hillman Cancer Center
Pittsburg, Pennsylvania

Keith Wonnacott, PhD
US Food and Drug Administration
Rockville, Maryland

James J. Yoo, MD, PhD
Wake Forest University School of Medicine
Winston-Salem, North Carolina

Contributors of Methods

Joseph H. Antin, MD
Dana-Farber Cancer Institute
Boston, Massachusetts

A. N. Balamurugan, PhD
Diabetes Institute for Immunology and Transplantation
University of Minnesota
Minneapolis, Minnesota

Hillary Bradbury, MT(ASCP)
OSU James Cancer Hospital and Solove Research Institute
Columbus, Ohio

Lizette Caballero, MT(ASCP)
Florida Hospital
Orlando, Florida

John Chapman, PhD
ThermoGenesis Corp
Rancho Cordova, California

Anna Chiou, MS
Biosafe
Eysins, Switzerland

Joy Cruz, CLS, MT(ASCP)SBB
University of California-San Francisco
San Francisco, California

Denise Cummings, RN
Beth Israel Deaconess Medical Center
Boston, Massachusetts

Sue Fautsch, BS, MT(ASCP)
University of Minnesota Masonic Cancer Research Center
Minneapolis, Minnesota

Deborah Lamontagne, MT(ASCP)
Beth Israel Deaconess Medical Center
Boston, Massachusetts

David Miller, MT(ASCP)
BioE, Inc
St Paul, Minnesota

Elsbeth Pirkl
Center for Molecular Biology
University of Heidelberg
Heidelberg, Germany

Shari Tyler Root, MT(ASCP)
BioE, Inc
St Paul, Minnesota

Leigh Ann Stamps, MT(AMT)
Sarah Cannon Blood and Marrow Transplant Program
Centennial Medical Center
Nashville, Tennessee

Linda Taylor, BS
CaridianBCT
Lakewood, Colorado

Table of Contents

SECTION II
Quality Assurance for Cellular Therapy Facilities 67

*Section Editors: Ellen Areman, MS, SBB(ASCP); Lizabeth Cardwell, MT(ASCP), MBA, RAC;
Karen Edward, BS, MT(ASCP); Cynthia Elliott, MT, HP(ASCP), CQA(ASQ); and
Michele W. Sugrue, MS, MT(ASCP)SBB*

9. Human Resources in the Cellular Therapy Facility 94

Brenda Alder, MS, MT(ASCP)SBB; Lizabeth Cardwell, MT(ASCP), MBA, RAC; Michele W. Sugrue, MS, MT(ASCP)SBB; and Ellen Areman, MS, SBB(ASCP)

10. Equipment Management in the Cellular Therapy Facility 112

Dave Krugh, MT(ASCP)SBB, CLS, CLCP(NCA)

SECTION VI

SECTION VIII
Section Editors: Ellen Areman, MS, SBB(ASCP), and Lynn O'Donnell, PhD

Preface

THIS BOOK IS THE RESULT OF CONTRIBU-
tions from a remarkable variety of sources.
First, we would like to thank the AABB Cellular
Therapy Committee for suggesting the project. In
addition, enormous gratitude is extended to those
who contributed methods, forms, or tables; these
attest to the quality of professionals in the field of
cellular therapy.

A Word on the Organization of Content

A glossary and a list of abbreviations are included
in this book. These are intended not to be comprehensive for the field of cellular therapy but to cover
those terms and abbreviations commonly used in
this book. Appendices related to specific chapter or
method content appear with the chapter immediately after the text and before any methods. Wherever methods were not submitted by the chapter
authors, the appropriate contributors are acknowl-
edged at the end of each chapter text before any
appendices and methods. The CD-ROM included
with the book offers all appendices and methods in
Microsoft Word format to allow the reader to cus-
tomize them for use as appropriate in his or her
facility. The methods are intended to serve as general outlines of procedures rather than as step-by-
step standard operating procedures. Specific company names may be mentioned merely for the convenience of the reader and should not be
considered endorsements of specific products or
manufacturers.

A Word from the Editor in Chief

When I first entered the field of cell processing
more than 20 years ago (although it was known as
"bone marrow processing" in those days), I never
anticipated the exciting future that lay ahead. The
cells that we processed came primarily from marrow, and investigators were just beginning to examine peripheral blood "stem" cells as another source
of hematopoietic cells for therapeutic use. Marrow
transplantation was an accepted, though high-risk,
therapy of last resort for patients with hematologic
malignancies and marrow failure—if the patient
wasn't too old and was fortunate enough to have an
HLA-identical sibling donor. Although some
visionaries may have started tossing around the
idea of a registry of HLA-typed unrelated volunteer
marrow donors, eventually to become the National
Marrow Donor Program (NMDP), not even the
most optimistic among them could have imagined
that in a short time more than a million people
would offer to donate their marrow and, later,
mobilized peripheral blood and lymphocytes to
strangers. In those days the only option for patients
not eligible for an allogeneic transplant was often a
dreadful treatment consisting of high-dose radiation or chemotherapy followed by a "transplant"
with autologous marrow that had previously been
collected and cryopreserved. The cell processing
laboratory staff not only processed, tested, and
froze the marrow, but was often expected to assist
with the marrow harvest procedure, thawing and
infusion.

Besides the procedures for concentration and cryopreservation of marrow cellular products that were performed in most cell-processing laboratories, investigators were starting to develop the forerunners of many of the "designer" cellular therapy products described in this volume. There were experimental protocols for purging residual cancer cells from autologous marrow and for depleting T-cells from allogeneic grafts. These were extraordinarily labor-intensive procedures that often employed toxic chemicals and pharmacologic agents. There were few assays available for demonstrating the purity or potency of manipulated cellular products. Although these attempts at marrow purification may have reduced the probability of relapse or graft rejection, the procedures themselves often increased transplant-related morbidity and mortality by delaying immune reconstitution or lengthening the period of marrow aplasia.

The cell-processing laboratories of 1987 were a far cry from the sophisticated facilities in operation today. Any but the most basic procedures were performed in research laboratories at academic medical centers. The clinical cell processing laboratory was usually staffed with a single technologist, who was often shared with another laboratory or the blood bank. There was not (and still is not, as of this writing) a formal training program for technical staff to learn this specialized work. The technical procedures were learned from more experienced people in other laboratories, with frequent frantic telephone calls to those mentors when something went wrong.

I had the good fortune to spend a short time at the beginning of my cell-processing career in a laboratory at Johns Hopkins that was operated single-handedly by Janice Davis, under Scott Rowley as the medical director. Within a few days I was supposed to be trained to operate a cell-processing laboratory by myself. I was amazed and a little intimidated by Janice's breadth of knowledge and by the variety and diversity of tasks she was able to perform. When I asked her who took over if she got sick, she told me, "I'm very healthy. I hardly ever get sick." And when I asked her for the name of a reference book or manual on cell processing, which I could purchase to keep in my lab, she just laughed. "There is no such book." she replied. That was when the idea took shape to put together the

original manual for cell-processing laboratories and the dedicated people who make them work.[1]

Looking back at the contents of that volume and then at this one, I realize what an incredible challenge the individuals performing this work have faced and continue to face as novel and increasingly complex cellular therapies move from bench to bedside. The development of tissue- and cell-based therapies for malignancies, regenerative medicine, and autoimmune diseases is occurring at a dizzying pace. Protocols involving selection, expansion, and combination of cells with other materials from a wide variety of sources are developed by basic scientists and often turned over to clinical laboratory scientists for translation and application. Along with developing and mastering complex cell-processing techniques, translational scientists must also develop and validate methods for determining the identity, purity, and potency of these unique and often poorly characterized products. And they must perform these procedures in compliance with regulatory requirements and professional standards that did not exist in 1987.

Although this book cannot possibly address all of the situations one might encounter in this rapidly expanding and unpredictable laboratory specialty, I hope it will provide some help in dealing with issues that may confront the staff of today's cellular therapy facility. At the rate at which new therapies and processes are being developed, I am sure it will not be another 20 years before an update to this volume will be needed.

A Word from the Associate Editor

I entered the field of cell therapy in 1994, after five years in a clinical hematology and transfusion medicine laboratory. It was late enough in the evolution of the field that I was able to learn many procedures from the work of pioneers like Ellen Areman, Janice Davis, and several of the other contributors to this project. But it was still early enough that peripheral blood stem cell therapy and other treatments that are routine in many cancer centers today were considered experimental, often requiring storage of autologous "back up" bone marrow collections for use if the cells failed to engraft. I will echo Ellen's remarks about the rapid advances of technology as well as the unpredictability and exponential growth potential of our field. I have had the joy and privilege to work with many passionate, diligent and motivated physicians, nurses, researchers and other technologists who patiently taught me things not found in textbooks or journal articles and helped me better understand hematopoietic cells and the people who donate and receive them. It is extraordinary to look back now and recall the number of bright lights in the cell therapy field with whom I have had the honor to interact over the years. I never would have predicted that I would work side-by-side in academic and research facilities as well as in professional organizations with those individuals whose accomplishments I so long admired, as well as brilliant young investigators who have gained my appreciation and respect. This project has been a great learning experience and I truly consider it an honor to have worked so closely with Ellen.

Ellen Areman, MS, SBB(ASCP)
Editor in Chief
Kathy Loper, MHS, MT(ASCP)
Associate Editor
July 2009

Reference

1. Areman EM, Deeg HJ, Sacher RA, eds. Bone marrow and stem cell processing: A manual of current techniques. Philadelphia: FA Davis, 1991.

About the Editors

Ellen M. Areman, MS, SBB(ASCP), is a Senior Consultant for the development of cellular biological products with the Biologics Consulting Group. Formerly, she served as a regulatory scientist and product reviewer at the US Food and Drug Administration (FDA), Center for Biologics Evaluation and Research, in the Office of Cellular Tissue and Gene Therapies. Before joining the regulatory community, she had spent over 15 years developing and managing cellular therapy laboratories in academic, government, and clinical centers. She is considered one of the pioneers in the field of cellular processing and graft engineering.

In the years before she joined FDA, Ms. Areman collaborated with numerous clinical and laboratory scientists as well as biotechnology companies in the development of new techniques for the manipulation of bone marrow, peripheral blood stem cells, umbilical cord blood, and lymphocytes. She has been involved in many aspects of the development, production, and quality control of cellular products and has published widely on such subjects as marrow and stem cell processing and transplantation; cell culture and expansion; immunotherapy; and cell cryopreservation and storage. She also edited the first manual of cell processing techniques, *Bone Marrow and Stem Cell Processing: A Manual of Current Techniques* (1995), which is still used as a reference in many laboratories throughout the world.

Ms. Areman received her Masters Degree in Experimental Pathology from Georgetown University and her Specialist in Blood Banking (SBB) certification from the National Institutes of Health.

Kathy Loper, MHS, MT(ASCP), currently serves as the Director of Cellular Therapies for AABB. She has been instrumental in expanding AABB's involvement in the field of cellular therapy and in the development of a wide variety of educational opportunities for cellular therapy professionals. Previously, she managed the Cell Processing and Gene Therapy Facilities at the Johns Hopkins Medical Institution, supporting these facilities in the performance of clinical and research aspects of cellular procurement, processing, and transplantation as well as innovative immunotherapies, including cancer vaccines.

Ms. Loper earned a Masters in Health Science Administration from Louisiana State University and is also certified as a medical technologist by the American Society of Clinical Pathologists. She is an active member of several professional organizations, including AABB and the International Society for Cellular Therapy, and has held numerous volunteer and committee positions in these and other professional societies.

Ms. Loper has authored numerous publications and presented at national and international meetings on both the technical and administrative aspects of cellular therapy.

Regulatory Considerations for Manufacturing Cellular Therapies in the United States

THIS SECTION PROVIDES A COMPREHEN-
sive overview of regulatory considerations for
the manufacturing of cellular therapies in the
United States. It reviews the regulatory history of
this still-evolving field and contains the most recent
advice from the US Food and Drug Administration
(FDA) for how to successfully prepare regulatory
submissions that describe the manufacturing, processing, and testing of cellular therapies. Academic
and industry experts who are experienced in preparing investigational new drug (IND) applications
and biologics license applications (BLA) for cellular
therapies offer their guidance on how best to interact with the FDA and to prepare the manufacturing
sections of regulatory submissions. Former FDA
staff members and consultants provide their expert
advice on the advantages and disadvantages of creating electronic regulatory submissions. They also
discuss how combination products containing cells
and medical devices (ie, tissue engineering products) are regulated by the FDA and areas where
additional clarification is needed. The critical role
played by professional societies in developing standards and providing accreditation for the cellular
therapy field is described and explained. Finally, a
listing of the Web sites of major regulatory bodies
and organizations active outside the United States
in the area of cellular therapies is provided as a
resource for the reader (see Appendix 1 at the back
of this book).

*Section Editors: Darin J. Weber, PhD, Senior Consultant, Biologics Consulting Group, Inc, Seattle, Washington, and Victoria A. Lake, BSc,
BA, RAC, Regulatory Affairs Director, Fred Hutchinson Cancer Research Center, Seattle, Washington*

The editors have disclosed no conflicts of interest.

In: Areman EM, Loper K, eds
Cellular Therapy: Principles, Methods, and Regulations
Bethesda, MD: AABB, 2009

◆◆◆ **1** ◆◆◆

A Brief History of FDA Regulation of Human Cells and Tissues

Liana Harvath, PhD

IN FEBRUARY 1997, THE FDA ANNOUNCED its "Proposed Approach to Regulation of Cellular and Tissue-Based Products."[1] This plan, a comprehensive, risk-based system of regulation for cellular and tissue-based products that range from conventional tissues to innovative cellular and gene therapy products, was finalized and became effective on May 25, 2005, as the rules for "Human Cells, Tissues, and Cellular and Tissue-Based Products (HCT/Ps)" in Title 21 of the Code of Federal Regulations (CFR), Part 1271. This chapter reviews the federal approach to cell and tissue product regulation, provides a brief history of events leading to the development of the "Proposed Approach to Regulation of Cellular and Tissue-Based Products," and discusses the progress made in implementing this regulatory approach.

Background

Legal Framework for Regulation of Biological Products

The federal Food, Drug, and Cosmetic Act (FD&C Act) and the Public Health Service (PHS) Act provide the legal framework for FDA regulation of bio-

logical products, including HCT/Ps. The FD&C and PHS Acts were preceded by the Biologics Control Act, passed by Congress on July 1, 1902, which authorized the Hygienic Laboratory of the Public Health and Marine Hospital Service [predecessor of the Center for Biologics Evaluation and Research (CBER), FDA] to issue regulations for all aspects of the commercial production of vaccines, sera, toxins, antitoxins, and similar products (see Table 1-1). The purpose of the Biologics Control Act was to ensure biological product safety, purity, and potency. The Biologics Control Act was authorized in response to an outbreak of tetanus, in 1901 in St Louis, MO, where 13 children died after receiving diphtheria antitoxin that was contaminated with tetanus, and in Camden, NJ, where 9 children died after they received tetanus-contaminated smallpox vaccine.[2]

Congress passed the PHS Act in 1944, which consolidated PHS laws. The Biologics Control Act was incorporated into Section 351 of the PHS Act as the "Regulation of Biological Products." Section 361 of the PHS Act authorized the enforcement of the control of communicable diseases. In 1955, the PHS biologics control function was expanded, and the regulation of biologics, which had been in the Laboratory of Biologics Control, was transferred to

Liana Harvath, PhD, Consultant, Liana Harvath, PhD, LLC, Rockville, Maryland

The author has disclosed no conflicts of interest.

Table 1-1. Federal Regulation of Biological Products

Year	Action	Purpose
1902	Biologics Control Act	A legislative framework was developed for the regulation of biologics and to protect Americans from unsafe products.
1938	The Federal Food, Drug, and Cosmetic Act	Biological products were considered to be drugs, and parts of the Federal Food, Drug, and Cosmetic Act concerning adulteration or misbranding were applied to biological products.
1944	The Public Health Service Act	The Laboratory of Biologics Control was authorized to license biological products as well as the establishments where the products were produced. The 1902 Biologics Control Act was incorporated into Section 351 of the Public Health Service Act, Regulation of Biological Products. Section 361 of the Public Health Service Act authorized enforcement of the Control of Communicable Diseases.
1970	The Pubic Health Service Act was modified to include "blood, blood components, and derivatives."	Regulatory oversight was increased for blood and blood products, leading to the licensing of interstate blood banks and the establishment of standards for the operation of all blood banks.
1993	Interim Rule for Human Tissue Intended for Transplantation[3]	The FDA required tissue banks to test donors of human musculoskeletal, ocular, or skin tissue for transplantation to protect the public health from transmission of human immunodeficiency virus infection and hepatitis infection. The Tissue Rule was finalized in 1997 and became 21 CFR Part 1270, Human Tissue Intended for Transplantation.[7]
1993	Application of Current Statutory Authorities to Human Somatic Cell Therapy Products and Gene Therapy Products; Notice[4]	Somatic cell therapy and gene therapy products are regulated by the FDA as biological products and are subject to applicable regulations of the Public Health Service Act and 21 CFR Part 312, Investigational New Drug Application.
1995	Draft Document Concerning the Regulation of Placental/Umbilical Cord Blood Stem Cell Products Intended for Transplantation or Further Manufacture Into Injectable Products [Docket 96N-0002][5]	The FDA proposed that autologous and allogeneic placental/umbilical cord blood cells intended for human administration for treatment, cure, diagnosis, or mitigation of disease or injuries be regulated by the FDA as licensed biological products.

(Continued)

Table 1-1. Federal Regulation of Biological Products (Continued)

Year	Action	Purpose
1996	Draft Document Concerning the Regulation of Peripheral Blood Hematopoietic Stem Cell Products Intended for Transplantation or Further Manufacture [Docket 96N-0026]	The FDA proposed that peripheral blood hematopoietic stem/progenitor cells intended for human transplantation be regulated by the FDA as licensed biological products.
1996	Guidance on Applications for Products Comprised of Living Autologous Cells Manipulated ex vivo and Intended for Structural Repair or Reconstruction [Docket 95N-0200][6]	The FDA provided guidance for the clinical investigation and use of living autologous cells manipulated ex vivo and intended for structural repair or reconstruction (MAS cells).
1997	Proposed Approach to Regulation of Cellular and Tissue-Based Products[1]	The FDA proposed a tiered approach to cell and tissue regulation with regulation focused on three general areas: 1) preventing the unwitting use of contaminated tissues with the potential for transmitting infectious diseases; 2) preventing improper handling or processing that might contaminate or damage tissues; and 3) ensuring that clinical safety and effectiveness are demonstrated for tissues that are highly processed, are used for other than their normal function (nonallogeneic function), are combined with nontissue components, or are used for metabolic purposes.
1998	Human Cells, Tissues, and Cellular and Tissue-Based Products; Establishment Registration and Listing; Proposed Rule[11]	The Final Rule was published January 19, 2001, and became 21 CFR Part 1271, Subparts A and B.[12]
1998	Request for Proposed Standards for Unrelated Allogeneic Peripheral and Placental/Umbilical Cord Blood Hematopoietic Stem/Progenitor Cell Products; Request for Comments [Docket 97N-0497][14]	The FDA requested comments and the submission of supporting clinical and nonclinical laboratory data to develop product standards to ensure the safety and effectiveness of minimally manipulated hematopoietic progenitor cells from unrelated donors of allogeneic peripheral or placental/umbilical cord blood.
1999	Suitability Determination for Donors of Human Cells, Tissues, and Cellular and Tissue-Based Products; Proposed Rule[15]	The Final Rule was published May 25, 2004, and became 21 CFR Part 1271, Subpart C. The effective date of implementation was May 25, 2005.[16]

Table 1-1. Federal Regulation of Biological Products (Continued)

Year	Action	Purpose
2001	Current Good Tissue Practice for Manufacturers of Human Cellular and Tissue-Based Products; Inspection and Enforcement; Proposed Rule[17]	The Final Rule was published November 24, 2004 and became 21 CFR Part 1271, Subparts D, E, and F. The effective date of implementation was May 25, 2005.[18]
2005	Human Cells, Tissues, and Cellular and Tissue-Based Products; Donor Screening and Testing, and Related Labeling; Interim Final Rule[19]	The FDA revised certain regulations regarding screening and testing of HCT/P donors and related labeling. The revisions were incorporated in the Final Rule.[20]
2006	Draft Guidance for Industry: Minimally Manipulated, Unrelated, Allogeneic Placental/Umbilical Cord Blood Intended for Hematopoietic Reconstitution in Patients with Hematological Malignancies[22]	The FDA provided recommendations that would allow a cord blood bank to apply for licensure of minimally manipulated, unrelated, allogeneic placental/umbilical cord blood for hematopoietic reconstitution in patients with hematological malignancies. The FDA invited comment to the Draft Guidance and held a public discussion on March 30, 2007, at the Cellular, Tissue, and Gene Therapies Advisory Committee meeting.
2007	Guidance for Industry: Regulation of Human Cells, Tissues, and Cellular and Tissue-Based Products; Small Entity Compliance Guide[21]	The FDA provided recommendations to help small-entity establishments that manufacture HCT/Ps better understand and comply with the regulatory framework of 21 CFR 1271.
2007	Guidance for Industry: Class II Special Controls Guidance Document: Cord Blood Processing System and Storage Container[23]	The FDA developed special controls to support the classification of a cord blood processing system and storage container as Class II devices.
2007	Draft Guidance for Industry: Cell Selection Devices for Point-of-Care Production of Minimally Manipulated Autologous Peripheral Blood Stem Cells[24]	The FDA proposed that when peripheral blood stem cells are recovered from a patient for autologous use in the same surgical procedure, and the peripheral blood stem cells are processed using a device that is approved or cleared for point-of-care indication, 21 CFR Part 1271 requirements do not apply to the facility performing the procedure. The devices are subject to the Food, Drug, and Cosmetic Act and FDA medical device regulations.

FDA = Food and Drug Administration; CFR = Code of Federal Regulations; MAS = manipulated autologous cells for structural use; HCT/Ps = human cells, tissues, and cellular and tissue-based products.

a Division of Biologics Standards, which became an independent entity within the National Institutes of Health (NIH).

The government further expanded biologics regulation because 290 cases of polio resulted when 94 vaccine recipients and 166 close contacts of vaccine recipients developed polio from Cutter Laboratories' vaccine, which was contaminated with live polio virus. In October 1970, the PHS Act was modified to include "blood, blood components, and derivatives" as biological products. The Division of Biologics Standards oversaw the control and release of biologics until 1972, when the division was moved from the NIH to the FDA and renamed the Bureau of Biologics. The move to the Bureau of Biologics in the FDA occurred because the NIH did not have an effectiveness review process equivalent to that performed for drugs at the FDA.

Regulatory oversight at the Bureau of Biologics was increased for blood and blood products. By 1973, the FDA regulated approximately 7000 blood collection facilities and required licensure of establishments that collected blood plasma by plasmapheresis. Good manufacturing practice standards were developed in 1975 for the operation of blood banks, and all registered blood establishments were required to test donors for hepatitis B virus. The PHS Act authorized the Laboratory of Biologics Control to license biological products and establishments and provided authority for the PHS, when necessary, to manufacture biological products.[2]

The FD&C Act was passed by Congress in 1938 to strengthen consumer protection from adulteration and misbranding of drugs and devices. Biological products were considered to be drugs under the FD&C Act, and the laws regarding adulteration and misbranding of drugs and devices were applied to biological products. The FD&C Act was enacted after 107 people died from consuming a misbranded commercial product (Elixir Sulfanilamide, S.E. Massengill, Bristol, TN) that had been made with diethylene glycol, a toxic solvent, instead of alcohol, the required solvent for the formulation.[2]

Events Leading to Tissue Regulation

From 1993 through 1996, the FDA released four documents concerning regulatory approaches to cellular and tissue products, ranging from musculoskeletal, ocular, or skin tissue (conventional tissue) for transplantation[3] to somatic cell therapy and gene therapy products,[4] and including placental/umbilical cord blood (UCB),[5] peripheral blood hematopoietic progenitor cell (HPC) products, and living autologous cells manipulated ex vivo and intended for implantation for structural repair or reconstruction.[6] The regulatory approaches for these products were developed to minimize the risks of transmission of communicable diseases from the human cells and tissues and to ensure the safety and effectiveness of cellular products that were processed or manipulated in a way that might alter their biological function.

Conventional Tissues

On December 14, 1993, the FDA published the Interim Rule on Human Tissue Intended for Transplantation[3], which became effective immediately. The interim rule was issued to protect public health from the transmission of human immunodeficiency virus (HIV) infection and hepatitis infection through transplantation of human tissue from donors known to be infected with or at risk for these diseases. Individuals involved in tissue banking testified before a Congressional Subcommittee on Regulation, Business Opportunities, and Technology of the Committee on Small Business (October 15, 1993) that human tissues from foreign sources were sold in the United States with little documentation concerning the source of the human tissue, the cause of death, the medical conditions of the donor, or the results of screening and testing. Investigations by the FDA confirmed that some human tissues available in the United States were obtained without adequate screening and testing to prevent the transmission of infectious diseases. In addition, the Centers for Disease Control and Prevention reported that HIV was transmitted through transplantation of some tissues in the early 1990s. These events led to the implementation of the interim rule. Four years later, after the FDA sponsored three public workshops and extended the public comment period for the interim rule, the final rule for Human Tissue Intended for Transplantation[7] was published on July 29, 1997, as 21 CFR Part 1270, Human Tissue Intended for Transplantation.

Somatic Cell and Gene Therapy Products

During the mid 1980s and early 1990s, the FDA received inquiries from manufacturers and clinical investigators concerning the regulatory pathway for somatic cell and gene therapy products. On October 14, 1993, the FDA published a notice that defined somatic cell therapy and gene therapy products and outlined the regulatory requirements for these biological products.[4] The FDA defined somatic cell therapy products as "autologous (ie, self), allogeneic (ie, intra-species), or xenogeneic (ie, inter-species) cells that have been propagated, expanded, selected, pharmacologically treated, or otherwise altered in biological characteristics ex vivo to be administered to humans and applicable to the prevention, treatment, cure, diagnosis, or mitigation of disease or injuries." Gene therapy products were defined as "products containing genetic material administered to modify or manipulate the expression of genetic material or to alter the biological properties of living cells." Somatic cell therapy and gene therapy products fell within the definitions of biological and drug products and, as such, the regulatory requirements of the PHS Act sections pertaining to biologics and drugs and the IND requirements of 21 CFR Part 312 were applicable to these products. Somatic cell and gene therapy products are subject to product licensure to ensure product safety, identity, purity, and potency and are subject to drug requirements such as conformity with current Good Manufacturing Practice (cGMP) regulations.

Autologous cultured chondrocytes (Carticel) became the first licensed somatic cell therapy product directly affected by the FDA's definition of a somatic cell therapy and the regulatory licensure requirements. Genzyme Tissue Repair began marketing Carticel in 1995 for the repair of "clinically significant, symptomatic, cartilaginous defects of the femoral condyle (medial, lateral or trochlear) caused by acute or repetitive trauma" according to an understanding that the FDA would not regulate the autologous cellular therapy. Shortly after the FDA informed Genzyme Tissue Repair that marketing approval for Carticel would be required, Genzyme Tissue Repair requested that the FDA clarify the product designation. The FDA notified Genzyme Tissue Repair that it could continue to market Carticel while jurisdiction was under con-

sideration and policy was under development. The FDA held a public hearing in November 1995 to discuss public health issues and concerns relating to the regulation of products that comprise living autologous cells that are manipulated ex vivo and intended for implantation for structural repair or reconstruction of the source tissue (*m*anipulated *a*utologous cells for *s*tructural use, or MAS cells).[8] In May 1996, the FDA issued guidance on applications for MAS cell products,[6] which stated that MAS cell products met the definition of somatic cell therapy products and required an IND exemption or FDA-approved license application. Carticel ultimately received FDA approval in August 1997 and became the first licensed somatic cell therapy product.

HPCs from Placental/Umbilical Cord Blood and Peripheral Blood

In the early 1990s, the FDA received inquiries from investigators who were engaged in establishing unrelated allogeneic UCB bank programs and from private citizens who were solicited by commercial UCB banks for speculative storage of newborn family members' UCB. Investigators asked if and how the FDA would regulate UCB banks. For example, would UCB banks be regulated as blood establishments, or was UCB viewed as an investigational product that required the submission of an IND application? Consumers asked the FDA whether promotional claims about UCB's curative properties were true and if the FDA reviewed UCB bank procedures.

Since 1995, the FDA has engaged in extensive public discussion regarding a proposed regulatory approach for UCB banking.[9] In December 1995, the FDA sponsored a public workshop with the National Heart, Lung, and Blood Institute (NHLBI) to discuss procedures for UCB collection and storage. The purposes of the workshop were to identify and discuss steps for collection, processing, and storage of UCB for transplantation and to determine what additional data were needed. At the workshop, the FDA released a draft document that outlined a regulatory strategy for UCB products for transplantation[5] and invited public comment on the draft document. The draft document proposed that autologous and allogeneic UCB intended for human administration for treatment, cure, diagnosis, or mitigation of disease or injuries be regulated by the FDA as licensed biological products.

During this period, the FDA was also considering a regulatory approach for HPCs obtained from peripheral blood. In February 1996, the FDA and the NHLBI cosponsored a public workshop to discuss procedures for the preparation, processing, and characterization of human peripheral blood HPCs for transplantation and to determine areas in need of further research. At the workshop, the FDA provided a draft document that proposed that peripheral blood HPCs intended for human transplantation be regulated by the FDA as licensed biological products.

From the information presented at these meetings and the comments received regarding the draft proposed regulatory approaches for UCB and peripheral blood HPCs, the FDA recognized a need to reconsider whether the concepts and procedures used to regulate traditional biological products were appropriate for regulation of peripheral and UCB HPC products. After consultation with representatives of the involved public, the FDA proposed a new regulatory framework for cellular and tissue-based products, which included UCB and peripheral blood HPCs.[1]

Proposed Approach to Regulation of Cellular and Tissue-Based Products

The FDA recognized the importance of developing a comprehensive, tiered, risk-based regulatory approach for a broad range of cellular and tissue-based products because the agency had traditionally used a fragmented regulatory approach for cellular products. The FDA announced its "Proposed Approach to Regulation of Cellular and Tissue-Based Products"[1] in February 1997, and it held a public meeting on March 17, 1997, to discuss and solicit information and views from the interested public. The proposed approach contained five public health and regulatory concerns: 1) prevention of transmission of communicable disease; 2) processing controls to prevent contamination of cells and to preserve their integrity and function; 3) clinical safety and effectiveness data requirements for cells that are from an unrelated allogeneic donor, manipulated (through processing that alters the

relevant functional characteristics of cells or tissues, such as cell expansion or genetic modification), used for other-than-normal function, or combined with nontissue components (including synthetic or mechanical components, drugs, or noncell or nontissue biologics); 4) labeling for proper product use that is clear, accurate, balanced, and not misleading; and 5) monitoring and communication with the industry through establishment registration and product listing with the FDA.

Under this risk-based system for regulating HCT/Ps, HCT/Ps that meet certain criteria would be regulated solely under Section 361 of the PHS Act and 21 CFR Part 1271, which focuses on preventing the introduction, transmission, or spread of communicable disease to the HCT/P recipient through donor eligibility and current good tissue practice requirements (see Table 1-2). Marketing of such products is permitted without clinical data or review of safety and efficacy. Other HCT/Ps, considered as higher-risk products, are regulated as biological products or medical devices, and evidence of their safety and effectiveness is required before they are marketed (Table 1-2).[10]

Implementing the Proposed Approach—The First 10 Years

From 1997 to 2007, the FDA published more than 23 documents related to implementation of the approach, including three proposed,[11,15,17] three final,[12,16,18] and two interim final tissue rules,[13,19] a request for proposed standards for unrelated allogeneic peripheral and UCB HPCs[14] (Table 1-1), and 16 guidance documents. Although the FDA intended to implement all three rules at the same time, some of the dates of implementation were delayed. In order to facilitate communication between tissue banks and the FDA, the first of the rules, which involved establishment and registration, was implemented before the other rules were finalized.

The first proposed rule, "Human Cells, Tissues, and Cellular and Tissue-Based Products; Establishment Registration and Listing" (registration rule), was published on May 14, 1998,[11] and the final registration rule was published on January 19, 2001.[12] The registration final rule set forth, in 21 CFR Part 1271, Subpart A, the definitions and general provisions pertaining to the scope and purpose of 21 CFR Part 1271, and in Subpart B, the registration

Table 1-2. Criteria Determining the HCT/P Regulatory Path

PHS Act Section 361, 21 CFR 1271	PHS Act Section 351, Regulation of Biological Products, Premarket Approval
To be regulated solely under Section 361 of the PHS Act and CFR Title 21 Part 1271, an HCT/P must meet all four criteria:	Sections 351 and 361 of the PHS Act and premarket approval authorities apply to HCT/Ps if they meet at least one of the following criteria:
1. Minimally manipulated. 2. Intended for allogeneic use only. 3. Not combined with a device or drug, except for sterilizing, preserving, or storage agents that do not raise clinical safety concerns. 4. Free of systemic effects and independent of the metabolic activity of living cells for its primary function, *unless* the HCT/P is for (a) autologous use, (b) allogeneic use in a first-degree or second-degree blood relative, or (c) reproductive use.	1. Manipulated such that biological or relevant functional characteristics of the cells or tissues are altered. 2. Genetically modified. 3. Expanded ex vivo. 4. Used for other-than-normal function of the HCT/P, or for structural tissue, used for a structural purpose in a location of the body where such functional purpose does not normally occur (non-allogeneic use). 5. Combined with a drug, device, or biological product that may raise clinical safety concerns. 6. Active systemically or dependent on the metabolic activity of the living cells for their primary function, *unless* minimally manipulated for (a) autologous use, (b) use in a first-degree or second-degree blood relative, or (c) reproductive use.

HCT/P = human cells, tissues, and cellular and tissue-based product; PHS = Public Health Service; CFR = Code of Federal Regulations.

and listing procedures. The registration rule was implemented in two stages: the first effective date in April 2001 pertained to conventional tissue establishments whose products were regulated under Section 361 of the PHS Act and 21 CFR Part 1270, and the second effective date in January 2004 pertained to establishments that manufactured HCT/Ps currently regulated as biological products, drugs, and devices, including HPCs from peripheral blood and UCB and reproductive cells and tissues.

The second proposed rule, "Suitability Determination for Donors of Human Cellular and Tissue-Based Products" (donor eligibility rule), was published on September 30, 1999,[15] and the final rule was published on May 25, 2004.[16] The donor eligibility rule set forth, in 21 CFR Part 1271, Subpart C, the provisions for screening and testing donors to determine their eligibility as donors. An interim final rule concerning donor screening and testing and related labeling was published and became effective on May 25, 2005. This interim final rule

revised certain regulations regarding the screening and testing of HCT/P donors and related labeling.[19] The FDA adopted the interim final rule as a final rule without change on June 19, 2007.[20]

The third proposed rule, "Current Good Tissue Practice for Manufacturers of Human Cellular and Tissue-Based Products; Inspection and Enforcement" (cGTP rule)[17] was published on January 8, 2001, and the final rule was published on November 24, 2004.[18] The cGTP rule set forth, in 21 CFR Part 1271, Subpart D, the cGTP requirements; in Subpart E, additional requirements for establishments described in 21 CFR Part 1271.10; and in Subpart F, the inspection and enforcement provisions for establishments described in 21 CFR Part 1271.10. The cGTP rule became effective on May 25, 2005. The FDA issued a "Small Entity Compliance Guide" in August 2007 to address questions and clarify issues regarding each of the tissue rules that comprise 21 CFR Part 1271.[21]

Regulation of Unrelated Allogeneic UCB and Peripheral Blood HPCs

In January 1998, the FDA published a request for proposed standards for unrelated allogeneic peripheral blood and UCB HPC products.[14] The public was invited to submit comments and clinical and nonclinical laboratory data and to support standards to ensure the safety and effectiveness of minimally manipulated HPCs derived from peripheral blood and UCB for unrelated allogeneic human transplantation. The standards-based approach to regulation of these unrelated allogeneic products was proposed because the products were actively used since the 1990s as alternatives to marrow HPCs, and investigators were convinced of their safety and effectiveness.

Many investigators voluntarily submitted IND applications to the FDA for unrelated UCB banking. The National Marrow Donor Program submitted an IND application covering its multicenter use

of peripheral blood HPCs in unrelated allogeneic transplantation programs. Data collected through the IND applications were to serve as the basis for UCB and peripheral blood HPC product standards. Proposed product standards were to include the criteria for acceptance of products, such as specifications for the volume, viable cell number, storage temperature limits, microbial or other contamination limits, and other relevant characteristics, such as CD34+ cell concentration. When UCB standards were developed, UCB banks could apply for a biological license for UCB by documenting that their bank met the established standards. In contrast, UCB or peripheral blood HPCs for autologous or related allogeneic transplantation would be regulated as tissue products under 21 CFR 1271 and would not require licensure (see Table 1-3).

Since December 1995, the FDA has facilitated the public exchange of information concerning UCB and peripheral blood HPC products by cosponsoring workshops with the NHLBI regard-

Table 1-3. Regulation of Minimally Manipulated Hematopoietic Progenitor Cells*

Source	Marrow	Peripheral Blood	Cord Blood
Autologous	No federal regulation	21 CFR 1271 applies, except Subpart C, Donor Eligibility, which is recommended but not required	21 CFR 1271 applies, except Subpart C, Donor Eligibility, which is recommended but not required
Related allogeneic (first-degree or second-degree blood relative)	No federal regulation	All subparts of 21 CFR 1271 are requirements	All subparts of 21 CFR 1271 are requirements
Unrelated allogeneic	Health Resources and Services Administration oversight (contract with the National Marrow Donor Program)	All subparts of 21 CFR 1271 are requirements; in addition, the FDA has requested product and establishment standards with eventual licensure as a biological product	All subparts of 21 CFR 1271 are requirements; in addition, the FDA has proposed product standards with eventual licensure as a biological product

*Hematopoietic progenitor cells that are more than minimally manipulated (eg, through ex-vivo expansion or genetic modification) are subject to investigational new drug requirements and licensure as biological products when intended for use as somatic cell or gene therapy products.
CFR = Code of Federal Regulations; FDA = Food and Drug Administration.

ing ethical, clinical, and scientific issues as well as providing periodic updates at the FDA Advisory Committee meetings.[9] In December 2006, the FDA published a draft guidance for public comment regarding proposed UCB product standards for minimally manipulated, unrelated, allogeneic UCB intended for hematopoietic reconstitution in hematological malignancies.[22] These proposed UCB product standards were discussed at the March 30, 2007, Cellular, Tissue, and Gene Therapies Advisory Committee meeting. Although the FDA has not yet provided a draft guidance concerning product standards for peripheral blood HPCs, it is likely that an opportunity will be provided for public comment about peripheral blood HPC product standards if and when they are developed. If product standards are not developed for unrelated allogeneic HPC products using this approach, the FDA may phase in the requirements for IND applications.

Future Directions

As new issues emerge, the FDA will continue to issue draft guidance, solicit public input, and develop final guidance to address regulatory issues. One area in need of attention involves the devices and associated technologies for HCT/P collection, storage, and processing. The successful development of devices and associated technologies is essential for continued progress in cellular therapies.

In 2007, the FDA released two documents concerning cell-processing devices: "Class II Special Controls Guidance Document: Cord Blood Processing System and Storage Container"[23] and a Draft Guidance on "Cell Selection Devices for Point-of-Care Production of Minimally Manipulated Autologous Peripheral Blood Stem Cells."[24] The recent guidance documents[23,24] focus on specific cellular product devices. It appears that the FDA is approaching cellular therapy device regulation on a case-by-case basis. Therefore, it is critical for device manufacturers to contact the FDA before moving forward with a regulatory application.

Several questions remain unanswered:

1. If a device is FDA approved or cleared for processing, storing, or collecting a product such as UCB, does the FDA require approval to market

the same device for bone marrow or peripheral blood HPC processing?

2. If so, do device manufacturers need to submit a 510(k) application to demonstrate substantial equivalence to the manufacturers' own predicate devices, or do manufacturers need to conduct clinical trials before marketing the devices?

3. How should cell-processing laboratories proceed if they use an FDA-approved device to process a different cellular product for which the device has not been approved or cleared?

These and other related questions need to be addressed by the FDA in the near future.

References/Resources

1. Food and Drug Administration. Proposed approach to regulation of cellular and tissue-based products. (February 28, 1997) Rockville, MD: CBER Office of Communication, Training, and Manufacturers Assistance, 1997.

2. Food and Drug Administration. CBER vision. Special commemorative issue. (July 1, 2002) Rockville, MD: CBER Office of Communication, Training, and Manufacturers Assistance, 2002.

3. Food and Drug Administration. Human tissue intended for transplantation; interim rule. Fed Regist 1993;58: 65514-38.

4. Food and Drug Administration. Application of current statutory authorities to human somatic cell therapy products and gene therapy products Docket No. 93N-0173. Fed Regist 1993;58:53248-51.

5. Food and Drug Administration. Draft document concerning the regulation of placental/umbilical cord blood stem cell products intended for transplantation or further manufacture into injectable products. Docket No. 96N-0002. Fed Regist 1996;61:7087-8.

6. Food and Drug Administration. Guidance on applications for products comprised of living autologous cells manipulated ex vivo and intended for structural repair or reconstruction. Docket No. 95N-0200. (May 1996) Rockville, MD: CBER Office of Communication, Training, and Manufacturers Assistance, 1996.

7. Food and Drug Administration. Human tissue intended for transplantation; final rule. Fed Regist 1997;62:40429-47.

8. Food and Drug Administration. Public hearing: Products comprised of living autologous cells manipulated ex vivo and intended for implantation for structural repair or reconstruction. Docket No. 95N-0200. Fed Regist 1995;60:36808-11.

9. Harvath L. Food and Drug Administration's proposed approach to regulation of hematopoietic stem/progenitor cell products for therapeutic use. Transfus Med Rev 2000;14:104-11.

10. Weber DJ. Navigating FDA regulations for human cells and tissues. BioProcess International 2004;2:22-6.

11. Food and Drug Administration. Human cells, tissues, and cellular and tissue-based products; establishment registration and listing; proposed rule. Fed Regist 1998;63:26744-55.

12. Food and Drug Administration. Human cells, tissues, and cellular and tissue-based products; establishment registration and listing; final rule. Fed Regist 2001;66:5447-69.

13. Food and Drug Administration. Human cells, tissues, and cellular and tissue-based products. Establishment registration and listing; interim final rule. Fed Regist 2004;69:3823-6.

14. Food and Drug Administration. Request for proposed standards for unrelated allogeneic peripheral and placental/umbilical cord blood hematopoietic stem/progenitor cell products; request for comments. Docket No. 97N-0497. Fed Regist 1998;63:2985-8.

15. Food and Drug Administration. Suitability determination for donors of human cellular and tissue-based products; proposed rule. Fed Regist 1999;64:52696-723.

16. Food and Drug Administration. Eligibility determination for donors of human cells, tissues, and cellular and tissue-based products; final rule. Fed Regist 2004;69:29786-834.

17. Food and Drug Administration. Current good tissue practice for manufacturers of human cellular and tissue-based products; inspection and enforcement; proposed rule. Fed Regist 2001;66:1508-55.

18. Food and Drug Administration. Current good tissue practice for manufacturers of human cellular and tissue-based products; inspection and enforcement; final rule. Fed Regist 2004;69:68612-88.

19. Food and Drug Administration. Human cells, tissues, and cellular and tissue-based products; donor screening and testing, and related labeling; interim final rule. Fed Regist 2005;70:29949-52.

20. Food and Drug Administration. Human cells, tissues, and cellular and tissue-based products; donor screening and testing, and related labeling; final rule. Fed Regist 2007;72: 33667-9.

21. Food and Drug Administration. Guidance for industry: Regulation of human cells, tissues, and cellular and tissue-based products (HCT/Ps); small entity compliance guide. (August 2007) Rockville, MD: CBER Office of Communication, Training, and Manufacturers Assistance, 2007.

22. Food and Drug Administration. Draft guidance for industry: Minimally manipulated, unrelated, allogeneic placental/umbilical cord blood intended for hematopoietic reconstitution in patients with hematological malignancies (December 2006) Rockville, MD: CBER Office of Communication, Training, and Manufacturers Assistance, 2006. [Available at: http://www.fda.gov/cber/gdlns/cordbld.pdf (accessed October 30, 2008).]

23. Food and Drug Administration. Guidance for industry: Class II special controls guidance document: Cord blood processing system and storage container. (January 2007) Rockville, MD: CBER Office of Communication, Training, and Manufacturers Assistance, 2007.

24. Food and Drug Administration. Draft guidance for industry: Cell selection devices for point-of-care production of minimally manipulated autologous peripheral blood stem cells. (July 2007) Rockville, MD: CBER Office of Communication, Training, and Manufacturers Assistance, 2007.

In: Areman EM, Loper K, eds
Cellular Therapy: Principles, Methods, and Regulations
Bethesda, MD: AABB, 2009

♦♦♦   **2**   ♦♦♦

The FDA Perspective on the Manufacturing, Production, and Processing of Regulated Cellular Therapies

Sarah Kennett, PhD; Cynthia Porter, PhD; Eda Bloom, PhD; and Keith Wonnacott, PhD

SOMATIC CELLULAR THERAPY IS THE administration to humans of autologous, allogeneic, or xenogeneic living cells that have been manipulated or processed ex vivo. The Food and Drug Administration (FDA) asserted jurisdiction over these products in 1993.[1]

Somatic cellular therapy products are drugs, biological products, and human cells, tissues, and tissue-based products (HCT/Ps) that are regulated under Section 351 of the Public Health Service (PHS) Act.[2-4] This means that somatic cellular therapies are subject to current good manufacturing practice regulations [cGMP; Code of Federal Regulations (CFR) Title 21 Parts 210 and 211],[5,6] biological product regulations (21 CFR 610),[7] and HCT/P regulations (21 CFR 1271),[8] including current good tissue practice and donor eligibility requirements.[9] The special concerns relevant to xenogeneic cells are not covered in this chapter, but further infor-

mation on the regulation of xeno-transplantation products can be found in FDA guidance[10] and on the FDA Web site.[11]

This chapter is intended to provide insight for navigating the regulations during the development of somatic cellular therapies for clinical use. The FDA has tried to facilitate an understanding of how the various regulations apply to cellular therapy products by issuing guidance documents that are both directly and indirectly relevant to cellular therapies. This chapter highlights some of the concepts in those guidance documents that address common challenges in cellular therapy product and process development.

Because the vast majority of cellular therapies are still investigational, the focus of this chapter is on product development rather than on product licensure. The primary focus is on the types of information that should be provided in the original

Sarah Kennett, PhD; Cynthia Porter, PhD; Eda Bloom, PhD (now deceased); and Keith Wonnacott, PhD, US Food and Drug Administration, Center for Biologics Evaluation and Research, Office of Cellular, Tissue, and Gene Therapies, Rockville, Maryland

The authors have disclosed no conflicts of interest.

submission, and common deficiencies are highlighted. After the general tips below, the sections that follow focus on specific issues and address many of the common manufacturing challenges encountered during product development.

General Tips

The following general tips for product development are helpful to remember regardless of the phase of development or the product being developed.

Tip 1: Be Data Driven

Unlike many research studies that are developed around good ideas, clinical research studies should be developed around good data. This is not true only of the proof-of-concept and pharmacology or toxicology data that support the clinical research, but also of the product development data that support manufacturing processes and controls. For example, answers to questions such as the following should be supported by data and not suppositions:

- Is the cellular starting material free of infectious viruses?

- Does the dose of irradiation render the cells replication-incompetent?

- Do the antibiotics in the culture media interfere with the sterility assay?

Data used to answer these questions should be complete and directly applicable to the specific product and manufacturing process, particularly if the plan is to cite publicly available data.

Tip 2: Provide Complete and Accurate Documentation

In addition to good data, good documentation is essential during product development. If documentation for investigational new drug (IND) or biologics license application (BLA) submissions is missing, incomplete, contradictory, or incorrect, the FDA is not able to make an independent assessment of the safety of a product. Complete, well-organized, and internally consistent data facilitate an accurate safety assessment.

Flowcharts, tables, and narrative descriptions are helpful and contribute to the clarity of submissions, but they should be supported with the

details. [Remember that in the process for IND applications, unlike that for National Institutes of Health (NIH) grant applications, there is no limit to the amount of detailed and relevant information that can be submitted.]

Using an organized format may be helpful in ensuring that all necessary information is included. For example, IND applications for somatic cell therapies should follow the same format and contain the same sections as IND applications for any investigational drug or biological product, as described in the IND regulations.[12] In addition, the organization and content of the chemistry, manufacturing, and controls (CMC) section within the IND application may follow the template described in the FDA guidance for cellular therapy reviewers.[13]

Tip 3: Be Informed

There are many resources available to sponsors who are developing cellular therapy products. Formal resources include the laws, regulations, and guidance documents. Many of the relevant resources can be found on the FDA Web site.[14] Additionally, the FDA staff participates in open public meetings and other forms of outreach to help inform the regulated community. Many of these presentations are easily accessible through the Internet.

Tip 4: Communicate with the FDA

The agency has a process for granting formal meetings.[15] There are several specified meetings, such as pre-IND meetings, end-of-Phase-II meetings, and pre-BLA meetings, but other formal meetings are also possible. In addition to formal meetings, reviewers at the FDA, when possible, try to answer questions as part of their outreach to sponsors.

Tip 5: Plan Ahead

Many of the problems sponsors may have with product development can be avoided by having a better understanding of their product earlier in the manufacturing process. For example, some characterization testing of a product may not directly affect safety and, therefore, may not be required by the FDA for early-phase studies. However, early product characterization testing, including tests for identity and potency, can help to avoid potential problems later in development.

Current Good Manufacturing Practices

Many academic institutions have recently built, or are interested in building, manufacturing facilities to support clinical research within the institution. It is not uncommon to hear that these new facilities are "good manufacturing practice" (GMP) facilities. In such cases, the term is used very narrowly—applying only to the design and function of the building and facility. However, cGMP includes much more than facility requirements. The subparts of the cGMP regulations are listed in Table 2-1, and "Buildings and Facilities" is only one of 11 subparts.

cGMPs should be considered from the beginning of a product's development. As mentioned previously, the Food, Drug, and Cosmetic Act (FD&C Act) requires all drugs and biologics to comply with cGMP.[16] The FDA has recently issued a draft guidance on cGMP for Phase I investigational products,[17] part of the agency's effort to develop an approach to implementing manufacturing controls during the early stages of development. The approach described in the draft guidance is in concert with the CBER's approach of taking into consideration the type of product and the stage of development in determining applicable cGMP.

Following are some of the recommendations of the draft guidance on cGMP for Phase I investigational products[17]:

- Use adequate quality control (QC) procedures, including well-defined written procedures, adequately controlled equipment, and accurately and consistently recorded data.

- Consider the risks posed by various aspects of the production environment that might adversely affect the quality of a product, and give thorough consideration to controls for aseptic processing, especially when the IND product is produced in a facility that was not expressly designed for that function.

- Use disposable equipment and disposable process aids, prepackaged water or validated water for injection, and presterilized containers.

- Use a closed system for manufacturing.

The information that is discussed in the following subsections of this chapter is designed to assist manufacturers in complying with regulatory requirements, including some of the cGMP regulations, and in demonstrating that the cellular therapy product is safe, pure, and potent. It is not intended to be an exhaustive discussion of the issues that make up cGMP and other regulations; rather, it is a selection of those issues that the FDA has observed to be common challenges for cellular therapy products.

Manufacture of the Cellular Therapy Product

Components and Materials

The manufacture of a cell therapy product that meets the standards set forth in FDA regulations necessitates beginning with safe and pure components and materials. This is often a challenge for cellular therapies, not only because of the risks

Table 2-1. Current Good Manufacturing Practice for Finished Pharmaceuticals (21 CFR Part 211)

Subpart A	General Provisions
Subpart B	Organization and Personnel
Subpart C	Buildings and Facilities
Subpart D	Equipment
Subpart E	Control of Components and Drug Product Containers and Closures
Subpart F	Production and Process Controls
Subpart G	Packaging and Labeling Control
Subpart H	Holding and Distribution
Subpart I	Laboratory Controls
Subpart J	Records and Reports
Subpart K	Returned and Salvaged Drug Products

associated with the cells themselves, but also because of the broad range of cytokines, growth factors, and other materials that are used for cell growth, cellular differentiation, or cellular activation. It is beneficial to include detailed information regarding components and materials in IND submissions to ensure adequate regulatory review. All materials used in the manufacture of the cell therapy product should be documented; the source and all testing should be noted.

Cellular Starting Material

Cells should be classified as autologous or allogeneic, and the tissue source, mobilization protocol, if appropriate, and collection method should be documented. Donor screening, safety testing, and any additional characterization should also be documented.

Donor screening and testing are essential for ensuring that the cellular starting material is safe; however, this is a common deficiency in many cellular therapy IND applications. For allogeneic cellular products, prospective donors must meet the eligibility requirements. A complete description of the testing and screening of the donors should be provided in IND submissions, and documentation of testing should be maintained in the study records.[9] Each prospective donor should be screened for high-risk behavior and tested for the following communicable disease agents and others as appropriate[18,19]:

- Human immunodeficiency virus, type 1 (HIV-1).
- Human immunodeficiency virus, type 2 (HIV-2).
- Hepatitis B virus (HBV).
- Hepatitis C virus (HCV).
- *Treponema pallidum* (syphilis).

In addition, specimens from donors of viable leukocyte-rich cells or tissues must be tested for the following cell-associated communicable diseases:

- Human T-cell lymphotrophic virus, type I (HTLV-I).
- Human T-cell lymphotrophic virus, type II (HTLV-II).
- Cytomegalovirus (CMV).

The FDA considers 1) risk of transmission, 2) severity of effect, and 3) availability of appropriate screening measures or tests as factors in determining whether a communicable disease not listed is relevant. West Nile virus, sepsis, and vaccinia are considered relevant diseases. Other communicable diseases or disease agents, such as Epstein-Barr virus (EBV), may be relevant, and sponsors should consult the appropriate regulations and guidances for more detailed information.[18-20]

The authors recommend that testing be performed using FDA-licensed, -approved, or -cleared donor screening tests when they are available.[21] Donors whose screening tests are reactive for HIV-1, HIV-2, HBV, HCV, HTLV-I, or HTLV-II should be excluded. Additional testing, including typing for polymorphisms and major histocompatibility complex (MHC) matching, should be included as appropriate. Detailed information on donor eligibility is available in an FDA guidance document.[20]

For autologous cell products, the FDA recommends that donors be tested for HIV-1, HIV-2, HBV, and HCV and that the medical history include questions pertaining to high-risk behavior for HIV and hepatitis. To ensure the safety of the recipient and of persons handling the product, autologous materials that are positive for specific pathogens and untested autologous materials should be labeled as such. In addition, the tissue culture methods used during the manufacture should be shown not to propagate viruses so that viruses are not delivered in increased titer back to the autologous recipient or spread to other persons.

In addition to safety testing, starting material characterization becomes important as products progress into the later stages of product development. There is often a great deal of heterogeneity in the starting cellular material. For example, cell number, phenotypes, activation status, or viability might differ among the starting materials obtained from different donors. Understanding heterogeneity is the first step to controlling it. The ability to control heterogeneity can become a problem in late-stage product development if heterogeneity affects the safety, purity, or potency of the product. Strategies for controlling heterogeneity can be designed and tested early in development if starting material characterization is initiated early.

It may be appropriate to use a cell bank system for some cellular therapy products, such as those that are produced repeatedly from the same cell source. These cell banks are often a two-tiered system composed of a master cell bank (MCB) and a working cell bank (WCB) derived from one or more vials of the MCB. Cells from the WCB are then used for the production of the cellular therapy product. One advantage of a cell bank system is the opportunity to characterize the cells in a methodical and detailed fashion. Cell bank systems should be documented thoroughly. Information regarding the history, source, derivation, characterization, and frequency of testing for each MCB and WCB should be provided. MCB characterization is often incomplete in original IND submissions, and the additional testing required can lead to long delays in the initiation of Phase I studies. The MCB characterization should include thorough testing to adequately establish the safety, identity, purity, and stability of the cells, as follows:

- Adventitious agent testing—bacteria, fungi, mycoplasmas, and viruses.

- Identity testing—genotypic, phenotypic, or other markers, including activity and maturation stage if appropriate.

- Purity—fraction of the cells displaying the identity markers, including identification of contaminating cells.

- Stability—genetic and phenotypic stability after passage and viability.

WCB characterization should include the following:

- Adventitious agent testing.

- Limited identity testing.

The cells should undergo viral testing, both in vitro (MCB, WCB, and a one-time test of the end-of-production cells, as appropriate) and in vivo (MCB). If there is not a two-tiered cell bank system in place, more detailed testing of the single-tier cell bank is necessary. Specifics of the testing will depend on the species of origin. If banked cells have been exposed to bovine, porcine, or other animal materials, such as porcine trypsin or fetal bovine serum (FBS), the cells should also be tested for bovine and/or porcine adventitious agents. If a feeder cell line is used, information describing the characterization of this cell line should be included. If the feeder line is of animal origin, the final product falls within the definition of a xenotransplantation product, and the relevant guidance document[10] should be consulted. Additional information regarding cell bank systems is available in FDA and International Conference on Harmonisation (ICH) documents.[22,23,24]

Other Materials

Certain materials, such as FBS, cytokines, and monoclonal antibodies, may be essential for cellular growth, differentiation, selection, purification, or other critical manufacturing steps but may not be intended to be part of the final product. Nevertheless, they can affect the safety, potency, and purity of the final product, especially by introducing adventitious agents. Providing a table that lists materials used in manufacturing and components found in the final formulation of the cell therapy product is a good way to ensure that the information is communicated clearly and consistently. The source, vendor, quality, and final concentration should be included. Whenever possible, FDA-licensed products should be used in the manufacturing process. If a material is not FDA approved (eg, research grade material), a certificate of analysis (COA) should be supplied, or if a master file exists in the FDA, a letter of cross-reference from the manufacturer should be provided, and additional testing may be important to ensure the safety and quality of the material. Limits should be established for the concentrations of all materials that may persist in the final product, and methods used to remove them should be provided.

Some materials that are frequently used in production of cellular therapies are the subject of specific regulatory concerns. Many of the potential concerns they raise can be avoided if the proper documentation is provided. However, when the supplier of the material has not performed all the required testing, additional testing is needed. The following are examples of these materials and the related regulatory requirements:

- Human serum albumin and other materials derived from human plasma should be documented to be FDA-licensed products, or documentation should be provided to demonstrate that appropriate donor eligibility criteria and appropriate production procedures have been followed. Additionally, a system should be in place to ensure that recalled lots are not used during the manufacture of the product.

- For animal-derived materials, the source species, supplier or vendor, country of origin, and stage of manufacturing (when appropriate) should be provided. Title 9 CFR 113.47 lists a number of viruses from bovine, caprine, ovine, porcine, and other species that may be of concern.[25] For example, porcine products should be documented to be free of porcine parvovirus. If a reagent is derived from bovine material, it is important to identify the bovine material; the source of the material; information on the location where the herd was born, raised, and slaughtered; and any information relevant to the likelihood that the animal may have ingested animal feed prohibited under 21 CFR 589.2000.[26] Bovine material may be introduced at different points in the production of a reagent, and the information described above should be provided for all bovine materials used.

- Information on the purification and testing of all monoclonal antibodies (mAbs) and growth factors (including cytokines) used in the manufacturing process should be provided. These products, when marketed for research purposes, may contain byproducts of the expression system, including endotoxin and adventitious agents, and some growth factors may be prepared using mAbs that have not been suitably tested for adventitious agents. Additional information is available in an FDA points-to-consider document.[27]

- Documentation of the source and adventitious agent screening of keyhole limpet hemocyanin (KLH).

In addition to the materials listed above, for which the introduction of adventitious agents is of great concern, antibiotics also generate regulatory concerns. FDA strongly encourages the use of antibiotic-free media because antibiotics may confound the results of sterility testing. (See "Microbiological Testing.") In addition, because some patients may be sensitive to penicillin, the FDA has recommended that beta-lactam antibiotics not be used during the manufacturing of therapeutic products for humans. If they are used, appropriate exclusion criteria and informed consent for the study should be addressed.

FDA recommends that a qualification program be established for all critical materials and that this program consist of appropriate safety tests, an anal-

ysis for purity, and a functional assay to ensure that these materials are performing as desired in the manufacturing process. These tests should be performed each time a new lot is qualified. Program functions may include testing each lot after receipt from the vendor or reviewing certificates of analysis supplied by the vendor that document all testing results. After the materials have been deemed adequate, they can be released for use in the manufacturing process.

Manufacturing Procedures

A common misconception among sponsors of cell therapy IND submissions is that the FDA is interested only in starting materials and final product testing and not in the details of manufacture. Given that for biological products in general, and cellular therapy products in particular, the manufacturing process itself plays a significant role in defining the product, the FDA requests detailed descriptions of all procedures used during the production and purification of the cellular therapy product.

To ensure product safety, the procedures, in addition to the assays used for product release testing, should be adequately developed by the time of an original IND submission, and their descriptions should be provided in that submission. When possible, a schematic of the production and purification process, in-process testing, and final product testing, with timing, should be provided. In order to monitor the product quality adequately during extended culture periods, FDA recommends that in-process testing be performed at various time points. This testing may include safety, product characterization, and purity of the cellular therapy product, including the types of cells present and percentage of each cell type. It is expected that the procedures used in manufacture will be refined during early-phase studies, but the manufacturing process should be well established before pivotal studies are initiated, and changes to the process should be minimized once the pivotal trials are initiated. Changes in manufacturing during or after the pivotal studies will require demonstration of product comparability. The clinical trial results could be confounded by manufacturing changes. Validation of analytical methods, systems processes, and facilities must be completed by the time of submission of a BLA.

Procedures describing the preparation of the autologous or allogeneic cells should include information about the method of cell collection, processing, and culture conditions. Cell numbers and concentrations or volumes of solution or medium should documented, as well as mechanical or enzymatic digestion steps or the use of a cell selection or separation device, including density gradients, magnetic beads, or fluorescence-activated cell sorting (FACS).

Systems for tracking, labeling, and segregation should be followed from collection of the cells until administration or other disposition of the product. Among cellular therapy products, descriptions of these systems are common omissions from the CMC section of IND submissions. The systems for tracking, labeling, and segregation should be designed to ensure unambiguously that a patient receives the correct cells. The labeling should include two unique patient-specific identifiers, and segregation procedures should be combined with appropriate cleaning and control procedures to prevent cross-contamination among products produced in the same facility.

Sterility, an important aspect of safety, is of great importance in cellular therapy manufacture. Because it is not possible to sterilize cellular therapy products before administration, documentation should be provided to demonstrate that aseptic processing steps are adequate. It may be beneficial to conduct a process simulation using bacterial growth media to demonstrate that processing is performed in a manner that will maintain sterility of an aseptically processed IND product. The following list provides an overview of aseptic processing concerns. More detailed information is available in an FDA guidance document.[28]

- Buildings and facilities: The manufacturing areas such as biological safety cabinets and clean rooms should be designed and controlled to ensure an aseptic environment.

- Personnel training, qualification, and monitoring: Personnel should be trained in proper aseptic techniques, clean room behavior, microbiology, hygiene, gowning, patient safety hazards posed by a nonsterile drug product, and written procedures that cover aseptic manufacturing area operations. These principles also apply to personnel who perform aseptic

sampling and microbiological laboratory analyses. A personnel monitoring program should be in place.

- Components and containers or closures: Components (including active ingredients and excipients) and any containers or closures that come in contact with the product should be sterile.

- Endotoxin control: Endotoxin in or on materials, containers, closures, and manufacturing equipment should be measured and controlled.

- Time limitations: Time limits should be established for each phase of aseptic processing, when appropriate, and these time limits should be supported by data.

- Laboratory controls: Environmental, microbiological, and particle monitoring should be performed in critical areas.

- Sterility testing: Accurate testing should be ensured. Important elements of testing include sample handling, control of the testing environment, understanding the test limitations, and investigating manufacturing systems following a positive test.

- Batch record review—process control documentation: All available batch records and data should be reviewed prior to the final release decision for an aseptically processed product and should include all in-process results, laboratory control results, environment and personnel monitoring data, and output data from support systems such as high-efficiency particulate air filtration (HEPA), heating, ventilation, and air conditioning (HVAC), and water for injection.

If irradiation procedures are used, the irradiation dose and qualification of equipment should be supported by data. For example, if irradiation is used to abrogate cell proliferation, documentation should be provided establishing that the dose of irradiation renders the cells replication-incompetent and that the cells maintain their desired characteristics. A description of the program for maintenance and calibration of the irradiator should also be provided.

Process timing can be critical in cellular therapy manufacturing. Storage time and conditions between cell collection and final harvest should be documented. Adequate procedures should be in place to ensure stability of the cellular product during fresh and frozen storage.

Both the procedures for preparing the product and the final product formulation are critical to product safety and quality. Information regarding these final steps, including centrifugation, buffers, and media used for washes, cell concentrations, and excipients, should be included in the IND submission. The storage and shipping conditions of cellular therapy products can be as varied as the products themselves, so it is important to properly define and document them. For example, if the final product is delivered to the clinical site frozen, shipping information and data to show that the product can be consistently thawed should be provided. Retention samples should be collected and properly stored. Retrospective analysis of retention samples may be very useful when unexpected situations arise. The FDA recognizes that for cellular therapy products, it might not be possible to follow all the requirements of 21 CFR 211 cGMP for reserve samples because of lot size and stability issues that would render the samples inadequate for future testing. It is expected that samples be retained, as appropriate to the product.

Product Specifications

Specifications are the quality standards (eg, tests, analytical procedures, and acceptance criteria) that confirm the quality of products and materials used in production. Specifications establish the set of criteria to which a product should conform to be considered acceptable for its intended use. Conformance to specification means that the material, when tested according to the listed analytical procedures, will meet the listed acceptance criteria. The specifications for cellular therapy products ensure the safety and consistency of the product. They should be based on experience with the specific product and similar products and may be refined as new data are collected. Various product specifications are discussed later in the chapter.

It is expected that certain specifications, such as those related to product safety, be in place before initiating Phase I clinical studies. As product development proceeds, additional specifications for product quality and manufacturing consistency should be implemented. Specifications for Phase I

studies should be based on data from lots used in preclinical studies and should include analytical procedures that are based on CFR methods or appropriate alternative methods. For Phase II, the specifications should be refined and tightened on the basis of data generated during Phase I. Phase III specifications should be based on further information collected during product development, and validation of analytical procedures should be ongoing or complete and consistent with data generated during clinical studies. For licensure, a complete set of specifications that is based on information collected during development using validated assays must be in place.[29]

Tests required for cellular therapy products include those for safety (microbiological testing, including sterility, mycoplasma, and adventitious viral agent testing, as appropriate), identity, purity (including endotoxin), potency, and other relevant parameters, such as viability. These tests will be discussed in further detail, and many are described in 21 CFR Part 610 and in FDA guidance documents.[6,7,13,17] Final product release specifications are a required component of a Phase I IND submission, although the actual specifications may evolve during product development. Specifications used for other intermediates should also be reported, as appropriate to the product. In-process testing should provide meaningful insight concerning process and product quality and should contribute to the safety and quality of the final product. All specifications should be clearly described in the IND submissions, and tabular format should be used when possible.

Testing of Cellular Therapies

The pharmaceutical industry, the FDA, and the ICH are exploring other manufacturing approaches that put more emphasis on process design and allow for more flexibility in product testing because testing alone cannot always be relied on to ensure product quality. Many of these concepts are applicable to the manufacture of cell therapies. Nonetheless, testing is an essential element in ensuring product quality.

Cellular therapies pose a number of challenges to final product testing. These challenges are often unique to cellular therapy. They may include the following:

- Short product shelf life due to cellular viability.

- Small sample volumes.

- Heterogeneous populations of cells.

- Variability in composition, activity, or potential of the cells.

- Inability to create appropriate reference materials.

- Complex or unknown mechanisms of action.

- Ability of the cells to differentiate after administration.

Because of these challenges, the FDA has tried to be flexible and innovative in how it applies the regulations for product testing. However, failure to provide procedures for adequate final product testing remains one of the primary deficiencies in new IND submissions. Table 2-2 describes the most common reasons that final product testing has been found deficient. This table highlights the challenges in applying final product testing regulations to cellular therapy products.

Recommendations for testing, including recommendations specific to testing during Phase I, are available in FDA guidance documents.[13,17] The FDA recognizes that for cellular therapy products at all phases, the lot size may be prohibitive for following test sample volume requirements given in CFR and USP test methods. It is expected that, for many products, approximately 10% of the product be allotted for sterility testing and that the amount used for other required lot release testing be adequate to provide valid results using the methods chosen.

Table 2-2. Common Product Testing Deficiencies

Test not performed

Inappropriate timing of sample collection

Inadequate description of test method

Unacceptable or unqualified test method

Inadequate or inappropriate specification

Microbiological Testing

Sterility (bacterial and fungal) testing. Sterility testing on the final product should be performed using the 14-day direct inoculation test method described in 21 CFR 610.12[30] or USP <71>.[31] Alternatively, an automated detection or other method that yields results equivalent to the method described in 21 CFR 610.12 may be used. Equivalency of an alternate testing method with the specified 14-day sterility test must be validated for licensure.[30-32] The method used for testing should be described in detail. Samples should include both cells and supernatant. Manufacturers of cellular therapies often use antibiotics during cell culture, but the presence of antibiotics in test samples may confound sterility results. Therefore, bacteriostasis and fungistasis testing, as described in USP <71>, should be performed to ensure that any residual antibiotic does not interfere with the sterility testing. It is important to note that samples for sterility testing should be obtained after final product manipulation, ie, after all washing procedures, and, preferably, as the final formulation. If the product is manipulated (eg, by washing or culture) after thawing or at any other time (eg, after transport to the study site), the sponsor should repeat the sterility testing. A "no growth" acceptance criterion is used for product release.

Cellular therapy products that are not cryo-preserved have short shelf lives. Therefore, the results of a full 14-day sterility assay on the final product may not be available before administration of the product. Whenever possible, a sample, including both cells and supernatant, should be taken for sterility testing approximately 48-72 hours before the final harvest or coincident with the last refeeding of the culture. An interim reading of this sterility test at the time of product release will contribute to a sterility determination. A rapid microbial detection test, such as a Gram's stain, should also be performed on the final product before administration, and these results will contribute to a sterility determination. A sterility test should also be performed on a sample of the final product, and both the in-process (48-72 hour) and the final product sterility test should be continued for the full 14-day culture.

A commonly overlooked piece of information that should be included in a cellular therapy IND submission is a positive sterility test action plan. Documentation of the procedures to be followed in the event that either of the 14-day sterility tests reveals that a contaminated product was administered to a patient should be in place before the initiation of clinical studies. These procedures should include physician and patient notification, identification and sensitivity testing of the contaminant, additional patient monitoring, investigation to determine potential sources of the contamination and corrective actions, and reporting of the incident to the institutional review board (IRB) and the FDA as an adverse event within 15 calendar days.

Mycoplasma testing. If product manufacture includes culture for more than 48 hours, the product should usually also be tested for mycoplasma contamination. Problems with mycoplasma testing seen by the FDA are similar to problems seen for sterility testing. Unlike sterility testing, mycoplasma testing should be performed on samples obtained before final manipulation (ie, on cells still in the culture medium, before final harvest and wash). Samples should include both cells and supernatant. The recommended testing procedure has been described in an FDA memorandum.[23] For products that must be administered before obtaining the results from mycoplasma culture testing, rapid mycoplasma detection assays (eg, PCR-based assays) may be performed. For licensure, equal sensitivity and specificity between the rapid assay and culture-based assay must be verified.[32]

Identity Testing

For licensed products, the identity of the final product must be verified by assays that will identify the product for proper labeling and will distinguish the product from other products being processed in the same facility.[33] Appropriate assays should be developed and used during product development. If an MCB is used in production, the identity of the MCB should also be verified, and if multiple cell lines are used, the testing should be capable of distinguishing between the cell lines. Assays that might be useful for identity testing include those for cell surface markers and those for genetic polymorphisms and MHC. Additional information regarding identity testing is available in FDA guidance.[34]

Purity Testing

Product purity can be defined as freedom from extraneous material, except that which is unavoidable in the manufacturing process.[35] Testing for purity includes assays for pyrogenicity or endotoxin, unintended cell populations (eg, distinguished by phenotypes), residual proteins or peptides used to stimulate or pulse cells, and materials used during manufacture, such as cytokines, growth factors, antibodies, and sera. Acceptance criteria should be established for known impurities. For example, limits should be set for unintended cell types in the final cellular product.

Any product intended for use by injection must be tested for pyrogenic substances.[36]

The specifics of endotoxin testing is another area commonly overlooked by sponsors of cell therapy IND submissions. Endotoxin testing using the limulus amebocyte lysate (LAL) assay method is adequate for early-phase clinical trials of cellular therapy products. Similar to samples for sterility testing, samples for purity testing should be taken from the final product, ie, following final manipulations. The acceptance criteria in the specifications for endotoxin testing must be set at or below the prescribed upper limits. The upper limit for endotoxin is 5 endotoxin units (EU) per kg of body weight per hour for parenteral drug, except for those administered intrathecally. Intrathecally administered drugs have a limit of 0.2 EU/kg body weight per dose.[38]

Potency Testing

Potency is the specific ability or capacity of the product to effect a given result, as indicated by appropriate laboratory tests or by adequately controlled clinical data obtained through the administration of the product in the manner intended.[39] Ideally, a potency assay is a quantitative in-vivo or in-vitro bioassay that measures biological function of the clinical mechanism of action. These may be by in vivo or in vitro tests.[40] If direct measure of a biological function is not feasible, data must be provided to justify use of a test or combination of tests to ensure product potency. The potency assay should be in place by the end of Phase II, and the assay must be validated for licensure.[29] Developing good potency assays can be challenging. Starting early and communicating with the FDA can help eliminate delays later in development.

Other Testing Concerns

Viability. For most cellular therapy products, the cells are intended to be viable. In some cases, cellular debris or cell clumping may affect the safety of the product. In all cases, viability is an important measure of product consistency. Therefore, a minimum viability release criterion should be established. It is recommended that this specification be at least 70%. If this level cannot be achieved, data should be submitted to support an appropriate level.

Cell count. A specification for the number of cells should also be established. In many cases, the total cell number defines the dose. In other cases, the dose may be defined by the number of cells of a specific cell type within the total cell population. In either case, there should also be specifications for the minimum number of viable and functional cells to be administered. Additional documentation should be provided regarding whether a maximum number or dose of cells to be administered has been established and the basis for this specification.

General safety testing. Cellular therapy products are exempt from general safety testing.[41]

Stability

The characteristics of the final cellular therapy product should remain within the specification limits until the product is administered to the patient. Stability testing ensures that products retain consistent safety, purity, and potency through the expiration date of the product. Documentation of stability testing will increase as product development proceeds. Stability testing in early phases of clinical trials should show that the product is sufficiently stable during intervals of holding and shipping and for the period required by the study (for cryopreserved products). During later phases, stability testing should be expanded to develop an expiration dating period for the product. By the end of Phase III, validation studies, including those using conditions that stress the system, should be completed.[42,43] During later development, or after licensure, it may be useful to develop formal stability protocols that are reviewed

by the FDA. These protocols may then be a basis for ongoing or recurring stability testing.

Results of stability studies, and the protocols used for the studies, should be provided in IND and BLA submissions.[43] The protocols should include analyses for product potency, product integrity, and sterility. In-process stability testing should be performed as appropriate (eg, prefreeze and post-thaw testing of cryopreserved cells used in the manufacturing process). Final product stability testing should demonstrate that product integrity, potency, and sterility have been maintained under the proposed shipping conditions, in addition to having been maintained under holding conditions. Further information regarding stability testing and protocols is available in ICH guidance documents.[44-47]

Validation in Manufacturing Cellular Therapy Products

All of the facilities, equipment, processes, systems, and methods used in the manufacture of cellular therapies should be shown to perform as expected. Validation of these parameters is required for licensure; the requirement for validation is set forth in the cGMP regulations for finished pharmaceuticals.[5,6] Validation is a documented program that provides a high degree of assurance that a specific process, method, or system will consistently produce a result meeting predetermined acceptance criteria. Validation provides documented evidence, acquired across the full range of operating conditions, that a process, method, or system does what it is supposed to do. It takes into account operating differences such as changes in operator, conditions, materials, or operating times, or other changes that might impact performance. Experience during development can often help to define those changes that are most likely to affect the product and thus inform the design of the validation studies. For products being manufactured for Phase I trials, recommendations on complying with the cGMP validation requirements have been described.[17]

Conclusion

This chapter has summarized current regulatory advice, regulations, and practices that pertain to the manufacture of cellular therapy products. However, as cellular therapy products are rapidly evolving, so must the regulation of these products. The reader is cautioned to investigate appropriate FDA Web sites to determine pertinent rules, guidance documents, and current practices.

References/Resources

1. Food and Drug Administration. Application of current statutory authorities to human somatic cell therapy products and gene therapy products. Fed Regist 1993;58:53248-51.

2. United States Code. Definitions. 21 U.S.C. Sec 321(g)(1). Suppl 4. Washington, DC: US Government Printing Office, 2000.

3. United States Code. Regulation of biological products. 42 U.S.C. Sec 262(a). Suppl 4. Washington, DC: US Government Printing Office, 2000.

4. Code of federal regulations. How does FDA define important terms in this part? Title 21 CFR Part 1271.3(d)(2). Washington, DC: US Government Printing Office, 2008 (revised annually).

5. Code of federal regulations. Current good manufacturing practice in manufacturing, processing, packing, or holding of drugs; general. Title 21 CFR Part 210. Washington, DC: US Government Printing Office, 2008 (revised annually).

6. Code of federal regulations. Current good manufacturing practice for finished pharmaceuticals. Title 21 CFR Part 211. Washington, DC: US Government Printing Office, 2008 (revised annually).

7. Code of federal regulations. General biological product standards. Title 21 CFR Part 610. Washington, DC: US Government Printing Office, 2008 (revised annually).

8. Code of federal regulations. Human cells, tissues, and cellular and tissue-based products. Title 21 CFR Part 1271. Washington, DC: US Government Printing Office, 2008 (revised annually).

9. Code of federal regulations. How do I determine if a donor is eligible? Title 21 CFR Part 1271.50. Washington, DC: US Government Printing Office, 2008 (revised annually).

10. Food and Drug Administration. Guidance for industry: Source animal, product, preclinical, and clinical issues concerning the use of xenotransplantation products in humans. (April 3, 2003) Rockville, MD: CBER Office of Communication, Training, and Manufacturers Assistance, 2003.

11. Xenotransplantation action plan. Rockville, MD: Food and Drug Administration, 2006.

12. Code of federal regulations. IND content and format. Title 21 CFR Part 312.23. Washington, DC: US Government Printing Office, 2008 (revised annually).

13. Food and Drug Administration. Guidance for FDA reviewers and sponsors: Content and review of chemistry, manufacturing, and control (CMC) information for human somatic cell therapy investigational new drug applications (INDs). (April 2008) Rockville, MD: CBER Office of Communication, Training, and Manufacturers Assistance, 2008.

14. References for the regulatory process for the Office of Cellular, Tissue, and Gene Therapies (OCTGT). Rockville, MD: Food and Drug Administration, 2007.

15. Food and Drug Administration. Guidance for industry: Formal meetings with sponsors and applicants for PDUFA products. (February 2000) Rockville, MD: CDER Office of Training and Communication and CBER Office of Communication, Training, and Manufacturers Assistance, 2000.

16. United States Code. Adulterated drugs and devices. 21 U.S.C. Sec. 351(a)(2)(B). Suppl 4. Washington, DC: US Government Printing Office, 2000.

17. Food and Drug Administration. Draft guidance for industry: INDs—approaches to complying with cGMP during Phase 1. (January 2006) Rockville, MD: CDER Office of Training and Communication and CBER Office of Communication, Training, and Manufacturers Assistance, 2006.

18. Code of federal regulations. Test requirements. Title 21 CFR Part 610.40. Washington, DC: US Government Printing Office, 2008 (revised annually).

19. Code of federal regulations. What donor testing is required for different types of cells and tissues? Title 21 CFR Part 1271.85. Washington, DC: US Government Printing Office, 2008 (revised annually).

20. Food and Drug Administration. Guidance for industry: Eligibility determination for donors of human cells, tissues, and cellular and tissue-based products (HCT/Ps). (February 2007) Rockville, MD: CBER Office of Communication, Training, and Manufacturers Assistance, 2007.

21. Code of federal regulations. What are the general requirements for donor testing? Title 21 CFR Part 1271.80(c). Washington, DC: US Government Printing Office, 2008 (revised annually).

22. Food and Drug Administration. International Conference on Harmonisation; guidance on viral safety evaluation of biotechnology products derived from cell lines of human or animal origin; availability. Docket No. 96D—0058. Fed Regist 1998;63:51074-84.

23. Food and Drug Administration. Memorandum: Points to consider in the characterization of cell lines used to produce biologicals. (July 12, 1993) Rockville, MD: CBER Office of Communication, Training, and Manufacturers Assistance, 1993.

24. Food and Drug Administration. International Conference on Harmonisation; guidance on quality of biotechnological/biological products: Derivation and characterization of cell substrates used for production of biotechnological/biological products; availability. Fed Regist 1998;63:50244-9.

25. Code of federal regulations. Detection of extraneous viruses by the fluorescent antibody technique. Title 9 CFR Part 113.47. Washington, DC: US Government Printing Office, 2008 (revised annually).

26. Code of federal regulations. Animal proteins prohibited in ruminant feed. Title 21 CFR Part 589.2000. Washington, DC: US Government Printing Office, 2008 (revised annually).

27. Food and Drug Administration. Points to consider in the manufacture and testing of monoclonal antibody products for human use. Docket No. 94-D—0259. (February 27, 1997) Rockville, MD: CBER Office of Communication, Training, and Manufacturers Assistance, 1997.

28. Food and Drug Administration. Guidance for industry: Sterile drug products produced by aseptic processing—current good manufacturing practice. (September 2004) Rockville, MD: CDER Office of Training and Communication and CBER Office of Communication, Training, and Manufacturers Assistance, 2004.

29. Code of federal regulations. Testing and release for distribution. Title 21 CFR Part 211.165. Washington, DC: US Government Printing Office, 2008 (revised annually).

30. Code of federal regulations. Sterility. Title 21 CFR Part 610.12. Washington, DC: US Government Printing Office, 2008 (revised annually).

31. United States Pharmacopeia. General chapter <71> sterility tests. USP 30. Rockville, MD: USP Convention, 2007.

32. Code of federal regulations. Equivalent methods and processes. Title 21 CFR Part 610.9. Washington, DC: US Government Printing Office, 2008 (revised annually).

33. Code of federal regulations. Identity. Title 21 CFR Part 610.14. Washington, DC: US Government Printing Office, 2008 (revised annually).

34. Food and Drug Administration. Guidance for industry: Human somatic cell therapy and gene therapy. (March 1998) Rockville, MD: CBER Office of Communication, Training, and Manufacturers Assistance, 1998.

35. Code of federal regulations. Purity. Title 21 CFR Part 610.13. Washington, DC: US Government Printing Office, 2008 (revised annually).

36. Code of federal regulations. Purity: Test for pyrogenic substances. Title 21 CFR Part 610.13(b). Washington, DC: US Government Printing Office, 2008 (revised annually).

37. United States Pharmacopeia. Chapter <151> pyrogen test. USP 30. Rockville, MD: USP Convention, 2007.

38. Food and Drug Administration. Guideline on validation of the limulus amebocyte lysate test as an end-product endotoxin test for human and animal parenteral drugs, biological products, and medical devices. (December 1987) Rockville, MD: CDER, Division of Manufacturing and Product Quality, and CBER, CDRH, and CVM, 1987.

39. Code of federal regulations. Definitions. Title 21 CFR Part 600.3(s). Washington, DC: US Government Printing Office, 2008 (revised annually).

40. Code of federal regulations. Potency. Title 21 CFR Part 610.10. Washington, DC: US Government Printing Office, 2008 (revised annually).

41. Code of federal regulations. General safety. Title 21 CFR Part 601.11(g)(1). Washington, DC: US Government Printing Office, 2008 (revised annually).

42. Code of federal regulations. Stability testing. Title 21 CFR Part 211.166. Washington, DC: US Government Printing Office, 2008 (revised annually).

43. Code of federal regulations. Application for biologics licenses; procedures for filing. Title 21 CFR Part 601.2. Washington, DC: US Government Printing Office, 2008 (revised annually).

44. Food and Drug Administration. International Conference on Harmonisation; final guidelines on stability testing of biotechnological/biological products; availability; notice. Docket No. 93D—0139. Fed Regist 1996;61: 36465-9.

45. Food and Drug Administration. International Conference on Harmonisation. Guidance for industry: Q1A(R2) stability testing of new drug substances and products. (November 2003) Rockville, MD: CDER Office of Training and Communication and CBER Office of Communication, Training, and Manufacturers Assistance, 2003.

46. Food and Drug Administration. International Conference on Harmonisation. Guidance for industry: Q1E Evaluation of stability data. (June 2004) Rockville, MD: CDER Office of Training and Communication and CBER Office of Communication, Training, and Manufacturers Assistance, 2004.

47. Food and Drug Administration. International Conference on Harmonisation; guidance for industry: Q1D Bracketing and matrixing designs for stability testing of new drug substances and products. (January 2003) Rockville, MD: CDER Division of Drug Information and CBER Office of Communication, Training, and Manufacturers Assistance, 2003.

In: Areman EM, Loper K, eds
Cellular Therapy: Principles, Methods, and Regulations
Bethesda, MD: AABB, 2009

◆ ◆ ◆   3

The Investigational New Drug Application

*David H. McKenna, Jr, MD; Victoria A. Lake, BSc, BA, RAC; and
Darin J. Weber, PhD*

BEFORE CLINICAL TRIALS WITH CELLU-lar therapies are initiated, an investigational new drug (IND) application needs to be filed with the Food and Drug Administration (FDA). Products requiring an IND application are subject to the applicable current good tissue practice (cGTP) and (more rigorous) current good manufacturing practice (cGMP) regulations [Section 351, Public Health Service Act (Biologic); Section 505, Food, Drug, and Cosmetic Act (Drug); and Code of Federal Regulations (CFR) Title 21 Part 312, Investigational New Drug Application].

Before IND application submission, a type B pre-IND meeting may be requested of the FDA.[1] This meeting (often a conference call) must be held within 60 days of the request from the IND sponsor, and the date must be determined within 14 days of receipt of the request. The FDA requires that a meeting packet be supplied to the agency at least 30 days before the meeting. This packet includes a table of contents, an agenda, lists of attendees and specific questions for the FDA, and supporting information. A meeting summary from the FDA usually follows within 30 days of the meeting. A type B pre-IND meeting is not required.

However, it is suggested that one be arranged if the product is novel or there are other concerns that have not already been addressed in existing guidance documents.[2] Avoidance of a clinical hold (discussed later) on an IND application is not guaranteed by a pre-IND meeting, but concerns identified during a pre-IND meeting often indicate whether there are important issues that should be resolved before the IND submission.

Overview

The IND application content and format are discussed in 21 CFR 312.23. For an initial IND application, a completed Form FDA 1571, "Investigational New Drug Application," must be submitted along with the following information:

- A table of contents.
- An introductory statement.
- A general investigational plan.
- An investigator's brochure (if not a sponsor-investigator IND application).
- The clinical protocols.

David H. McKenna, Jr, MD, Scientific and Medical Director, Molecular and Cellular Therapeutics, University of Minnesota, St Paul, Minnesota; Victoria A. Lake, BSc, BA, RAC, Regulatory Affairs Director, Fred Hutchinson Cancer Research Center, Seattle, Washington; and Darin J. Weber, PhD, Senior Consultant, Biologics Consulting Group, Inc, Seattle, Washington

D. McKenna has disclosed a financial relationship with BioE, Inc. V. Lake and D. Weber have disclosed no conflicts of interest.

Manufacturing Process Flowchart

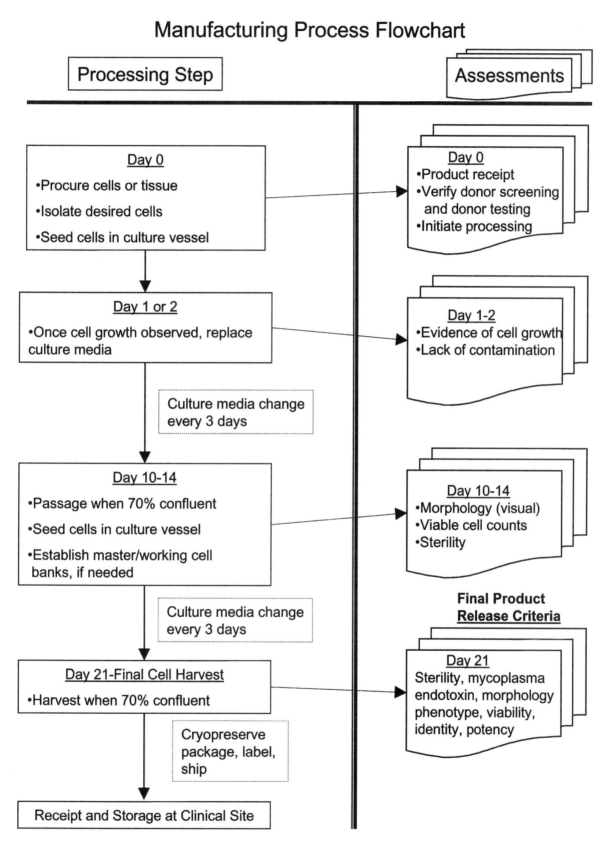

Figure 3-1. Sample flow diagram for cell processing and testing.

- A completed Form FDA 1572, which includes investigator data, facilities data, and institutional review board (IRB) data.
- The chemistry, manufacturing, and controls (CMC) information.
- The pharmacology and toxicology data.
- A record of previous human experience.
- Any other additional necessary information.

The FDA reviews the IND application on the basis of the best available science.[3] Upon receipt, the FDA issues an acknowledgment letter that provides the IND number and working title. The FDA review team typically consists of a product reviewer, who examines product safety and manufacturing issues; a pharmacology and toxicology reviewer, who examines the supporting preclinical studies; a clinical reviewer, who examines the proposed clinical study design and analysis; and a regulatory project manager, who is responsible for the IND administrative management. Reviewers with additional expertise may be assigned to review the IND submission.

The emphasis of the IND review is on data that demonstrate product safety, provide basic product characterization information, address product manufacturing and quality issues, establish appropriate product release testing specifications, and ensure that there is a strong scientific rationale for the clinical development program that is supported by informative preclinical studies. FDA reviewers have 30 days from the date of receipt to review the IND submission and determine whether the IND application may proceed or will be placed on clini-cal hold. Typically, one or more of the FDA reviewers contacts the IND holder by phone to discuss any outstanding issues and determine if they can be resolved before the 30-day review period expires. The clinical trial may commence upon notification from the FDA or once 30 days have passed from the date of receipt of the application at the FDA. If the FDA requests more information from the IND holder, the study may be placed on clinical hold until the FDA receives an acceptable response. In the event of a clinical hold decision, the FDA sends the IND holder a letter detailing the basis for the clinical hold and the specific information that is needed to remove the hold. The letter also contains a variety of non-hold-related, reviewer comments, which should be addressed as product development continues but which do not need to be addressed for the clinical hold to be removed.

Once the IND study is allowed to proceed, the FDA expects the study to be conducted in an appropriate manner that includes informed consent and a clinical monitoring program. Adequate records must be kept, and adverse events must be reported to the FDA as required. Any amendments to product manufacturing or the clinical trial must be submitted to the FDA. Furthermore, if the amendment is considered major (eg, dose change or substantial alteration to manufacturing), the modification should not be implemented before receipt and acknowledgement by the FDA. In some cases, it may be appropriate to discuss the proposed changes with the assigned FDA reviewers before the

Table 3-1. Sample Table for Materials Used During Manufacturing

Component or Material	Vendor	Source	Grade	Certificate of Analysis Available?
Culture medium	Company XYZ	Synthetic	Cell culture	Yes
Fetal bovine serum (FBS)*	Company 123	Bovine	Cell culture	Yes
Growth Factor X[†]	Company ABC	Recombinant	Cell culture	Yes
Dimethylsulfoxide	Company DEF	Synthetic	Cell culture	Yes

*FBS will be sourced from vendors who obtain FBS from low-risk countries as required in 9 CFR Part 94.18.

[†]Cross-reference letter to BB-Master File #XXXXX provided in (IND application) Appendix.

Table 3-2. Sample Table for Product Release Testing

Test	Typical Test Method	Typical Specification
Compliance with cGMP Requirements		
Sterility	USP <71> or 21 CFR 610.12	Negative
Mycoplasma	Culture method*	Negative
Purity (pyrogenicity)	(Limulus amebocyte lysate) endotoxin	<5 EU/kg (non-intrathecal) <0.2 EU/kg (intrathecal)
Identity	Not specified	Product specific[†]
Potency (functional assay)	Not specified	Product specific[†]
Viability	Not specified; propidium iodide or Trypan Blue	Product specific[†]; minimally >70%; lower with justification
Cell dose	Not specified; manual or automated cell counter	Product specific[†]; specific number depends on dosing indicated in clinical protocol
Potency	Not specified; secretion of a biologically relevant factor or marker	Product specific[†]; for early-phase clinical studies, a specification of "for information only" is acceptable
Characterization of Desired Therapeutic Cells		
Specific marker A	Not specified; flow cytometry, immunohistochemistry, PCR	Product specific[†]; often a minimum percentage of detectable expression
Specific marker B	Not specified; flow cytometry, immunohistochemistry, PCR	Product specific[†]; often a minimum percentage of detectable expression
Specific marker C	Not specified; flow cytometry, immunohistochemistry, PCR	Product specific[†]; often a minimum percentage of detectable expression
Characterization of Other Cellular Constituents		
Specific marker D	Not specified; flow cytometry, immunohistochemistry, PCR	Product specific[†]; often a maximum percentage of detectable expression
Specific marker E	Not specified; flow cytometry, immunohistochemistry, PCR	Product specific[†]; often a maximum percentage of detectable expression
Specific marker F	Not specified; flow cytometry, immunohistochemistry, PCR	Product specific[†]; often a maximum percentage of detectable expression

*Testing recommended at cell harvest.
[†]To be developed by product manufacturer.
cGMP = current good manufacturing practice; EU = endotoxin units per kilogram; PCR = polymerase chain reaction.

information is submitted to the IND file at the FDA.

Finally, a detailed annual report must be submitted to the FDA within 60 days of the anniversary date of the IND submission. This report is divided into two main sections: 1) individual study information; and 2) summary information. The individual study information typically includes a brief summary of each study being conducted under the IND application and information on the study progress, enrollment, and clinical results, if available. The summary information includes tabular summaries of adverse events, patient withdrawals, and manufacturing changes or information. For cellular therapies, the FDA also requests that a lot release table be included in the annual report. This table details the lot release information for each lot of the cellular therapy product, such as cell count, viability, and sterility testing results.

Chemistry, Manufacturing, and Controls Section

The CMC section of the IND application details the manufacturing of the cellular therapy product and, as such, is the primary focus of the remainder of this chapter. Product manufacturing, characterization, and testing information, including lot release specifications, are included in the CMC. A flow diagram is helpful in outlining the cell manufacturing process (see Fig 3-1), and summary tables should be created that describe the materials and reagents used during manufacturing as well as in-process and final product lot release testing (see Tables 3-1 and 3-2).

The amount of information included in the CMC section depends on the phase of the clinical trial (see 21 CFR 312.21), the source of the cellular materials (eg, autologous, allogeneic, or xenogeneic), and the complexity of the manufacturing process.[4] Sufficient information should be submitted to ensure the proper identification, quality, purity, and potency of the cellular therapy product.

A team approach to writing the CMC works well and ideally involves the laboratory and medical directors, principal investigators, manufacturing technical staff, and quality assurance (QA) or regulatory staff. All of the aforementioned parties bring valuable contributions to the effort.

Many FDA documents offer guidance for writing CMC sections for cell therapies.[5-10] The 2008 Guidance for Reviewers,[8] as well as documents referenced therein, is particularly helpful because it outlines the approach recommended to FDA reviewers of CMC sections of cellular-therapy-related submissions. It may be used as the framework for the CMC section, with other documents.[5-7,9,10] Appendix 3-1 offers a sample outline of a standard operating procedure for completing the CMC section of a cellular therapy IND application.

References/Resources

1. Food and Drug Administration. Guidance for industry: Formal meetings with sponsors and applicants for PDUFA products. (February 2000) Rockville, MD: CBER Office of Communication, Training, and Manufacturers Assistance, 2000.
2. Weiss KD. The biological pre-IND meeting. Rockville, MD: CDER, 2004.
3. Fink DW. Embryonic stem cell-based therapies: US-FDA regulatory expectations. Rockville, MD: CBER, 2007.
4. Weber DJ. Manufacturing considerations for clinical therapies derived from stem cells. Methods Enzymol 2006;420:410-30.
5. Food and Drug Administration. Memorandum: Points to consider in the characterization of cell lines used to produce biologicals. (July 12, 1993) Rockville, MD: CBER Office of Communication, Training, and Manufacturers Assistance, 1993.
6. Food and Drug Administration. Guidance for industry: Content and format of investigational new drug applications (INDs) for Phase I studies of drugs, including well-characterized, therapeutic, biotechnology-derived products. (November 1995) Rockville, MD: CDER Office of Training and Communication and CBER Office of Communication, Training, and Manufacturers Assistance, 1995.
7. Food and Drug Administration. Guidance for industry: Guidance for human somatic cell therapy and gene therapy. (March 1998) Rockville, MD: CBER Office of Communication, Training, and Manufacturers Assistance, 1998.
8. Food and Drug Administration. Guidance for FDA reviewers and sponsors: Content and review of chemistry, manufacturing, and control (CMC) information for human somatic cell therapy investigational new drug applications (INDs). (April 2008) Rockville, MD: CBER Office of Communication, Training, and Manufacturers Assistance, 2008.

9. Food and Drug Administration. Draft guidance for industry: INDs—approaches to complying with cGMP during Phase I (January 2006) Rockville, MD: CDER Office of Training and Communication and CBER Office of Communication, Training, and Manufacturers Assistance, 2006.

10. Cellular, Tissue and Gene Therapies Advisory Committee, Food and Drug Administration. FDA briefing document: Potency measurements for cellular and gene therapy products. (February 9, 2006) Rockville, MD: FDA, 2006.

Appendix 3-1. Sample Outline for Preparing the Chemistry, Manufacturing, and Controls Section of an Investigational New Drug Application

Description

This is an outline of one approach to preparing a chemistry, manufacturing, and controls (CMC) section of an investigational new drug (IND) application. It is based on Food and Drug Administration draft guidance.[1]

Outline

I. *Product Manufacturing and Characterization Information*
    A. General description of product
        1. Cell type, derivation
        2. Processing laboratory, address:
            - Accreditations
            - Reference type V master file (MF) for facility (if filed)
    B. Procurement
        1. Type of starting material
            - Peripheral blood mononuclear cells, cord blood, marrow, tumor, cell line, other
        2. Collection site
        3. Overview of process
    C. Infectious disease testing and prevention of cross-contamination
        1. Donor suitability according to current good tissue practice
        2. Medical history
        3. List of testing performed on donor
        4. Quarantine if positive infectious disease result
        5. Outline of process if product with positive result is to be infused
    D. Cell processing
        1. Description of processing methods
        2. Flow diagram outlining processing and testing

    E. Reagents
        1. Table indicating materials or components, manufacturer, and status [with reference to certificates of analysis (COAs), MFs and other IND submissions (if related), and FDA-approval if approved]
        2. Human serum albumin (HSA) (from certified countries)
        3. Include COAs for all reagents

II. *Product Testing*
    A. Microbial testing
        1. Sterility testing (bacterial or fungal culture)
            - Test method (eg, United States Pharmacopeia [USP], automated)
            - Time points tested (eg, final product, in-process), number of days culture is held)
        2. Mycoplasma testing
            - Test method [eg, polymerase chain reaction (PCR), culture]
            - Time points tested (eg, final product, in-process), number of days culture is held
            - Indication that sample for testing will include cells
        3. Gram's stain
            - Reference to donor infectious disease testing (Section I-C above)
    B. Identity
        Labeling, segregation, any test methods employed (eg, HLA, ABO typing)
    C. Purity
        1. Constitution of final suspension (eg, washed cells in 5% HSA)

2. Analysis (eg, flow cytometry, endotoxin)

D. Potency

Analysis (eg, flow cytometry as in-vitro surrogate, other in-vitro functional assays, in-vivo assessment)

E. Additional testing
  1. Viability
     - Method (eg, microscopy, flow cytometry)
     - Time points tested
  2. Cell dose
     - Method (eg, hematology analyzer)
     - Actual doses (range)
     - Minimum dose to allow for infusion
  3. Other
     - Retain aliquot

III. *Product Release Criteria Testing*

Table with lot release testing, including assay, method, specification, and location of testing if not in cell-processing laboratory

IV. *Product Stability*

A. Stability testing to support post-production clinical use

B. State of final product (eg, fresh, cryopreserved) and transit time and conditions

V. *Other Issues*

A. Product tracking
  1. Labeling according to standards and regulations
  2. Unique identifiers (number, name)

3. Process of confirmation of identity before administration
4. Segregation system

B. Labeling
  1. According to standards and regulations
  2. Additional items on label
  3. Include "Caution: New Drug— Limited by Federal Law to Investigational Use" according to 21 CFR 312.6
  4. Attach sample label or hangtag

C. Container or closure
  1. Bags, tubing sets, flasks, etc, used in processing
  2. Indication of compatibility with cells

D. Environmental impact

"The sponsor claims categorical exclusion [under 21 CFR 25.31(e)] for the study under this IND. To the sponsor's knowledge, no extraordinary circumstances exist."

E. Validation and qualification of the manufacturing process and facility
  1. Indicate process validation performed before clinical use; summary of validation may be included
  2. Reference facility MF, if on file

Reference/Resource

1. Food and Drug Administration. Draft guidance for reviewers: Instructions and template for chemistry, manufacturing, and control reviewers of human somatic cell therapy investigational new drug applications; availability. (August 18, 2003) Rockville, MD: CBER Office of Communication, Training, and Manufacturers Assistance, 2003.

In: Areman EM, Loper K, eds
Cellular Therapy: Principles, Methods, and Regulations
Bethesda, MD: AABB, 2009

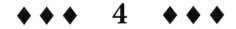

4

Biologics License Applications for Cellular Therapies

Elizabeth Smith

SOMATIC CELLULAR THERAPIES ARE REGulated under Section 351 of the Public Health Service (PHS) Act. The PHS Act requires individuals or companies (ie, the manufacturers) to obtain permission from the United States Food and Drug Administration (FDA) to introduce a biological product into interstate commerce within the United States. This request for permission comes in the form of a biologics license application (BLA), as described in the Code of Federal Regulations (CFR), Title 21, Part 601. Upon approval of the BLA, the FDA's Center for Biologics Evaluation and Research (CBER) issues a license for the production and sale of the biological product. Such license constitutes a determination that the establishment and the product meet the requirements set forth in the applicable regulations governing the quality, safety, purity, and potency for a licensed biologic.

This chapter provides an overview of the process for submitting a BLA, including meetings with the FDA, application fees, review timelines, and other administrative information relating to a BLA submission. In addition, Appendix 4-1 provides an outline for a sample table of contents to illustrate the general organization and format of the BLA.

Pre-BLA Submission Activities

It is recommended that applicants maintain frequent and meaningful contact with their FDA reviewers throughout the development program. To avoid potential delays in the BLA filing and ultimately to obtain licensure more rapidly, the information in the investigational new drug (IND) application should be kept as current as possible. It is important for applicants to stay abreast of the regulations and guidelines for somatic cell therapies as they continue to evolve. Updating the chemistry, manufacturing, and controls (CMC) section of the IND application to reflect the "to-be-licensed" process before submitting the BLA, when possible, provides the FDA reviewers with an opportunity to comment on the adequacy of the CMC section for the product in the context of the development stage (eg, Phase II or post-Phase III). It also provides the sponsor with an opportunity to resolve potential issues before the clinical trials are complete and the BLA is submitted. It is often very difficult to make changes in the manufacturing process and product specifications once the clinical trials are complete.

Elizabeth Smith, Vice President, Quality and Regulatory Affairs, Dendreon Corporation, Seattle, Washington

The author has disclosed a financial relationship with Dendreon Corporation.

Before submitting the BLA, the sponsor should request a pre-BLA meeting with the FDA to discuss the proposed format and content of the BLA. It is recommended that the meeting be held sufficiently in advance of the proposed filing date to provide adequate time to address concerns that may arise during the pre-BLA phase. FDA has established procedures for FDA staff[1] and guidance for sponsors for the conduct of meetings.[2]

There are three types of meetings with sponsors: Type A, necessary meetings to discuss issues that are impeding further development of the product (eg, clinical holds); Type B, meetings at predefined milestones in development (eg, pre-IND, end-of-Phase II); and Type C, all other meetings. A pre-BLA meeting is considered a Type B meeting.

Usually, the FDA grants a single pre-BLA meeting unless the topics to be covered exceed the scope of what can be accomplished in a single meeting. Once a complete meeting request is submitted, the pre-BLA meeting is scheduled within 60 days of the request. The pre-meeting materials must be received by the FDA no later than 4 weeks before the meeting; otherwise, the meeting will be rescheduled. The meeting materials should include the following:

- Product name.
- Product type or structure (eg, autologous cell therapy pulsed ex vivo with peptides).
- Proposed indication.
- The type of meeting (eg, Type B).
- General purpose or context for the meeting.
- Specific objectives and key outcomes for the meeting (eg, reach agreement on the proposed format and content for the BLA).
- Proposed agenda with estimated time for each item.
- Specific questions (eg: Does the FDA agree that for the purpose of Product X, the drug substance and drug product are the same and the CMC information will be included only in the drug product section of the BLA? Is the proposed preclinical data package sufficient to support licensure?).
- Clinical data summary (as appropriate).
- A summary of the safety and efficacy data intended to support approval for the proposed indication. A tabular summary of the clinical studies conducted to date, their status, and the

study report format is useful. The summary should be clear about which studies will be submitted and whether the reports will be full clinical study reports, abbreviated reports, or synopses. The proposed format and content of the integrated summary of safety and integrated summary of efficacy should be discussed, particularly if departure from the guidance is proposed. It is also important to discuss the plans for providing raw data [SAS files (SAS Institute, Cary, NC)] and to obtain agreement on the scope and format of raw data for submission. For example, it may be necessary to submit raw data from radiological imaging studies, and such a submission must be coordinated carefully with FDA.

- Preclinical data summary (as appropriate).
- A tabular summary of the nonclinical pharmacology or toxicology studies intended to support licensure.
- CMC information (as appropriate).
- A summary of the "to-be-licensed" manufacturing process and release specifications, describing changes, if any, from the process used for clinical trials to that proposed for licensure. There must be agreement on the approach for demonstrating comparability.
- A list of all individuals, including their titles, who will attend the proposed meeting from the sponsor's organization.
- A list of FDA staff (or staff from other disciplines) requested by the sponsor to participate in the proposed meeting.

After the meeting, the FDA will provide minutes that describe the agreements and issues to be resolved as well as any items that require action. It is recommended that the sponsor also generate minutes and submit them to the FDA, particularly if there is not concordance in the conclusions between the sponsor and the FDA. Usually, the FDA is willing to have follow-up teleconferences to address any unresolved questions from the initial meeting. Clear documentation of these discussions is critical.

The following are additional presubmission considerations:

- Does the product qualify for fast track designation?[3] If so, this must be considered before the BLA is filed.

- Will the facilities be ready for a preapproval inspection (PAI) at the time of the initial BLA filing?
- Will the BLA be submitted on paper, electronically, or both?

Fees

The Prescription Drug User Fee Act (PDUFA), initially enacted in 1992 and reauthorized in 2002 and 2007, set forth a requirement for the sponsor of the BLA to pay "user fees" to the FDA. In exchange for "user fees," the FDA establishes performance goals for (among other things) the timely review of new and supplemental license applications. Fees are assessed for initial applications, supplemental applications, establishments, and products. Table 4-1 summarizes the user fees for each category for Fiscal Year 2008.[4] User fees change with each fiscal year and are communicated to industry through the Federal Register and the FDA Web site.

User fees may be waived or reduced under certain circumstances [Food, Drug, and Cosmetic Act, Section 736(d)], including situations when:

- A waiver is necessary to protect public health.
- The fees present a significant barrier to innovation because of limited resources or other circumstances.
- The fees exceed the present and future costs of FDA's review of the application.

Table 4-1. User Fees by Category[4]

Fee Category	Fiscal Year 2008 Fee Rate
Applications requiring clinical data	$1,178,000
Applications not requiring clinical data	$ 589,000
Supplements requiring clinical data	$ 589,000
Establishment fees	$ 392,700
Product fees	$ 65,030

- The entity submitting the BLA has fewer than 500 employees, including affiliates.
- The application is for a designated orphan drug.

Reference should be made to the draft guidance for obtaining a user fee waiver or reduction. Useful information, including announcements regarding current user fees, can be located on the FDA Web site and by contacting the PDUFA staff at the FDA.

The user fee payment is due at the time of the initial filing. If the application is being submitted in a "rolling" fashion as permitted under fast track designation, the fees are due with the first rolling submission. If the BLA is refused for filing, the applicant is refunded 75% of the user fee. Establishment and product fees are assessed annually for licensed products only.

Review Timelines

The FDA has established procedures for the administrative processing and review of the BLA, which include target time frames for these activities, including communication with the applicant. Figure 4-1 highlights the FDA's key administrative and communication activities associated with an original BLA.

The PDUFA review clock establishes target review times by which the FDA takes action on an application. Review timelines for BLAs vary depending on whether the submission is the original BLA or a supplement, and whether the application has been given priority or standard review status. Priority designation is granted to biologics that, if approved, provide a significant improvement in the safety or effectiveness of the treatment, diagnosis, or prevention of a serious and life-threatening disease. Under the PDUFA, the FDA's goal is to take action within 10 months from the date of submission for a standard original BLA, and 6 months from the date of submission for a priority-designated application. Supplemental BLA review times depend on the type and scope of the supplement.

Once the application is received, the FDA reviews it to determine whether it will be accepted or refused; the latter case is described as "refusal to file" (RTF). The BLA may be refused for filing if information has been omitted that is required

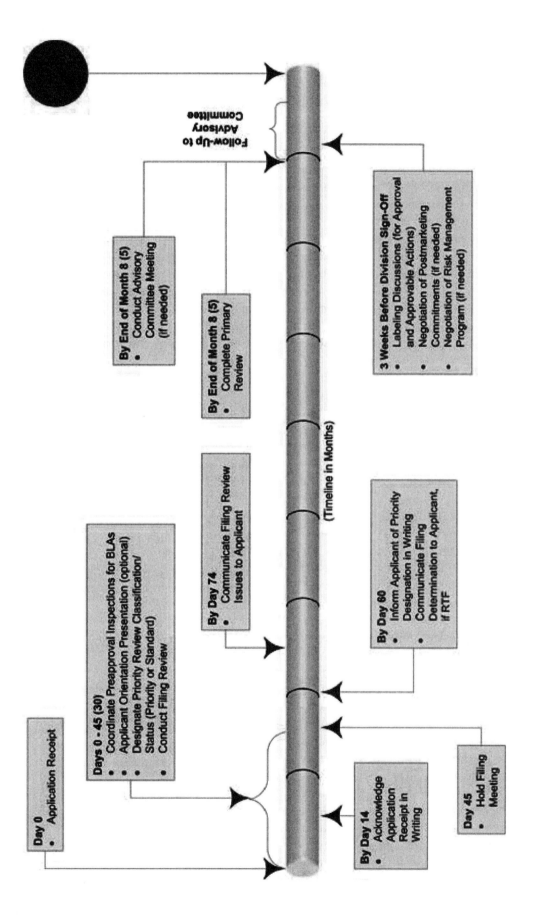

Figure 4-1. Processing and review timeline for biologics license applications. The number in parentheses indicates modification of timeline for priority status reviews.
BLA = biologics license application; RTF = refusal to file; PDUFA = Prescription Drug User Fee Act.

under 21 CFR 601.2 or necessary for performing a substantive review. More specifically, applications may be refused for filing for many reasons, including the following:

- Inadequate organization of either the paper or electronic submission.
- Failure of the electronic submission to meet the technical requirements for filing (eg, SAS dataset cannot be opened, the hyperlinks and bookmarks are inoperable, or information is not located in the proper folders).
- Missing protocols or reports.
- Data tabulations or listings are not interpretable.
- Missing financial disclosures or statements of compliance.
- Omission of critical analyses as planned in clinical studies.
- Inadequate assays for determining safety, purity, or potency.

The FDA completes its review for filing within 45 days after receipt of the BLA, and it communicates the filing status to the sponsor in writing within 74 days after receipt of the BLA. If the BLA is refused for filing, the applicant may decide to file the BLA over protest.[5]

During the review, the FDA may contact the applicant by phone or in writing with requests for information necessary to conduct the review. These communications are termed "information requests" and do not constitute an action that stops the review clock. In addition, FDA may provide the applicant with a "discipline review" letter. The discipline review letter conveys early concerns to the applicant from a given review discipline (eg, CMC review). The user fee review clock is not stopped for discipline review letters.

Applicants are encouraged to respond to information requests or discipline review letters as quickly as possible to keep the review moving efficiently. Responses are submitted as amendments to the BLA. The potential impact to the review clock is assessed with each amendment. The FDA may decide to review the amendment in the current review cycle or wait to review it in the next review cycle. During the last 3 months of the review clock, amendments to the BLA are classified as either major or minor. Submission of major amendments during the last 3 months results in an extension of the review clock by 3 months.

On or before the PDUFA date, the FDA takes action on the application so that the PDUFA goal can be met. Such action may be an approval or a "complete response." If the application is approved, the applicant receives its license, which is the final action on the original application.

A complete response indicates that the FDA has completed its review of the application, and deficiencies must be addressed before further action is taken. At this point, the review clock is stopped until the BLA is amended. The complete response letter identifies each deficiency to be addressed. The applicant may then amend the BLA to address the deficiencies, and a new review clock is established according to the scope of the information necessary to address the deficiencies. Amendments to the BLA in response to a complete response letter are classified as Class I or Class II resubmissions, after which the review clock restarts. Class I resubmissions are given a 2-month review clock, and Class II resubmissions are given a 6-month review clock.

The applicant may also withdraw the BLA.

Several factors play a role in whether the BLA is reviewed successfully in a single review cycle. Some of the factors are within the control of the applicant:

- A well-organized and complete submission.
- Pre-approval inspection preparedness.
- Electronic vs paper submissions.
- Early identification and communication of issues to allow sufficient time for resolution.
- Timely follow-up to the FDA's requests for information.

For a comprehensive sample outline of a BLA, see Appendix 4-1.

References/Resources

1. Food and Drug Administration. Manual of standard operating processes and procedures. SOPP 8101.1: Scheduling and conduct of regulatory review meetings with sponsors and applicants. (May 18, 2007) Rockville, MD: CBER, 2007.
2. Food and Drug Administration. Guidance for industry: Formal meetings with sponsors and applicants for PDUFA products. (February 2000) Rockville, MD: CBER Office of Communication, Training, and Manufacturers Assistance, 2000.
3. Food and Drug Administration. Guidance for industry: Fast track drug development programs—designation,

development, and application review. (July 2004) Rockville, MD: CDER and CBER, 2004.

4.   Food and Drug Administration. Prescription drug user fee rates for Fiscal Year 2008. Fed Regist 2007;72:58103-6.

5.   Food and Drug Administration. Manual of standard operating processes and procedures. SOPP 8404.1: Issuance and review of responses to information requests and discipline review letters to pending applications. (June 11, 2002) Rockville, MD: CBER, 2007.

Appendix 4-1. Sample Outline for the Content and Organization of a Biologics License Application

The organization and content of a biologics license application (BLA) are described in the Code of Federal Regulations (CFR), Title 21, Part 601 and outlined in Food and Drug Administration (FDA) Form 356h. Form FDA 356h is available in PDF format.[1]

Format

All initial and supplemental BLA submissions must be accompanied by a completed Form FDA 356h. Form FDA 356h lists 20 items, and each item refers the applicant to the pertinent regulation. These 20 items serve as the backbone of the table of contents or "index" of the submission.

The applicant may choose to use the common technical document format rather than the BLA format as an alternative approach. However, to ensure that the application is acceptable for filing and to avoid any confusion with the administrative processing of the application, the applicant should reach agreement with the FDA on the proposed organization of the content and structure of the submission.

Content

Item 1: Index

The index includes a comprehensive table of contents for the entire submission. If the BLA is electronic, the index serves as the roadmap for navigating the submission so that any section of the BLA may be accessed from this single location.

Item 2: Labeling

Labeling regulations are set forth under 21 CFR 201 and 610, and such labeling is reviewed and approved for licensed biologics. The BLA contains the following draft labeling:
- Draft carton and container labels.

- Draft package insert (no annotation).
- Any studies performed for label comprehension or trade name review.

Once the draft labeling texts (labels, cartons, and package insert) are approved, the final labeling is submitted under the BLA. Labeling submissions, including draft and final labeling, are accompanied by a completed Form FDA 2567.[2]

Item 3: Summary

The summary is a required section of the BLA. It is typically read early in the review of the BLA and is referenced considerably. This section is a comprehensive and factual summary of the cellular therapy and is designed to provide the reviewers of all disciplines a broad understanding of the product and the technical aspects supporting its licensure. The section, which is typically 50 to 200 pages in length, is organized according to 21 CFR 314.50(c), unless an alternative is agreed to by the FDA in advance. Helpful guidance is available,[3] although it is not specific to cellular therapies because the same principles apply for organization and general content for all BLAs. Summary tables, figures, and process flow diagrams should be used where possible to facilitate review. It is also useful, particularly if the application is provided electronically, to cross-reference the technical section of the BLA that contains the detailed information.

The following is a sample table of contents for the summary, which is based on FDA guidance (similar tables of contents appear under other items). While this general outline conforms to the guidance, it may be suitable to modify it to accommodate particular nuances of the proposed cellular therapy and the types of studies to be submitted in support of licensure. It is highly recommended that significant deviations from the guidance be discussed in advance with the FDA to avoid potential refusal-to-file (RTF) issues.

3.0 Overall Summary
    3.1 Annotated Package Insert
    3.2 Pharmacologic Class, Scientific Rationale, Intended Use, and Potential Clinical Benefits
    3.3 Foreign Marketing History
    3.4 CMC
        The format of the chemistry, manufacturing, and controls (CMC) summary will likely need to be customized for the proposed biologic according to the type of therapy, its method of manufacture, and testing. "Drug substance" applies to the biologically active component of the cell therapy, and "drug product" refers to the final product that is formulated and ready for delivery to the patient.
        3.4.1 Drug Substance
            3.4.1.1 General Information (names, codes, and composition)
            3.4.1.2 Manufacturer
            3.4.1.3 Characterization
            3.4.1.4 Method of Manufacture
            3.4.1.5 Process Controls and Process Validation
            3.4.1.6 Specifications and Methods
            3.4.1.7 Stability
        3.4.2 Drug Product
            3.4.2.1 Composition and Dosage Form
            3.4.2.2 Manufacturer
            3.4.2.3 Specifications and Methods
            3.4.2.4 Container or Closure System
            3.4.2.5 Stability
            3.4.2.6 Investigational Formulations
    3.5 Nonclinical Pharmacology and Toxicology Summary
    3.6 Human Pharmacokinetic and Bioavailability
    3.7 Microbiology
        This section applies only to anti-infective agents.
    3.8 Clinical Data Summary and Results of Statistical Analyses
        3.8.1 Clinical Pharmacology
        3.8.2 Overview of Clinical Studies
        3.8.3 Controlled Clinical Studies
        3.8.4 Uncontrolled Clinical Studies

        3.8.5 Other Studies
            3.8.5.1 Published and Unpublished Studies
            3.8.5.2 Foreign Marketing
        3.8.6 Safety Summary
            3.8.6.1 Adverse Reactions
            3.8.6.2 Clinical Laboratory Data
            3.8.6.3 Serious and Clinically Important Events
            3.8.6.4 Deaths
            3.8.6.5 Dose
            3.8.6.6 Intrinsic and Extrinsic Factors
            3.8.6.7 Overdosage and Drug Abuse Potential
        3.8.7 Conclusions and Benefit/Risk Relationship and Proposed Postmarketing Studies

Item 4: Chemistry

Item 4 contains a complete description of the chemistry, manufacturing, and control information for the cellular therapy. It details the method of manufacturing, from the control and qualification of source materials to final formulation and delivery to the patient. Process flow diagrams, which are accompanied by narratives with sufficient detail for the reviewers to understand the process, are included in this section. It may be necessary to add additional major sections to the sample table of contents to accommodate the specific cellular therapy.

4.0 Chemistry
    4.1 Chemistry, Manufacturing, and Controls Information
        4.1.1 Drug Substance
            4.1.1.1 General Information (nomenclature and general properties)
            4.1.1.2 Manufacture
                – Identification and responsibilities
                – Floor diagrams
                – Other products in the same facility
                – Contamination precautions
            4.1.1.2.1 Description of Manufacturing Process and Process Controls
                – Flow charts
                – Process narratives

Item 5: Nonclinical Pharmacology and Toxicology

Item 5 includes study reports for all nonclinical pharmacology and toxicology studies performed to assess the mode of action, in-vitro effects, and safety of the cellular product. The nature of many cellular therapies does not lend them to traditional pharmacology and toxicology. For example, studies to evaluate absorption, metabolism, and excretion of cellular therapies would not apply in most cases. The specific nonclinical assessments required to support licensure are typically discussed with the FDA during the development process and at the pre-BLA meeting. Justification for not performing traditional nonclinical studies is also provided in this section, if applicable.

5.2.5   Reproductive and Developmental Toxicity
5.3   Local Tolerance
5.4   Other Toxicity Studies (eg, antigenicity, immunogenicity, or mechanistic studies)
5.5   Statement of Compliance

Item 6: Human Pharmacokinetic and Bioavailability Studies

In most cases for cellular therapy products, human pharmacokinetic and bioavailability studies will not apply. In these instances, a statement is to be included in item 6 indicating that these studies are not applicable or not required for the proposed biologic and a brief rationale is to be provided. If any human pharmacokinetic or bioavailability studies were performed, the following format applies:

6.0   Human Pharmacokinetic and Bioavailability Studies
   6.1   Tabulated Summary of Studies
   6.2   Summary of Data and Overall Conclusions
   6.3   List of All Formulations Used in Clinical Trials
   6.4   Analytical Methods
   6.5   Individual Study Reports
   6.6   Literature Review

Item 7: Microbiology

7.0   Microbiology
   Not applicable. This section applies only to anti-infective agents.

Item 8: Clinical Data

8.0   Clinical Data
   8.1   Overview of Clinical Studies
      8.1.1   Tabular Listing of All Clinical Studies
   8.2   Clinical Pharmacology
   8.3   Controlled Clinical Trials
      8.3.1   Clinical Study Reports
         8.3.1.1   Study 1 Final Report
         8.3.1.2   Study 2 Final Report
   8.4   Uncontrolled Clinical Trials
      8.4.1   Clinical Study Reports
         8.4.1.1   Study 3 Final Report
   8.5   Integrated Summary of Efficacy

      8.5.1   Background
         8.5.1.1   Overview
         8.5.1.2   Proposed Indication
         8.5.1.3   Rationale for Integration
         8.5.1.4   Abbreviations and Definitions of Terms
      8.5.2   Study 1 Efficacy Summary
         8.5.2.1   Introduction
         8.5.2.2   Baseline Demographics
         8.5.2.3   Efficacy Results
      8.5.3   Single-Agent Efficacy
      8.5.4   Analysis of Dose Response
      8.5.5   Evidence of Long-Term Effectiveness, Tolerance, or Withdrawal Effects
      8.5.6   Efficacy in Special Populations
         8.5.6.1   Gender
         8.5.6.2   Ethnicity
         8.5.6.3   Age
         8.5.6.4   Other Subgroups
      8.5.7   Discussion
      8.5.8   Conclusions
   8.6   Integrated Summary of Safety
      8.6.1   Background
         8.6.1.1   Overview
         8.6.1.2   Proposed Indication
         8.6.1.3   Rationale for Integration
         8.6.1.4   Abbreviations and Definitions of Terms
      8.6.2   Study 1 Safety Summary
         8.6.2.1   Baseline Demographics
         8.6.2.2   Summary of Exposure
         8.6.2.3   Summary of Adverse Events
            8.6.2.3.1   Most Frequent Adverse Events
            8.6.2.3.2   Discussion of Key Adverse Events
            8.6.2.3.3   Serious Adverse Events
               8.6.2.3.3.1   Deaths and Discontinuations
            8.6.2.3.4   Clinical Laboratory Abnormalities
      8.6.2.4   Single-Agent Safety Summary
      8.6.2.5   Analysis of Dose Response
      8.6.2.6   Drug-Drug Interactions
      8.6.2.7   Long-Term and Withdrawal Effects
      8.6.2.8   Pharmacologic Properties or Other Properties of Interest
   8.7   Summary of Benefits and Risks

Item 9: Safety Update

The safety update is submitted as an amendment 4 months after the initial submission of the BLA (or 3 months for priority applications) to update the pending application with new safety information that may reasonably affect the contraindications, warnings, precautions, or adverse reaction statements in the draft labeling. Other safety updates may be requested at other times by the FDA. The safety update may not be required for certain biologics and should be discussed with the FDA at the pre-BLA meeting.

Item 10: Statistics

This is a copy of item 8 and contains all specific information necessary for the statisticians to conduct their review and reanalysis, such as data definition files, SAS transport files, and programs.

Item 11: Case Report Tabulations

This section contains the tables and data listings for the required studies and tabulations of safety data for all studies.

Item 12: Case Report Forms

Unless other arrangements have been made with the FDA, this section contains complete case report forms (CRFs) for all subjects who died, experienced a serious adverse event (SAE), or dropped out of the study because of an adverse event. The FDA may request copies of CRFs for other subjects at any time during the review. It is therefore useful to discuss with the FDA at the pre-BLA meeting which CRFs should be included with the initial submission.

Item 13: Patent Information

Provide a listing of all patents for the proposed biologic.

Item 14: Patent Certification

Does not apply to biologics.

Item 15: Establishment Description

15.0 Establishment Description[5]
 15.1 Facility Overview
 15.2 Water Systems

  15.2.1 General Description
  15.2.2 Validation Summary
  15.2.3 Routine Monitoring Program
 15.3 Heating, Ventilation, and Air Conditioning
  15.3.1 General Description
  15.3.2 Validation Summary
  15.3.3 Routine Monitoring Program
 15.4 Computer Systems
 15.5 Contamination and Cross-Contamination Precautions
  15.5.1 Cleaning Procedures and Validation
   15.5.1.1 Dedicated Equipment
   15.5.1.2 Shared Equipment
  15.5.2 Containment Procedures

Item 16: Debarment Certification

Item 17: Field Copy Certification

Does not apply to biologics.

Item 18: User Fee Cover Sheet (Form FDA 3397)

Item 19: Financial Information (Financial Disclosures)

Item 20: Other

References/Resources

1. Food and Drug Administration. Form 356h: Application to market a new drug, biologic, or an antibiotic drug for human use. Rockville, MD: CDER, 2005.
2. Food and Drug Administration. Form 2567: Transmittal of labels and circulars. Rockville, MD: CBER, 2005.
3. Food and Drug Administration. Guideline for the format and content of the summary for new drug and antibiotic applications. (February 1987) Rockville, MD: CDER, Office of Training and Communication, 1987.
4. Food and Drug Administration. International Conference on Harmonisation: Guideline for industry: Structure and content of clinical study reports; ICH E3. (July 1996) Rockville, MD: CDER Office of Training and Communication, 1996.
5. Food and Drug Administration. Guidance for the submission of chemistry, manufacturing, and controls information and establishment description for autologous somatic cell therapy products. (January 1997) Rockville, MD: CBER Office of Communication, Training, and Manufacturers Assistance, 1997.

In: Areman EM, Loper K, eds
Cellular Therapy: Principles, Methods, and Regulations
Bethesda, MD: AABB, 2009

◆◆◆ 5 ◆◆◆

Electronic Submissions of Cellular Therapy Investigational New Drug and Biologics License Applications

Daniel P. Offringa

THIS CHAPTER PRESENTS A HIGH-LEVEL overview of electronic submissions to the Center for Biologics Evaluation and Research (CBER) that involve cellular therapy products. For detailed information, refer to the cited guidance documents.

Brief History

The early electronic submissions in the mid-to-late 1990s varied widely in content and quality. They sometimes even required their own hardware platforms for review. In an effort to standardize submissions, the Food and Drug Administration (FDA) issued the first guidance documents for electronic submissions in 1999. These guidance documents covered both general considerations (revised in 2003) and the submission of various types of premarket approval applications, including biologic license applications (BLAs) and new drug applications (NDAs).[1,2] In 2002, CBER-specific guidance was issued for the electronic submission of investigational new drug (IND) applications.[3] Most recently, the FDA issued guidance in conjunction with the International Conference on Harmonisation of Technical Requirements for Registration of Pharmaceuticals for Human Use (ICH) that outlines the electronic common technical document (eCTD) format, which can be used for IND applications, license applications, and submissions to regulatory authorities in the European Union and Japan.[4-6]

Advantages of Electronic Submissions over Paper

Electronic submissions cost more to prepare than paper, but they offer multiple advantages, such as the following:
- Increased efficiency of FDA review by offering quick navigation through the submission by

---

Daniel P. Offringa, Consultant, The Biologics Consulting Group, Inc, Alexandria, Virginia

The author has disclosed no conflicts of interest.

means of bookmarks and hyperlinks, searchable documents, the ability to compare multiple versions of documents (eg, clinical protocols and product labeling), and cut-and-paste functionality for formulating review.

- Instant reviewer access to entire IND applications and BLA submissions throughout their lifecycle, including all amendments. Paper submissions to a reviewer, in contrast, can take several days to access.
- Faster industry response to questions and requests from the FDA because companies also have access to the electronic document.
- Expedited delivery to the FDA through the Electronic Submissions Gateway (ESG). The ESG is a portal that allows industry to securely transmit regulatory submissions to the FDA via the Internet. More detail can be found on the ESG Web site (http://www.fda.gov/esg).

Initial Considerations

Submission Format

The first consideration when planning an electronic submission is deciding on the format. The CBER allows electronic submissions in the traditional formats, in accordance with the 1999 electronic BLA (eBLA) and 2002 electronic IND (eIND) guidances,[2,3] or in the eCTD format. The traditional formats have a structure that follows the organization of FDA Forms 1571 (IND) and 356h (BLA), and they employ portable document format (PDF) table of contents (TOC) documents for submission navigation. As the name implies, eCTDs are based on the CTD structure and replace PDF TOCs with extensible markup language (XML) files (also referred to as an XML backbone). The XML backbone is a text file that is used by an eCTD viewing application to present a TOC view of the submission.

The main reasons for choosing a traditional format are familiarity and a smaller initial software investment. On the other hand, the eCTD format is preferred by the FDA and is accepted internationally. In addition, content from an eCTD IND application can be leveraged for an eCTD BLA.

When a sponsor is planning a first electronic submission, the FDA requests that the applicant submit a sample of the electronic document in advance. The sample is reviewed by the electronic submission staff at the FDA, who notify the sponsor of any issues that need to be addressed and resolved.

Software

Regardless of the chosen format, it is recommended that PDF tools be purchased to aid in the preparation of an electronic submission. These tools can automate the creation of bookmarks and hyperlinks, perform link audits, and provide an overview of the document information fields for multiple PDFs. For eCTDs, a publishing tool should also be purchased. Publishing tools can be desktop or server based and may include the option to integrate with an electronic document management system (EDMS). The cost of publishing tools varies depending on the type selected, with desktop solutions being the least expensive. An EDMS is useful for electronic submissions but is certainly not required. In lieu of purchasing an EDMS, good document management can also be achieved by following standard operating procedures (SOPs) and instituting access controls on the file system.

Document Formatting

Formatting for PDF documents is specified in detail in the general considerations guidance document.[1] This guidance addresses topics such as font size, page margins, and resolution for scanned documents.

Document Granularity for eCTD Submissions

Document granularity refers to the CTD section level at which separate documents are submitted. For example, Section 2.5 (Clinical Overview) is submitted as a single document. The specifications are outlined in detail in the ICH M4 organization guidance.[6] However, the FDA provides flexibility in granularity beyond that mentioned in the guidance, especially for IND applications. The proposed granularity of the electronic submission should be discussed with the FDA.

Building the Submission

Converting to PDF

When converting source documents (eg, Microsoft Word documents) to PDF, it is important to follow the specifications (eg, font embedding and image compression) in the general considerations guidance.[1] It is also important to confirm that the documents included are compatible with Adobe Acrobat 5.0 (PDF version 1.4) for archival purposes.

Traditional Format

For traditional electronic submissions, files and folders are organized as outlined in the guidance documents.[2,3] PDF TOCs are used for navigation throughout the submission and are created at several levels. The highest-level TOC is called the "roadmap" and summarizes the history of the submission. Bookmarks and hyperlinks are provided to the original submission and all amendments.

The next level is the main TOC, which lists and provides bookmarks and hyperlinks to the items contained in individual submissions. It is organized according to the item listings on FDA Forms 1571 and 356h.

The last level is the item TOC, which provides links to the files submitted for a particular section [eg, Chemistry, Manufacturing, and Controls (CMC)].

eCTD Format

As mentioned previously, the eCTD format replaces PDF TOCs with an XML backbone. The publishing tool automatically creates the submission structure by using predefined specifications and metadata (eg, sponsor name, product, and modules being submitted) supplied by the user. The result is a skeleton that contains placeholders for the eCTD section documents. The actual submission is then built by adding documents to the appropriate locations. The publishing tool automatically updates the XML backbone as content is added. For clinical and nonclinical study reports, separate XML files called study tagging files (STFs) are created, which contain study metadata and tie together study reports submitted as multiple documents. Detailed information regarding STFs can be found in the implementation document.[7]

Bookmarking and Hyperlinking PDFs

This step is performed once documents have been added to the submission folder structure to ensure that links between files function correctly. For documents with a TOC, a bookmark and hyperlink are created for each item in the TOC. If there is no TOC, bookmarks for each heading are provided if the document is more than several pages long. Hyperlinks are also created throughout the body of the document for references to items that appear on another page or to external documents (eg, tables, figures, and references). Once all hyperlinks have been created, they are converted to blue text. Documents with bookmarks are set to open with the bookmark pane visible.

Finalizing the Submission

PDF Audit

Once all the submission files are in place and the hyperlinking is complete, it is a good idea to perform a link audit with a PDF tool to confirm that there are no broken links. If any broken links are discovered, the tool identifies the links and corresponding files. Broken links most often occur when a file is moved or renamed after a link has been created. PDF tools are also useful for checking or setting the document information fields and for confirming that PDF files are optimized.

eCTD Validation

A number of these PDF auditing functions may also be performed by using the eCTD publishing tool validation procedures. In addition, the validation removes unused placeholders from the submission structure and confirms that the submission complies with eCTD specifications. Having a validated submission ensures that it will load correctly into the FDA eCTD viewing system.

Submission

Electronic submissions can be sent on media (eg, CD or DVD) or through the ESG. Media submissions should be accompanied by a paper cover letter and an FDA Form 1571 or 356h. ESG submissions require prior registration. Information regarding the registration process can be found on the ESG Web site [http://www.fda.gov/esg].

References/Resources

1. Food and Drug Administration. Guidance for industry: Providing regulatory submissions in electronic format—general considerations. (October 2003) Rockville, MD: CBER Office of Communication, Training, and Manufacturers Assistance, 2003.

2. Food and Drug Administration. Guidance for industry: Providing regulatory submissions to the Center for Biologics Evaluation and Research (CBER) in electronic format—biologics marketing applications. (November 1999) Rockville, MD: CBER Office of Communication, Training, and Manufacturers Assistance, 1999.

3. Food and Drug Administration. Guidance for industry: Providing regulatory submissions to CBER in electronic format—investigational new drug applications (INDs). (March 2002) Rockville, MD: CBER Office of Communication, Training, and Manufacturers Assistance, 2002.

4. Food and Drug Administration. Guidance for Industry: Providing regulatory submissions in electronic format—Human pharmaceutical product applications and related submissions using the eCTD specifications. (April 2006) Rockville, MD: CBER Office of Communication, Training, and Manufacturers Assistance, 2006.

5. International Conference on Harmonisation of Technical Requirements for Registration of Pharmaceuticals for Human Use. ICH M2 Expert Working Group: Electronic Common Technical Document specification version 3.2. (February 04, 2004) Geneva, Switzerland: ICH, 2008. [Available at http://estri.ich.org/eCTD/ (accessed October 31, 2008).]

6. Food and Drug Administration. Guidance for Industry: Granularity document. Annex to M4: Organization of the CTD. (October 2005) Rockville, MD: CBER Office of Communication, Training, and Manufacturers Assistance, 2005.

7. Food and Drug Administration. FDA implementation of study tagging file v2.2. (August 2005). Rockville, MD: CBER, 2005.

In: Areman EM, Loper K, eds
Cellular Therapy: Principles, Methods, and Regulations
Bethesda, MD: AABB, 2009

♦♦♦ **6** ♦♦♦

Cellular Therapies Regulated as Combination Products

Joyce L. Frey-Vasconcells, PhD

CELLULAR THERAPIES COME IN MANY different forms and are delivered in many different ways. In some instances, living cells are seeded on natural or synthetic biomaterials (through tissue engineering) and implanted into patients or applied topically, such as with skin replacement products. In other cases, the only means for delivering a cellular therapy is through a specialized delivery system, such as a catheter. The Food and Drug Administration (FDA) refers to such products as "combination" products because the biomaterials or the delivery system are often regulated as medical devices themselves. Thus, bringing together a biological product (cells) and a medical device (biomaterials or a catheter) is combining two products normally regulated separately. This chapter explains what combination products are, identifies ways to determine how cell-based combination products are regulated by the FDA, and identifies challenging issues with these products that require further clarification from the FDA.

What Is the Definition of a Combination Product?

As defined in the Code of Federal Regulations (CFR), Title 21, Part 3.2(e), combination products include the following:

- A product composed of two or more regulated components (eg, drug and device, biologic and device, drug and biologic, or drug, device, and biologic) that are physically, chemically, or otherwise combined or mixed and produced as a single entity.

- Two or more separate products packaged together or as a unit and composed of drug and device products, device and biological products, or biological and drug products.

- A drug, device, or biological product packaged individually that, according to its investigational plan or proposed labeling, is intended for use only with an approved specified drug, device, or biological product, where both are

Joyce L. Frey-Vasconcells, PhD, Executive Director, Pharmanet Consulting, Washington, District of Columbia

The author has disclosed no conflicts of interest.

required to achieve the intended use, indication, or effect and where, upon approval of the proposed product, the labeling of the approved product would need to be changed, eg, to reflect a change in intended use, dosage form, strength, route of administration, or significant change in dose.

- Any investigational drug, device, or biological product packaged individually that, according to its proposed labeling, is for use only with another specified investigational drug, device, or biological product, where both are required to achieve the intended use, indication, or effect.

Who Determines Which Center Will Have Review Responsibility for a Combination Product?

Because combination products consist of two or more separately regulated products, it is not always clear which organizational component within the FDA would have primary jurisdiction for the premarket review and regulation of these products. In 1990, Congress passed the Safe Medical Devices Act, which implemented Section 503(g) of the Food, Drug, and Cosmetic Act (FD&C Act). This section specified how the FDA would determine the primary jurisdiction for combination products and enhanced the efficiency of agency management and operations by providing procedures for determining which agency component will have primary jurisdiction where the jurisdiction is unclear or in dispute. The Safe Medical Devices Act indicated that designation of the agency organizational unit should be based on the primary mode of action (PMOA) of the product. However, the act did not define PMOA. Therefore, the process of center assignment was not always transparent to sponsors.

In addition, procedures for identifying the designated agency component were based on intercenter agreements that describe the allocation of responsibility for broad categories of products. However, these agreements were written in 1991, and many novel products were not envisioned and therefore are not part of the intercenter agreements. Moreover, in 2003, several biological product classes were transferred from the Center for Biologics

Evaluation and Research (CBER) to the Center for Drug Evaluation and Research (CDER).[1] Therefore, a procedure for requesting a designation of an agency component with primary jurisdiction was developed and is outlined in 21 CFR 3.7. However, because of the lack of statutory definition for PMOA, there was still much confusion in center assignment and inefficiency in the review process for combination products.

In 2002, the Medical Device User Fee and Modernization Act mandated the establishment of the Office of Combination Products (OCP) within the Office of the Commissioner to coordinate the review of combination products. The OCP was established on December 24, 2002. Its primary function is to work with the three medical product centers and industry regarding the regulation of combination products. However, the review and development of regulatory policy are still the responsibility of the individual centers. OCP responsibilities include making jurisdictional determinations; overseeing the coordination of premarket review; ensuring consistent and appropriate postmarket regulations; developing policy, guidance, and regulations in conjunction with the centers; serving as a resource for industry and the FDA review staff; and resolving review timeliness disputes. The OCP's objective is to ensure that the regulation of combination products is clear, consistent, appropriate, predictable, and transparent. For further information and guidance on combination products and the OCP, see the OCP Web site.[2]

Can the Applicant Determine Which Center Will Review the Product?

In some cases, it is very clear that the mode of action of the combination product stems from the drug, biologic, or device. For example, cells used for cardiac repair using a cardiac catheter would be regulated through the biologic regulations by CBER because the mode of action of the therapy is the cells used, and the delivery device is the cardiac catheter. The OCP has posted the jurisdictional decisions on its Web site.[3] Some examples from the Web site are listed in Table 6-1. Because most of these products are still investigational, the FDA can describe them only in general terms. This can be

Table 6-1. Examples of How Some Medical Products Containing Living Cells Are Regulated[3]

Combination Cellular and Device Products Regulated by the Center for Biologics Evaluation and Research as Biological Products

- Cellular transplant for diabetes treatment
- Autologous cellular product and delivery device
- Autologous cells and scaffold for orthopedic use
- Autologous cells and scaffold for organ replacement
- Device and biologic to separate stem cells for reinfusion after chemotherapy
- Cultured bone marrow cells and bone void filler with handling agent for immunotherapy
- Autologous chondrocytes and scaffold for repair of cartilage defects
- Autologous mesenchymal cells and scaffold for diaphragm repair

Combination Cellular and Device Products Regulated by the Center for Devices and Radiological Health as Medical Devices

- Dental implant coated with autologous cells
- Bone void filler with blood component to act as matrix and enhance handling properties

helpful if the product in development is similar to precedent products.

In other cases, intercenter agreements may be used to determine which center will review a product. However, it is important to keep in mind the limitations of these agreements. If the sponsor knows the PMOA of the product, it is possible to determine through these agreements to which center the product may go. When it is difficult to determine the product's most important therapeutic action, a request for designation (RFD) should be made through the OCP. This request can go through an informal or formal process. When the FDA has experience with similar types of products, it is possible to request an informal determination either by phone or e-mail. However, it is important to understand that the informal determinations are not binding on the agency. In other cases, a formal RFD should be made. This process is described in the sections that follow.

How Does the Applicant Request Designation of A Combination Product?

The process for requesting designation is outlined in 21 CFR 3.7, and additional details are provided in an FDA guidance document.[4] Although the RFD process is voluntary, it should be undertaken for any product for which jurisdiction is unclear or in dispute. An RFD is usually submitted by a sponsor, but if an application has been submitted to a center and there is disagreement internally about the identity of the lead center, a staff member of the center can request designation by the OCP. The request should be submitted before an application is filed for premarket review and must contain sufficient information for the OCP to make a determination. The submission cannot be more than 15 pages long and should adequately address the following key questions (again, see guidance document for additional details[4]):

- What is the product?
- In what way will the product be used?
- How does the product work?
- What is the product's most important therapeutic action?
- What is the basis for the PMOA determination? (Data are often helpful.)
- How does the sponsor think the product should be assigned? Why? (An assignment algorithm can be used if appropriate.)

Once a submission is received by the OCP, staff members review the submission for completeness and file the submission within 5 working days, at which time they notify the sponsor of the filing date. The OCP determines which centers review the application in conjunction with the OCP. The FDA has 60 days from the filing date to issue a letter outlining the designation determination and reason. If the FDA does not issue the letter by day 60, the sponsor's recommendation of the agency component with primary jurisdiction becomes the designated agency component.

What Criteria Does the OCP Use to Make the Designation Determination?

For combination products, the primary jurisdiction for premarket review and regulation is outlined in Section 503(g)(1) of the FD&C Act. This provision states that assignment to the lead center is based on a determination of the PMOA. In the Federal Register (August 25, 2005), the FDA published a final rule defining PMOA.[5] The rule became effective November 23, 2005. This rule defines PMOA as "the single mode of action of a combination product that provides the most important therapeutic action of the combination product." The most important therapeutic action is the mode of action expected to make the greatest contribution to the overall intended therapeutic effects of the combination product. In some cases, it is not possible to determine the PMOA. In these situations, the final rule describes an algorithm that the FDA uses to make the center assignment. The next step is to determine the assignment of similar products that raise similar questions regarding safety and effectiveness with respect to the combination product. When there are not similar products, the final step is to identify which center has the most expertise related to the most significant safety and effectiveness questions raised by the combination product.

What Regulations Need Clarification from the FDA?

When a combination product is being developed, it is sometimes difficult to understand and determine which regulations apply. The regulations that apply to biologics and drugs are different from those that apply to devices. For example, drugs and biological products must be manufactured under current good manufacturing practice (cGMP; see 21 CFR 210 and 211), whereas devices are manufactured under quality system regulations (QSRs; see 21 CFR 820). Because of the difference in the regulations, the following areas are of most concern to manufacturers and need clarification from the FDA:

- Which manufacturing regulations (cGMP or QSRs) apply?
- What are the necessary postmarketing reporting requirements?
- How many applications should be submitted for marketing?
- When is cross-labeling required?

Good Manufacturing Practice

The FDA has issued a draft guidance outlining the similarities between good manufacturing practice (GMP) and QSRs[6] and indicated that parallel systems are not necessary for manufacturing combination products. However, each constituent part is subject to its governing regulations (GMP or QSRs) before the products are combined. During and after the combination [21 CFR 3.2(e)(1) or (e)(2)], both regulations apply. However, compliance can be achieved by using either set of regulations (GMP or QSR) and paying special attention to key areas. The draft guidance document provides a table (Table 6-2) that describes how to achieve compliance.

In addition, in April 2006, the OCP announced plans for proposed rule-making to clarify and streamline GMP requirements for combination products, as described in the draft guidance document. The proposed rule would provide a flexible quality management regulatory framework for a quality system (QS) program under one set of regulations. The sponsor could apply GMP or QSRs provided that the system incorporates select, key provisions from the regulations pertaining to the other part of the combination product. It is important to check the OCP Web site for updates of this proposed rule [http://www.fda.gov/Combination Products/default.htm].

Postmarket Adverse Event Reporting

The FDA has issued a concept paper and requested comments on postmarket safety reporting require-

Table 6-2. Key Current Good Manufacturing Practices to Consider During and After Joining Copackaged and Single-Entity Combination Products[6]

If the Operating Manufacturing Control System Is Relevant to CFR Part 820 (QSR)		If the Operating Manufacturing Control System Is Relevant to CFR Part 210 or 211 (cGMP)	
Carefully Consider These cGMP Requirements	Title	Carefully Consider These QSRs	Title
§ 211.84	Testing and approval or rejection of components, drug product containers, and closures	§ 820.30	Design controls
§ 211.103	Calculation of yield	§ 820.50	Purchasing controls
§ 211.137	Expiration dating	§ 820.100	Corrective and preventive actions
§ 211.165	Testing and release for distribution		
§ 211.166	Stability testing		
§ 211.167	Special testing requirements		
§ 211.170	Reserve samples		

CFR = Code of Federal Regulations; QSR = quality system regulation; cGMP = current good manufacturing practice.

ments. Currently, manufacturers are required to report adverse events according to the provision that is associated with the marketing application for that combination product. For example, if the combination product was approved or cleared under the device regulations, the postmarket reporting requirements would come from the medical device reporting (MDR) regulations under 21 CFR Part 803. If the combination product was approved under the biologic or drug regulations, the postmarket reporting requirements would come from 21 CFR 314.80. However, there are clear differences between the two provisions:

- **Device malfunction reporting** [21 CFR 803.3 (r)(2)(ii) and 21 CFR 803.20]: In addition to the reporting of device malfunctions associated with a death or serious injury, the MDR regulation also requires reporting of device malfunctions where no death or serious injury occurred but when such device or similar device marketed by the manufacturer would be likely to cause or contribute to a death or serious injury if the malfunction were to recur. Requirements for reporting for drugs and biological products do not include an analogous statement.

- **5-Day MDR reporting** [21 CFR 803.10(c)(2) (i)]: The MDR regulation requires reporting, within 5 days, of 1) any reportable event that necessitates remedial action to prevent an unreasonable risk of substantial harm to the public health and 2) any MDR reportable event for which the FDA has made a written request for the submission of a 5-day report. There is no such provision in the drug and biologic reporting requirements.

- **Drug and biological product "alert" reporting** [21 CFR 314.80(c)(1) and 600.80(c)(1)]: For drugs and most biological products, postmarket safety reporting emphasizes adverse events that are both serious and unexpected. Although device safety reporting requires reporting of any serious injury within 30 days, the reports would not necessarily flag an event as both serious and unexpected, and their deadline is twice as long as the earlier alert reporting period of 15 days.

- **Blood-related deaths** (21 CFR 606.170): The biological product regulations require reports of a blood-related death to be submitted to CBER as soon as possible (eg, by phone, fax, or e-mail), and a written report to be submitted within 7 days of the death. The FDA believes that for some blood-containing combination products regulated under the device or drug provisions of the act, early notification of blood-related deaths may be necessary to ensure consistent and appropriate postmarket regulation.

The FDA is considering how it can supplement the reporting requirements to adequately monitor and assess the risks of combination products.[7]

Number of Marketing Applications

Even though the PMOA determines the lead center, it does not dictate what type of marketing application is submitted. Depending on the type of combination product, the approval, clearance, or licensure may require a single application or separate applications for the separate constituents of the combination product. The FDA has found that one application is usually sufficient for most combination products. However, a sponsor may elect to submit two applications. For example, there may be some advantages for marketing authorization under a particular type of application (eg, new drug product exclusivity, orphan drug benefits, or proprietary data protection when two firms are involved). In other cases, the FDA may determine that two marketing applications are necessary. Following is a list of other examples in which two applications may make sense:

- When regulatory provisions are necessary that are not available under the lead application.
- Where constituents are separate and complex products.
- Where constituents have uses beyond the combination.

- When a biologics license application (BLA) for further manufacture is appropriate.
- When labeling changes for an approved product are necessary.
- When regulatory consistency is needed.

The FDA has issued a concept paper on this subject and has actively sought input from stakeholders.[8]

Cross-Labeling

One of the FDA's most important functions is to ensure adequate and clear labeling so that physicians and patients have a clear understanding of not only when to use a product but also how to use the product in a manner that minimizes medical risks. In developing a combination product, the combination product manufacturer must consider how the product will be labeled. In some cases the two constituent parts may need separate labeling to minimize the risks. The following are situations in which cross-labeling may be important:

- Product A enhances the safety or effectiveness of product B.
- Product A uses product B in a new route of administration.
- Product A uses product B for a new indication or a new patient population.
- Product A is a new component of a previously approved combination product.
- Labeling of product A and product B will be inconsistent in the same way.
- Labeling of product A and product B will be contradictory.

The use of two products together when labeling is inconsistent or contradictory may cause confusion for the end user and may cause harm. However, one of the most significant labeling issues arises in cases when there is no ongoing relationship between two companies. Company A may use company B's product to develop a combination product without discussion with company B. When the FDA takes steps to approve company A's combination product, the FDA would realize that company B needs to change the label of its product. Without a relationship between the two companies, company B may decide that it does not want to change the label because of financial costs or liability issues. In such a case, the pathway to enable company A to obtain approval of the combination product while ensuring adequate regulatory oversight is not always clear. In some cases, the FDA will not approve the product in the interest of protecting the public health. On May 10, 2005, the FDA in conjunction with the Drug Information Association held a workshop to discuss this issue.[9]

Conclusion

There are many developmental and regulatory challenges in developing a combination product. The FDA has issued a guidance document describing some of the early development considerations for combination products.[10] The manufacturer must consider the complexity of the product and understand that its development will involve individuals from different scientific disciplines and different regulatory backgrounds. There are issues related to communication and the potential for one company to work with another. With regard to the regulatory environment, many of the issues have been outlined in this chapter. Developers need to understand how their products will be regulated, the regulatory requirements and pathway, who the FDA participants will be, the differences between centers, and the potential differences in regulation in other countries. Combination products are complex, but they hold much potential benefit to public health. Careful thought, cooperation, and a defined developmental pathway are necessary for these products to be a success.

References/Resources

1. Food and Drug Administration. Transfer of therapeutic biological products to the Center for Drug Evaluation and Research. Rockville, MD: Office of Combination Products, 2008.
2. Food and Drug Administration. Office of Combination Products. Rockville, MD: Office of Combination Products, 2008.
3. Food and Drug Administration. Jurisdictional determinations. Rockville, MD: Office of Combination Products, 2008.
4. Food and Drug Administration. Guidance for industry and FDA staff: How to write a request for designation (RFD). (August 2005) Rockville, MD: Office of Combination Products, 2005.
5. Code of federal regulations. Definition of primary mode of action of a combination product. Title 21 CFR Part 3. Fed Regist 2005;70:49848-62.
6. Food and Drug Administration. Guidance for industry and FDA: Current good manufacturing practice for combination products (draft guidance). (September 2004) Rockville, MD: Office of Combination Products, 2004.
7. Food and Drug Administration. Postmarket safety reporting for combination products. Rockville, MD: Office of Combination Products, 2008.
8. Food and Drug Administration. Number of marketing applications for a combination product. Rockville, MD: Office of Combination Products, 2008.
9. Food and Drug Administration. Proceedings of the Drug Information Association and the Food and Drug Administration cross labeling workshop: Combination products and mutually conforming labeling, Bethesda, MD, May 10, 2005. Rockville, MD: Office of Combination Products, 2005.
10. Food and Drug Administration. Guidance for industry and FDA staff: Early development considerations for innovative combination products. (September 2006) Rockville, MD: Office of Combination Products, 2006.

In: Areman EM, Loper K, eds
Cellular Therapy: Principles, Methods, and Regulations
Bethesda, MD: AABB, 2009

◆◆◆ **7** ◆◆◆

Standards and Accreditation for Cellular Therapies

Carolyn A. Keever-Taylor, PhD

FROM THE BEGINNING OF REGULATORY efforts in cellular therapies by the Food and Drug Administration (FDA), professional societies with a focus in this area appreciated the need for oversight and took the lead in developing programs not only to help their members comply with the anticipated regulations but also to promote a high quality of practice in the field. These efforts included the development of standards and the establishment of voluntary accreditation programs that were in harmony with governmental regulations and at the same time designed to address the unique aspects of cellular therapy products. The professional societies most active in this area include AABB, the American Society for Blood and Marrow Transplantation (ASBMT), the American Association of Tissue Banks (AATB), and the International Society for Cellular Therapy (ISCT). These societies, including the accreditation program created by ASBMT and ISCT in the Foundation for the Accreditation of Cellular Therapy (FACT), have sought and established an ongoing dialog with the FDA to provide input into the regulatory process as it continues to move forward.

More recently, standard-setting groups, namely, the College of American Pathologists (CAP) and The Joint Commission, that had historically focused on hospitals and clinical testing laboratories have broadened their standards to include aspects of cellular therapy processing. The standard-setting efforts have largely encompassed all cellular therapy product sources, including autologous products, and the establishment of umbilical cord blood (UCB) banks. This chapter describes general aspects of the standard-setting process, the different standard-setting groups, and their accreditation processes.

Cellular Therapy Product Standards

One of the challenges in developing cellular therapy product standards is the variety of donor types (eg, autologous, related, or unrelated) and tissue sources (eg, hematopoietic or nonhematopoietic) that support this type of therapy. Further differences among products arise for tissue and cell-based products: some are banked and others are

Carolyn A. Keever-Taylor, PhD, Director, BMT Processing Laboratories, and Professor of Medicine, Division of Neoplastic Diseases, Medical College of Wisconsin, Milwaukee, Wisconsin

The author has disclosed no conflicts of interest.

fresh or are directed donations. One reason for the proliferation of standards is the need to address the unique aspects of the different types of cellular therapy products and the activities required for their recovery or collection and their processing, distribution, banking, and use (transplantation or infusion). The FDA has focused its good tissue practice (GTP) regulations on the safety of cellular therapy products, specifically on the potential of these products to transmit communicable diseases. However, the voluntary standard-setting groups have sought to cover more broadly other aspects of program operations that also affect product quality and function. As a result, the field now has multiple sets of standards that have overlapping as well as unique content.

The requirement of a comprehensive quality system (QS), along with that of process control, is common to all of the current standards that apply to cellular therapy products. The emphasis within the standards has been on the desired endpoint, with fewer details about how to attain that endpoint. Therefore, most of the standard-setting groups also provide written guidance on how to comply with given standards, or they provide guidance through their central offices. Adherence to a given set of standards is voluntary, whereas the need to abide by governmental laws and regulations is not. The standard-setting process is ongoing, and regular updates and revisions are made to ensure that the standards meet the changing requirements of the field. In all cases, standards require that facilities abide by applicable laws and regulations should standards differ from those regulations.

The decision to adopt a given set of standards and to seek accreditation is based on several factors, which include 1) the activities of the facility (eg, types of products processed and product testing), 2) the organizational structure of the facility (eg, freestanding structure or part of a hospital or academic department), and 3) insurance or cooperative group requirements. Cost may also be an issue because fees are assessed to cover the expense of the accreditation process.

A brief history and description of the standard-setting groups involved with cellular therapy in North America and their accreditation processes follow. More information can be obtained at each organization's Web site, as listed in Table 7-1.

AABB

AABB has a long history of standard-setting for blood components and first included requirements relating to hematopoietic progenitor cell products (HPCs) in 1991 as part of the 14th edition of *Standards for Blood Banks and Transfusion Services*. In association with the increase in regulatory focus on cellular therapy, AABB published a set of dedicated standards covering the collection and processing of HPC products, *Standards for Hematopoietic Progenitor Cells*, in 1996. Laboratories were first accredited under these standards shortly thereafter. In the early-to-mid-1990s, UCB was becoming more widely used as a source of HPCs for transplant, and UCB banks were being established. To address the unique aspects of the banking of UCB HPC products, AABB published a dedicated volume, *Standards for Cord Blood Services*, in 2001. Subsequently it was determined that there was a need for standards that addressed issues unique to cells that were not of HPC origin, such as pancreatic islets. However, rather than develop a third set of standards, the AABB Board of Directors decided to include all three areas in a single set of standards titled *Standards for Cellular Therapy Product Services*, the first edition of which was published in 2004.

The current AABB standards are organized according to a set of quality system essential (QSE) elements common to all standards published by AABB. Topic areas include the following 10 elements: 1) organization, 2) resources, 3) equipment, 4) customer and supplier issues (agreements), 5) process control, 6) document and records, 7) deviations and nonconforming products or services, 8) assessments (internal and external), 9) process improvement, and 10) safety and facilities. The AABB standards focus on processing activities but also include requirements related to the recovery or collection of the cellular therapy product and activities surrounding product infusion and patient outcome. The AABB standards have an 18-month review cycle, and the committee charged with standards review and revision includes a public representative and representatives from the FDA and other related professional societies and organizations. The wide range of representation is designed to keep the AABB standards in harmony with other standards and with regulations. Draft standards are

Table 7-1. Accreditation and Standard-Setting Groups

Group	Cellular Therapy Focus	Standards	Accreditation Duration	Web Site for Documents
AABB*	Collection, cord blood banking, cellular product processing, storage, and distribution	*Standards for Cellular Therapy Product Services*	2 years	http://www.aabb.org/ (order form)
AATB*	Retrieval, tissue processing, storage, or distribution of tissue	*Standards for Tissue Banking*	2 years	http://www.aatb.org/ (order form)
CAP*	Product testing (eg, microbiology, flow cytometry, hematology), collection, processing, storage, and distribution of HPCs and tissue	*Standards for Laboratory Accreditation Laboratory Accreditation Manual* General and specific laboratory checklists	2 years; self-assessment during the off-cycle year	http://www.cap.org/ (free to download)
FACT*	Clinical program, collection, cord blood banking, cellular product processing, storage, and distribution	FACT-JACIE *International Standards for Cellular Therapy Product Collection, Processing, and Administration* FACT-NetCord *International Standards for Cord Blood Collection, Processing, Testing, Banking, Selection, and Release*	3 years	http://www.factwebsite.org/ (free to download)
The Joint Commission†‡	Medical facility issues, CT product testing, acquisition, receipt, storage; and storage and distribution of tissues within a facility	*Comprehensive Accreditation Manual for Laboratory and Point-of-Care Testing*	2 years	http://www.jointcommission.org/ (order form)
NMDP§	Unrelated products, including donor screening, collection, distribution, cord blood banking, processing	National Marrow Donor Program *Standards*	3 years; provide documentation yearly	http://www.marrow.org/ABOUT/Providing_Hope/NMDP_Network/Maintaining_NMDP_Standards/ (free to download)

*Voluntary. AABB accreditation is required for institutional members. FACT accreditation is required for some cooperative group transplant trials and by some insurance providers.

†Required. Hospitals must be Joint-Commission-accredited (or equivalent) for all other standard-setting groups.

‡The American Osteopathic Hospital Association Healthcare Facilities Accreditation Program is considered to be an equivalent hospital and laboratory accrediting organization by the Centers for Medicare and Medicaid Services.

§NMDP membership is required for access to its unrelated donors. NMDP requires AABB or FACT accreditation for participating cord blood banks. NMDP requires CAP certification for microbiology testing laboratories.

AATB = American Association of Tissue Banks; CAP = College of American Pathologists; FACT = Foundation for the Accreditation of Cellular Therapy; JACIE = Joint Accreditation Committee of the International Society for Cellular Therapy and the European Group for Blood and Marrow Transplantation; NMDP = National Marrow Donor Program.

published on the AABB Web site for public comment before final committee review, legal review, AABB board approval, and publication. A document is posted at the AABB Web site that contains questions and answers that have arisen for a given edition of standards to serve as guidance for compliance.

Because AABB is an accreditation body, its policies are consistent with internationally accepted standards published by the International Organization for Standardization (ISO).[4] The initial accreditation process starts with a self-assessment that uses a customized accreditation tool developed from the standards to cover the specific activities of the facility. This self-assessment along with other supporting documentation is provided to the AABB National Office for review before the site visit is scheduled. Once the submitted documents are reviewed and accepted, the facility is visited by a lead AABB assessor, accompanied by one or more trained volunteer assessors with expertise specific to the facility's activities. As of 2007, accreditation site visits are unannounced but conducted within a specified calendar quarter according to the accreditation cycle. Before leaving the site, the assessor provides a summary report that details the findings, to which the facility must respond within 30 days with any appropriate corrective actions. Questions concerning the intent of the standards are referred to the AABB Standards Committee for resolution. In cases in which nonconformances might affect patient care, documentation that corrective actions have been implemented is required. The AABB Board of Directors awards a 2-year accreditation that covers the facility's assessed activities. A repeat on-site assessment and reapproval is required by the end of the 2-year cycle.

Accreditation is offered to both domestic and international facilities. AABB lists accredited facilities on its Web site.

Foundation for the Accreditation of Cellular Therapy

In 1996, the two professional societies that focus on HPC therapy, ISCT and ASBMT, sponsored FACT, a free-standing organization, to develop standards and a voluntary accreditation program. The first edition of the FACT *Standards for Hematopoietic Progenitor Cell Collection, Processing and Trans-*

plantation was published in 1996. Similar to the AABB standards, the first edition focused on the collection, processing, and clinical use of HPC products. In conjunction with NetCord, the international UCB banking arm of EuroCord, and the international registry for the European Group for Blood and Marrow Transplantation (EBMT), FACT developed a separate series of standards, the *International Standards for Cord Blood Collection, Processing, Testing, Banking, Selection and Release*, which were first published in 2000. Unlike AABB, FACT has determined that it is more efficient to keep the banking aspects of HPCs separate from the processing and transplantation aspects that are covered by the cellular therapy standards.

The Joint Accreditation Committee of ISCT and EBMT (JACIE) was established in 1999 to address the need for standards and accreditation in the European Union. For this purpose, JACIE adopted the first edition of FACT standards in its entirety. The FACT-JACIE collaboration evolved from a joint review in 2002 to active participation by JACIE in standards development by the third edition of the standards, published in 2006. These standards are now titled *FACT-JACIE International Standards for Cellular Therapy Product Collection, Processing and Administration*.

The FACT-JACIE cellular therapy standards include three parallel sections that cover the clinical transplant program, the collection programs (marrow and apheresis), and the processing facility. Both HPC products and therapeutic cell products are covered. The current standard-setting process involves an initial review and revision of each section by separate clinical, collection, and laboratory working groups. The resulting document is further reviewed by a standards steering committee, which is composed of the chair and cochair of each of the separate working groups along with the chair of the overall standards edition and representatives from the FACT central office. Draft standards are made available for public review and comment, followed by a final steering committee review, legal review, FACT board approval, and, finally, publication. The FACT standards review cycle is now every 3 years, and the UCB banking standards and cellular therapy products standards are offset by 1 year. The Cellular Therapy Products Standards Steering Committee and each of the working groups include one or more representatives from JACIE, along with volunteers who have recognized expertise in each of the sections for which they are responsible. Likewise, the Cord Blood Banking Standards Committee is composed of FACT and NetCord representatives with expertise in UCB banking. At each level of review, current regulations and other existing standards are considered, to promote harmonization.

The FACT standards are similar in content to those developed by AABB but also include patient care standards, reflecting the belief that accreditation must assess the clinical aspects of transplantation as well as collection and laboratory practices. Each of the major sections of the standards requires a comprehensive quality management program and includes facility design and operations; policies and procedures; donor evaluation, selection, and management; recordkeeping; labeling; processing; storage; transportation; the release and distribution of cellular therapy products; adverse event reporting; auditing; and outcomes analysis.

To be eligible for FACT accreditation, clinical programs must use collection facilities and laboratory facilities that comply with FACT standards. Facilities that meet the requirements specified in the FACT standards regarding training and experience initiate the accreditation process by completing a self-assessment, using a checklist derived from the FACT standards and providing supporting documentation to the FACT accreditation office. After review and approval of the submitted materials, an inspection team of trained volunteers is assigned, and an inspection date is scheduled with the facility.

FACT inspection teams are composed of one or more individuals with recognized expertise in each of the areas to be inspected. Collection, processing, and clinical facilities can be accredited separately. The number of inspectors assigned is based on the complexity of the program (eg, number of clinical sites or number of collection sites). A designated team leader oversees the on-site visit. At least three inspectors are required for a typical transplant program that consists of a clinical program, a collection facility (usually marrow and apheresis), and a processing facility.

Inspections usually require a single day, although if there are multiple sites, the inspection may extend over 2 days. UCB bank inspections usually require 1.5 days because of the need to visit multiple collection sites. The facility is provided with a preliminary verbal report at the end of the site visit, and a written report follows after review by the FACT Accreditation Committee. On the basis of the inspection findings, the facility may be granted accreditation immediately or may be required to respond with a plan to correct deficiencies, to provide evidence that significant deficiencies have been corrected, or, if serious issues arise, to undergo a focused reinspection of the area of concern. The FACT board grants final approval and accreditation. Facilities successfully completing this process are approved for 3 years. Renewal of accreditation requires repeat inspection.

To date, FACT has accredited 153 HPC facilities in North America, including 8 in Canada, along with 15 UCB banks, 9 of which are outside the United States. JACIE has a separate accreditation program with a process that is similar to that of FACT. JACIE inspections are performed in the language of the applicant facility. FACT accreditation is required by a number of cooperative groups (eg, Eastern Oncology Group and the Children's Oncology Group) before a facility may participate in transplant clinical trials and by several insurance providers for a facility to be considered as a transplant center of excellence.

American Association of Tissue Banks

The AATB has established standards that focus on the safety and optimal clinical performance of banked tissue. The AATB first published draft guidelines for tissue banking in 1977 and published the first edition of standards in 1984. The AATB accreditation program was established in 1985. A standards committee within AATB oversees regular updates to the program that correspond to AATB's most recent standards, now published in their 12th edition. In addition to an accreditation program, AATB has a program for the training and certification of tissue banking personnel.

The overall content of the AATB standards is similar to that described for FACT and AABB and includes standards for operations, the need for a quality program, and process controls. The AATB standards focus on the donor or family consent process, donor screening and testing, and the recovery, banking, and distribution of tissues. The standards do not include requirements for the clinical programs using the recovered cells and tissues. Changes to standards may occur between editions and are reviewed and approved by the AATB Board of Governors and communicated to the membership through the *AATB Bulletin*.

Organizations that bank tissue, including those associated with assessing donor suitability, tissue recovery, processing, storage, labeling, and distribution of cells or tissue are eligible for accreditation. Also eligible are tissue distribution intermediaries (agents who acquire and store cells or tissue for further distribution) and tissue dispensing services (facilities that receive, maintain, and deliver tissues to the ultimate user for transplantation or research). If a tissue bank does not perform a given activity or service, the provider of that activity or service to the tissue bank must meet applicable AATB standards.

At the time of application for accreditation, a facility completes and submits a self-assessment using an audit form and preinspection checklist obtained from the AATB executive office. An individual not directly responsible for the activity being audited must perform the preinspection audit. The AATB checklist must be cross-referenced to the location within the tissue bank's policies and procedures that proves compliance. Once the initial application is reviewed and approved, an on-site inspection is scheduled, and the facility must provide its entire standard operating procedures manual for review by an independent inspector hired by the AATB. An average scheduled inspection occurs over 2 days. The inspection period can be extended by a day or more, depending on the number of tissue banking activities performed by the bank or because of a finding by the inspector. A preliminary inspection report is provided to the tissue bank at the end of the site visit. Inspection reports are reviewed and evaluated by the accreditation program manager in consultation with the inspectors. The report is then reviewed by the AATB Accreditation Committee, who will determine if the tissue bank is in compliance with AATB standards, determine the need for corrective actions, or require a repeat inspection if serious deficiencies are found. Final review and approval are granted by the AATB Board of Governors on the basis of recommendations made by the accreditation committee.

Accreditation is awarded for 3 years for the services that are provided (eg, recovery, processing, storage, distribution, and/or research) and includes references to specific tissue types associated with those services (eg, musculoskeletal, cardiac, vascular, skin, and/or reproductive). Yearly documentation of continued compliance in the form of an annual survey and self-assessment is required. Unannounced repeat inspections to verify performance may occur.

To date, the AATB has accredited tissue banks in the United States and Canada, and listings of accredited tissue banks can be accessed at the AATB Web site (see Table 7-1).

National Marrow Donor Program

The National Marrow Donor Program (NMDP) was established by Congress in 1986 to facilitate the matching of potential bone marrow recipients with unrelated donors.[5] NMDP activities now include coordination of the collection and distribution of marrow, apheresis, and cord blood products from unrelated donors.

Congress also mandated that the NMDP establish criteria for centers that participate in the program in the form of standards. NMDP standards separately address the requirements for the participation of 1) donor centers (recruitment, screening, and HLA typing of unrelated donors), 2) UCB banks (that have at least 100 HLA-typed products banked), 3) apheresis centers (stimulated and unstimulated peripheral blood cells), 4) collection centers (bone marrow), and 5) transplant centers. The NMDP requires that its members implement quality standards, standards for tissue typing, informed consent of donors, donor advocacy, donor selection criteria to protect the donor and prevent the transmission of communicable disease, and procedures to ensure the proper collection and transportation of HPC products. The NMDP standards outline only the most basic guidelines to achieve the program's goals in these areas but do serve as a standard of care for patients.

The NMDP requires AABB or FACT accreditation for UCB banks and also requires that transplant centers and hospitals affiliated with collection centers have Joint Commission or equivalent accreditation. Laboratories that provide services required by the NMDP must have Clinical Laboratory Improvement Amendments (CLIA) certification or CAP accreditation. The NMDP Standards

Committee reviews the standards on a 2-year cycle and makes changes as needed to remain up to date with regulations and the standards of other organizations. Revised draft NMDP standards are available for public comment before review and final acceptance by the NMDP Board of Directors.

The NMDP does not accredit facilities; rather, it grants membership for qualified facilities. For each NMDP center type, an application is submitted that includes a series of questions designed to document adherence to the participation criteria and standards. NMDP staff members review the documents and assist the center if the documentation needs clarification before formal review by the NMDP Membership Committee. The NMDP Executive Committee issues membership approval. No on-site inspection is required except for UCB banks. At the time of this writing, NMDP holds an IND exemption for unrelated UCB transplantation and, therefore, has an oversight role for the facilities involved. For UCB banks, a 1.5-day, on-site inspection by two or three NMDP staff members is performed, which includes visits to collection sites.

Once membership is awarded, facilities must provide yearly documentation of compliance and undergo announced on-site data audits every 3 or 4 years. UCB banks are reviewed on a more frequent schedule, and the audit includes review of procedures and operations.

College of American Pathologists

CAP has a long history of standard-setting and accreditation of clinical laboratories that perform diagnostic testing. CAP has general laboratory standards as well as specific standards for laboratory specialty areas. Checklists derived from the CAP standards are used for the accreditation process. The Transfusion Medicine Checklist includes standards specific to the collection, transport, processing, storage, and administration of cellular therapy products, including HPCs, as well as standards applicable to tissue banks for the storage and issue of tissues other than HPCs.

In addition to the accreditation program, CAP provides an extensive proficiency testing program for specialty areas. For laboratories that test specified analytes, participation in a CAP-provided or a CAP-approved proficiency program is a requirement of CAP accreditation. In all cases, laboratories must participate in some form of proficiency testing, whether internal or external. Proficiency programs tailored for progenitor cell processing and UCB testing are now available, and although these are not on the CAP list of required analytes, they would satisfy the general requirement for proficiency testing.

The CAP *Standards for Laboratory Accreditation*, the *Laboratory Accreditation Manual*, and the checklists are available for downloading at the CAP Web site (see Table 7-1). The checklists include items derived from the standards that are intended to assess compliance, along with notes, commentary, and references to provide guidance on how to achieve compliance. Laboratories seeking CAP accreditation must comply with applicable items from the Laboratory General Checklist as well as the checklists of the appropriate specialty areas. For the most part, if a cellular therapy laboratory complies with AABB, FACT, or AATB standards, the requirements of the CAP standards will also be met, although some details may vary. Laboratories that operate within a hospital or blood center may be able to apply for CAP accreditation as a limited-service laboratory under the umbrella of the parent hospital's clinical laboratory.[6]

When applying for initial CAP accreditation, the laboratory must indicate the specialty areas for which it is seeking accreditation (eg, transfusion service, flow cytometry, or hematology) and must use the Master Activity Menus to identify the tests or activities performed. A complete version of the current CAP inspection checklists will be provided with the initial applications packet. A customized checklist that contains only the relevant items that will be reviewed is provided before the inspection and upon application for reaccreditation. Self-completed preinspection checklists do not need to be returned to the Laboratory Accreditation Program Office.

An inspection team is assigned according to the specialty areas to be inspected, and an on-site inspection is scheduled. As of 2006, CAP inspectors must undergo specific training before performing an inspection. Laboratory inspections usually occur over 2 days. At the end of the inspection, a written report of the findings is provided to the facility.

Responses to cited deficiencies are required within 30 days of the inspection. Once all responses are received and deficiencies are corrected or disputes resolved, the appropriate CAP regional commissioner awards accreditation for 2 years. A self-inspection using an updated checklist is performed at the beginning of the second year and is provided to CAP, along with a plan to correct deficiencies. Reaccreditation site visits must occur within a 30-day period before the facility's accreditation anniversary date. Unannounced inspections may occur.

The Joint Commission recognizes CAP accreditation, as do many state laboratory certification programs. CAP has accredited more than 6000 laboratories worldwide.

The Joint Commission

Since 1979, part of The Joint Commission mission to improve the safety and quality of public health care has included the development of standards and the accreditation of hospital laboratory services. This activity was extended to freestanding laboratories in 1995. Laboratories are accredited using standards contained in the *Comprehensive Accreditation Manual for Laboratory and Point-of-Care Testing (CAMLAB)*, which can be obtained through the Joint Commission Web site (see Table 7-1). Joint Commission standards address the results that a laboratory should achieve but do not specify the methods by which that should be accomplished. In general, Joint Comission standards have a strong focus on laboratory safety, quality control, and proficiency testing. Standards related to the acquisition, receipt, storage, and distribution of tissues and cell products are now included. These standards extend to tissue banks as well as to cellular therapy laboratories that process tissue of HPC origin.

Laboratory surveys are generally conducted separately from other parts of the health-care organization. However, laboratory-specific elements included in the parent organization survey may be reviewed with the parent survey. The laboratory surveys are conducted by experienced medical technologists, who are employed and trained by The Joint Commission. Since 2004, Joint Commission surveys have used a method that traces patients through the care, treatment, and services they receive. Following the survey, the organization receives a report that includes any findings and requirements for improvement. The organization

must address all issues by providing evidence of standards compliance before accreditation is awarded.

Participation in a Centers for Medicare and Medicaid Services (CMS) proficiency testing program for all regulated tests is required to achieve and maintain accreditation. Accreditation is awarded for 2 years. The Joint Commission Laboratory Accreditation Program is recognized by CMS as meeting the requirements of CLIA, so a separate CLIA inspection is not required. Although The Joint Commission recognizes CAP accreditation in lieu of a laboratory survey, dual accreditation is not granted. However, CAP-accredited laboratories do not need to complete the intracycle Periodic Performance Review, which is required of laboratories that are accredited by The Joint Commission alone to support continuous compliance to standards.

Joint Commission surveys may be announced or unannounced. The organization has accredited nearly 2000 organizations that provide laboratory services, including nearly 3200 laboratories certified according to CLIA.

Standards Harmonization

The number of independent, standard-setting organizations in the United States and Europe, along with the national and international regulations that control cellular therapy products, has led to instances in which standards and regulations within or between countries are not in harmony. For HPC products alone, data from the World Marrow Donor Association (WMDA), of which the NMDP is a member, indicate that in 2005 nearly 40% of unrelated products were shipped internationally, clearly indicating the need for global standards in this field. The World Health Organization (WHO) has endorsed the effort for harmonization through a series of meetings to address relevant issues in the field.[7,8] The WHO efforts have started with guidelines designed to ensure uniform product safety requirements.[8]

In 2006, an attempt was initiated by the Alliance for Harmonization of Cellular Therapy Accreditation (AHCTA) to establish an ongoing dialog between organizations for the harmonization of standards and regulations. The AHCTA comprises representatives from AABB, ASBMT, EBMT, ISCT, JACIE, FACT, NetCord, and WMDA (see http://www.ahcta.org). The objective of AHCTA is to create a single set of quality, safety, and professional requirements for cellular therapy products, including HPCs, that covers all aspects of the process from assessment of donor eligibility to transplantation and clinical outcome. To achieve this objective, AHCTA strives to establish a collaborative environment for the drafting of complementary standards and guidelines. The ambitious, but highly desirable, goal is to have a global set of standards that can be used by the cellular therapy professional community and the regulatory authorities. For this goal to be achieved, regular communication on all relevant issues affecting cellular therapy guidelines is required. The partnership of the regulatory authorities in the application of the resultant global standards is essential to their successful adoption. To facilitate this goal, AHCTA endeavors to inform and support these authorities in the area of cellular therapy regulation. At the time of this writing, the first issue to be addressed by AHCTA is the development of minimum import and export requirements.

ISBT 128 for Cellular Therapy

Clerical errors remain a common cause of confusion and concern in the practice of cellular therapies. The high incidence of imported and exported products further adds to this issue because of the differences in language. In cooperation with the International Council on Commonality in Blood Banking Automation (ICCBBA), cellular therapy organizations formed an advisory group to develop a global standard for cellular therapy product terminology, coding, and labeling. The group was established in 2005 and includes representation from the following organizations: the AABB, ASBMT, American Society for Apheresis (ASFA), EBMT, FACT, ICCBBA, International Society of Blood Transfusion (ISBT), ISCT, ISCT Europe, JACIE, NMDP, and WMDA.

The group developed uniform terminology, definitions, and labeling requirements and published an implementation plan.[9,10] At the time of this writing, both the AABB and FACT require the use of the ISBT 128 proper names, and the *Circular of Information for the Use of Cellular Therapy Prod-*

ucts (Circular) also incorporates this terminology. A US consensus group was formed to develop labels meeting US-specific requirements. It is expected that the standard-setting organizations will gradually require implementation of the terminology and ultimately the full coding system. An updated list of product names and definitions, as well as registered facilities and vendors, may be found at the ICCBBA Web site (http://www.iccbba.org).

In concert with the harmonization effort, the International Cellular Therapy Coding and Labeling Advisory Group developed an implementation plan for the uniform labeling of cellular therapy products. This effort included the development of a common terminology and a coding system based on the ISBT 128 labeling standards.[9] A plan for the introduction of ISBT 128 in cell processing laboratories was recently published.[10]

The effort to establish a global core set of labeling standards that serves as the basis for more specific standards required by a given organization is under way. Individuals can help facilitate harmonization by becoming familiar with existing standards and responding to postings of draft standards and regulations during the public or member comments period.

Circular of Information

In an effort to standardize labeling and comply with regulatory and voluntary requirements, the *Circular* was developed and is revised and updated every 2 years by a multi-organizational work group. Participants include AABB, AATB, America's Blood Centers (ABC), the American Red Cross (ARC), ASBMT, ASFA, CAP, FACT, ICCBBA, ISCT, NMDP, FDA, the Health Resources and Services Administration (HRSA), JACIE, and NetCord. The *Circular* is intended to be an extension of the cellular product label. Each processing or issuing facility is encouraged to provide more facility- or product-specific information along with the product. The *Circular* has evolved to include international representation, and efforts to align terminology with the ISBT 128 nomenclature have increased its usefulness. Not all products are covered, and some facility modification is expected. The *Circular* is designed to accompany products, to be available to healthcare personnel who administer the products, and to be available to patients, upon request.

Achieving Accreditation

Cellular therapy has become an increasingly regulated field. This increased regulation has resulted in the proliferation of overlapping sets of standards. Which standards are best for a given facility and what accreditations should be sought? Most facilities want, or may be required, to be accredited by more than one organization. For tissue banks, AATB accreditation is more comprehensive than CAP or JCAHO alone. Facilities involved primarily or exclusively in cellular therapy products of HPC origin might seek AABB or FACT accreditation. AABB institutional members are required to be accredited under AABB standards. However, because FACT separately accredits clinical transplant programs, a number of cooperative groups, multicenter clinical trials, and insurance providers require FACT accreditation. To be FACT accredited, clinical programs must use collection and processing facilities that meet FACT standards, necessitating that they be part of the inspection process, even though formal accreditation is not required. In the United States, processing facilities, UCB banks, or tissue banks that provide product testing (eg, white blood cell counts or flow cytometry) may need to be certified according to CLIA in the future to be able to charge for these services. Sponsored clinical trials commonly require that testing used for product release be performed by laboratories certified under CLIA, or in some cases CAP-accredited laboratories, to standardize the quality of the testing. Hospital-based processing or collection facilities may seek accreditation by The Joint Commission for their testing or cell-processing activities. NMDP membership is required for any HPC-processing facility that is part of a clinical program that performs unrelated donor transplantation.

For the most part, the standards of these various organizations are in agreement but have a different focus or level of detail that requires the facility to be familiar with each set of standards before seeking accreditation. During the accreditation process, preparation is essential. It is helpful to use checklists or other tools made available to facilities before inspection to identify the documentation required to demonstrate compliance. Facilities should ensure that the necessary records are readily available during the inspection and be prepared for both announced and unannounced inspections. Maintaining systems in accordance with standards requires as much effort as establishing them initially. It is the responsibility of all involved personnel to ensure that standards are followed. Universally, the standard-setting organizations require that the specific activities performed by these facilities adhere to federal, state, or local regulations, but adherence to any given set of standards may not assure compliance with the regulations. Therefore, despite achieving potentially multiple accreditations, the facility must still be aware of and comply with applicable governmental regulations. However, this process is less onerous for laboratories that have achieved and maintained voluntary accreditation.

References/Resources

1. Food and Drug Administration. Proposed approach to regulation of cellular and tissue-based products. [Docket No. 97N-0068]. (February 28, 1997) Rockville, MD: CBER Office of Communication, Training, and Manufacturers Assistance, 1997.
2. Food and Drug Administration. Current good tissue practice for human cell, tissue, and cellular and tissue-based product establishments; inspection and enforcement; final rule. Fed Regist 2004;69:68611-88.
3. Food and Drug Administration. Human cells, tissues, and cellular and tissue-based products; establishment registration and listing; final rule. Fed Regist 2001;66: 5447-69.
4. International Organization for Standardization. ISO/IEC Guide 17025:2005. General requirements for the competence of testing and calibration laboratories. Geneva, Switzerland: ISO, 2005.
5. United States Code. National Bone Marrow Donor Registry. 42 U.S.C., Chapter 6A, Subchapter II, Part I, §274k. Washington, DC: US Government Printing Office, 1986.
6. Sharkey F, ed. Laboratory accreditation manual. Northfield, IL: College of American Pathologists, 2007:78-9.
7. World Health Organization. Report: First global consultation on regulatory requirements for human cells and tissues for transplantation, Ottawa, 29 November to 1 December 2004. Geneva, Switzerland: WHO, 2005. [Available at http://whqlibdoc.who.int/publications/2005/9241593296.pdf (accessed October 31, 2008).]
8. World Health Organization. Aide-mémoire on key safety requirements for essential minimally processed human cells and tissues for transplantation. Geneva, Switzer-

land: WHO, 2006. [Available at http://www.who.int/transplantation/AM-SafetyEssential%20HCTT.pdf (accessed October 31, 2008).]

9. Ashford P, Distler P, Gee A, et al. Standards for the terminology and labeling of cellular therapy products. Transfusion 2007;47:1319-27.

10. Ashford P, Distler P, Gee A, et al. ISBT 128 implementation plan for cellular therapy products. Transfusion 2007;47:1312-8.

Quality Assurance for
Cellular Therapy Facilities

◆ ◆ ◆

WIKIPEDIA, THE INTERNET ENCYCLO-pedia, at one point defined *quality* as the "non-inferiority, superiority, or usefulness of something."[1] That definition is certainly too broad and general to describe quality in the context of a cellular therapy (CT) product or facility. Perhaps the American Society for Quality (ASQ) comes closer by defining it as "1. the characteristics of a product or service that bear on its ability to satisfy stated or implied needs; 2. a product or service free of deficiencies."[2] That same organization defines *quality assurance (QA)* as "all the planned and systematic activities implemented within the quality system [QS] that can be demonstrated to provide confidence that a product or service will fulfill requirements for quality."[2] On the other hand, ASQ defines *quality control (QC)* as "the operational techniques and activities used to fulfill requirements for quality."[2] ASQ further says, "Often, however, 'quality assurance' and 'quality control' are used interchangeably, referring to the actions performed to ensure the quality of a product, service, or process."[2]

The QA program provides the tools for ensuring that all systems and elements affecting the quality of the product are functioning as expected and can

Section Editors: Ellen Areman, MS, SBB(ASCP), Senior Consultant, Biologics Consulting Group, Inc, Alexandria, Virginia; Lizabeth Cardwell, MT(ASCP), MBA, RAC, Principal, Compliance Consulting, Seattle, Washington; Karen Edward, BS, MT(ASCP), Regulatory/Quality Systems Consultant, Advanced Cell and Gene Therapy, LLC, New York, New York; Cynthia Elliott, MT, HP(ASCP), CQA(ASQ), Consultant, CT Auditing and Compliance Services, LLC, Sugar Hill, Georgia; and Michele W. Sugrue, MS, MT(ASCP)SBB, Coordinator, Research Programs, Division of Hematology/Oncology, Department of Medicine, University of Florida and Shands Hospital , Gainesville, Florida

The editors have disclosed no conflicts of interest.

be relied upon to do so. It should consist of an overarching set of coordinated measures designed to direct and control an organization to continually improve the effectiveness and efficiency of its performance. The role of QA is to provide consistency and satisfaction in terms of methods, materials, and equipment, and it affects all activities of the organization at every interface, from identification of customer requirements to customer satisfaction with the organization's output.

A successful QA program has the following features:

- Describes the quality policy and quality objectives of the organization.
- Includes mechanisms to ensure that QA activities are carried out as defined.
- Provides a basis of communication to prevent staff from having to search out, guess at, or remain ignorant of processes.
- Ensures manufacturing consistency when personnel leave or join the organization.
- Provides guidance or a source for internal audits and assessments.

Organizations that have requirements to establish, implement, and maintain a quality program include those that provide accreditation for CT facilities, such as the AABB, the Foundation for the Accreditation of Cellular Therapy (FACT), the Joint Accreditation Committee of the International Society for Cellular Therapy and the European Group for Blood and Marrow Transplantation (JACIE), the International Organization for Standardization (ISO), and NetCord; those that regulate CT manufacturers, such as the European Medicines Agency (EMEA), the Food and Drug Administration (FDA), Health Canada, and the Therapeutic Goods Administration (TGA); and those that provide and monitor donor registries, such as the National Marrow Donor Program (NMDP) and the World Marrow Donor Association (WMDA).

Whereas QA is a system for assuring the consistent production of a product or service that meets specific criteria, QC provides the means for measuring aspects of the product or service to determine whether the QA criteria are being met. QC activities are tailored to evaluate individual processes to ensure that the final product meets the required specifications.

Origins of Quality Concepts

Records as far back as the 13th century describe the organization of craftsmen into cooperative groups called guilds. One purpose of these guilds was to set standards for their craft to ensure a consistent level of quality. After the Industrial Revolution, the factory system of individual product inspection during manufacturing took the place of the craftsmanship model and continued up to World War II. During the production of wartime materials, it became obvious that inspection of every item produced in a factory was slowing down production and limiting factory output. The military devised and implemented sampling techniques to replace individual product inspections.

After World War II, the concept of total quality management (TQM) as a means of "building in" quality was adopted in Japan and subsequently in the United States. The idea of preventing inferior manufacturing by improving processes rather than detecting it by inspection continues to dominate, although the TQM terminology may have fallen out of favor. Organizations continue to implement novel quality systems and tools to improve the quality of their output.[3]

The nongovernmental ISO was founded in 1946 with members from 25 countries to develop a common set of manufacturing, trade, and communications standards. ISO is composed of representatives from each associated country and acts as a consortium with strong links to many governments. As of 2003, the organization had 147 members. Because of quality problems in many British high-tech industries, such as munitions production during World War II, the British government decided to require factories to follow documented manufacturing procedures and improve record-keeping to ensure that the procedures were being followed. The British standard became known as BS 5750 and was considered a management standard because it did not specifically describe the manufacturing process but, rather, how to manage it. In 1987, the British government persuaded ISO to adopt BS 5750 as an international standard, which became "ISO 9000." It consists of 3 models for QA requirements at various stages of production. ISO 9000 is the foundation for a quality management system, ensuring that information is recorded and systems are in place to capture and standardize manufacturing and other processes.[4]

Although many autologous and allogeneic hematopoietic progenitor cell (HPC) transplants were performed from the 1960s to the 1980s, no federal agencies or professional organizations were promulgating quality standards or requirements for the HPC products. Evaluation of CT manufacturing quality was primarily related to assessing the product characteristics before and after processing. Even without regulations or standards to guide them, many laboratories implemented systems and processes that were expected as part of a clinical laboratory environment. Such systems involved properly documenting procedures; monitoring equipment; ensuring sterility of supplies and reagents; using, when possible, sterile materials approved for human use; using mechanisms to properly identify donor, recipient, and product; maintaining trained and competent staff; and performing clinical outcome analysis.[5]

Cellular Therapy Today

The quality requirements implemented for blood during the 1990s were the basis for many of the current CT quality management and manufacturing practices. These requirements were especially relevant during the early years of clinical CT, when many products were manufactured and issued by blood banks and transfusion medicine departments.

During the early part of the 1990s, the FDA began publishing recommendations for QS documentation for blood establishments and, in July 1995, published the Guideline for Quality Assurance in Blood Establishments.[6] Many of the principles adopted by the FDA were based on ISO 9000 standards,[7] and the document became the foundation for establishing QA in blood banks. This guidance document provides the requirements for establishing a quality program for a blood bank and the oversight of this program within a facility.

Several organizations offer voluntary accreditation programs that are based on their own standards and requirements, which usually address the development of and adherence to quality standards.

The AABB was originally founded to support and encourage blood research, to promote the exchange of scientific information, and to develop standards of practice for blood banks. In 1991, the 14th edition of *Standards for Blood Banks and Transfusion Services* introduced a section devoted to bone marrow processing. The AABB began conducting voluntary accreditation of HPC facilities in 1996 with the publication of its first edition of *Standards for Hematopoietic Progenitor Cells*, which included a requirement for a documented quality program. Because of the uniqueness of each CT product as well as the potential for international members, AABB updated its quality program requirements in 2000 to be aligned with ISO 9000:1994 quality requirements. ISO9000:1994 emphasized QA by means of preventive actions, instead of mere inspection of the final product, and continued to require evidence of compliance with documented procedures. Cord blood, in 1996, and somatic cell therapies, in 2002, were added to the accreditation menu. AABB CT standards, now in the *Standards for Cellular Therapy Product Services*, are updated every 18 months.

The International Society for Cellular Therapy (ISCT) was established in 1992 (then known as the International Society of Hematotherapy and Graft Engineering, or ISHAGE) to represent technologists, scientists, and physicians who worked in the area of hematopoietic stem cell graft manipulation. ISCT developed the first draft of the "Standards for Hematopoietic Cell Collection and Processing."

The American Society for Blood and Marrow Transplantation (ASBMT) was formed in 1993 as a professional organization that represented physicians and investigators involved in the clinical conduct of HPC transplantation. The society developed the first draft of the "Clinical Standards for Hematopoietic Cell Transplantation."

In December 1994, ISCT and ASBMT merged their standards into a single document, which covered all aspects of hematopoietic CT (collection, processing, and transplantation). The two societies established FACT to develop a voluntary inspection and accreditation program that was based on the joint standards of ISCT and ASBMT. The first edition of FACT standards was published in 1996 and also contained a requirement for a quality management plan at all stages of transplantation: clinical, collection, processing, and administration.

In 2000, recognizing the global impact of cord blood banking and transplantation, FACT partnered with NetCord, an international network of nonprofit public cord blood banks, to establish international standards for cord blood collection, processing, testing, banking, unit selection, and release, as well as requirements for a quality management plan.

On February 28, 1997, the FDA published an announcement to inform the public of its intention to regulate cellular and tissue-based products. The FDA proposed an approach in which the regulatory oversight is proportional to the risk to the product recipient.[8]

On May 25, 2005, the FDA published the last of a series of regulatory documents for cellular and tissue-based products, which included procedures for registration and listing, donor eligibility, and current good tissue practice (cGTP).[9] This document specifies that any establishment performing any steps in manufacturing "must establish and maintain a quality program" [Code of Federal Regulations (CFR) Title 21, Part 1271.160] "designed to prevent, detect, and correct deficiencies that may lead to circumstances that increase the risk of introduction, transmission, or spread of communicable diseases" [21 CFR 1271.3(hh)].

This section focuses on the development and use of systems, processes, and tools that enable an organization to recognize and correct events and trends that can negatively affect the products or services it provides. These systems should enable the entity to continuously maintain and improve the quality of its output, meeting the needs and expectations of its customers. The material provided here is intended to serve as a starting point for developing a quality program.

The chapters were compiled by QA experts who reviewed current requirements and trends. The chapters are not meant to be comprehensive for the subject matter. The design or revision of an individual quality program will depend on items such as upper management commitment, the specific CT products manufactured, the manufacturing scheme, resources, organizational complexity, voluntary standards, and governmental regulations.

References/Resources

1. Wikipedia. Quality. San Francisco, CA: Wikimedia Foundation, 2008. [Available at http://en.wikipedia.org.]
2. American Society for Quality. Basic concepts: Glossary. Milwaukee, WI: ASQ, 2008. [Available at http://www.asq.org/glossary/q.html (accessed November 20, 2008).]
3. American Society for Quality. Basic concepts: The history of quality—overview. Milwaukee, WI: ASQ, 2008. [Available at http://www.asq.org/learn-about-quality/history-of-quality/overview/overview.html (accessed June 18, 2009).]
4. International Organization for Standardization. The ISO story. Geneva, Switzerland: ISO, 2008. [Available at http://www.iso.org/iso/about/the_iso_story/ (accessed November 20, 2008).]
5. Areman EM, Deeg HJ, Sacher RA. Bone marrow and stem cell processing: A manual of current techniques. Philadelphia: FA Davis, 1992:9-10.
6. Food and Drug Administration. Guideline for quality assurance in blood establishments. Docket No. 91N-0450. (July 11, 1995) Rockville, MD: CBER Office of Communication, Training, and Manufacturers Assistance, 1995.
7. Nevalainen DE, Lloyd HL. ISO 9000 quality standards: A model for blood banking? Transfusion 1995;35:521-4.
8. Food and Drug Administration. Proposed approach to regulation of cellular and tissue-based products. (February 28, 1997) Rockville, MD: CBER Office of Communication, Training, and Manufacturers Assistance, 1997.
9. Code of federal regulations. Human cells, tissues, and cellular and tissue-based products. Title 21 CFR Part 1271. Washington, DC: US Government Printing Office, 2004 (revised annually).

In: Areman EM, Loper K, eds
Cellular Therapy: Principles, Methods, and Regulations
Bethesda, MD: AABB, 2009

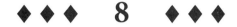

8

Quality and Process Control

Lizabeth Cardwell, MT(ASCP), MBA, RAC, and Michele W. Sugrue, MS, MT(ASCP)SBB

QUALITY CONTROL (QC) OF CELLULAR therapy (CT) products can be defined as operational techniques and activities used to monitor and eliminate the causes of unsatisfactory performance at any stage of a process. In addition, QC serves as a significant component of any process control program.

Regulatory requirements for QC include those enforced by individual states as well as those enforced by federal agencies, such as the Food and Drug Administration (FDA) and the Centers for Medicare and Medicaid Services (CMS), and the Clinical Laboratory Improvement Amendments (CLIA). Voluntary standards also define requirements for QC—eg, the standards of The Joint Commission, the AABB, the Foundation for Accreditation of Cellular Therapy (FACT), the College of American Pathologists (CAP), and the International Organization for Standardization (ISO).

QC programs must be sufficiently comprehensive to ensure that all of the factors related to the manufacturing of human cells, tissues, and cellular and tissue-based products (HCT/Ps) function as expected. QC processes can usually be applied to all types of cellular product manufacturing facilities regardless of size or complexity.

Quality Control Process Model

Applying the model published by Berte[1] and defining the key steps, one may generate a QC process for use within the CT processing facility. The key steps of the process (see Fig 8-1) are as follows:

1. Define where QC is required.
2. Review and approve the defined program.
3. Perform testing.
4. Evaluate results.
   a. If results are acceptable, continue to Step 5.
   b. If results are unacceptable:
      i. Evaluate and perform corrective action.
      ii. Retest and determine the acceptability of the results.
5. Document results and retain records.

Lizabeth Cardwell, MT(ASCP), MBA, RAC, Principal, Compliance Consulting, Seattle, Washington, and Michele W. Sugrue, MS, MT(ASCP)SBB, Coordinator, Research Programs, Division of Hematology/Oncology, Department of Medicine, University of Florida and Shands Hospitals, Gainesville, Florida

The authors have disclosed no conflicts of interest.

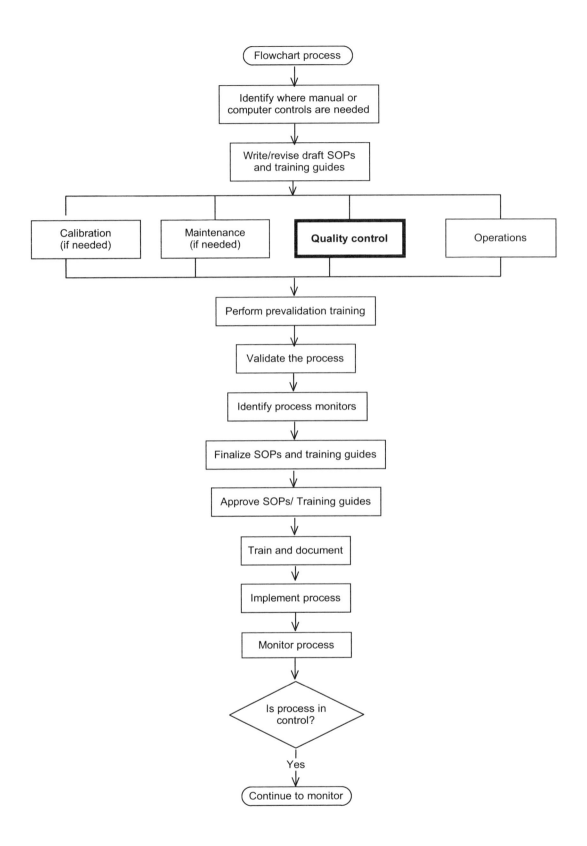

Figure 8-1. Process control flowchart. (Adapted with permission from Berte.[2])
SOP = standard operating procedure.

Quality Control Documentation and Records

All QC programs must create records and documentation that follow institutional guidelines as well as established regulations and standards. A QC program, like any other process in a CT processing or manufacturing facility, must have documentation that will define objectives as well as the course of action and interpretation of results. Process control of QC documentation should be a reflection of the following:

1. Policies related to QC must be written to state the intent of the facility to meet requirements, regulations, and standards as they apply to that facility.
2. Processes related to QC are written descriptions of how a facility will implement all applicable regulations, requirements, and standards.
3. Standard operating procedures (SOPs) and test methods are written instructions to carry out measurements of QC and include all information required for proper performance of the task.
4. Worksheets or forms may be used, in paper version or in validated computer systems, to record testing results. Worksheets should include the identity of personnel performing the testing, the outcome of testing, the interpretation of results, and the date and time when testing is performed.
5. Schedules of QC testing should be established to meet or exceed all requirements, regulations, and standards. It is not unusual for QC programs to need to accommodate overlapping regulations and standards. Table 8-1[3] provides a list of suggested QC performance intervals.
6. Review of QC results must be performed and documented promptly. Unacceptable results must be investigated and corrective action documented and implemented. Follow-up QC must be performed to ensure that testing results meet acceptable criteria.

Quality Control Inputs

Reagent and supply QC is a required element of consistent quality through process control. The ultimate goal of reagent and supply QC is to ensure that the materials are functioning properly, as recommended by the manufacturer, on each day of use. QC should apply to all steps that employ reagents and supplies, as follows, beginning with receipt of the items in the laboratory and ending with the final disposition of the CT product:

1. **Receipt.** Upon receipt, variables that could affect the function and stability of reagents and supplies must be checked and documented. An example of a supplies log is shown in Appendix 8-1.
2. **Storage.** Once the reagents and supplies have been accepted into inventory, proper storage as recommended by the manufacturer must be maintained to avoid degradation or alteration.
3. **Usage.** When reagents and supplies are received, it may be necessary to perform QC testing of new lot numbers to ensure their proper function before use.
4. **Identity.** Although certificates of analysis or package inserts from reagent manufacturers may provide documentation of QC testing, the CT facility must determine its own policy and define criteria for acceptability. This may involve in-house testing for identity and stability of the material. The quality assurance (QA) program is responsible for defining the schedule of testing. Factors that may impact schedules include frequency of use, operating hours of the laboratory, personnel changeover during standard operation, and potential for contamination and deterioration.
5. **Disposition.** It is postulated that the ultimate measure of reagent and supply performance may be the ability of the CT product to provide expected clinical function within an expected period. Patient outcome should be tracked as one measure of product quality. However, so many variables affect the clinical course of a CT recipient that most facilities depend on surrogate measures. Post-processing or post-thaw in-vitro analyses, such as cell viability, cell recovery, colony formation, bag integrity, and sterility, are frequently used as quality indicators.

Additional information regarding the QA of materials can be found in Chapter 11.

Equipment

All equipment used in the collection, processing, and testing of CT products must be traceable and must undergo scheduled performance of QC pro-

Table 8-1. Suggested Quality Control Performance Intervals for Common Cellular Therapy Laboratory Equipment*

Equipment	Frequency of Quality Control
Thermometers (compare to NIST certified or traceable)	
• Liquid in glass	• Annually
• Electronic	• As specified by manufacturer
Timers/clocks	Twice yearly
Pipette calibration	Quarterly
Sterile connecting device	
• Weld check	• Each use
• Function	• Annually
Microhematocrit centrifuge	
• Timer check	• Quarterly
• Calibration	• Quarterly
• Packed cell volume	• Annually
Cell Counters/Hemoglobinometers	
• Each use	• Day of use
• Calibration	• As specified by manufacturer
Apheresis equipment	
• PM Checklist requirements	• As specified by manufacturer
• Day of use requirements	• As specified by manufacturer
Dry shipper	
• Requalify	• Quarterly or as specified by manufacturer
Waterbath	
• Temperature sensor	• Annually
Centrifuge	
• RPM or RCF (*g*)	• Quarterly
• Timer	• Quarterly
• Temperature	• Quarterly
Balances/scales	Semiannually
Biological safety cabinet	
• Checklist requirements, including smoke test and airflow and recertification	• Semiannually or as recommended by manufacturer
Liquid nitrogen storage tank	
• Level/temperature	• Daily or weekly as indicated by qualification
Alarm monitoring system	
• Test—alarm and notification	• Quarterly
• Back up of data	• Semiannually
Cell washer	
• PM Checklist requirements	• As specified by manufacturer
• Day of use requirements	• As specified by manufacturer
Microscope	Annually
Tissue culture incubator	Semiannually
Specialized laboratory equipment	As specified by manufacturer
Controlled-rate freezer	
• Temperature probe calibration (vs NIST thermometer and graph parameters)	• Quarterly
• Other maintenance	• As specified by manufacturer

*The frequencies listed above are suggested intervals, not requirements. For any new piece of equipment, installation, operational, and performance qualification must be performed. Depending on qualification parameters, quality control may be performed at a greater frequency initially while a performance track record is established. At a minimum, the frequency must comply with the manufacturer's suggested intervals and should be performed after repair. If no such guidance is provided, the intervals in this table would be appropriate to use. Other basic laboratory equipment, including refrigerators and freezers, may also be used but are not included here.
NIST = National Institute of Standards and Technology; PM = preventive maintenance; RPM = revolutions per minute; RCF = relative centrifugal force (*g*).

cedures. Accompanying records must be properly maintained and thus serve as a critical part of the quality program. At a minimum, the frequency of equipment QC review should be as described in the equipment operator's manual or, more often, as appropriate for facility use. The accuracy and reproducibility of QC test results must be evaluated frequently to determine that the equipment used in the CT processing facility is functioning properly. QC for equipment applies in the following areas:

Installation. Before routine use, equipment for the manufacture of CT products must be properly installed and qualified.

Calibration. Calibration is a technique for measuring the performance of an instrument against an accurate standard. The schedule of calibration may vary from one instrument or piece of equipment to another and depends on applicable regulatory requirements, usage, and the manufacturer's recommendation.

Safety. Not only is a safety program for equipment critical in a properly functioning facility, but it is also required by the Occupational Safety and Health Administration (OSHA). Elements that should be included in an instrument safety program are electrical functions, cleaning (decontamination), and practical instructions to avoid injury.

Operation. Evaluation of all equipment must be performed to ensure that all functions are operating effectively. Such evaluations must be carried out before equipment is placed into service, periodically during use, and after repairs. Establishment of scheduled QC testing must meet or exceed the manufacturer's recommendations and must fulfill all requirements defined by accrediting and regulatory agencies.

Corrective Action. Any piece of equipment not meeting the specification set by the manufacturer or by its qualification in the laboratory must be removed from operation until corrective action is performed and documented.

Additional information concerning QA of equipment is presented in Chapter 10.

Methods

Methods are systematic instructions and techniques for performing a task, including all associated documents and records. The type of QC program needed for methods used in a cellular product facility depends on the specific functions performed. Examples of measures of QC for CT production are sterility testing, cellular functionality, completeness of records, and document control.

Personnel

Quality analysis of personnel is initiated when a potential staff member is considered for employment and that person's qualifications are evaluated. Once an individual is employed by the facility, proper training and verification of competency by qualified personnel are required before the employee is permitted to perform assigned tasks. These steps are necessary to ensure that processes are performed as expected and in a consistent manner and that they result in an acceptable outcome. Further discussion of human resources can be found in Chapter 9 of this section.

Trends

Evaluating information gathered from testing, outcome analyses, and proficiency surveys and comparing the information to pre-established acceptable criteria are important components of QC. Whether the facility is examining analyte results for a trend or monitoring unsatisfactory documentation retention, corrective action is required and must be documented. In addition, follow-up measures that verify the facility's ability to meet acceptable criteria must be taken.

Change Control

From a QA perspective, the foundation for a good change control system is complete documentation of the production process, including all equipment, instruments, materials, systems, and software used for CT product manufacturing. Management of change in the CT facility requires adequate document control, purchasing control, and maintenance tracking systems. In addition, staff must be trained in the importance of and the procedure for correctly documenting any changes to the production process, equipment, instruments, systems, and software used for the manufacture of CT products. Adequate documentation requires a team of individuals committed to maintaining process control.

The team needs to understand the intent of regulations, standards, and guidance regarding change control as well as the intent of organizational systems, SOPs, and forms developed to appropriately and consistently document changes. Such training and understanding are especially needed if a cellular product is being used under an investigational new drug (IND) exemption. Before any changes are implemented in product manufacturing, the regulatory implications of the changes must be discussed with the research team's regulatory representative to determine the content and timing of institutional review board (IRB) and FDA notification.[5] Important changes may require validation, an IND amendment, and possibly FDA consultation and approval before implementation. Certain document changes that affect the process and materials must also include regulatory representative assessment before approval. The regulatory representative is an important member of the change control cross-functional team.

An SOP must be in place that directs the purchasing of any equipment, instruments, reagents, supplies, systems, or software to be used for the process or product. The SOP will direct the purchasing staff to order only those items that conform to the required specifications, usually instructing that no substitutions be made without written permission from an authorized individual.

The specifications, purchasing documentation, and information on replacement parts for equipment should be located in the file specific to the type of equipment. This information forms the foundation or starting point for change control. Even a small replacement part in an instrument such as a centrifuge can cause a change in the performance of the device. A change control SOP with an accompanying form should address the activities required to evaluate the change effect, to document the change, and to address the calibration, reverification, or validation of the equipment or system after the change.

The evaluation of the appropriate verification or validation of the change to equipment, instrumentation, systems, or software requires a cross-functional team. The team will determine whether the maintenance, part change, model change, or version change will affect the function and, in turn, potentially affect the product character or quality. If necessary, a validation protocol will need to be

generated, approved, and successfully executed before use of the system or equipment for further CT manufacturing or monitoring. Appendix 8-2 provides an example of a change-control form.

Process Verification and Validation

The FDA regulatory requirements for process verification and validation are described in numerous sections of the Code of Federal Regulations[6-10] (CFR; emphasis below added):

- Section 1271.220(c): "You must ensure…that each in-process HCT/P is controlled until the required inspection and tests or other *verification* activities have been completed."
- Section 1271.220(d)(2): "When you use a published *validated* process, you must *verify* such a process in your establishment."
- Section 1271.230(a): "Where the results of processing described in §1271.220 cannot be fully *verified* by subsequent inspection and tests, you must *validate* and approve the process according to established procedures."
- Section 211.110(a): "…Control procedures shall be established to monitor the output and *validate* the performance of those manufacturing processes that may be responsible for causing variability…."

Although the terms "verification" and "validation" are often used interchangeably, they have different meanings. The classic regulatory definition of process validation is "establishing documented evidence which provides a high degree of assurance that a specific process will consistently produce a product meeting its pre-determined specifications and quality attributes."[5] Verification, however, is "confirmation by examination and provision of objective evidence that specified requirements have been fulfilled."[5] Table 8-2 illustrates some differences between the validation and verification processes.

Validation strategy should be considered during process development. Systematic collection of data during development is used to establish acceptance criteria for validation studies. Effective, successful validation requires adequate development. It is inappropriate to continue development activities within the scope of the process validation. If the validation does not meet its predetermined accep-

Table 8-2. Differences between Validation and Verification

Validation	Verification
Ensures that a process will consistently produce a product that meets predetermined specifications.	Confirms that specified requirements have been fulfilled. Results are compared to predetermined acceptance criteria (or reference material).
Shows the reproducibility and robustness of the process.	Tests or inspects to see if a product meets criteria.
Extends system wide and covers worst-case conditions.	Might require sample sizes that limit product availability. May be destructive.
Is repeated enough times to provide adequate documentation that the system performs effectively, reproducibly, and robustly.	Occurs repeatedly (as in a test method).

tance criteria, it has failed, and appropriate investigation, corrections, justifications, and possible revalidation must be considered and documented.

During data collection and process development, consideration should be given to the type of CT product, the limits and attributes of the production process, and the regulatory strategy appropriate for the product. The level of resources dedicated to process validation with processing limits testing will be a corporate strategy issue. A validation master plan (VMP) can reflect the strategy for validations throughout the CT facility. Part of the strategic thought should include which validations will be done before implementation, which validations will be done concurrent to the production process, and which validations will be conducted retrospectively as data review.

From the QA perspective, all validation protocols must fulfill the following requirements:
- Be generated with appropriate acceptance criteria.
- Be reviewed and approved by technical and quality staff before execution.
- Be executed without major deviations and meet acceptance criteria.
- Be reported promptly, in documents reviewed and approved by technical and quality staff.
- Be maintained and archived in controlled documents.

The process validation protocol document may contain the production batch record, which may include details of worst-case excursions or limits for the process documented by redline or other means. The number of times the process will be executed and the excursions for each process run

should be documented. The acceptance criteria for each process validation run may be listed in their own section of the validation protocol or may be referenced to the data collection forms. The second option is especially useful when the protocol is large and the data collection forms are many. Appendix 8-3 provides an outline for a validation protocol document.

Process Simulation

Process simulation (also known as media fill) is a type of process validation that is designed to demonstrate the following:
- That the process and the personnel performing the process can produce an aseptic product, even with the maximum number of interventions.
- That personnel are adequately trained in the aseptic processes.
- That the environment where aseptic production occurs is appropriate.
- That gowning practices are adequate.

Process simulation validation is especially important for cellular products manufactured by aseptic processing and delivered to the patient immediately after collection or processing. Because there is no time to wait for full-term sterility test results (verification) before product administration, a process simulation validation provides a greater degree of confidence that the process can deliver uncontaminated cellular products.

Process simulation is designed to simulate the complete CT production process, usually by substituting a microbial culture medium for the actual product and materials. Aseptic processing is discussed further in Chapter 14 of this section.

Product Changeover (Line Clearance)

Although no specific FDA regulations pertain to product changeover or line clearance, the main reason for publication of the good tissue practice (GTP) regulations (21 CFR 1271) was to prevent contamination and release of contaminated CT products. These requirements are similar in intent to those required by 21 CFR 211 for the segregation, cleaning, and monitoring of material, equipment, and systems. In the biologics and pharmaceutical processes, the term "line clearance" traditionally describes the activities involved in changing a work area and the associated equipment between the preparation of product batches.

SOPs that address product changeover should be designed and implemented to prevent contamination by infectious agents and cross-contamination between different lots of the same or different CT products. Segregation of products can be accomplished temporally or spatially, and, in either case, SOPs need to be generated to provide consistent direction to operators. In both cases, sufficient segregation and labeling must be maintained when different products are processed using the same pieces of equipment (eg, centrifuges, biological safety cabinets, or incubators) and the same operators. A determination of the adequacy of segregation will depend on the risk factors for contamination (open system), the extent of labeling of the product, the equipment labeling, and the training and competence of the laboratory staff.

Any shared equipment or space must receive extensive cleaning between preparation of different products and between separate steps of the production process. At a minimum, the biological safety cabinet must be cleaned using recommended procedures after processing of each lot is completed. The cleaning SOPs must define routine sanitization procedures that include escalating routines for specified intervals (before and after each process, weekly, monthly, and quarterly) and sanitizing agent rotation, as applicable. Appendix 8-4 provides an example of a product changeover or line clearance form.

Product Segregation

It is especially important to have adequate segregation and cleaning procedures if animal products (such as fetal bovine serum) or viral constructs (in gene therapy) are used in proximity to other cell-processing operations and materials. Performing gene therapy work in the same environment as other cell processing is not recommended and is generally unacceptable. Separate production suites should be established with appropriate environmental controls. The air flow in the viral-processing suites should be of negative pressure in relation to the surrounding environments to prevent contamination of those areas. The cleaning procedures used in gene therapy suites should be validated to prove clearance of the potentially contaminating agents.

Personnel traffic, process steps, and materials flow should be considered to help establish segregation of products and processes. A one-way processing direction will keep reagents used upstream from contaminating downstream events. Having separate gowning and de-gowning rooms will decrease the risk of contaminated clothing and the risk of the staff's contaminating the clean gowns or gloves in the gown-in area. A "pass-through," with or without high-efficiency particulate air (HEPA) filtration, to pass the completed closed product out of the production environment, is often used to prevent contamination. Removal of all materials, components, tools, and waste from the production areas between product lots is essential to effective product changeover. If operators are not required to leave the processing area after working with a product, to de-gown, and then to re-gown, other specific changes of gloves, gowns, and sleeves must be observed and documented before they begin work on another product. SOPs should be generated to address the product changeover process: 1) cleaning or sanitizing the processing room and equipment following any process, 2) protecting the area and equipment from contamination between processing operations by limiting access, and 3) inspecting and verifying the cleanliness and organization of the area immediately before use.

Donor Eligibility

Donor eligibility (DE) is the subject of Subpart C of the CFR regulations for HCT/Ps (21 CFR 1271). This subpart describes the regulatory requirements for implementing donor screening and testing for relevant communicable disease agents and diseases and must be followed for allogeneic donors of cells or tissue used in CT products.

The QA function for a cell-processing establishment must generate, approve, implement, and maintain standard procedures to address the steps involved in donor eligibility determinations. Accordingly, the regulations describe the need for screening (21 CFR 1271.75), for testing (21 CFR 1271.80 and 1271.85), and for a responsible person [21 CFR 1271.3 (t)] with knowledge, skills training, and authorization to assess and determine DE using the available information. All the available DE information must be documented by using an established summary of records form, which is described in 21 CFR 1271.55(a)(3). The responsible person evaluates all medical record screening and test results before making the final DE determination. The determination must include the name of the responsible person and the name and address of the establishment making the determination. The summary of records must accompany the CT product at all times once eligibility has been determined.

The logistics for defining, documenting, and implementing the DE procedures and accompanying forms are greatly affected by the number of entities that are involved in the determination. The establishments or departments involved in determining DE must be included in designing and documenting the DE process. For example, the cell or tissue donation is not acquired at the cell-processing establishment. The cell or tissue recovery location may be a different part of the same medical center or may be a separate, distantly located establishment. The separation by responsibility and space complicates the review of medical records and, depending on the type of donation, may complicate the speedy acquisition of the appropriate samples for DE testing.

The cellular product manufacturing establishment must have a cooperative and contractual agreement with each donation or collection site to provide the required donor information. The manufacturer has ultimate responsibility to ensure the safety of the product and must ensure that contractors also comply with the applicable regulations. Product manufacturers must have procedures that describe how to control and audit contractors to fulfill this responsibility.

The DE screening process is based on a review of the donor's records and an interview for risk factors and clinical evidence of relevant communicable diseases and potential disease agents. In the case of umbilical cord blood, the mother of the donor is the subject of the donor screening and testing. The screening process must be followed for live and deceased cell and tissue donors. If medical records are unavailable, the CT establishment must have other means of ensuring DE. All the processes for donor screening must be delineated in SOPs and documented on the summary of records form.

In the United States, donors of cellular products for allogeneic use must be tested for the following, at a minimum:

- Human immunodeficiency virus, types 1 and 2.
- Hepatitis B virus.
- Hepatitis C virus.
- *Treponema pallidum.*

Any donors of viable, leukocyte-rich cells or tissue must be reviewed and tested for human T-cell lymphotropic virus. For many CT products, donors are also tested for cytomegalovirus. Donors of reproductive cells or tissue require screening and testing for evidence of chlamydia and gonorrhea. The regulations provide for an abbreviated screening in the case of a donor's additional donation within 6 months of the original DE determination. "The abbreviated procedure must determine and document any changes in the donor's medical history since the previous donations that would make the donor ineligible, including relevant social behavior" [21 CFR 1271.75(e)].

The CT production facility must test or arrange for the testing of donor samples for relevant communicable diseases. For products distributed in the United States, it is the responsibility of the manufacturer of the CT product to contract with, audit, and verify that the testing establishment is certified to perform such testing on human specimens under CLIA (or equivalent standards as applicable), uses FDA-licensed, -approved, or -cleared donor screening tests, and performs the tests in accordance with the package insert. If the FDA-licensed screening tests are not available, as is the case for chlamydia and gonorrhea, the FDA-licensed test for "asymptomatic, low-prevalence population" [21 CFR 1271.80(c)] is used. If the collection is from cadavers, tests specifically labeled for cadaveric samples must be used when available.

Recovery or Collection (See also Section V)

Donor Identification

No single step in cell or tissue procurement is more critical than accurate identification of the donor. Collection facilities usually require that two trained individuals confirm the identity of the donor. This practice extends beyond product labeling to include confirmation of physicians' orders and signatures of the informed consent. Any discrepancy must be resolved before the collection procedure is initiated.

In addition, before collection of umbilical cord blood, identification of not only the donor (infant) but also the mother (birth, biologic, or surrogate) and the associated placenta is necessary.

Before collection of cells or tissues from a cadaveric donor, the type of donor (heart-beating or nonheart-beating) must be confirmed as specified by the protocol in use.

Supplies, Reagents, Equipment, and Environment

Each collection facility, whether it is an apheresis center, a surgical operating room, or a delivery suite, must maintain safe, sanitary operations in regard to staff, donor, and cell or tissue integrity. Areas for procurement, donor examination and evaluation, supplies, and equipment storage must be appropriately sized, defined, and controlled.

Supplies, reagents, and equipment for the recovery process must be stored and used according to the manufacturer's recommendations and facility SOPs. Materials should be inspected before use to confirm that they meet acceptance criteria. Collection facilities should be able to document and track all critical materials used in the collection of cells and tissues.

Collection Methods and Aseptic Technique

Collection methods should be approved, verified, and performed according to written procedures. Critical to the collection method is the prevention of microbial contamination of cellular products. Staff training must include proper aseptic technique in the collection of the various types of cells and tissues recovered. Acceptance criteria must be defined for each collection procedure.

Labeling

The procedure for the labeling of samples, cellular or tissue collections, and containers must prevent misidentification or mislabeling. All labels and transportation containers must meet governmental regulatory requirements and the standards of accrediting organizations and must permit product tracking. Special processes must be in place for the proper documentation and labeling of contaminated or nonconforming recovered cells or tissue, as well as their shipping or transportation containers.

Documentation and Records

Documentation related to collection facilities and their functions includes keeping records such as the following:
- Donation process records, which note the unique identifier, date and time of collection, name and address of the collection facility, details of collection, identification of responsible staff, and review signature.
- Donor evaluations.
- Donor eligibility records.
- Informed consent records.
- Physicians' orders for collection.
- Records of errors, accidents, and adverse events related to the cell or tissue collection.
- Distribution records.
- QC records.

Staff Qualifications, Including Collection Facility Director

Personnel qualifications and training must be determined for each task performed within the facility. Collection facility directors and medical directors must meet defined regulatory and medical standard requirements. Staff competency training and continuing education documentation, both periodic and ongoing, must be maintained for all personnel. Maintenance of staff competencies often presents challenges when procurement is infrequent. Techniques to assess competency may include mock collections or written examinations.

Personnel responsible for the procurement of cord blood often perform collection techniques at distant facilities, which presents unique issues for assessing competency. Evaluation of competency is critical to ensure the collection of cord blood products that meet acceptable criteria for banking.

Product Outcome and Audits

Assessment of quality and integrity as well as the performance of outcome analysis are important to the collection facility. Proficiency measurements may include testing for microbial contamination and cellular analyses. The outcomes analysis may include engraftment parameters.

Collection facilities should have established timetables for the performance and review of audits, which can be used to recognize trends, document problems, and identify improvement opportunities.

Deviations, Nonconformances, and Adverse Events

Procedures must be in place to ensure the recognition, assessment, investigation, and monitoring of deviations, nonconformances, and adverse events related to cell and tissue recovery. The procedures should address issues specific to donors, recipients, and CT products. Method 8-1 provides an example of a procedure for maintaining a corrective and preventive action (CAPA) program.

Tracking and Traceability

A cornerstone of good manufacturing practice (GMP) is the traceability of all incoming and outgoing materials. Traceability is especially important for materials and components that become part of the product or that directly contact the product during the manufacturing process. A discussion of QA of supplies and materials is provided in Chapter 11.

For CT product manufacturing, the primary raw material is the donated cells or tissue. Controlled procedures and forms for identifying the primary raw material should be implemented. In many cases, adequate documentation will require collaboration with the facility contracted to provide the cellular or tissue materials. The collection or recovery establishment must have its own SOPs to describe the recovery processes and methods for positive identification and labeling of the raw material cells or tissues, or it must be contractually committed to and trained for using the procedures provided by the product manufacturer.

CT products must be entirely traceable from the donor to the "consignee or final disposition" and from the "consignee or final disposition" backwards to the donor (21 CFR 1271.290). Unique identifying numbers or codes (also called lot or batch numbers) must be assigned, and the material or product and all accompanying paperwork must be labeled with the lot numbers. An SOP and number log must be available to define and track the lot numbers assigned.

The lot numbers should appear on all records associated with the processing or production steps. The identity code must not include the donor, patient, or subject name; social security number; or medical record number unless the donation is an autologous donation, a directed reproductive tissue donation, or a directed donation made by a first- or second-degree blood relative.

The procedures and forms for tracking cellular products may differ slightly according to the type of raw material, the processing activities, and the final manufactured product. An example of a product tracking form is shown in Appendix 8-5.

Storage Controls

Safety/Tamper Controls and Segregation

Process controls addressing all aspects of CT product safety must be in place to ensure the well-being of products during all phases of storage, from the point of collection to the stage of final distribution. Only authorized personnel should have access to cell-processing and storage areas. In addition, storage devices should be equipped with tamper-evident seals and controlled-entry systems.

Addressed within the procedures for CT product storage control must be a system to minimize contamination and cross-contamination of HCT/Ps and their exposure to materials that may adversely affect their stability and integrity. Such efforts may include outer protective coverings, liquid nitrogen vapor-phase frozen storage, segregation of potential contaminating products, and single-product storage containers designed for liquid product storage. Maintaining sanitary conditions of all storage devices is critical to the safe storage of CT products.

Storage Specifications, Conditions, and Duration

For each type of CT product that a facility collects, manufactures, and distributes, procedures must be in place to establish the duration and conditions for storage. Temperature ranges for each type of product must be defined and verified or validated to maintain viability and function and to minimize the opportunity for growth of infectious agents. The length of storage and the expiration date, if applicable, should be included as part of the CT product specification. The duration of storage applies not only to cryopreserved final products but also to products in the liquid phase, following collection, during processing, during and after culture, and after thawing.

Temperature Controls, Monitors, and Equipment Validation

Controls for adequate temperature maintenance and monitoring during the storage period are essential in the procedure for CT product storage. Because of the crucial nature of the storage temperature in either the liquid or vapor phase of nitrogen, procedures and records should be in place to ensure and document that proper levels of liquid nitrogen are maintained. The storage equipment must undergo qualification that documents its ability to activate an alarm system when temperature deviations occur. Equipment procedures should be immediately available to instruct personnel in sustaining storage temperatures. The alarm system must enable the notification of appropriate personnel on a 24-hour basis, allowing for adequate response time and documentation. Alarm

conditions are considered deviations and, as such, require appropriate action documentation.

Inventory Control, Prevention of Mix-Ups, and Records

Processes within a CT product facility must be conducted in a way that prevents potential product identification errors. Facilities can prevent identification errors by controlling the manner in which products are labeled and placed into inventory. The location of each product and its associated sample aliquots must be maintained in an inventory system. This system must be operational at all times and, if computer-based, have adequate validation and backup procedures in place. Access to this system should be limited to key personnel.

Transportation Controls

Labeling and Packaging

Once a CT product is approved for transportation, process control policies must be in place to make certain that both labeling and packaging practices meet federal, state, and local regulations and accrediting standards, if required. These practices must define the use of validated packaging containers and labels. The transportation containers should be demonstrated to prevent leakage, maintain a specific defined temperature, and withstand other physical stresses during distribution.

Modes and Monitoring

Selection of appropriate modes of transportation is of the utmost importance in ensuring safe delivery. Only qualified couriers should handle CT storage devices. All efforts should be made to minimize transportation time. The transportation systems in place should allow for alternate transportation plans in emergencies. Temperature monitoring must be implemented as part of the transportation controls. It is important that the appropriate records accompany CT products during transportation, but all efforts should be made to maintain the confidentiality of the donor and recipient.

Chain of Custody and Tamper Control

Process controls that guarantee an unbroken chain of custody with tamper-proof protection are integral to reliable CT product transportation. Each stage of transport should be documented by the signature of the parties who have contact with the product. The chain of custody becomes part of the product record.

Nonconformances and Deviations

In the event that a product does not meet release criteria, processes must be in place to allow nonconforming products to be transported in accordance with all applicable requirements and regulations.

Receipt, Predistribution Shipment, and Distribution of HCT/Ps

Receipt

Within a facility, processes must be established to ensure that, upon arrival, incoming CT products are inspected and accompanying records are reviewed before the products are determined to be acceptable. These processes may distinguish between products that require further manipulation and those that arrive ready for storage or administration. In either case, conditions during transportation, container integrity, and visual inspection details should be documented according to establishment acceptance criteria. Furthermore, accompanying records and labels should include a distinct identification code attached to the product container, statements of DE, and a summary of the records used to make the eligibility determination. Finally, records that address source material, collection date, receiving personnel, and product inspection, as well as other requirements of 21 CFR 1271 and appropriate accrediting organization standards, must be re-viewed and maintained.

Processes must address the verification of acceptance criteria and the actions to take when these criteria are not met. These actions may include repeat testing or additional testing, placing the product in quarantine, or discarding the product. Procedures should be established for proper segregation of quarantined products and for notification of appropriate parties regarding products from ineligible donors.

Predistribution

Predistribution refers to the transportation or shipment of CT products that have not completed quality verification on the basis of pre-established criteria that may include DE requirements. In these cases, it is incumbent on the shipping facility to establish and maintain process controls that address the methods of properly shipping quarantined products, as well as the manner in which transportation compliance would be fulfilled.

Distribution

Process controls are critical in ensuring the distribution of CT products that meet release criteria. Before distribution, both donor processing and product information must be reviewed in the context of institutional acceptance and release criteria. As previously noted, predistribution is acceptable if adequate controls are implemented.

Donor Criteria

Applicable regulations and standards for donor acceptability must be addressed in the acceptance and release criteria. Such items as informed consent, DE, donor selection, and collection orders (when applicable) should be reviewed before product release.

Final Processing and Testing Criteria

Process control includes review of the final label, donor and product testing results, and processing reports.

Criteria for Release to Recipient

Product release criteria should include a request for the product or an order for administration; satisfactory labeling; product inspection; recipient identification; the test results for each test required for release, including acceptability determination and documentation of personnel reporting test acceptance; availability for release; and accompanying records or statements.

Controls must address the failure to meet release criteria and the requirement for exceptional release. Defining criteria for these cases is critical and should be included in the program SOPs. In general, nonconforming products should not be released for clinical use. However, in some extraordinary circumstances, the patient's needs may outweigh the risks. In such cases, the facility must adequately document the reason for release and obtain necessary signatures for approval. Reports that document the nonconformity must be created and completed with a description of the patient outcome and problem resolution.

Product Administration

Whether the patient care facility that administers the CT product is adjacent to or remote from the manufacturing site, it must still abide by applicable regulations and standards and maintain process control mechanisms for notification and reporting of adverse events and outcomes. These systems must define methods by which this information is relayed to the manufacturer and to relevant regulatory agencies and the action taken upon notification.

Acknowledgments

Method 8-1 was submitted by Tara Sadeghi, BS, Regulatory Compliance/Quality Assurance Coordinator, Cell Therapy Laboratory and Cord Blood Bank, MD Anderson Cancer Center, Houston, Texas.

References/Resources

1. Berte LM. Quality manual preparation workbook for cellular therapy product services. Bethesda, MD: AABB Press, 2005:29-33.
2. Berte L, ed. A model quality system for the transfusion service. Bethesda, MD: AABB, 1997.
3. Roback JD, Combs MR, Grossman BJ, Hillyer CD, eds. Technical manual. 16th ed. Bethesda, MD: AABB, 2008.
4. Ziebell L, Kavemeier K, eds. Quality control: A component of process control in the blood bank and transfusion service. Bethesda, MD: AABB Press, 1999.
5. Food and Drug Administration. Guideline on general principles of process validation. (May 1987) Rockville, MD: CDER Office of Compliance, 1987.
6. Code of Federal Regulations. Human cells, tissues, and tissue-based products. Title 21, CFR Part 1271. Washington, DC: US Government Printing Office, 2008 (revised annually).
7. Code of Federal Regulations. Title 42, CFR Part 74. Washington, DC: US Government Printing Office, 2008 (revised annually).
8. Code of Federal Regulations. Laboratory requirements. Title 42, CFR Part 493 to end. Washington, DC: US Government Printing Office, 2008 (revised annually).
9. Code of Federal Regulations. Biologics. Title 21, CFR Parts 600-680. Washington, DC: US Government Printing Office, 2008 (revised annually).
10. Code of Federal Regulations. Drugs: General. Title 21, CFR Parts 200-299. Washington, DC: US Government Printing Office, 2008 (revised annually).
11. Food and Drug Administration. Draft guidance for reviewers: Instructions and template for chemistry, manufacturing, and control reviewers of human somatic cellular therapy investigational new drug applications; availability. (August 18, 2003) Rockville, MD: CBER Office of Communication, Training, and Manufacturers Assistance, 2003.
12. FACT-JACIE international standards for cellular therapy product collection, processing, and administration. 3rd ed. Omaha, NE: Foundation for the Accreditation of Cellular Therapy and the Joint Accreditation Committee of ISCT and EBMT, 2006.
13. International Standard ISO 9001: Quality systems—model for quality assurance in design, development, production, installation, and servicing. In: ISO 9000 quality management compendium. 6th ed. Geneva, Switzerland: ISO, 1996.
14. Keever-Taylor CA. Process control: Application to the cell processing laboratory. Cytotherapy 2002;2:63-73.
15. Nunes E, Motschman T. Regulations A to Z for blood and HCT/Ps. 8th ed. Bethesda, MD: AABB Press, 2008.
16. Food and Drug Administration. Proposed approach to regulation of cellular and tissue-based products. (February 28, 1997) Rockville, MD: CBER Office of Communication, Training, and Manufacturers Assistance, 1997.
17. Code of federal regulations. Revision of laboratory regulations (Clinical Laboratory Improvement Amendments of 1988). Title 42, CFR Parts 493.801 through 493.807. Washington, DC: US Government Printing Office, 2008 (revised annually).
18. Padley D, ed. Standards for cellular therapy product services. 3rd ed. Bethesda, MD: AABB, 2008.
19. Weber, DJ. Biosafety considerations for cell-based therapies. BioPharm International 2004;7:48-55.
20. Weber DJ. Navigating FDA regulations for human cells and tissues. BioProcess International 2004;2:22-6.
21. Areman EM, Deeg HJ, Sacher RA, eds. Bone marrow and stem cell processing: A manual of current techniques. Philadelphia: FA Davis, 1992.

Appendix 8-1. Incoming Critical Supplies Log

NA = Not Applicable
A = Acceptable   U = Unacceptable
Qty. = Quantity

Month/Year _____

Item	Manufacturer	Lot #	Expiration Date	Qty. Received	Date Received	Visual Inspection		Staff Initials	Review of Package Insert (Initial/Date)	Certificate of Analysis Supplied (Yes/No)	Dept.
						A	U				
						A	U				
						A	U				
						A	U				
						A	U				
						A	U				
						A	U				
						A	U				
						A	U				

Department Head Review/Date _____

Quality Review/Date _____

Appendix 8-2. Sample Change-Control Form

CHANGE PROPOSAL FORM *Section I (to be filled out by Initiator)*		
Equipment or System Name:	Change Form No.	
Equipment # (if available)		
Initiator:	Dept.:	
Reason for Change: *(routine maintenance or repair)*		
Describe Scope of Work: *(what will be done and equipment affected)*		
List All Documents Affected by the Proposed Change: *(document changes may be required)*		
Signature:	Date:	

Section II (to be filled in by Quality Assurance and Regulatory Affairs)

QA/Regulatory Evaluation		Yes	No
Do regulatory filings require amendments or supplements?			
Is validation, qualification, or certification required? Which one: _____			
Does the change require FDA approval?			
Approval - I have reviewed the proposal and approve the change:			
Mfg. Signature:	Date:		
Signature:	Date:		
Signature:	Date:		
Signature:	Date:		
Signature:	Date:		
Implementation of the Change			
The change has been authorized and assigned to the following individual(s):			
Implementation Plan: *(describe how the work will be accomplished, estimated cost and expected completion date)*			

Section III (to be filled in by QA)

Follow Up		Yes	No
All documents affected have been modified to reflect the change.			
The scope of work described in Section II has been completed.			
The change has been implemented according to plan. If no, describe:			
Final Review and Approvals			
Mfg. Signature:	Date:		
QA Signature:	Date:		
Regulatory Signature:	Date:		
Comments:			

FDA = Food and Drug Administration; QA = quality assurance.

Appendix 8-3. Document Format for General Process Validation Protocol

1. Approval signature page.
2. Objective: "To gather and document evidence that . . . verifies that . . . performs in compliance with . . . and results in an HCT/P that meets acceptance criteria."
3. Scope: "This protocol identifies the necessary steps/operations to perform . . . ."
4. System description: A general description of the HCT/P production process, which might include a flowchart.
5. Responsibilities: Identifies the departments responsible for initiation, review, approval, execution, and report generation.
6. Execution of operational qualifications: More specific assignment of responsibility for completion of the various data collection forms.
7. Documentation requirements: Outlines the good documentation practices that will be used and the process for handling deviations or exceptions.
8. Acceptance criteria: Lists the acceptance criteria or references where acceptance criteria can be found (eg, on data forms).
9. Protocol exceptions/resolution: Provides the forms used to make comments and document deviations.
10. Reports/data forms designed to collect and analyze the data.

HCT/P = human cells, tissues, and cellular and tissue-based product.

Appendix 8-4. Product Changeover Record

Part Number/Description:	Room Number:
Lot Number:	Production Date:

Criteria	Conforms (Check one)		Signature	
			Operator	Verifier
1. Verify scheduled room cleaning has been performed.	Yes ☐	No ☐		
2. Have all of the documents from the previous process been cleared from the area?	Yes ☐	No ☐		
3. Have all of the materials from the previous process been cleared from the area?	Yes ☐	No ☐		
4. Have all horizontal surfaces been cleaned before staging materials: BSC, equipment, tables?	Yes ☐	No ☐		
5. Are all of the correct documents present?	Yes ☐	No ☐		
6. Are all of the materials (part numbers/lot numbers) listed on the Batch Record present?	Yes ☐	No ☐		
7. Are all of the materials labeled properly and legibly with a release sticker, part number, lot number, and description?	Yes ☐	No ☐		
8. Where applicable, are all of the materials labeled properly and legibly with expiration date?	Yes ☐	No ☐		

Comments: any "No" reply must be addressed and comments made.

BSC = biological safety cabinet.

Appendix 8-5. Sample Product Tracking Form

Product Tracking Form	
This form is used to document transfer from the cellular therapy laboratory (CTL) to the patient infusion site. Transport of the cellular product between consignees is documented in compliance with good manufacturing practice and good tissue practice requirements to ensure adequate tracking and traceability.	
Recipient (Patient) Information (completed by CTL)	Product Information (completed by CTL)
Recipient Location:	Product Identifier:
Recipient Name:	Product Volume (mL):
Recipient Identifier:	Product Expiration Date/Time:
Visual Inspection of the Product (completed by CTL) *The product has been visually inspected for container integrity, product color, and turbidity.*	Product Label Verification (completed by CTL) *Recipient and product identity have been compared with source documents provided to the CTL and have been found to agree.* **Requires double sign-off.**
Visual Inspection of the Product: Acceptable Not Acceptable	*Signature/Date/Time:*
If not acceptable, notify laboratory supervisor before transport.	*Signature/Date/Time:*
Donor Eligibility Statement as required by the Food and Drug Administration (21 CFR 1271, Subpart C).	

- The donor of this cellular therapy product has been medically screened for relevant communicable diseases and meets eligibility criteria.
- The donor of this cellular therapy product is negative or nonreactive for relevant infectious disease tests. The following testing has been performed in a laboratory certified under CLIA: HBsAg, anti-HBc, anti-HIV 1/2, anti-HCV, anti-HTLV-I/II, STS, HIV NAT, HCV NAT, and HBV NAT.
- Final donor eligibility has been completed and the donor has been determined to be eligible. Donor eligibility was determined by [*insert organization name*].

Recipient (Patient) Identification Check Before Injection (completed by clinical staff)
Recipient and product identity have been confirmed from the product label, patient wristband, and product tracking form and have been found to agree with one another. **Requires double sign-off.**

Signature: Dept: Date/Time:

Signature: Dept: Date/Time:

CLIA = Clinical Laboratory Improvement Amendments; HBsAg = hepatitis B surface antigen; anti-HBc = antibody to hepatitis B core (antigen); anti-HIV 1/2 = antibody to human immunodeficiency virus, types 1 and 2; anti-HCV = antibody to hepatitis C virus; anti-HTLV-I/II = antibody to human T-cell lymphotropic virus, types I and II; STS = serologic test for syphilis; NAT = nucleic acid testing; HBV = hepatitis B virus; GMP = good manufacturing practice; GTP = good tissue practice.

Method 8-1. Maintaining a Corrective and Preventive Action Program

Purpose

To provide a description of the system for documenting corrective and preventive actions (CAPAs) within facility quality and regulatory systems and to ensure that resolution is obtained for such actions, to prevent occurrence or recurrence of potentially adverse actions or events. All CAPAs are subject to management review.

Responsibility

All personnel: Responsibilities include initiating a request for a CAPA for any quality or regulatory system when potential for an adverse action is seen and implementing CAPAs when requested by management. A request for corrective or preventive action for any quality or regulatory system can be made by any employee.

Management personnel: Responsibilities include reviewing and approving CAPAs that fall within the scope of their management and providing adequate resources (financial, personnel, time, and training) for implementing approved CAPAs.

Quality assurance (QA) personnel: Responsibilities include management of the CAPA program and approval or rejection of CAPA plans as well as the review, tracking, and approval of the implementation of CAPAs.

Definitions

- A *CAPA* is a corrective or preventive action.
- A *corrective action* is an action that is or will be taken to immediately correct an issue.
- A *preventive action* is an action that is or will be taken to minimize the potential for the occurrence or recurrence of an existing or potential issue.

Procedure

A. *General*
   1. A CAPA form (see Fig 8-1-1) is initiated for the following purposes:
      a. To document an action or event that potentially affects the quality or regulatory compliance of a facility material or process.
      b. To ensure that an action or event that potentially affects the quality or regulatory compliance of a facility material or process is made visible within the quality system in order to resolve the action or event and prevent recurrence.
      c. To provide for a mechanism for resolution.
   2. A request for a CAPA for any quality or regulatory system can be made by any facility employee.
   3. Any notification received by the QA group that indicates a quality or regulatory system within the facility or a vendor thereof is in need of nonroutine review, investigation, revision, or evaluation may be documented on a CAPA form.
   4. The following are situations that require the generation of a CAPA record:
      a. Any situation in which a facility employee observes an activity that may cause concern that a process may be inadequate, unclear, misleading, or noncompliant with regulations.
      b. Feedback that indicates unsatisfactory practices by a vendor that could have an impact on activities of the facility.
      c. Feedback that indicates unsatisfactory practices by a facility employee or department regarding regulated activities.
      d. Results from activities of an audit (internal or external).
      e. Results from activities associated with a deviation from normal processes, or trends of deviations, that require nonroutine follow-up and possible CAPAs.
      f. Results from activities associated with a product complaint, or trends of complaints, that require nonroutine follow-up and possible CAPAs.

CORRECTIVE AND/OR PREVENTIVE ACTION RECORD

Section A: Initiation

CAPA #   Response Due Date:

Initiated by: Dept: Date Initiated:

Assigned to: Dept: Date Assigned:

Brief Description:

Type of Action To Be Taken:

_____

Responsible Person: _____Date: _____
QA: _____Date: _____

Section B: Investigation

Description of Investigation:

Determination of Cause:

Proposed Action Plan:

Responsible Person: _____Date: _____
QA: _____Date: _____

Section C: Outcome and Implementation

Outcome of Investigation:

Verification of Cause:

Actions Implemented and Completed:

Responsible Person: _____Date: _____
QA: _____Date: _____

Figure 8-1-1. Sample corrective and preventive action form.

g. A notice of information concerning analytical release data or stability testing data, or trends of data, that may require nonroutine follow-up and possible CAPAs.

h. Results from activities of management review and compliance meetings that require CAPAs.

B. *Initiation Procedure*

1. A CAPA record is initiated by the generation of the appropriate CAPA form.

2. The action should be assigned by QA personnel to the person responsible for ensuring the CAPA is completed.

3. A response due date must be assigned by QA personnel.

4. A brief description of why the CAPA has been initiated should be given.

5. The suggested type of action must be assigned.

6. Once a CAPA has been initiated, the following must be notified:

    a. The QA group.

    b. The persons to whom the CAPA resolution has been assigned and their manager.

    c. Any other affected personnel.

C. *Investigation Procedure*

1. The need for a CAPA is reviewed and determined on a case-by-case basis. Discussions regarding the determination involve the initiator of the request, the management of the affected department, and QA personnel. Any determination and the rationale for the determination are to be documented on the CAPA form.

2. The cause of the issue should be determined during discussions. If no assignable cause is discovered, sufficient explanation should be given regarding how this determination was reached.

D. *Action Plan Procedure*

1. Once the need for a CAPA is determined, an action plan should be decided on by the management of the department requiring implementation and the QA department and should be documented.

2. Corrective Action

    a. The immediate action to be taken in order to correct the issue is described.

The action should be readily identifiable as correcting the issue and should be able to be appropriately and clearly documented.

b. The CAPA record should identify how the action will correct the issue. If no action is required, the rationale that supports this conclusion should be explained.

3. Preventive Action

a. The CAPA record should describe the action to be taken to minimize the potential for occurrence or recurrence of an issue or potential issue. The action may involve additional training or a change in a process or system and should be able to be appropriately and clearly documented.

b. The CAPA record should identify how the action will minimize the potential for occurrence or recurrence of an issue or potential issue. If no action is required, the CAPA record should explain the rationale that supports this conclusion and what steps will be taken to ensure tracking of the issue or potential issue.

4. Approval of the proposed CAPA is demonstrated by the signature of the management of the department requiring implementation and of QA personnel in the appropriate section describing the action to be taken on the CAPA form.

a. Approval by the management of the department requiring implementation signifies the following:

    • Acceptance of the CAPAs to be taken as reasonable and achievable.

    • Assurance that appropriate personnel will be assigned to implement or coordinate the implementation of the CAPAs.

b. Approval by QA personnel signifies the following:

    • The management of the department requiring implementation and QA personnel are in agreement about the appropriateness of the actions to be taken.

- All foreseeable quality issues are adequately addressed by the action.

5. Approval of the proposed CAPA is to be reported to the initiator of the request, the management of any department involved with implementation, the QA department, and all other personnel who are otherwise responsible for managing the CAPA resolution.

E. *Closure Procedure*

1. Upon completion of the implementation of the action, the person assigned to the implementation must sign and date the CAPA record with the completion date and forward the CAPA record to the QA department for review and closure.

2. Closure of a CAPA resolution is signified by the signature of QA personnel.

    a. Evidence of completion of a CAPA resolution is documented and reviewed by QA personnel.

    b. Attachments to the form for review must be included as necessary.

c. The date of completion of the CAPA resolution is recorded.

d. The signature of QA personnel for the closure of a CAPA resolution signifies satisfactory implementation and documentation of the CAPA.

F. *QA Oversight*

1. QA personnel track all CAPA activities.

    a. The QA CAPA database is reviewed periodically to determine the status of all open CAPA resolutions.

    b. Updates are given at routine management meetings regarding the following:

    - The status of all open CAPA resolutions.
    - The closing of any CAPA resolutions.
    - Trends discovered in CAPA resolutions.

    c. The CAPA program and QA oversight of the CAPA program are subject to management review.

In: Areman EM, Loper K, eds
Cellular Therapy: Principles, Methods, and Regulations
Bethesda, MD: AABB, 2009

◆◆◆ **9** ◆◆◆

Human Resources in the Cellular Therapy Facility

*Brenda Alder, MS, MT(ASCP)SBB; Lizabeth Cardwell,
MT(ASCP), MBA, RAC; Michele W. Sugrue, MS, MT(ASCP)SBB;
and Ellen Areman, MS, SBB(ASCP)*

EVERY ACTIVITY PERFORMED IN THE CELlular therapy (CT) facility requires knowledgeable, conscientious, and trained individuals to ensure quality throughout the manufacturing process. The diversity of tasks and responsibilities can stretch the available resources, often requiring cross-training of staff. In a small facility, the same people may be responsible for collection, processing, and testing of products. Such tasks as cleaning and environmental monitoring may also fall on the technical staff. Because of high demand for skilled staff and lack of formal training programs, it is often difficult to recruit experienced personnel, making training and competency review critical aspects of human resources development in a CT program.

Personnel Requirements and Selection

Each CT facility should have a mechanism for providing an adequate number of qualified personnel to perform, verify, and manage all activities within the facility safely, effectively, and efficiently. Such details should be outlined in a facility policy that defines the roles of executive management as well as the duties of the operations or laboratory director; medical director; supervisory, technical, and quality staff; and other employees in the organization. Appendix 9-1 provides an example of the personnel policy of a hospital CT facility.

Job descriptions should be available for all positions that involve processes and procedures that affect the quality of CT products. These job descriptions should clearly define the qualifications, responsibilities, and reporting relationships of each position, especially those needed to perform critical tasks. (See Appendices 9-2 and 9-3 for examples of job descriptions.) The personnel selection process should consider the applicant's qualifications for a particular position as determined by education, training, experience, certifications, and licensure. For quality control (QC) laboratory test-

Brenda Alder, MS, MT(ASCP)SBB, Quality Assurance and Standards Coordinator, Northside Hospital, Atlanta, Georgia; Lizabeth Cardwell, MT(ASCP), MBA, RAC, Principal, Compliance Consulting, Seattle, Washington; Michele W. Sugrue, MS, MT(ASCP)SBB, Coordinator, Research Programs, Division of Hematology/Oncology, Department of Medicine, University of Florida and Shands Hospital, Gainesville, Florida; and Ellen Areman, MS, SBB(ASCP), Senior Consultant, Biologics Consulting Group, Inc, Alexandria, Virginia

The authors have disclosed no conflicts of interest.

ing staff, the requisite personnel qualifications must be compatible with regulatory requirements such as those established under the Clinical Laboratory Improvement Act (CLIA) as well as with any state or local regulations.

Training

Once an employee is hired, he or she must be properly trained in the CT facility's policies and procedures. In addition to receiving training to perform the specific tasks and procedures required for the position, staff should also receive adequate orientation and instruction in the areas of safety, quality, aseptic technique, computer operation, security, and confidentiality. The position-specific phase of training should encompass the operational issues defined for the new employee's work area. Training must be provided for each procedure for which the employee has responsibility to ensure that new staff members are competent to perform their duties and responsibilities independently. There should be written criteria for staff eligibility to perform training, and this eligibility should be documented. Time frames for completion of training should be defined.

Facility policy should also require training before the introduction of a new process, test, or service, and documentation that employees are competent to perform the new task should be available. All employees should have the opportunity to ask questions and seek additional help, clarification, or training for any procedure or operation for which they are responsible at any time during their tenure. Appendix 9-4 provides an example of a form used to document training in a hospital CT facility.

Training focused on the requirements for CT products regulated under the Food and Drug Administration (FDA) current good tissue practice (cGTP) requirements in the Code of Federal Regulations (CFR), Title 21, Part 1271 should be performed and documented for staff involved in the production of those CT products. The training program should provide staff with an understanding of the regulatory basis for the facility's policies and procedures and should train them in facility-specific applications of the cGTP requirements. This training should be provided at regular intervals that are defined in facility policy to ensure that the staff remain familiar with regulatory requirements.

Competency

Facility policies and procedures should describe and define the process and criteria for determining competence, and all training should be documented, reviewed, and recorded. The facility should have written policies that define expectations for staff competency evaluations, including a definition of minimum acceptable performance, and remedial measures for providing a means for staff to meet the minimum performance criteria. Competency evaluations for all staff involved in the manufacture of CT products must be regularly scheduled and can include a combination of written evaluations; direct observation of activities; review of work records or reports, computer records, and QC records; testing or processing of unknown samples; and evaluation of the employee's problem-solving skills. Competency assessments do not always need to be targeted at individual tests or procedures performed by the employee, but can be grouped together to assess like techniques or methods. Appendix 9-5 provides an example of a competency assessment policy, and Appendices 9-6 and 9-7 provide examples of competency assessment forms for a hospital CT facility.

Proficiency Testing

In addition to the use of controls and standards, proficiency testing (PT) is performed to ensure the adequacy of analytical methods, procedures, and equipment and the competency of personnel. Regular participation in a PT program provides verification of laboratory competency and shows a commitment to the maintenance and improvement of performance. It demonstrates that analytical procedures are under control and gives analysts confidence that the service that they provide will withstand scrutiny. PT may be divided into two groups: external (supplied by an outside provider) and internal (manufactured and tested exclusively within a facility).

PT is an essential component of a quality program and is required by many regulatory and accrediting agencies. To maintain CLIA certification, for instance, a laboratory must participate in a PT program approved by the Centers for Medicare and Medicaid Services (CMS) for the methods the laboratory uses that fall under CLIA regulations. In cellular product manufacturing facilities, analyses that fall under regulatory statutes differ from laboratory to laboratory and depend on which tests are performed by personnel. For example, the analysis of CD34+ cell enumeration (flow cytometry) on product or patient samples may be performed by the staff at one cell-processing facility, but by a separate laboratory at another facility.

External Proficiency Testing

PT evaluates a laboratory's analytical performance in comparison to other laboratories, reference standards, or reference laboratories. It serves as an external verification of the quality of a laboratory's results. Monitoring trends in PT results allows the laboratory to identify potential problems related to imprecision, equipment drift, systematic error, and human error.

PT programs provide laboratories with samples containing specified and characterized material. The laboratory analyzes the samples, as part of its routine testing program, and reports the results to the PT program. The PT program analyzes results from numerous participating laboratories and reports the results. The laboratory receives a report from the PT program that shows how closely its results agree with the accepted value and the values achieved by other laboratories. When necessary, the participating laboratory can then take appropriate action to improve performance.

Identifying appropriate external PT providers to meet the needs of the cellular-processing facility can be difficult because procedures and analytes may not yet be commonplace in clinical laboratory testing. Some vendors now offer PT samples and programs that mimic hematopoietic progenitor cell products and allow for integration into the daily operation of a cellular therapy processing facility. Analyses include nucleated cell counting, cellular viability determination, and colony-forming unit identification or enumeration. Although some of these analyses are ungraded, they provide an opportunity to anonymously compare the performance of a laboratory against similar facilities.

Internal Proficiency Testing

Alternative methods to assess test performance are a viable option and can serve as a valuable self-monitoring tool when external PT is not available. Often a laboratory may use internal PT for assessing the performance of staff to determine competency. For analyses in which technologist subjectivity is involved in determining results, internal PT can provide documentation of reproducibility among staff. The same performance objectives should apply as for external PT programs.

Objectives for Proficiency Testing

In facilities that subscribe to external PT programs or perform internal PT, processes and procedures must be in place to ensure that the testing is performed in a consistent manner that will attain the desired outcome and the most accurate result. A designated staff member should be given the responsibility to monitor compliance and ensure that PT is performed according to instructions. All PT results should be communicated to the staff, and all unacceptable results, whether internal or external, require investigation and corrective action.

Corrective Action in Proficiency Testing

A process control mechanism should be adopted as a standard operating procedure (SOP) for corrective action. Corrective action is required whenever an incorrect response is obtained, including all test results obtained when pre-established acceptance criteria are not met. An example of this mechanism is the following:

1. The responsible staff member reviews the PT results with the individual who performed the test to determine possible reasons for the error.
2. The responsible staff member reviews the written test procedure and QC guidelines with the testing personnel.
3. The responsible staff member observes the individual while he or she repeats the test procedure using the sample on which the incorrect result was obtained. If the sample is unavailable, other samples with a known value may be tested.

4. All retesting, review, and corrective action must be documented.

Proficiency Testing Records

A separate file for PT results and evaluations should be maintained. All records should be filed for the required retention period as defined by regulatory agencies and accreditation standards, including any data, investigation, and corrective action reports related to PT.

Continuing Education

Each facility should define in its policies the amount and type of annual continuing education hours required for each CT position, taking into consideration any state or accreditation requirements that apply. Continuing education hours should be documented. Appendix 9-8 provides an example of a continuing education policy.

Appendix 9-1. Sample Policy for Personnel, Training, and Competency

I. **Purpose:** To give an overall description of how the cellular therapy (CT) facility provides adequate personnel, training, competency, and evaluations. To define the qualifications required for the medical director and other personnel responsible for the CT facility.

II. **Policy**

A. *Personnel*

1. The quality program includes the following:
   a. Definition of staffing needs.
   b. Definition of the process for hiring qualified (by education or experience) individuals.
   c. Provision of initial and ongoing training.
   d. Assessment of individual competence at specified intervals.
2. Staffing details are as follows:
   a. Hours of operation: [describe]
   b. Extended or weekend hours: May be required as needed.
   c. CT staff are available 24 hours a day, 7 days a week, 52 weeks per year.
   d. Minimum number of staff: [detail]
   e. Maximum number of staff: [detail]
3. General job descriptions are provided below and include appropriate and defined qualifications for each position. Each staff member maintains a copy of his or her job description in a personnel binder.
4. Refer to the competency assessment (Appendix 9-5) and continuing education (Appendix 9-8) policies also.

B. *Training, Competency, and Evaluations*

1. Documented processes for training include ongoing identification, design, delivery, and evaluation of all staff training needs.
2. Records of training for job-related tasks and competence assessment are kept in the individual employee personnel files. The evaluation and documentation of staff competence initially and at appropriately defined intervals are described in detail in the competency assessment policy. Retraining needs are also identified and addressed appropriately in the competency assessment policy.
3. Performance appraisals are completed after the first 90 days of employment, and yearly once training is complete. The performance review is based on job accountabilities, objective measures, and predefined standards. Documentation is kept in the individual employee's personnel file.
4. Designated laboratory staff can be qualified as trainers to verify the competency of other employees once they themselves have demonstrated competency in a particular task.
5. CT management can authorize other CT staff to review and sign CT documents (eg, forms, records, or worksheets) as needed.
6. The employees of the CT facility are required to complete continuing education hours annually as specified in each job description.

III. **General Job Descriptions**

A. *Medical and Laboratory Directors*

1. The CT facilities are under the direction of a medical director (with MD credentials) and a laboratory director (MD or PhD), who supervise all medical and technical policies, administra-

tive operations, medical procedures, validation studies, and compliance with standards and regulations for the facility. If both areas are overseen by one director, that individual must be an MD.

2. The medical or laboratory director has training and experience in CT processing and infusion of CT components.

3. The medical or laboratory director prescribes tests and procedures for measuring, assaying, and monitoring properties of the cell products that are essential to the evaluation of their safety and usefulness.

4. Precollection evaluation of prospective HPC donors is under the direction of the medical director and those the medical director designates.

B. *CT Facility Supervisor*

1. The CT facility supervisor must possess the licenses and registrations required by state and local authorities and must have at least 5 years of experience in cell processing. The supervisor, under the direction of the medical and laboratory directors, oversees the technical operations related to the provision of products and services.

2. The supervisor is responsible for the following:
   a. Reporting to the medical director and other upper management personnel.
   b. Management of all technical staff, which includes responsibility for scheduling and performance reviews.
   c. Ensuring that the technical staff is capable and trained appropriately.
   d. Supervising and reviewing training and competency assessments.

C. *Quality Improvement and Standards Coordinator*

1. The quality improvement and standards coordinator must possess the licenses and registrations required by state and local authorities and must

have at least 5 years of experience in cell processing. The coordinator must also have at least 2 years of experience in all aspects of departmental standard operating procedures (SOPs), compliance with regulatory standards, and training and competency documentation. This person reports to the executive management.

2. The quality improvement and standards coordinator is responsible for the following:
   a. Exercising control in all matters related to compliance with professional standards as well as with applicable federal, state, and local regulations.
   b. Recommending corrective action or making changes in the quality system when appropriate.
   c. Reviewing and approving quality and technical policies, processes, procedures, and quality audits.

D. *CT Facility Specialist*

1. The CT facility specialist must possess the licenses and registrations required by state and local authorities and a minimum of 2 years of clinical laboratory experience, 1 year of which is preferably CT processing experience.

2. The CT facility specialist must possess the following:
   a. Good communication and interpersonal skills and the ability to work well as part of a team.
   b. The ability to prioritize required duties and responsibilities, define problems, collect data, establish facts, draw valid conclusions, and interpret instructions furnished in written, oral, diagram, or schedule form.
   c. The training and competence to process, cryopreserve, and distribute CT products.
   d. Documentation of education, training, and experience.

Appendix 9-2. Sample Job Description for Cellular Therapy Specialist

Position Title

Cellular Therapy Specialist—Hematopoietic Progenitor Cell (HPC) Transplant Program

Occupational Summary

Functions as a member of the transplant team by assisting in the coordination, development, and implementation of the technical section of the cellular therapy (CT) transplant program. Performs and assists with complex procedures such as HPC collection and processing, concentration, purging, selection, cryopreservation, thawing, and infusion, according to approved clinical protocols.

Primary Duties and Responsibilities

1. Processes autologous and allogeneic HPCs, as requested by the physician in accordance with developed procedures and protocols. Is able to work without supervision. Performs calculations during processing to assess product yields. Uses aseptic technique while performing all cell processing procedures. Investigates and resolves any problems with procedures or processes.

2. Develops techniques for processing HPCs. Performs validation processes on new instrumentation and equipment.

3. Communicates with physicians, transplant nurses, and transplant coordinators to schedule apheresis (HPC-A) collections, marrow harvests, HPC infusions, and to report daily processing yields. Participates in multidisciplinary meetings to review and assess patient status and issues concerning patients or donors. Assists physicians and data managers in accessing processing information for unrelated donor registry documentation.

4. Assists the marrow harvest team in the collection and filtering of marrow from normal donors and autologous patients in the operating room.

5. Identifies and transfers frozen HPCs from the storage freezer to the transport container. Ensures the secure transportation of HPCs to the designated location. Is responsible for patient and component verification for the infusion of stem cell products. Thaws the cryopreserved HPCs and assists the nursing and medical staff during the infusion or transplantation of the HPCs or marrow.

6. Collects and labels required laboratory samples. Creates and maintains accurate and complete charts of patient and donor laboratory results, consents, prescriptions, processing worksheets, and cryopreservation and infusion records. Performs internal assessments and develops outcome analysis forms for review by the medical director.

7. Develops, prepares, and updates policies and procedures according to Foundation for the Accreditation of Cellular Therapy (FACT), AABB, Joint Commission, Food and Drug Administration (FDA), and/or state regulatory guidelines. Implements and follows policies and procedures. Participates in the review of treatment protocols and procedures.

8. Performs quality control and preventive maintenance on instrumentation and equipment in the CT laboratory. Maintains records of all maintenance performed.

9. Monitors and maintains a secure storage depository for cryopreserved HPCs. Performs inventory review of cryopreserved HPCs.

10. Practices proper safety techniques in accordance with hospital and departmental policies and procedures. Immediately reports any mechanical or electrical equipment malfunctions, unsafe conditions, or employee, patient, or visitor injuries or accidents to management.

Additional Duties and Responsibilities

Performs other duties as assigned by CT laboratory management or medical director. The above statements are intended to describe the general nature and level of work performed by staff assigned to this classification. They are not to be construed as an exhaustive list of all job duties performed by the staff so classified.

License or Certification Required

State or national certification as applicable (specify).

Knowledge, Skills, and Abilities Required

Experience

1. Experience as a medical technologist.
2. Minimum of 5 years of clinical laboratory experience.
3. HPC processing experience.

Language Skills

1. Excellent communication and interpersonal skills.
2. Ability to effectively present information and respond to questions from managers, clients, customers, and the general public.
3. Ability to read, analyze, and interpret periodicals, professional journals, technical procedures, or governmental regulations.

4. Ability to write reports, action plans, business correspondence, policies, and procedures.

Mathematical Skills

Ability to perform advanced mathematical calculations.

Reasoning Ability

1. Ability to make independent decisions within established parameters.
2. Ability to prioritize required duties and responsibilities.
3. Ability to define problems, collect data, establish facts, and draw valid conclusions.
4. Ability to interpret instructions furnished in written, oral, diagram, or schedule form.
5. Ability to solve practical problems and deal with concrete variables in situations in which only limited standardization exists.

Attitudes and Behaviors

1. Ability to adjust to changes in schedules, working hours, and procedures. Position may require extended hours at intervals.
2. Willingness to interact with donors, patients, and family members.

Working Conditions

Possible exposure to infectious diseases, hazardous chemicals and materials, needle sticks, blood, and body fluids.

Appendix 9-3. Sample Job Description for Quality Assurance Specialist

Position Title

Quality Assurance Specialist—Cellular Therapy

Occupational Summary

Responsible for policy and procedure preparation, maintenance, and oversight. Responsible for regulatory readiness and compliance with relevant standards and regulations.

Primary Duties and Responsibilities

1. Responsible for all regulatory compliance tasks and functions: reviews, revises, and updates operational policies. Completes applications and coordinates correspondence with outside agencies and accrediting bodies.
2. Participates in development and maintenance of a quality control program. Reviews and compiles summary reports and data.
3. Coordinates quality improvement activities and plans and makes regular reports to directors, hospitals, and other agencies as appropriate.
4. Identifies staff training needs and participates in the training of staff.
5. May assist directors and data managers in system design for the documentation, collection, processing, and evaluation of databases for registry compliance and clinical outcome review.
6. Coordinates departmental quality improvement plans and reporting with the hospital-wide plan and objectives, including patient satisfaction, clinical outcome, and cost reduction.
7. Demonstrates the hospital value statements.
8. Works with the cellular therapy laboratory supervisor and specialists to ensure a complete and efficient integration of daily operations, quality control, regulatory compliance, and quality improvement planning.

9. Participates in evaluating and selecting external providers of technical or professional services, such as reference laboratory testing or consulting.

Additional Duties and Responsibilities

Performs other duties as assigned by supervisor.

License or Certification Required

State or national certification as applicable (specify).

Knowledge, Skills, and Abilities Required

Experience

1. Bachelor of science in medical technology, biological science, or a related field.
2. Minimum of 5 years of experience in HPC collection, processing, infusion, and/or patient management.
3. Minimum of 2 years of experience in all aspects of departmental policies and regulatory compliance.
4. Minimum of 2 years of experience in training and competency assessment and documentation.
5. Proficiency in the use of computers.
6. Proven coordination, team, leadership, and service skills.

Language Skills

1. Excellent oral and written communication skills.
2. Ability to effectively present information and respond to questions from managers, clients, customers, and the general public.
3. Ability to read, analyze, and interpret periodicals, professional journals, technical procedures, or government regulations.

4. Ability to write reports, action plans, business correspondence, policies, and procedures.

Mathematical Skills

Ability to perform advanced mathematical calculations.

Reasoning Ability

1. Ability to interpret instructions furnished in written, oral, diagram, or schedule form.

2. Ability to solve practical problems and deal with concrete variables in situations in which only limited standardization exists.

Attitudes and Behaviors

Ability to adjust to changes in schedules, working hours, and procedures. Position may require extended hours at intervals.

Working Conditions

Possible exposure to infectious diseases, hazardous chemicals and materials, needle sticks, blood, and body fluids.

Appendix 9-4. Sample Cellular Therapy Facility Training Checklist

Employee: _____

#	Items Reviewed	Trainee Initials	Trainer Initials	Date of Satisfactory Performance
1	**Media Preparation**			
	Marrow Harvest			
	Cryopreservation Media			
	Handling Dimethyl Sulfoxide			
	Overnight Storage			
	Operation of Cell Selection Device			
2	**Product Manipulation—Bone Marrow**			
	Concentration or Buffy Coat			
	RBC Reduction			
	Plasma Depletion and Washing			
	Unrelated Donor Registry Products			
	Preparation for Transport			
	Database Use and Documentation			
3	**Product Manipulation—Peripheral Blood**			
	Concentration			
	Peripheral Blood Cell Selection			
	Allogeneic Donor Leukocytes (CD3) by apheresis and whole blood			
	Database Use and Documentation			
4	**Cryopreservation**			
	Sample Aliquots			
	Bone Marrow			
	Peripheral Blood Progenitor Cells			
	Donor Leukocytes (CD3)			
	CD34+ Selected Cells			
	Database Use and Documentation			
5	**Thawing, Infusion, and Transport**			
	Identification of HPCs for Infusion			
	Issue of HPCs			
	Thawing of HPCs			
	Thawing of Cord Blood			
	Thawing of CD34+ Selected Cells			
	Infusion of HPCs			
	Transportation of HPCs within the Facility			
	Transportation of HPCs to Other Facilities			
	Transportation of Registry Products			
	Return of HPCs			
	Database Use and Documentation			

Lab Supervisor or Designee Review:_____Date:_____

Appendix 9-5. Sample Competency Assessment Policy

I. **Purpose**
To provide guidelines for assessing and documenting employee competence.

II. **Materials and Equipment Needed**
Competency form—cellular therapy (CT) laboratory specific.

III. **Policy**
 A. *Frequency of Competency Assessment*
 1. Competency will be assessed before assuming duties, as needed following implementation of new methods or systems, and in conjunction with the annual performance evaluation.
 2. The CT facility supervisor or designee will identify procedures or equipment that require new, ongoing, or more intensive assessment.
 B. *Methods of Competency Assessment*
 1. Direct or verbal observations documented by the supervisor or other designated person.
 2. Review of completed documents (eg, processing, test results, event management reports, or adverse reaction reports).
 3. Use of a mock sample.
 4. Written or oral tests.
 5. Other methods designed by the supervisor.
 C. *Responsibility for Competency Assessment*
 1. The medical director (or the equivalent) will review and approve the annual competency of each employee. The medical director may help identify opportunities for improvement, develop action plans, and set educational goals for the laboratory.
 2. The CT supervisor or designee will do the following:

 a. Help identify or develop areas for ongoing competency assessment.
 b. Identify opportunities for improvement and develop action plans and education goals for the laboratory.
 c. Assess employee skills.
 d. Work with employees to improve competence and skills as needed.
 e. Review and sign each employee's annual competency summary.
 3. The employee will do the following:
 a. Assist with peer review as assigned.
 b. Review competency assessment plans and meet all deadlines for completion of the competency assessment.
 c. Complete personal competency assessment documentation and review performance with the supervisor.
 d. Comply with training or skill improvement requirements as defined by the supervisor or medical director, if indicated.
 D. *Documentation of Competency Assessment*
 1. The employee personnel files will be used to store completed competency documentation.
 2. **Competency Assessment Checklists.** Checklists are completed for each staff member upon demonstration of competency in the subject area. Once competency is demonstrated, the employee is approved to perform the task. If an employee does not document competency in an assigned area, the employee is not qualified to perform work in that area until the competency has been documented.
 3. **Competency Retraining.** If at any time the employee does not successfully complete the competency test or demonstration, the employee is retrained

and must successfully repeat the demonstration. Problem areas and potential areas for improvement are documented, and a corrective action plan is developed by the supervisor and reviewed with the employee before the annual evaluation. An employee who does not meet competency requirements for specific areas may be restricted by a corrective action plan. Continued or recurrent competency failures may be used for reassignment, disciplinary action, or termination.

4. **Approved Trainers.** Cellular therapy facility staff who have previously demonstrated competency in a specific area may verify the competency of other employees in that area.

IV. References/Resources

1. Wright D. The ultimate guide to competency assessment in health care. 3rd ed. Minneapolis, MN: Creative Health Care Management, Inc, 2007.
2. FACT-JACIE international standards for cellular therapy product collection, processing, and administration. 3rd ed. Omaha, NE: Foundation for the Accreditation of Cellular Therapy and the Joint Accreditation Committee of ISCT and EBMT, 2006.
3. Padley D, ed. Standards for cellular therapy product services. 3rd ed. Bethesda, MD: AABB, 2008.
4. Code of federal regulations. Human cells, tissues, and cellular and tissue-based products. Current good tissue practice. Title 21 CFR Part 1271, Subpart D. Washington, DC: US Government Printing Office, 2008 (revised annually).
5. Code of federal regulations. Subpart H: Participation in proficiency testing for laboratories performing non-waived testing. Title 42 CFR Parts 493.801 through 493.807. Washington, DC: US Government Printing Office, 2008 (revised annually).

Appendix 9-6. Sample Cellular Therapy Facility Competency Assessment Checklist

Peripheral Blood Stem Cell Concentration

Employee:_____ Date:_____

#	Items Reviewed	Performed Correctly? Check Appropriate Box	
		Yes	No
1	Ensures stem cell evaluation packet is completed properly?		
2	Determines when the collection process for hematopoietic progenitor cells from apheresis (HPC-A) will conclude?		
3	Assigns stem cell collection number correctly?		
4	Generates labels correctly?		
5	Orders blood cultures, blood type, flow analysis, or other testing correctly?		
6	Obtains correct blood type accession label from the laboratory?		
7	Labels all samples correctly?		
8	Cleans the biological safety cabinet correctly?		
9	Records lot numbers of supplies used?		
10	Primes COBE 2991 correctly?		
11	Installs tubing set correctly?		
12	Verifies information on HPC-A collection label attached to the product?		
13	Collects samples for cell counts correctly?		
14	Uses and discards needles and sharps correctly?		
15	Operates COBE 2991 correctly to concentrate HPC-A?		
16	Performs calculations correctly?		
17	Maintains aseptic technique correctly?		
18	Completes HPC-A worksheet correctly?		
19	Is competent to perform HPC-A concentration?		

/ /

_____
Trainer signature   Employee signature   Date

If not competent, correction plan recommended: _____

Correction plan completed: / /
_____
                 Trainer signature   Employee signature   Date

Comments: _____

_____

◆

Appendix 9-7. Sample Competency Assessment Form

Competency Assessment Form for (List Job Title)   Cellular Therapy Specialist

Employee Name   **Assigned Work Area**

This form is to be completed by the employee. For each of the competency statements listed below, the employee may select the method of verification he or she would like to use for validation of his or her skill in that area. See the method of verification for details on completion. When this form is complete, submit it to the area supervisor, as indicated.

Competency	Method of Verification	Date Completed
Technical Domain		
Donor eligibility (DE) determination. Understands the hospital, Food and Drug Administration (FDA), AABB, and Foundation for the Accreditation of Cellular Therapy (FACT) regulations and procedures governing the determination of donor eligibility for cellular therapy (CT) donors.	Complete the designated CT laboratory DE case study.	
	Create a case study for determining DE for autologous donors.	
	Review three FDA ineligible donor files and list the factors contributing to the DE determination.	
Complete *two* of the verification methods.	Read and discuss the DE and good tissue practice PowerPoint presentations.	
Biohazard labeling. Understands the types of biohazard labels and their use in labeling products that meet the biohazard criteria.	Complete the designated CT laboratory biohazard labeling case study.	
	List the specific sections in all CT laboratory standard operating procedures (SOPs) that discuss biohazard labeling.	
	Create a biohazard labeling case study.	
Complete *two* of the verification methods.	List and discuss all sections of Code of Federal Regulations (CFR) Title 21, Part 1271 that reference biohazard labeling.	

Communicable disease transmission by human cellular and tissue-based products (HCT/Ps). Understands the FDA definition of "relevant communicable disease and disease agents (RCDADs)" and the screening tests used to detect RCDADs and other communicable diseases.	Complete the Infectious Disease Marker Training Test.
	List the 21 CFR Part 1271 references for the communicable diseases that the FDA requires testing for on HCT/P donors.
	List the infectious disease markers that are required by the transplantation program at the hospital for determining DE.
Complete *two* of the verification methods.	
Critical Thinking Domain	
HCT/P deviation reporting. Understands the critical thinking decisions for determining when deviation reporting to the FDA is required.	Complete an FDA HCT/P deviation form for the recipient of a CT product. Use the example of a donor who had a risk factor documented on the donor history questionnaire that was not acknowledged by the collection staff; thus, the product was collected and distributed without the correct biohazard labeling on the bag.
	List the CT laboratory SOP that defines the types of deviations to report through the CT laboratory event management system. Then run a report in event management and identify the five most common deviations reported by the CT laboratory for 1/1/08 to 12/31/08.
	Complete the "HCT/P Deviation Reporting" section of the designated case study.
Complete *one* of the verification methods.	
CT review. Understands the processes of stem cell collection, processing, storage, and transplantation. Review critical aspects of CT and the different types of stem cell transplantation.	Complete all review questions in the online course "Basic Cellular Therapy" produced by the AABB and COLA. There are review questions at the end of each module with feedback mechanisms on where to go in the review material to gain more information on a particular topic.
	Prepare a PowerPoint presentation that describes the basics of CT collection, processing, transplantation, and storage.
Complete *one* of the verification methods.	
Interpersonal Domain	
Communication and time management. Understands the necessity to communicate effectively and manage multiple projects.	☐ Print three e-mails in which you were communicating necessary information to keep other employees or departments informed.

(Continued)

Appendix 9-7. Sample Competency Assessment Form (Continued)

Competency	Method of Verification	Date Completed
Interpersonal Domain (Continued)		
Complete *one* of the verification methods.	☐ Type a description of your daily priorities and how you can manage your time effectively.	
	☐ Provide a copy of a transcript of attendance at one of the following classes: ☐ Mentor training ☐ Workplace conflict ☐ Communication basics	
	☐ Write a summary of a situation in which you participated (or print an e-mail if documented as such) in which you either solved a problem or prevented a problem from occurring.	
	☐ Participate in a hospital volunteer program and provide written evidence.	

This section is to be completed by the supervisor:

With consideration of the employee's performance and competency assessment, this employee is competent to perform the role of

_____ in _____.   ☐ YES (may work independently)

(job class and and title)   (assigned work area)   ☐ NO (requires supervision)

Action Plan:

Employee Signature: _____ Date: _____

Supervisor Signature: _____ Date: _____

Appendix 9-8. Sample Policy for a Continuing Education Program

I. **Purpose**

To provide a policy that describes the requirements of and documentation for continuing education and training for employees of the cellular therapy (CT) facility to keep staff abreast of the new developments in the area of hematopoietic stem cell collection, processing, and transplantation.

II. **Procedure**

A. *Continuing Education*

1. Every year, each employee of the CT facility is required to complete the following minimum continuing education requirements:
   a. Full-time employees: 15 hours.
   b. Part-time employees: 10 hours.
2. The continuing education requirements will be relevant to the employee's job description. Either interdepartmental in-services or attendance at a function outside the facility can meet the requirement. Examples include the following:
   a. Supervisory courses.
   b. Quality assurance courses.
   c. Presentations at interdepartmental in-services.
   d. Attendance at professional meetings (eg, AABB, ISCT, FDA, or ASH).
   e. Audioconferences.
   f. Programs or guest speakers.
   g. Meeting presentations.
   h. Article reviews.
3. Continuing education hours are awarded as hours of time spent in each endeavor or as allotted by the organization holding the meeting.

B. *Documentation of Continuing Education*

1. Documentation of attendance can include the following:
   a. Certificate of attendance. This certificate usually will display the credits earned.
   b. Publication presentation (copy of abstract or article).
2. Documentation that involves speakers, other presentations, or an article review will be recorded in the employee's continuing education file.
3. All supporting documentation that is received from attendance will be placed in the employee's competency notebook.
4. Employees will have an annually updated Record of Mandatory Education form in their individual notebooks.
5. The CT facility laboratory supervisor or designee will annually review the employee's continuing education file and notebook for completion.

III. **Notes**

Annual continuing education requirements will be completed before the employee's yearly evaluation.

IV. **References/Resources**

1. FACT-JACIE international standards for cellular therapy product collection, processing, and administration. 3rd ed. Omaha, NE: Foundation for the Accreditation of Cellular Therapy and the Joint Accreditation Committee of ISCT and EBMT, 2006.
2. Padley D, ed. Standards for cellular therapy product services. 3rd ed. Bethesda, MD: AABB, 2008.

In: Areman EM, Loper K, eds
Cellular Therapy: Principles, Methods, and Regulations
Bethesda, MD: AABB, 2009

◆◆◆ 10 ◆◆◆

Equipment Management in the Cellular Therapy Facility

Dave Krugh, MT(ASCP)SBB, CLS, CLCP(NCA)

AN EVER-INCREASING VARIETY OF LABO-ratory equipment and instrumentation has been developed or adapted for use in the manufacture of cellular therapy (CT) products. These devices range in complexity from basic centrifuges to complex cell sorters. One thing all of them have in common is the need for appropriate selection and proper qualification before being used in the manufacturing process. Once the equipment has been installed and qualified, preventive maintenance (PM) and quality control (QC) schedules must be created and rigorously followed to ensure continued acceptable performance. A procedure that outlines steps to follow when the equipment is out of control or fails to operate properly must also be in place before the use of a new piece of equipment can be authorized. Depending on the application of the equipment, the CT laboratory or manufacturer may be required to demonstrate compliance with a number of regulations and standards.

A rigorous and well-designed quality program must include standard operating procedures (SOPs) to control, qualify, calibrate, maintain, clean, sanitize, and monitor critical equipment, ie,

equipment that has a reasonable potential to affect cell products, processes, or services. Method 10-1 provides a sample policy and procedure for equipment selection, and Method 10-2 provides a sample procedure for equipment management.

Equipment Qualification

The first step in equipment management is qualification. Equipment qualification is usually broken down into four key elements: design qualification (DQ), installation qualification (IQ), operational qualification (OQ), and performance qualification (PQ).

Design Qualification

DQ defines the operational and functional specifications for the equipment by detailing the decisions made in the selection of the device manufacturer or supplier, including vendor qualification (Table 10-1). Depending on the equipment characteristics, vendor qualification can be relatively straightforward for off-the-shelf equipment with no modifications, or it can be much more complex for

Dave Krugh, MT(ASCP)SBB, CLS, CLCP(NCA), Clinical Instructor, Department of Pathology, College of Medicine and Public Health, and Clinical Program Manager, The Ohio State University—The James Cancer Hospital and Solove Research Institute, Columbus, Ohio

The author has disclosed no conflicts of interest.

Table 10-1. Design Qualification Components

- Definition of functional specifications to ensure that the equipment is appropriate for the designated use and within the manufacturer's specifications.
- Definition of operational specifications to ensure that measuring and testing are within manufacturer's specifications.
- Cost.
- Warranty—terms and length.
- Maintenance or service—contract, availability, cost, and turnaround time. Will facility personnel be able to perform maintenance, or must maintenance be performed by outside vendors?
- Regulatory status (eg, FDA 510(k) cleared).
- Vendor reputation—reliability, customer, or technical support.
- Change control—how software updates, recalls, and notifications are provided.
- Installation requirements—physical space, plumbing and electrical requirements, alarms, computer hardware and software, and temperature and humidity requirements.
- Installation assistance—installation qualification, operational qualification, and calibration certificates are provided.
- Training—availability, on-site options, and cost.

customized equipment or computer software. Vendor qualification should incorporate equipment development, validation, and support (Table 10-2).

Installation Qualification

IQ ensures that the equipment is received as specified in design qualification, that it is properly installed, and that the environment is suitable for the operation and use of the equipment. Installation qualification may be performed by the vendor or user.

Operational Qualification

OQ ensures that the equipment will function in the facility environment according to specifications when operated under normal conditions. Features of OQ include the type and number of samples required, the frequency of testing, types of reference equipment required, and statistical methods used to interpret the data. Equipment is typically placed into service after OQ, which may be performed by the vendor or user.

Performance Qualification

PQ ensures that the equipment consistently performs according to established specifications for its routine use. Elements of PQ may include testing in parallel with a comparable instrument, repeatability and robustness of equipment when operated under varying conditions and by different operators, and testing parameters that tend to drift. It also includes review of calibration, PM, and QC to ensure that fluctuations in equipment performance are negligible.

Table 10-2. Important Questions for Equipment Vendor Qualification

- Does the vendor have a documented and certified or accredited quality system?
- Are equipment hardware and computer software developed and validated according to the manufacturer's standard operating procedure and applicable regulatory or accreditation standards and guidelines?
- Is the vendor able to make product development and validation records accessible to regulatory or accreditation organizations?
- Does the vendor provide a statement that the equipment meets customer specifications?
- Is a customer feedback and response system in place for reporting problems or requesting equipment enhancements?
- Does the vendor provide assistance in installation qualification and operational qualification?
- Is a change-control system in place to notify users of changes?

Requalification

Requalification is required when there are changes to equipment configuration that may affect performance (eg, significant repair or movement) or notable changes in equipment performance or in CT product quality. Appendix 10-5 provides an example of an equipment requalification checklist.

Equipment Quality Control

Master Equipment List

A master equipment list containing at least the following information about each piece of equipment should be maintained:
- Unique identifier.
- Designation (critical or noncritical).
- Calibration requirements.
- QC requirements.
- PM requirements.
- Date of purchase.
- Date put into service.

Calibration and Quality Control

Equipment that requires calibration or QC must be clearly identified, and SOPs must be developed that address the frequency of these activities (eg, before initial use or after repair and at prescribed intervals), the method, acceptance criteria, documentation, corrective action, and the use of certified equipment. After calibration or QC, equipment should be protected from unauthorized adjustments and improper handling, maintenance, and storage.

Documentation of calibration, PM, and QC must be accessible to staff to ensure that defined parameters are maintained during use. A process must be in place to follow when equipment is found to be out of calibration. This process should include investigation of 1) the validity of a previous inspection or calibration, 2) test results, and 3) CT products manufactured by using the faulty equipment.

Out-of-Service or Malfunctioning Equipment

An SOP is also needed for dealing with equipment that has malfunctioned or has been taken out of service. Such a procedure should include notification and documentation of the equipment malfunction, replacement with alternative equipment, follow-up equipment calibration, and requalification, as applicable.

Preventive Maintenance

A written SOP must be established and implemented for equipment PM to prevent malfunction, equipment contamination, and product cross-contamination. The SOP should include 1) cleaning and maintaining equipment, 2) line clearance, 3) the removal or obliteration of previous batch identification, 4) the protection of clean equipment from contamination, 5) inspection of cleanliness prior to use and 6) the use of equipment logs and worksheets. Equipment maintenance logs should include such information as the action, date, and time performed; the identification of the individual performing the task; the CT product and lot number, if applicable, and review by the designated supervisor. At a minimum, equipment must be maintained according to manufacturing or operational instructions.

Records Review

Records of equipment used during procurement, processing, storage, and distribution must be maintained to ensure identification and the ability to recall CT products associated with specific equipment, if necessary.

Computer-Controlled Equipment

In addition to the SOPs previously described, computer-controlled equipment requires defined SOPs for at least the following:
- System maintenance and operation.
- System security.
- The display and verification of data before final acceptance.
- The authorization process for additions or alterations.
- Document modification.
- Backup data storage with a validated retrieval process.
- An alternative process for continued operation during computer downtime.

Acknowledgments

Method 10-1 was submitted by Hillary Bradbury, MT(ASCP), and Dave Krugh, MT(ASCP)SBB, CLS, CLCP(NCA), The Ohio State University— The James Cancer Hospital and Solove Research Institute, Columbus, Ohio.

References/Resources

1. Padley D, ed. Standards for cellular therapy product services. 3rd ed. Bethesda, MD: AABB, 2008.

2. FACT-JACIE international standards for cellular therapy product collection, processing, and administration. 3rd ed. Omaha, NE: Foundation for the Accreditation of Cellular Therapy and the Joint Accreditation Committee of ISCT and EBMT, 2006.

3. Code of federal regulations. Title 21 CFR Parts 211, 600, 820, and 1271. Washington, DC: US Government Printing Office, 2008 (revised annually).

4. Food and Drug Administration. Guidance for industry: Guideline on general principles of process validation. (May 1987) Rockville, MD: FDA, 1987.

Appendix 10-1. Critical Equipment Selection Form

Description of equipment:	Intended use: Product- or process-specific? ☐ **Yes** ☐ **No** ☐ Storage ☐ Processing ☐ Transport ☐ Measuring/Testing ☐ Monitoring ☐ Other:	
Define equipment specifications: *(continue on back if necessary)* **Functional**	**Operational**	
List top two choices: *(attach additional choices if necessary)*	Model#: Manufacturer: Supplier:	Model#: Manufacturer: Supplier:
Meets defined specifications? (Attach details) Functional: Operational:	☐ Yes ☐ No ☐ N/A ☐ Yes ☐ No ☐ N/A	☐ Yes ☐ No ☐ N/A ☐ Yes ☐ No ☐ N/A
Cost of equipment:		
Warranty: Define terms and length		
Maintenance or service: Describe contract, availability, cost, TAT		
Regulatory: Describe regulatory status, IDE or IND use, process validation, and manufacturer or distributor experience in the cellular therapy field.		
Reputation: Describe reliability, customer service, and technical support.		
Change control: Are software updates, recalls, and notification provided?		
Installation requirements: List physical space, plumbing, electrical, alarms, hardware or software, humidity, and temperature requirements.		
Installation assistance: Are installation and qualification, IQ and OQ documents, and calibration certificates provided?		
Training: Describe the availability, the cost, and whether it is provided on site.		
Pros: List other positive features.		
Cons: List other negative features.		

Appendix 10-1. Critical Equipment Selection Form (Continued)

Final selection of equipment:	
Supervisor approval:	Date:
Director approval:	Date:

TAT = turnaround time; IDE = investigational device exemption; IND = investigational new drug.

Appendix 10-2. Equipment Qualification Form

Manufacturer:	Model Number:	Serial Number:
Intended Use or Function:		☐ **Critical** (perform IQ, OQ, and PQ) ☐ **Noncritical** (perform IQ only)
Date Received:	Cellular Therapy (CT) Facility Identifier:	Clinical Engineering Identifier:

Requires Associated Process Validation? ☐ Yes ☐ No
Validation Title and Number:

Installation Qualification	N/A (Initials)	Date Performed	Initials
Inspect packaging for problems during shipment. Ensure that correct items have been received.			
Unpack equipment (on loading dock for large items) and inspect it for damage, missing parts and documents, or other unacceptable conditions. Contact the manufacturer to report problems.			
Place sign prominently on equipment stating: "Do Not Use. Qualification in Progress."			
Clinical engineering (CE) personnel: Check electrical safety, assign CE identifier, apply CE inventory label, and update CE inventory.			
Disinfect all inner and outer surfaces of equipment according to SOP.			
Review all manuals and documentation accompanying equipment.			
Assemble and install equipment, according to manufacturer's instructions.			
Perform installation checks. *Attach documentation of results.*			
Verify that equipment powers up and performs basic functions at startup.			
Verify all connections (plumbing, gas, and electrical) are correct and function properly. List connections:			
Perform checks indicated in the equipment or IQ or OQ manual provided by the manufacturer.			
Verify that computer hardware and software are installed properly.			
Verify that critical parameters of the equipment have been calibrated correctly. List reference instruments in the "Comments" section. List parameters:			
Verify that the calibration certificate has been received and is acceptable.			
Perform an alarm test to ensure that equipment audible and visual alarms activate appropriately.			
Verify any other basic initial specifications not already tested (eg, space and access). List:			
Assign an equipment identifier and label the equipment with the identifier.			
Add equipment to the equipment inventory list and indicate whether QC or PM is required.			
Perform initial training on use of the equipment (by manufacturer if possible).			
Submit the warranty card and establish an equipment file that contains the purchasing documents, manuals, warranty, selection documents, etc.			

Appendix 10-2. Equipment Qualification Form (Continued)

Comments:

Supervisor or Director Approval/Date: ☐ PASS ☐ FAIL

_____/_____

Final Specifications

Functional Specifications: Operational Specifications:

List tests to verify each specification under "Verify specifications" in the OQ or PQ sections, as appropriate. Submit form to the CT laboratory director for approval of the specifications, the OQ or PQ test plan, and the implementation plan.

Director Approval/Date: _____

Operational Qualification: ☐ N/A for noncritical equipment	N/A (Initials)	Date Performed	Initials
Set equipment to normal operating parameters (eg, date, time, temperature control set points, alarm set points, LN_2 level, and CO_2 percentage). List parameters:			
Verify specifications. Describe the test plan and attach a summary of the results.			
Connect critical equipment to the CT laboratory alarm systems. By:			

(Continued)

Appendix 10-2. Equipment Qualification Form (Continued)

Comments:

CT Laboratory Director Approval/Date: ☐ **PASS** ☐ **FAIL**
_____/_____
Comments:

Performance Qualification: ☐ N/A for noncritical equipment	N/A (Initials)	Date Performed	Initials
Verify specifications. Describe the test plan and attach a summary of the results.			
Following implementation, review QC/PM records and the equipment malfunction forms to ensure that fluctuations in performance are negligible and that QC and PM activities are adequate. List period of time for review (eg, 3 months, 1 year):			

Comments:

Appendix 10-2. Equipment Qualification Form (Continued)

CT Laboratory Director Approval/Date: ☐ PASS ☐ FAIL

_____/_____

Comments:

Implementation Plan: Implement after: ☐ IQ ☐ OQ ☐ PQ	**N/A** (Initials)	**Date Performed**	**Initials**
Establish or revise CT laboratory SOPs and forms for use and QC/PM schedules.			
Contact CE personnel to update their inventory with the appropriate maintenance information.			
Conduct staff education and training.			
Remove the sign that states: "Do Not Use. Qualification in Progress" from the equipment.			
Transfer the products or reagents into the equipment. List specific instructions:			

Date Placed into Service:

IQ = installation qualification; OQ = operational qualification; PQ = performance qualification; N/A = not applicable; SOPs = standard operating procedures; CE = clinical engineering; PM = preventive maintenance.

Appendix 10-3. New Equipment Qualification Checklist

Equipment Number	Equipment Name

Items	Date Completed
	Tech Initials
Initial Equipment Receipt	
1. Unpack equipment.	
2. If capital equipment, request an asset tag.	
3. Verify that all parts, manuals, and shipping logs have been received.	
4. Send warranty information back to company.	
5. Submit documentation to Document Control.	
Installation	
1. Attach the equipment identification number and "not in service" sign.	
2. Notify facilities for the initial setup, placement, gas, and electrical hookup.	
3. Ensure that the equipment functions within the manufacturer's guidelines (eg, assembly, electrical checks, initial setup, alarms verification, and calibration).	
4. Request an equipment connection to the continuous alarm system, if applicable.	
5. Record the installation date in the equipment logbook.	
6. Submit all documentation to the quality assurance (QA) department and to the manager, supervisor, or designee for review.	
Standard Operating Procedure (SOP) and Database	
1. Resolve all material safety data sheet (MSDS), hazard, and safety issues.	
2. Review regulations and standards for applicable regulations.	
3. Initiate or revise the equipment SOP.	
4. Create an equipment activity summary or QC log sheets.	
5. Request that document control personnel update the equipment database.	
6. Ensure that QA personnel and the manager, supervisor, or designee review updated equipment database before implementation.	
Equipment Use	
1. Personnel training completed and documented.	
2. Ensure that manager, supervisor, or designee approve equipment for use.	
3. Remove the "not in service" sign and give it to the document control personnel, who update the database with the current "in use" status.	
Manager or Supervisor Review *(signature and date):*	
QA Personnel Review *(signature and date):*	

Appendix 10-4. Equipment Activity Log

Equipment Number	Equipment Name

If a piece of equipment is not used for a time, record the specific dates that it was not used and the reason in the Comments field.

Dates	Activity Performed	Comments	Initials	Review (Initials/Date)

Appendix 10-5. Equipment Requalification Checklist

Equipment Number	Equipment Name

Items	Date Completed
	Tech Initials
Equipment Receipt from Service Provider	
1. Ensure that equipment is labeled with the calibration or preventive maintenance (PM) date, service provider, next due date or expiration date, and equipment number.	
2. Submit all repair and service reports, the calibration certification, and other documentation to the manager, supervisor, or designee for review *before* the service provider leaves the premises.	
Documentation	
1. Obtain the master equipment file (MEF) and logbook from document control personnel.	
2. Record maintenance, repair, and calibration activities on the equipment activity log.	
3. Submit the MEF, if necessary, and logbook to the manager, supervisor, or designee for review.	
4. Receive notification from the manager, supervisor, or designee that the equipment is approved for use and submit all documentation to quality assurance (QA) personnel for review.	
5. Perform any startup procedures appropriate to the equipment.	
6. Clean equipment according to the applicable standard operating procedure (SOP) before use.	
7. Remove the "not in service" sign and give it to document control personnel, who update the database with the current "in use" status.	
Manager or Supervisor Review *(signature and date):*	
QA Personnel Review *(signature and date):*	

Method 10-1. Selecting and Qualifying Equipment

Purpose

To provide instructions for ensuring that all equipment used in the cellular therapy (CT) facility is selected and qualified for its intended use and that it meets specified requirements.

Summary

Critical equipment is defined as any device that has a reasonable potential to affect the quality of cellular therapy products, processes, or services. These devices are selected following a process that starts with the definition of the equipment's intended use and its required functional and operational specifications. Installation qualification (IQ) is performed on all equipment to ensure that it meets the specifications of the CT facility and is properly installed in the facility environment. Critical equipment also undergoes operational qualification (OQ) and performance qualification (PQ) to ensure that it will function consistently according to appropriate specifications during routine use.

Policies and Procedures

A. *General Policy*
   1. All equipment in the CT facility is assigned a unique identifier.
   2. All equipment must be calibrated, maintained, monitored, and used within appropriate environmental conditions according to the manufacturer's instructions and in accordance with applicable standards and regulations.
   3. All equipment should be identified on an inventory list that indicates whether equipment is critical or noncritical and whether it requires quality control (QC) or preventive maintenance (PM). This list should be reviewed annually by management and updated as new equipment is added.

B. *Policy for Selection of Critical Equipment*
   1. Equipment is determined to be critical if it has a reasonable potential to affect the quality of cellular therapy products, processes, or services. This determination is made by management before the purchase of a new piece of equipment.
   2. Most equipment for processing and storage, and some equipment for testing and transport, is considered critical equipment.
   3. The selection of new critical equipment is documented on a critical equipment selection form (Appendix 10-1).
   4. When possible, the CT facility will select critical equipment that has been approved or cleared by the Food and Drug Administration (FDA) for the intended use. If such equipment is not available, it must meet one of the following criteria:
      a. It must be used in an institutional review board (IRB)-approved research study under an FDA-sanctioned investigational device exemption (IDE) or investigational new drug (IND) application.
      b. It must undergo process validation by the CT facility.
      c. It must be recognized and established in the CT field as acceptable for the intended use. Depending on the device, process validation may still be necessary.
   5. Specifications for Critical Equipment
      a. General specifications
         • General specifications should be defined before purchase according to the level of risk to the quality of cellular therapy products, processes, or services associated with the device's not performing as expected. Initial specifications should be defined as completely as possible before selection.

- General specifications may be based on specifications reported by manufacturers.
- General specifications may vary according to the intended use of the device.
- General specifications may be further defined following receipt of critical equipment.

  b. Functional specifications
  - Equipment must be able to perform the specific functions required for the intended use.
  - Specific functions may be required for equipment to perform appropriately in nonroutine situations or worst-case scenarios, such as power outages.

  c. Operational specifications
  - Equipment operates in a specific manner, interfacing with technologists and the physical environment. Understanding how the equipment operates can be helpful in selecting equipment, but the details may not need to be specified.
  - Specific operational requirements may be necessary in some situations and, therefore, need to be specified prior to selection.

  d. Critical equipment candidates are identified and evaluated to determine how well each meets the defined specifications.

6. Management reviews the final equipment selection and gives approval to purchase the equipment.

C. *Policy for Qualification of Equipment*

1. Qualification of new equipment is documented on an equipment qualification form (Appendix 10-2).
2. All equipment must be qualified for its intended use. For critical equipment, this includes establishing that it is able to meet defined specifications after proper installation.
3. The CT facility supervisor or director determines whether the equipment requires an associated process validation.

4. Equipment qualification includes IQ, OQ, PQ, and an implementation plan.
   a. IQ establishes that the equipment is received as specified, that it is properly installed, and that the facility environment is suitable for its operation and use.
   b. OQ demonstrates that critical equipment will function according to the established specifications in the facility environment.
   c. PQ demonstrates that critical equipment consistently performs according to established specifications for its routine use.
   d. The implementation plan provides instructions for placing equipment into service, including the addition of equipment to standard operating procedures (SOPs) and QC and PM schedules, staff training, and the transfer of products, if appropriate.

5. The plan for each portion of the qualification process must be developed in advance and must be approved by management.
6. OQ and PQ are usually not required for noncritical equipment.
7. Once IQ for critical equipment has been completed, the initial functional and operational specifications established during equipment selection are reviewed and the specifications to be verified in OQ and PQ are finalized.
8. A plan for specific tests to verify that the equipment operates according to the finalized specifications is developed. The following considerations should be included in the development of the test plan:
   a. The type and number of samples required to verify acceptable operation.
   b. The frequency of testing.
   c. Which users are adequately trained to perform tests.
   d. What reference equipment is required.
   e. What statistical methods should be used to evaluate test results.
   f. Whether some tests are more appropriately performed as part of PQ.

9. Any worst-case-scenario testing is typically performed during OQ.

10. Noncritical equipment is placed into service upon completion of IQ. Critical equipment is typically placed into service upon completion of OQ. However, critical equipment that requires more extensive qualification may be qualified during PQ.

11. Any specifications that were not tested during OQ are tested during PQ. These may include specifications such as the following that relate to the consistency of operation during routine use:
    a. Parallel testing (eg, split samples) studies between the new equipment and reference laboratories or currently used equipment.
    b. The testing of the repeatability or robustness of equipment when it is operated under varying routine conditions (eg, different shifts or technologists).
    c. The testing of parameters that tend to drift.

12. Requalification is required after changes to equipment configuration that may affect performance—for example, after a significant repair, movement, or modification of equipment, but not after routine PM or a minor repair. Requalification may also be necessary when there is a notable change in equipment performance or in product quality.

D. *Selection of Critical Equipment Procedure*
   When the need to purchase a new piece of equipment is identified, it must be designated "critical" or "noncritical." If management determines that the equipment will be considered "critical equipment," a critical equipment selection form should be completed as follows:
   1. Provide a brief description of the critical equipment that is needed and check the appropriate box to indicate its intended use, including whether the specific products or process is critical to the intended use.
   2. List the initial functional and operational specifications for the critical equipment.

3. In the following situations, it may be acceptable to have only one candidate device and to abbreviate the selection process:
   a. Emergency replacement of a failed device.
   b. The purchase of the same model of an existing device.
   c. The purchase of specialized, one-of-a-kind equipment.

4. Evaluate each candidate to determine how well each meets the defined specifications and check the appropriate box next to "Meets defined specifications?"

5. Provide a brief description for each of the following additional considerations, if applicable:
   a. The cost of the equipment. Obtain a quote from the manufacturer for the purchase price of the equipment, including any required accessories (eg, platform divider for LN_2 freezer).
   b. Warranty. Determine which items (eg, parts or labor) have a warranty and the length of the warranty.
   c. Maintenance or service. Determine if a maintenance or service contract is available from the manufacturer and, if so, the associated cost and approximate time it will take for the technician to make a service call. Determine the hours that technical service is available.
   d. Regulatory status. Determine if the equipment is cleared or approved by the FDA for the intended use, whether an IDE or IND application or a process validation will be required, or whether the equipment is established in the CT field for the intended use.
   e. Reputation. Evaluate the manufacturer's reliability in terms of quality, customer service, and technical support. Contact other users of the equipment, if possible.
   f. Change control. Determine if the manufacturer will provide software updates or notification of product recalls.

g. Installation requirements. Determine the equipment's installation requirements in terms of physical space, plumbing, electrical, alarms, computer hardware or software, humidity, and temperature.

h. Installation assistance. Determine if the manufacturer performs installation or qualification and provides IQ or OQ documents or calibration certificates.

i. Training. Determine if the manufacturer provides any type of training on the use of the equipment, either on site or at an alternate location and, if so, the associated cost.

j. Pros and cons. List any other positive or negative features.

6. On the basis of all of the information obtained, determine which candidate device best meets the needs of the organization. List the final equipment selection on the critical equipment selection form and submit the form to management for review and approval for purchase.

E. *Qualification of Equipment Procedure*

1. When a new piece of equipment is received, initiate an equipment qualification form (Appendix 10-2). List the manufacturer, model number, serial number, date received, and a brief description of the intended use or function, and check the appropriate box to indicate whether this equipment is considered "critical."

2. Submit the equipment qualification form to management for decisions regarding the following:
   a. Whether an associated process validation is required.
   b. Which procedures are required for IQ.
   c. How a plan for implementation of noncritical equipment should be defined.

3. Installation Qualification
   a. Inspect equipment upon receipt for problems during shipment, and compare the equipment with the purchase order to ensure that the correct items were received.

b. Unpack and inspect equipment to ensure that there are no signs of damage or other unacceptable conditions and that all parts and documents were received (eg, operating manuals, maintenance instructions, and calibration certificates). Immediately contact the manufacturer to report damage or other problems.

c. Prominently label equipment with a sign that reads, "Do Not Use. Qualification in Progress."

d. Arrange for the following steps to be performed by the appropriate department:
   • An electrical safety inspection of the equipment.
   • The assignment of an organizational equipment identifier.
   • The application of the inventory label to the equipment.

e. Review all manuals and documentation that accompany the equipment for items relating to equipment operation and function.

f. Disinfect all inner and outer surfaces of the equipment before use, as appropriate.

g. Perform installation or assembly according to the manufacturer's instructions. (This step may be performed by a manufacturer's or vendor's representative.)

h. Perform installation checks and verify basic equipment functions. These checks may include the following:
   • Verifying that equipment powers up and performs basic functions at startup.
   • Verifying that all connections (ie, plumbing, gas, and electrical) are correct and function properly.
   • Performing checks indicated in the equipment or IQ or OQ manual provided by the manufacturer.
   • Verifying that computer hardware or software is installed properly.
   • Verifying that critical parameters of the critical equipment have been

calibrated correctly (eg, temperature, CO_2, or rpm).

- Verifying that the certificate of calibration was obtained and is acceptable.
- Performing alarm testing to ensure that equipment alarms (eg, audible) activate appropriately.
- Verifying any other basic initial specifications that have not already been tested (eg, whether the equipment fits in the intended space, is accessible by staff, and does not restrict passageways).

i. Verify that a unique identifier has been assigned and that the equipment identifier label is prominently displayed.

j. Enter the equipment into the equipment inventory and indicate whether the equipment is critical or noncritical and whether it requires calibration, QC, or PM.

k. Familiarize the staff with the equipment by demonstration and, if indicated, arrange for staff training, either on site or at an outside facility.

l. Submit the equipment warranty form to the manufacturer.

m. Establish a new equipment file, which contains the operator's manual, a copy of the invoice or purchase order, a copy of the warranty form, equipment qualification form and associated installation records, and critical equipment selection form.

n. Submit the completed equipment qualification form to management for review and approval of IQ.

o. Upon approval of IQ, place noncritical equipment into service according to the implementation plan on the equipment qualification form.

4. For critical equipment, consult with management and complete the information on the equipment qualification form:

a. List all functional and operational specifications to be verified in OQ and PQ. Include specifications defined during equipment selection that were not verified in IQ and any additional specifications.

b. List the specific OQ and PQ tests to be performed to verify that the equipment operates according to specifications. Each specification must be tested, although more than one specification may be verified by a single test.

c. List the plan for implementation of the equipment.

d. Submit the equipment qualification form to management for approval of specifications, the OQ or PQ test plan, and the implementation plan.

5. Operational Qualification

a. Set the equipment to normal operating parameters (eg, date, time, temperature control set points, alarm set points, LN_2 level, and CO_2 percentage).

b. Perform all OQ tests to verify that equipment operates properly. Connect the equipment to the central alarm systems, if applicable.

c. Attach the results of OQ to the completed equipment qualification form, and submit the form to management for review and approval of OQ.

d. If the equipment is to be implemented upon approval of OQ, place the equipment into service according to the implementation plan.

6. Performance Qualification

a. Perform any PQ tests to verify that the equipment performs the procedure properly as indicated on the equipment qualification form. Attach the results and submit the form to management for approval before implementation.

b. If the equipment was not placed into service during OQ, place equipment into service according to the implementation plan.

c. Following implementation, review the equipment QC and PM records and the equipment malfunction forms to ensure that any fluctuations in equipment performance are negligible and that PM and QC activities are adequate.

   d. Attach the results of PQ to the completed equipment qualification form and submit the form to management for review and approval of PQ.

7. Implementation plan

   a. Incorporate the required PM, QC, and instructions for use into the SOPs, forms, and schedules. Contact the appropriate departments to update their inventory with the appropriate maintenance information.

   b. Train operators on the appropriate use of the equipment and educate them on any new or revised SOPs, forms, etc.

   c. Remove the sign that reads: "Do Not Use. Qualification in Progress" from the equipment.

   d. Transfer products or reagents into the equipment, if applicable, according to the implementation plan.

Records

Inventory and equipment forms are reviewed by the appropriate management staff and maintained in the relevant equipment files.

Anticipated Results

Appropriate selection and qualification of equipment.

Related Documents

Appendix 10-1. Critical Equipment Selection Form.
Appendix 10-2. Equipment Qualification Form.

References/Resources

1. Padley D, ed. Standards for cellular therapy product services. 3rd ed. Bethesda, MD: AABB, 2008.
2. FACT-JACIE international standards for cellular therapy product collection, processing, and administration. 3rd ed. Omaha, NE: Foundation for the Accreditation of Cellular Therapy and the Joint Accreditation Committee of ISCT and EBMT, 2006.
3. Huber L. In search of standard definitions for validation, qualification, verification, and calibration. LabCompliance, 2001. [Available at http://www.labcompliance. com/solutions/free_literature.aspx?sm=b_d (accessed December 23, 2008).]
4. Huber L. Equipment qualification in practice. LabCompliance, 2001. [Available at http://www.labcompliance.com/solutions/free_literature.aspx?sm=b_d (accessed December 23, 2008).]
5. Huber L, Welebob L. Selecting parameters and limits for equipment operational qualification. Accreditation and Quality Assurance 1997;2:316-22.

Method 10-2. Equipment Management

Purpose

To provide a description of the overall system for managing equipment for a cellular therapy (CT) facility to ensure that each piece of equipment is installed, operated, maintained, and repaired as intended by the manufacturer and according to standard operating procedures (SOPs), and that the appropriate documentation is maintained.

- This procedure applies to equipment used to perform the manufacturing and testing of CT products.
- This procedure does not address the operation and maintenance requirements for individual equipment items. Refer to the specific equipment SOP for individual equipment details.

Materials and Equipment

1. Equipment logbook.
2. Master equipment file (MEF).

Policies and Procedures

A. *Master Equipment Database*

A master equipment database is maintained to track pertinent information for each piece of equipment. The following information should be on file for each item:
- Equipment number.
- Equipment name.
- Equipment description.
- Model number.
- Serial number.
- Manufacturer.
- Vendor.
- Power supply requirements.
- Emergency backup power required.
- Ownership.
- Location.
- Facility identification .
- Maintenance provider.
- Maintenance contact information.
- Maintenance phone number.
- Receipt date.

- Usage status.
- Designation:
  - Critical.
  - Noncritical.

B. *Master Equipment File*

1. An MEF for a specific piece of equipment is initiated at the time of equipment receipt.
2. MEFs are maintained in an area accessible to the laboratory personnel who will be using the equipment. Document control personnel are responsible for the management of the files.
3. Each MEF should include the following sections:
   - Purchase information.
   - Installation information.
   - New equipment qualification checklist (see Appendix 10-3).
   - Operator manual.
   - Maintenance, calibration, and repair documentation.
   - Service provider contact information.
   - Quality control (QC) records (eg, temperature charts and daily start-up records).

C. *Equipment Status*

1. In use.
   a. When equipment is "in use," an equipment activity log (Appendix 10-4) should be maintained in the equipment logbook for documentation of all preventive maintenance (PM) and service activities.
   b. Routine cleaning and QC should be performed on "in use" equipment, and the activities should be recorded on the applicable QC worksheet or equipment activity log.
   c. If the equipment status changes from "in use" to "not in service," as in the case of equipment sent out for repair,

the equipment status changes should be documented on the equipment activity log and applicable equipment shutdown procedures performed.

2. Not in use.
    a. Equipment may require a state of use that includes regular PM or calibration but no regularly scheduled cleaning or daily QC. This state is referred to as "not in use." All equipment considered "not in use" is labeled with a "not in use" sign that displays the date the equipment was removed from use.
    b. If the equipment status changes to "in use," equipment requalification must be performed and an equipment requalification checklist (Appendix 10-5) completed.
3. Not in service.
    a. When equipment is "not in service," maintenance of the equipment activity log and applicable QC worksheets is not required.
    b. If the equipment status changes from "not in service" to "in use," the equipment status change is documented on the equipment activity log, and any applicable equipment startup checklist is completed.

D. *Equipment Logbooks*
1. When an equipment SOP is approved, an equipment logbook is assembled with the specific documentation for that piece of equipment:
    a. Equipment activity summary: A summary of the QC, PM, and calibration activities that must be performed for each equipment item or category.
    b. Equipment QC logs, if applicable.
    c. Equipment activity log: Used for each equipment item to log all activities described in the applicable equipment SOP.
2. Equipment logbooks should be stored in close proximity to the applicable equipment.

E. *Equipment Qualification*
A new equipment qualification or equipment requalification checklist is initiated and completed for each newly received piece of equipment, equipment returned from repair or maintenance, or equipment being put into use from "not in use" status.

F. *Equipment Receipt*
1. All newly received equipment initiates a new equipment qualification checklist.
2. A unique equipment number is assigned according to the facility numbering system.
3. An MEF and an equipment logbook that contains the received paperwork are created.

G. *Installation*
1. A new equipment qualification checklist is completed as installation steps are performed.
2. Facility staff or a service provider install equipment, which may include uncrating, assembly, electrical checks, initial setup, alarm verification, and calibration, depending on the manufacturer's requirements.
3. If the equipment requires continuous monitoring, it should be connected to a central alarm system.
4. Installation information is recorded in the equipment logbook on the equipment activity log.

H. *Validation*
Equipment validation is performed according to the applicable master validation plan.

I. *Initiation of Equipment SOPs*
1. If a new piece of equipment does not have an existing SOP, one must be created. If the new piece of equipment replaces or supplements current equipment, the appropriate SOP should be reviewed and revised, if needed. The operator's manual should be used as a reference when the equipment SOP is written.
2. An equipment activity summary should be prepared for each item or category of equipment. The operator's manual should be used as a reference. The equipment activity summary should be included as an appendix to the new equipment SOP.
3. If daily QC monitoring is required, a daily QC log should be created and included as an appendix to the new equipment SOP.

J. *Yearly Equipment QC, PM, and Calibration Schedule*
The new equipment item should be added to the yearly QC, PM, and calibration schedule.

K. *Training*
1. Employees who will use a piece of equipment must read and sign the appropriate SOPs before training.
2. If required, a manufacturer's technical representative may train employees in the operation of certain equipment. The company that performs the training should provide documentation that is maintained in the employee's training and competency file.
3. If a manufacturer's technical representative does not perform the training, the facility manager, supervisor, or a designee is responsible for training employees on equipment operation and maintenance and for completing training documentation.

L. *Initiation of Equipment Use*
When employee training has been performed and documented, the equipment is ready for its intended use.

M. *Cleaning*
1. Laboratory personnel or a qualified service provider perform routine equipment cleaning according to the applicable equipment procedure.
2. Cleaning activities are documented on the equipment activity log or QC logs located in the equipment logbook.

N. *PM and Calibration*
1. Qualified service providers or trained CT facility staff perform PM and calibration activities according to the applicable equipment SOP.
2. PM and calibration activities should be scheduled with the appropriate service provider. Current contact information should be kept in the MEF.
3. If the equipment requires removal for PM or calibration, the date of the equipment removal and any other pertinent information must be documented.
4. All pieces of equipment should be labeled with the following information after the service is performed:
   a. Calibration or PM date.
   b. Service provider.
   c. Next calibration due or expiration date (applies only to items that have a calibration expiration date and will be dis-

carded upon expiration, eg, thermometers).
   d. Equipment identification number.
5. The service provider should provide a calibration certificate or other documentation that indicates that the appropriate service was performed and that the piece of equipment is ready for use.
6. The maintenance and calibration activities should be recorded. If the equipment is returned from being removed for PM or calibration, the maintenance and calibration activities should be recorded and submitted for review.

O. *Malfunction and Repair*
1. If a piece of equipment malfunctions, the appropriate service provider should be contacted to schedule repair.
2. If the equipment cannot be used and is determined to be "not in service," appropriate personnel should be notified regarding appropriate backup equipment or procedure availability.
3. If the piece of equipment is being removed for repair, the date of the equipment removal and any other pertinent information should be recorded on the equipment activity log in the applicable equipment logbook.
4. If the piece of equipment is being serviced on site, the service provider should service the equipment promptly.

P. *Recordkeeping*
MEFs and equipment logbooks along with their contents should be maintained indefinitely.

Q. *Document Review*
1. Equipment records should be periodically reviewed to ensure that the necessary QC and cleaning procedures were performed.
2. The quality assurance (QA) unit should perform a periodic internal audit of the equipment management system.

Expected Results

All equipment must be operated according to the manufacturer's instructions, facility equipment operation, and maintenance SOPs. All activities should be recorded on appropriate forms and entered into appropriate electronic databases.

Related Documents

Appendix 10-3. New Equipment Qualification Checklist.
Appendix 10-4. Equipment Activity Log.

Appendix 10-5. Equipment Requalification Checklist.

Reference/Resource

1. Code of federal regulations. Title 21 CFR 211 Parts 160, 211.194, 820.72, and 1271.200. Washington, DC: US Government Printing Office, 2008 (revised annually).

In: Areman EM, Loper K, eds
Cellular Therapy: Principles, Methods, and Regulations
Bethesda, MD: AABB, 2009

◆◆◆   **11**   ◆◆◆

Quality Assurance of Supplies and Materials for Cellular Therapy Facilities

Marcia Swearingen, MS, MT(ASCP)SBB

THE MANUFACTURE OF A CELLULAR THERapy (CT) product requires strict attention to quality, from the collection of the source cells or tissue through processing, storage, and distribution. The materials and services used to produce the therapeutic product are critical to its safety and effectiveness. The manufacturers of CT products must be certain that these materials and services meet the specifications they have set. Various mechanisms have been used for oversight of suppliers and vendors, but frequently the most useful mechanism is an actual visit to the supplier's facility to observe and audit the supplier's procedures.

Whether the cellular product is classified as a high-risk biologic ("351" product) or a lower-risk human cellular or tissue-based product ("361" product), the manufacturer of the product is responsible for its safety when it is used as intended. If the cellular material is collected or recovered by another facility and transported to the manufacturing facility, the manufacturer should be familiar with the practices of the collecting facility and be confident that it is in compliance with all relevant regulations and standards. Materials that come in contact with or become a part of a cellular product during collection, manufacture, or storage must be of the highest grade available and must be qualified to demonstrate that they meet the requirements of the CT manufacturer.

Agreements

Each CT processing or manufacturing facility should have a process in place for preparing and maintaining agreements with providers of critical supplies and services as well as with customers for which the program provides CT products or services. These agreements should clearly identify the customer needs and expectations for products and services in a formal document. Those customer requirements should then be incorporated into the product service specifications. Feedback and review of the agreement should be performed routinely, and changes should be made as needed and approved. The following are some examples of agreements that might be considered for a CT program:

Marcia Swearingen, MS, MT(ASCP)SBB, Director of Laboratory Services, San Diego Blood Bank, San Diego, California

The author has disclosed no conflicts of interest.

- Vendor contracts.
- Materials and service contracts with service providers such as the following:
  - Cord blood collection centers.
  - Apheresis centers.
  - Courier services.
  - Infectious disease testing laboratories.
  - Microbiology testing laboratories.
- Physician group orders.
- Product storage agreements.
- Product disposition agreements.
- Informed consent of the donor or patient.

Customer and Supplier Relations

A quality program should have a well-defined process to control critical supplies and customer agreements. The first step in this process is to identify the materials and services considered to be critical in a given program. It is easiest to determine what is critical by evaluating each process or procedure and listing items that affect the quality of the product or service. Critical supplies and services are those that are involved in manipulating, coming in contact with, or testing the cellular product. Table 11-1 provides examples of critical equipment services, materials, and testing.

Supplier Qualification

Critical supplies and services identified in a CT program should be obtained from suppliers that have been qualified on the basis of facility requirements. Each facility should clearly define its expectations for the suppliers and should evaluate them according to such factors as performance, availability, delivery, cost, and support. A system should be set up to qualify the suppliers, provide the documentation, and periodically review whether the suppliers have met the requirements as agreed. Appendix 11-1 provides an example of a supplier qualification survey, a quick reference of qualification guidelines in each category—critical equipment, services, materials, and testing. Facilities can qualify suppliers by such mechanisms as vendor surveys, problem histories, reference surveys, and site visits and audits. Once a supplier has been qualified, the company should be added to a master list for quick reference, updates, and additions. Periodic evaluation of the supplier's performance helps to ensure the supplier's continued ability to meet requirements and specifications.

Table 11-1. Examples of Critical Equipment, Services, Materials, and Testing

Why Critical?	Supplies	Activities
Used to manipulate the cells	(Equipment) Centrifuges Freezers Biological safety cabinets Cell washers	(Services) Preventive maintenance Calibration services Facility cleaning Irradiation Transportation
Come in contact with the cells	(Materials) Anticoagulants Diluents Media Reagents Growth factors and cytokines Cryoprotectants Bags (eg, for transfer, culture, and storage) Tubes	(Testing) Infectious disease testing HLA testing Microbial testing Flow cytometry Colony-forming assays Cell characterization Other release assays and quality control testing

Receipt, Inspection, and Testing of Supplies

A process should be in place to evaluate incoming materials before their acceptance or use. For cellular products regulated as biologic drugs ("351" products), the Code of Federal Regulations (CFR) Title 21, Part 210.3 requires that the facility define acceptance criteria and develop procedures to control material that does not meet specifications. In addition, current good tissue practice (cGTP) requires that materials used in the production of HCT/Ps be sufficiently controlled and verified to meet specifications [ie, 21 CFR 1271.260(a) and 1271.210].

Each organization needs to have a system that allows materials to be brought into the system when they are received at the facility. The warehouse log or database should provide a method to record and trace received materials and inspect, sample, or test them as appropriate to ensure that they meet specifications. The log or database should enable immediate access to at least the following information: materials that have been received; materials that have been qualified, verified, and released; materials that have been rejected; the quantity and location of materials in storage; storage conditions; and whether a certificate of analysis (COA) was included. The materials log or database can also provide a method of documentation for renewal of supplier agreements. Item numbers, lot numbers, and expiration dates of each item should be recorded in the materials database as well as in the processing or manufacturing record for each cellular product. This information can be critically important for rapid identification of affected CT products in the event of a recall.

Validated assays should be used when available to test materials that require identity testing or lot-to-lot equivalence evaluation.

If a problem is encountered during the receipt and verification process, the shipment should be quarantined to prevent inadvertent use of unqualified material. Incoming material that does not meet specifications should be reported to quality assurance personnel and to the supplier. Corrective action may include return of the material to the vendor or destruction of the material.

For security and hygienic purposes, access to warehouse and materials storage areas should be strictly controlled and not directly accessible from outside the facility or from administrative space. The storage area should be free of extraneous and unrelated items to facilitate location of the stored articles when requested. Items considered critical should be protected and strictly controlled as a risk management measure. If labels or stickers are used to identify the status of materials, they should have an explicit purpose and be properly completed.

Facilities should have a procedure for responding to manufacturer or FDA recall of materials used in the production of cellular products. In addition to removing those materials from use in CT production, the facility may need to develop a testing program for stored or banked cellular products that were manufactured using these materials to determine whether they can continue to be made available for clinical use. By recording the lot numbers of all materials used in the production of each CT product, CT facilities can perform look-back procedures and can notify the appropriate parties when necessary to protect the health and safety of product recipients. [See Appendix 8-1 (Chapter 8) for a sample log of incoming critical supplies.]

Appendix 11-1. Supplier Qualification Survey

Supplier name: _____

Address: _____

Contact name and telephone: _____

Product or service provided: _____

Critical (circle one)	**Equipment**	**Service**	**Material**		**Testing**
Supplier is...					
Registered or licensed by the FDA			Y	N	NA
Certified under CLIA			Y	N	NA
State licensed			Y	N	NA
Compliant with GMPs			Y	N	NA
Accredited (by AABB, ASHI, FACT, ISO, or CAP)			Y	N	NA
Specify:_____					
The supplier will or does...					
Have a quality plan in place			Y	N	NA
Provide MSDS			Y	N	NA
Provide a certificate of analysis			Y	N	NA
Notify the customer of changes or problems			Y	N	NA
Have a formal recall process			Y	N	NA
Have a customer complaint and resolution process			Y	N	NA
Agree to on-site audits			Y	N	NA
The equipment and testing supplier will or does...					
Use or provide equipment cleared under 510k			Y	N	NA
Provide SOP assistance			Y	N	NA
Provide a validation plan			Y	N	NA
Validation recommendations			Y	N	NA
Test plans			Y	N	NA
Provide training support			Y	N	NA
Training assistance on site			Y	N	NA
Training tools			Y	N	NA
Reagents or materials for training			Y	N	NA
Provide documentation					
Installation qualification and checklist			Y	N	NA
Preventive maintenance plan and checklist			Y	N	NA
Postmaintenance calibration and checklist			Y	N	NA

FDA = Food and Drug Administration; CLIA = Clinical Laboratory Improvement Amendments; GMP = good manufacturing practice; ASHI = American Society for Histocompatibility and Immunogenetics; FACT = Foundation for the Accreditation of Cellular Therapy; ISO = International Organization for Standardization; CAP = College of American Pathologists; MSDS = material safety data sheet; SOP = standard operating procedure.

In: Areman EM, Loper K, eds
Cellular Therapy: Principles, Methods, and Regulations
Bethesda, MD: AABB, 2009

◆ ◆ ◆   12   ◆ ◆ ◆

Documents and Records

Betsy W. Jett, MT(ASCP), CQA, CQM/OE(ASQ)

FOR THE PURPOSE OF STANDARDS SETTING, AABB defines "documents" as written or electronically generated information, including materials such as quality manuals, policies, processes, procedures, agreements, contracts, labels, and forms. It defines "records" as information captured in writing or electronically that provides objective evidence of activities that have been performed or results that have been achieved.[1] Similar definitions are used in the family of quality management systems standards of the International Organization for Standardization (ISO) commonly referred to as "ISO 9000."[2] The distinction between documents and records is that documents provide information to guide or instruct the reader as to what should happen, and records provide information about what actually did happen. A blank form is considered a document by AABB because it instructs the user as to what data should be recorded. Once those data are recorded, the completed form becomes a record. The completed form may include data such as direct observations, results, and signatures that tell the reader if and how an activity was performed and what was achieved.

Documentation as a Value-Added Activity

ISO 9000 standards describe the value of documentation as enabling "communication of intent and consistency of action."[2] Good documentation helps an organization accomplish its operational and quality goals in a way that conforms to regulatory, accreditation, and customer requirements. It facilitates the uniform training of staff. It provides a means to ensure that processes are repeatable and traceable, and it provides objective evidence of process performance and outcomes. Finally, it allows the effectiveness of operational and quality management systems to be evaluated so that the performance of those systems can be improved.[2]

Many of the documents and records required in cellular therapy (CT) programs are dictated by regulatory agencies and accrediting organizations such as the Food and Drug Administration (FDA),[3-6] the Centers for Medicare and Medicaid Services (CMS),[7] the Occupational Safety and Health Administration (OSHA),[8] the AABB,[1] and the Foundation for the Accreditation of Cellular Ther-

Betsy W. Jett, MT(ASCP), CQA, CQM/OE(ASQ), Chief Operations Officer, Department of Transfusion Medicine, National Institutes of Health, Bethesda, Maryland

The author has disclosed no conflicts of interest.

apy (FACT).[9] CT programs should carefully review relevant regulations and standards when setting up document and records systems to identify externally mandated requirements.

In addition, CT programs should define their own internal requirements for documents and records on the basis of their unique operational and quality management system needs. It is often difficult for organizations to identify what documents need to be created and maintained and what level of detail is sufficient to ensure the effectiveness of their operational and quality management systems without burying themselves in paperwork. Documentation should be a value-added activity. Documents and records should be created where there is an identified need and should be retained only for as long as they are still useful. During the design of any new process, the organization should define the record that will be needed to provide evidence that the process and its outputs meet specified requirements. An important aspect of creating value-added documents and records is to establish a process for how they will be accessed and communicated to those who need to know the information.

Characteristics of an Effective Document

Documents provide guidance and instructions to facilitate sound decision-making and to help ensure that work processes are performed correctly and consistently. The ability of the reader to easily understand the information presented in the document is critical to its effectiveness. The information should be presented in a way that avoids ambiguity. Documents must be kept up to date so that the information presented reflects the organization's current approved policies and procedures.

Plain Language

The Plain Language Action and Information Network provides guidelines for writing effective documents.[10] Documents that are written using plain language tend to be more precise, are more likely to express exactly what was intended, and result in improved reader comprehension. The following are some basic principles of plain language writing:

- Identify your audience and write with that audience in mind.
- Organize material with useful headings that meet the needs of the audience.
- Include only one issue in each paragraph.
- Use short sentences. Two lines long should be the average.
- Keep the subject, verb, and object close together in a sentence.
- Place the main idea before any exceptions and conditions in a sentence.
- Use common words. Avoid noun strings.
- Use the active voice for verbs and avoid turning verbs into nouns.
- Use examples.
- Use tables, vertical lists, or illustrations to present complex information.
- Minimize cross-references.

Instructional Documents

To be effective, instructional documents should be written and presented in a way that promotes accurate comprehension at a reasonable reading speed. Often, a combination of text and diagrams is used. Four cognitive processes are thought to contribute toward successful completion of written instructions[11]:

1. Forming a mental picture or idea of how the procedure should be completed.
2. Encoding the procedure by identifying and memorizing the steps involved.
3. Performing self-checks during the procedure to verify that it is being performed correctly
4. Self-correcting mistakes that were identified during the self-checks.

The following tips for the development of "read-to-do" documents accommodate these cognitive processes[11]:

- Explain the purpose and the intended outcome at the beginning of the procedure. A short paragraph and a picture may be appropriate.
- Break the procedure out into a list of separate, executable actions. Group or outline tasks in complex procedures according to when they occur in the procedure, and use natural breaking points.
- Number each step.
- Separate text that gives advice and warnings from text that describes the action in each step.

- Use a sentence structure that puts the action before any conditions (eg, say, "Clamp the tubing when all of the plasma is expelled," not "When all of the plasma is expelled, clamp the tubing").
- Use a sentence structure that puts the outcome before the action (eg, "Prepare a 4-lead harness using a sterile connecting device," not "Using a sterile connecting device, prepare a 4-lead harness").
- Use pictures and diagrams to illustrate what the outcome of an activity should look like.
- Provide self-checks at natural breaking points or critical steps in the procedure that allow the reader to pause and verify what has been done so far.
- Include instructions for how to correct common problems in the procedure.
- Test the effectiveness of the written procedure before it is implemented. Test it on someone who was not involved in writing it and who has limited experience in performing it.

Forms

Forms should be designed to be user-friendly and to facilitate the creation of accurate and complete records. Clear and succinct form headings and instructions assist the user in recording the right information. The size of data entry fields should allow the user to record the amount of data required by using a font size that is comfortable to read. The visual design of the form should be considered. Effective use of white space and placement of information affect the user's experience and ability to complete the form accurately and quickly. For example, the placement of data entry field labels and descriptors in Web-based forms influences the way that the user interacts with an online form.[12] The alignment of labels and data entry fields affects the time it takes to complete the form and the effort required to understand the information presented.

Document Management

A well-designed document management system provides a structure for the creation, maintenance, archiving, and destruction of documents according to the business, quality, and legal needs of an organization. The system should be designed to ensure that documents in use by the organization are comprehensive, current, and available. Important aspects of a well-structured document management system are described in the following paragraphs.

Document Development and Maintenance

Documents should be reviewed and approved before they are put into use to ensure that they meet the needs of the organization and comply with applicable regulations, standards, and organizational policies. Once put into use, documents should be reviewed and updated to ensure that they continue to meet the needs of the organization and reflect current policies and procedures. Changes should be reviewed and the document revised and re-approved if changes are significant. A document history or audit trail should allow the reader to see what changes have been made and when.

Identification and Version Control

Documents and their revisions should be easily identifiable so that the correct document and version are used. Copies of obsolete documents should be retrieved and archived or destroyed to prevent their inadvertent use.

Access

Current approved documents should be readily available to authorized staff at the time and location in which they will be used.

Retention

Documents should be retained according to the requirements of regulatory and accrediting agencies and for as long as they are useful to the organization. Obsolete documents that provide context for the accurate interpretation of records should be retained for as long as the records that they relate to are retained.

Destruction

Documents should be destroyed in a way that prevents inadvertent use and protects the interests of the organization. Any copies of documents should be destroyed at the same time as the original, at the end of the defined retention period.

Characteristics of an Effective Record

A record is created whenever data or information is captured and stored in written or electronic format. Effective records are easy to read, self-explanatory, and unambiguous. Forms used to capture data should be user-friendly to facilitate the creation of accurate and complete records.

To the extent possible, a record should be self-explanatory, that is, it should not require a separate document for the information to be used and its meaning interpreted. Records should include units of measure, normal ranges, and other descriptors as appropriate to orient the reader and facilitate interpretation of the data.

Records should be created in a way that eliminates ambiguity. Clear definition of the data that make up the record helps to eliminate the risk of misidentification and misinterpretation.

Record Management

Record management includes all of the activities and controls that are put in place to ensure that records are complete, accurate, and preserved for as long as they are still useful to the organization. Important aspects of a well-structured record management system are described in the following paragraphs.

Record Content

The organization should consider several factors when deciding what information must be recorded and preserved. Government regulations and professional accreditation standards require that certain records be created and retained for a specified period. Other data may be important to the organization for the following purposes:

- To successfully complete a process.
- To provide good service and patient care.
- To assist co-workers and other health-care professionals in delivering services or patient care.
- To ensure continuity if the individual is unable to complete an activity once it has been started.
- To provide for supervisory oversight.
- To support training.
- To provide for quality monitoring, evaluation, and improvement.

- To protect the legal and ethical interests of the organization, the donor, and the patient.
- To provide the documentation required for reporting to outside entities.

Record Creation and Alteration

Data should be recorded immediately or as soon as possible after being created (eg, through direct observation, measurement, calculation, or completion of a step in processing). This principle is fundamental to ensuring that records are accurate and complete.

Records should be legible and indelible. Once a record is created, any alterations, including the addition, modification, or removal of information, should be clearly documented in a way that permits the reader to see the original data, the change made to the record, who made the change, and the date and time that it was changed. For future use, it may be helpful to record the rationale for the change if it is not obvious to the reader and the information is important.

Records should be proofread for errors to the extent possible. Processes that rely on transcription, manual data entry, or duplication of data are highly vulnerable to errors. When possible, the original record should be the final record.

Confidentiality and Security

Measures that ensure the confidentiality and security of records are important to preserve the privacy of individuals, promote trust, and protect the organization's business interests and assets. Records with sensitive and personally identifiable information are often protected by two levels of physical or electronic security.

The record management system must protect both physical and electronic records from inadvertent and unauthorized disclosure. It must also protect them from physical damage, alteration, or destruction. Organizations typically create copies of both electronic and physical records and store those copies in a location and manner that will preserve the information if the original records are inadvertently damaged or destroyed.

The records management system should include guidelines and procedures for release of information upon request as well as in emergency situations in which the information may have critical importance for the safety and welfare of an individual.

The U.S. Department of Health and Human Services regulatory requirements for the privacy and security of health-care records are described in the Code of Federal Regulations (CFR) Title 45, Part 164.[13]

Access

Records should be organized in a logical manner for efficient retrieval and stored in a location that allows for timely retrieval.

It is important to pay attention to how records are grouped. For example, information about a donor and recipient on the same physical record may be problematic if one of these individuals requests access to his or her records and the other individual's information is not redacted. The same consideration should be given for records that contain information about more than one family member.

Context

Information contained in records may require context so that it is interpreted correctly because its relevance and meaning may change over time. It is important to retain the context of the information that is stored for long periods to prevent the misuse and misinterpretation of data in a way that could cause harm. For instance, the procedure used to perform a test and the normal range in use at the time may determine the relevance of a test result when it is being used in decision-making or evaluation many years after the test result was generated.

Retention

Records should be retained as specified by legal, regulatory, and organizational requirements. In the absence of specific guidelines, the organization must weigh the risks of retaining records (such as inadvertent disclosure, use of obsolete or outdated information, cost of storage) against potential benefits (such as the availability of information important to the patient or as legal evidence).

Destruction

Original records and all copies of the records should be destroyed in a way that preserves the privacy and rights of individuals. Agreements with outside suppliers who provide record storage, transportation, and destruction services should specify requirements for maintaining security and confidentiality.

The destruction of electronic records is accomplished by destroying the media or by permanently erasing the electronic data. Verifying that all copies of electronic data have been destroyed can be difficult because they can easily be copied for backup and data analysis. The organization's record management system should provide for the control of data backup media and data extraction requests.

Summary

In conclusion, the effective management of documents and records is vital to ensuring that work processes are performed accurately and consistently, to preserving the organization's information assets, to protecting the interests of the patient, and to providing for organizational accountability and performance improvement.

References/Resources

1. Padley D, ed. Standards for cellular therapy product services. 3rd ed. Bethesda, MD: AABB, 2008.
2. American National Standards Institute, International Organization for Standardization, American Society for Quality. ANSI/ISO/ASQ Q9000—2000: Quality management systems—fundamentals and vocabulary. Milwaukee, WI: American Society for Quality, 2000.
3. Code of federal regulations. Human cells, tissues, and cellular and tissue-based products. Title 21, CFR Part 1271. Washington, DC: US Government Printing Office, 2008 (revised annually).
4. Code of federal regulations. Current good manufacturing practice for finished pharmaceuticals. Title 21, CFR Part 211. Washington, DC: US Government Printing Office, 2008 (revised annually).
5. Code of federal regulations. Electronic records; electronic signatures—scope and application. Title 21, CFR Part 11. Washington, DC: US Government Printing Office, 2008 (revised annually).
6. Code of federal regulations. Investigational new drug application. Title 21, CFR Part 312. Washington, DC: US Government Printing Office, 2008 (revised annually).
7. Code of federal regulations. Laboratory requirements. Title 42, CFR Part 493. Washington, DC: US Government Printing Office, 2008 (revised annually).

8. Code of federal regulations. Occupational safety and health standards. Title 29, CFR Part 1910. Washington, DC: US Government Printing Office, 2008 (revised annually).

9. FACT-JACIE international standards for cellular therapy product collection, processing, and administration. 3rd ed. Omaha, NE: Foundation for the Accreditation of Cellular Therapy and the Joint Accreditation Committee of ISCT and EBMT, 2006.

10. Plain Language Action and Information Network. Federal plain language guidelines. Plain 2005. [Available at http://www.plainlanguage.gov/howto/guidelines/bigdoc/TOC.cfm (accessed December 19, 2008).]

11. Burnham C. Improving written instructions for procedural tasks. Working papers. Berkeley, CA: National Center for Research in Vocational Education, 1992.

12. Wroblewski L. Best practices for form design. IA Summit 2007. LukeW Interface Designs, 2007. [Available at http://www.lukew.com/resources/articles/WebForms_Luke W.pdf (accessed December 19, 2008).]

13. Code of federal regulations. Security and privacy. Title 45, CFR Part 164. Washington, DC: US Government Printing Office, 2008 (revised annually).

In: Areman EM, Loper K, eds
Cellular Therapy: Principles, Methods, and Regulations
Bethesda, MD: AABB, 2009

◆ ◆ ◆   13   ◆ ◆ ◆

Audits of Cellular Therapy Facilities

Sharon E. Tindle, MS

QUALITY AUDITS ARE A MEANS OF MONI-toring the quality management system of the cellular therapy (CT) facility. A quality audit is defined as a documented, independent inspection and review of a facility's activities. The purpose of a quality audit is to verify, by examination and evaluation of objective evidence, the degree of compliance with those aspects of the quality program under review.[1,2] Quality audits are performed at defined intervals and evaluate the quality management system by assessing policies and procedures for compliance with applicable regulations and standards and also by assessing the actual process and results against the written policies and procedures.

Depending on the function of the facility, quality auditing in the United States may be required by government agencies such as the Food and Drug Administration (FDA)[3,4] as well as some state departments of health. Other accrediting and professional organizations also require quality auditing in their standards: the AABB,[1] the Foundation for the Accreditation of Cellular Therapy (FACT) and NetCord,[2] The Joint Commission,[5] the College of American Pathologists (CAP),[6] the International Organization for Standardization (ISO),[7] and the Clinical and Laboratory Standards Institute (CLSI).[8]

External Audits

External audits include inspections and surveys performed by regulatory and accrediting organizations not affiliated with the facility being assessed. Many organizations now conduct unannounced inspections. Facilities should have policies and procedures in place that describe how to manage unannounced assessments. These policies and procedures should address at least the following:

- Key personnel to be notified.
- Provisions for the inspection team's work space.
- Responsibilities of individual staff members.

Proficiency testing (PT) is another method of external auditing and is designed to ensure the adequacy of testing methods and equipment as well as the competency of the personnel who perform the testing.[2] PT is usually described as a means of determining laboratory testing performance by using interlaboratory comparisons, in which a PT program periodically sends multiple specimens to members of a group of laboratories for analysis or identification.[6] The program compares each laboratory's results with those of other laboratories in the group or with an assigned value. PT results must then be reviewed, and test outcomes must be presented to staff.[1,2] PT failures must be investigated and corrective actions taken as appropriate.

Sharon E. Tindle, MS, Stem Cell Laboratory Manager, St. Vincent's Comprehensive Cancer Center, New York, New York

The author has disclosed no conflicts of interest.

Internal Audits

The purpose of an internal audit is to verify that a quality management program is in place and to determine whether the quality system and processes related to CT products comply with facility requirements. For facilities subject to FDA regulations, internal audits must assess core current good tissue practice (cGTP) requirements, as defined in the Code of Federal Regulations (CFR).[3]

Determining the effectiveness of the quality program provides an opportunity to review processes, recognize problems, detect trends, and identify areas for improvement. Audits are also used to check any previously identified nonconformance or procedure changes and to assess how effective the changes have been. Internal audits help a facility prepare for external audits. When all these actions are performed appropriately, there should be no surprises when an external auditor comes to the facility.

At a minimum, procedures should be in place for performing the following tasks related to the internal quality audit:

- Scheduling.
- Preparing.
- Conducting.
- Documenting.
- Reviewing.
- Reporting.

Having these procedures in place ensures that the audits are completed routinely by using consistent processes. Although it may not be required that every activity be assessed during every internal audit, each activity should be audited at least once in the audit cycle, usually annually. Depending on the regulations or standards under which the facility operates, specific auditing schedules and procedures may be required. High-risk areas should be audited more often to ensure conformance. A targeted audit can also be performed if a particular problem has arisen, to establish the source of the problem and document any corrective actions.

An example of an internal audit standard operating procedure (SOP) is shown in Method 13-1.

Audit Schedule

Audits should be planned on the basis of the importance of the activity to the quality of the product or service. Particular attention should be paid to critical control points in the processes being audited. For example, audits can focus in depth on one quality system (process or focused audit) or take a more comprehensive view of all the quality systems (system audit). A process audit focuses on a specific process within a system or a specific area within a process. A system audit examines the interaction of the processes that make up a system. Audits can include routine scheduled quality indicators and PT results. For collection facilities, audits should include evaluation of, at a minimum, the documentation of proper donor eligibility determination, the maintenance of sterility, and the meeting of collection criteria. Transplant programs should periodically audit such information as patient outcome, donor screening, testing, engraftment, and treatment-related mortality.[2] Processing and manufacturing facilities should audit quality control (QC) testing results such as cell counts, viability, flow cytometry, microbial contamination, and other product testing. These facilities should also audit their production, storage, and shipping records to ensure accuracy and completion as well as to discover deviations and nonconformances.

Audit Management and Review

The audit plan should define responsibilities, including who will perform the audit and how it will be performed, who will review the results and determine what actions are needed, and how executive management will be informed of the audit process and results.

The auditing plan should also include procedures for dealing with any nonconformances found during the audit. The audit results and any corrective and preventive actions must be communicated to the appropriate staff. The action plan should include a description of the corrective action and a date for it to be completed. After an adequate time is allowed for change implementation, follow-up action is needed to verify and document that corrective actions and preventive actions have been implemented and that these actions are effective.

Auditor Qualification and Training

Audits should be conducted by individuals who have sufficient expertise to identify problems but who are not solely responsible for the process being audited so that the assessor is not auditing his or her own work. Auditor training is recommended, and a formal auditing procedure will assist in keeping the audits uniform.

Auditors should be trained to use appropriate open-ended questions and to not make assumptions without evidence. They should have the following skills:

- Good observational skills and the ability to report factual information.
- Good interpersonal skills, being able to put the auditee at ease and to remain calm when dealing with difficult personalities.
- Good listening skills, encouraging the auditee to talk and being flexible in following where the questions lead, but remaining focused on what is being audited.
- A positive attitude and the ability to note successes as well as problems, emphasizing that the purpose of the audit is not to place blame but to correct problems.

Auditing Methods

There are many methods of performing audits that can be used in various combinations, depending on the requirements of the situation. Methods may include personnel interviews, direct observation, and the review of records and SOPs.

- The approach of observing and asking questions verifies that the written policy or procedure is being followed, that outcomes for any problem areas identified through the quality management process have been adequately investigated and resolved, and that previously cited deficiencies have been corrected.
- Personnel can be asked questions about the procedures being performed. Using open-ended or hypothetical questions (who, what, when, where, why, and how) and asking personnel to show something in response to questions will provide more information than "yes" or "no" questions elicit. The auditor should emphasize to personnel who are being interviewed or are

providing other information that the purpose of the audit is not to look for problem areas so that punitive measures can be taken, but rather to look for evidence that processes are working appropriately and to take advantage of opportunities for improvement.

- Direct observation allows the assessor to verify that SOPs are being followed and to watch for potential problems. Practices that deviate from documented policies and procedures should be noted by the assessor.
- Records, documents, worksheets, and computer reports can be reviewed for completeness and accuracy. SOPs can be reviewed to ensure that they are available to staff, that the version being used is up to date and has been reviewed appropriately, and that SOPs are in compliance with regulations. Documentation of corrective actions for previous deficiencies can be reviewed to ensure that appropriate and effective actions have been implemented.

Auditing Resources

Many resources are available that can be helpful in developing an auditing program. The AABB Web site (www.aabb.org) gives examples of how some facilities have organized their auditing programs with assessment tools and commendable practices. The CLSI Web site (www.clsi.org) offers guidelines that relate to quality management systems. The American Society for Quality Web site (www.asq.org) also provides references for how to conduct an audit.

References/Resources

1. Padley D, ed. Standards for cellular therapy product services. 3rd ed. Bethesda, MD: AABB, 2008.
2. FACT-JACIE international standards for cellular therapy product collection, processing, and administration. 3rd ed. Omaha, NE: Foundation for the Accreditation of Cellular Therapy and the Joint Accreditation Committee of ISCT and EBMT, 2006.
3. Code of federal regulations. Title 21, CFR Parts 16, 1270, and 1271. Washington, DC: US Government Printing Office, 2008 (revised annually).
4. Code of federal regulations. Title 21, CFR Part 820. Washington, DC: US Government Printing Office, 2008 (revised annually).

5. Comprehensive accreditation manual for hospitals. Oakbrook Terrace, IL: The Joint Commission, 2008.

6. Commission on Laboratory Accreditation. Laboratory general checklist. Northfield, IL: College of American Pathologists, 2006.

7. ISO 9001:2000: Quality management systems—requirements. Geneva, Switzerland: International Organization for Standardization, 2000.

8. Application of a quality management system model for laboratory services: Approved guideline GP26-A3. Wayne, PA: Clinical and Laboratory Standards Institute, 2004.

Method 13-1. Internal Audits for the Cellular Therapy Facility

Purpose

To provide instructions for performing internal quality assessments that encompass personnel, reagents, equipment, product quality, patient outcome, and quality improvement. Internal assessments are conducted to verify whether the quality system and the collection, processing, storage, distribution, and administration of hematopoietic progenitor cell (HPC) products and the provision of related services comply with requirements and to determine the effectiveness of the quality program.

Schedule

Routine assessments are performed quarterly, but assessments may be performed more frequently if a problem is noted. Indicators that are monitored continuously are discussed in weekly quality assurance (QA) meetings, and summary reports are reviewed in quarterly transplant QA meetings. These indicators include precollection peripheral blood CD34/mL, postprocessing product CD34/kg, the efficiency of the collection procedure (peripheral blood to final product), sterility, adverse reactions, and technical problems.

Background

A "life of a product" assessment is a systematic examination that is performed at defined intervals and with sufficient frequency to determine whether activities associated with HPC products comply with requirements and standard operating procedures (SOPs) and are suitable for achieving defined objectives. All procedures involved in the life of a specific product, from the initial scheduling of the patient or donor to the final disposition of the product, including quality assessments of personnel, reagents, and equipment used in the procedures, are audited.

Procedure

1. Select the personnel who will perform the assessment. Audits should be conducted by an individual who is not solely responsible for the process being audited so that the assessor is not auditing his or her own work.
2. Randomly select three products processed within the 3 months before the current date. At least one of the three products should have been administered to qualify for the assessment.
3. For each of the products, review the apheresis unit patient and donor files for completeness, including documentation for donor selection and approval, catheter placement, the apheresis procedure, patient care, adverse reactions, and product disposition.
4. For each of the products, review the stem cell laboratory patient and donor files for completeness, including the documentation for processing and infusion procedures, technical problems, and adverse reactions.
5. Review the daily quality control (QC) records for all reagents and equipment used in processing and storage, including documentation for quality control on the day of processing.
6. Review the training and competency records of apheresis unit and progenitor cell laboratory personnel performing the procedures.
7. If any failure to meet requirements is noted, select and audit an additional three examples.
8. Communicate the results of the assessment to the appropriate staff. Management is responsible for any corrective actions, if necessary.
9. Take prompt corrective action on nonconformances found during the assessment. Document follow-up action to verify and record the implementation and effectiveness of the corrective action and preventive action taken.
10. Present reports of the assessment to the medical director, who is responsible for the final

review of all internal quality assessments and corrective actions.

References/Resources

1. Code of federal regulations. Current good tissue practice for human cell, tissue, and cellular and tissue-based product establishments; inspection and enforcement; final rule. Title 21, CFR Parts 16, 1270, and 1271. Washington, DC: US Government Printing Office, 2008 (revised annually).

2. New York State Department of Health. Stem cell banks. Title 10, Subpart 58-5. Albany, NY: New York State Registry, 2004.

3. Padley D, ed. Standards for cellular therapy product services. 3rd ed. Bethesda, MD: AABB, 2008.

4. FACT-JACIE international standards for cellular therapy product collection, processing, and administration. 3rd ed. Omaha, NE: Foundation for the Accreditation of Cellular Therapy and the Joint Accreditation Committee of ISCT and EBMT, 2006.

In: Areman EM, Loper K, eds
Cellular Therapy: Principles, Methods, and Regulations
Bethesda, MD: AABB, 2009

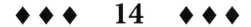

14

Maintaining Safety in Cellular Therapy Facilities through Quality Assurance

Florinna Estioco Dekovic, MT(ASCP)BB, CQA(ASQ)

CELLULAR THERAPY (CT) FACILITIES ARE special, often unique, work environments that may pose a variety of risks to those who work in them as well as to the products manufactured. For the health and well-being of cellular manufacturing staff, safety measures must be implemented to minimize risks and provide security in the facility. These measures are best developed and written in tandem with the quality program. They include mechanisms for preventing cross-contamination of products and personnel and implementation of safe procedures for equipment use. A firm control of the manufacturing environment is ideally supplemented by a suitably designed facility that has appropriate engineering features and judicious environmental management oversight. Additionally, people working with infectious agents or potentially infected materials must be made aware of possible hazards and must be trained and proficient in the methods required for handling such material. This chapter presents practical examples, explanations, and useful audit checklists for meeting safety requirements and provides information that can be integrated into facility standard operating procedures (SOPs).

The Facility Designed for Security

A facility designed with security and safety in mind contributes to workers' protection, which in turn enables them to concentrate on their work with the confidence that they are not subject to illness or injury from dangers in the workplace. A handful of problems that may appear to be trivial to management can significantly affect either the quality of a cellular product or staff performance.

The US Food and Drug Administration (FDA) in its good manufacturing practice (GMP) regulations [Code of Federal Regulations (CFR) Title 21, CFR Part 211.42(c)] states that "Operations shall be performed within specifically designed areas of adequate size. There shall be separate or defined areas or such other control systems to prevent con-

Florinna Estioco Dekovic, MT(ASCP)BB, CQA(ASQ); UCSF GMP Laboratory Operations and Quality Assurance Manager; University of California-San Francisco; San Francisco, California

The author has disclosed no conflicts of interest.

tamination and mix-ups during manufacturing."[3] State and regional authorities as well as accrediting bodies such as the Foundation for the Accreditation of Cellular Therapy (FACT) and AABB may also specify workplace requirements to maintain the safety of staff and the integrity of products. From a safety point of view, practical necessities such as ample lighting, satisfactory worktable space, ergonomically designed computer stations, lab chairs, and comfortable benches at the biological safety cabinets (BSCs) are sometimes overlooked. Other sensible amenities include a suitable hand-washing station, adequate and convenient lavatories, and a gowning area near staff lockers.

Safe movement and flow of both materials and personnel through a facility must also be well thought out. For example, current desirable cleanroom designs allow staff, management, and other spectators to observe manufacturing areas from a segregated vantage point of glass corridors or window partitions. Such an arrangement provides an environmentally controlled boundary between the manufacturing and observation areas. A flow-through map of the facility helps staff to navigate the different functional spaces in a manner that minimizes the introduction of contaminants.

Access to rooms for gowning and de-gowning, processing, preservation, and storage should be limited to authorized personnel. Gowning rooms should provide privacy with hanging ceiling curtains or cubicle rooms for changing.

For facilities that work with open systems, airlock corridors with interlocking doors between classified cleanrooms provide an additional layer of environmental security. Through the use of an electronic card system, the interlocking doors limit entry and exit from critical rooms while facility personnel with authorized access are able to traverse critical areas in a controlled manner.

It is helpful to develop a facility checklist for individual operations to determine if manufacturing spaces meet the requirements for cellular products. An operational checklist may be used as a training tool for new staff and for subsequent auditing purposes.

Personal Hygiene Practices

Contamination control through personal hygiene practices should be observed in any type of laboratory. By far, people who enter and use the processing laboratories contribute the most contamination in a facility. Even the most immaculately groomed individuals generate a shower of particles from their skin, hair, and clothing. Typical lab barrier clothing alone is not enough to maintain low emission of particulates. Perfume, aftershave products, hair chemicals, makeup, and even breath contribute to adverse airborne materials. Certain activities such as smoking, changing contact lenses, brushing and combing one's hair, or applying cosmetics should be strictly forbidden in processing facilities. Cleanroom personnel hygiene rules are further listed in Table 14-1.

Table 14-1. Personnel Hygiene Rules for Working in Cleanrooms

1. Avoid the use of perfumes, hair spray, aftershaves, and heavy makeup.
2. Wear clean, unstarched, low-shedding garments.
3. Be clean-shaven or use beard covers with facemasks.
4. Completely cover the hair with a head covering or cleanroom bouffant. Tie long hair before donning bouffant. Double the hair cover if hair is thick.
5. Thoroughly wash and dry hands before donning gloves.
6. Step on the tack mats at least three times before putting on shoe covers. Ideally, have a pair of clogs or shoes for wearing only in the cleanrooms. No open-toe shoes or sandals are permitted.
7. Use an individual locker to store personal belongings and street clothes.
8. Request duty outside the laboratory or in another nonmanufacturing area when suffering from a viral or bacterial infection.
9. Strictly follow the gowning procedure posted in the gowning room, and use a floor-length mirror to confirm proper gowning.
10. Avoid touching, rubbing, and scratching exposed areas of the body after gowning.

Protection of Personnel in the Cellular Manufacturing Facility

Despite the seemingly straightforward nature of gowning and de-gowning, these tasks, if improperly performed, together with less-than-acceptable aseptic technique, may contribute to out-of-specifications (OOS) incidents in a cellular-processing facility.

Special barrier clothing known as personal protective equipment (PPE) traps and holds particles emitted by the user, protecting the cellular product from contamination by the manufacturing staff. Moreover, PPE protects workers from exposure to potentially infectious cellular products as well. Gowning practices and the use of PPE in a cellular manufacturing facility must be validated, followed, and monitored for compliance. Such disposable PPE as lab coats, gloves, shoe covers, face covers, and head covers must be readily available for staff, trainees, service vendors, and visitors. PPE specific to cleanrooms must be worn in classified rooms. Staff must remove their PPE when entering non-controlled areas or when leaving the manufacturing facility. When staff leave for a brief period, policy should require that they remove and discard PPE and re-gown with a new set of PPE before re-entering the classified areas.

New employees should receive appropriate training related to all aspects of facility safety, especially the use of PPE and adherence to sterile techniques. Correct gowning practice can be facilitated with a series of pictures or diagrams in the gowning areas. These aids are simple to create with the current computer programs available to laboratory personnel. A brief training video of gowning and de-gowning procedures is another useful tool for ensuring compliance for both staff and visitors before entering the cleanrooms.

Other topics that should be included in the employee safety orientation are blood-borne pathogens, biohazardous waste disposal, the use of hazardous materials, radiation safety (when appropriate), the packing and transportation of biohazardous materials, protocol to follow for medical emergencies, and procedures for fires and natural disasters. A personnel safety checklist is provided in Table 14-2.

Aseptic Technique

For protection of both staff and the manufactured product, it is important to train personnel in aseptic technique. "Aseptic" means "without organisms." The practices that help to reduce and prevent the risk of contamination during processing and handling of cellular materials are collectively referred to as "aseptic technique." Because CT products cannot be sterilized or tested for every conceivable infectious agent, personnel must be proficient with procedures for preventing the transfer of organisms to or from the cellular material. The set of such procedures includes some or all of the following: removing or killing microbial organisms from hands and materials, using sterile objects and processing materials, and reducing the

Table 14-2. Personnel Safety Checklist

1. Maintain a staff signature sheet that is up to date and readily available for inspectors.
2. Develop an emergency action plan (EAP).
3. Keep emergency phone numbers readily accessible and in the EAP.
4. Encourage personnel to become familiar with the layout of the facility and the closest exits to each staff member.
5. Enforce compliance with the visitor sign-in and sign-out log.
6. Be sure the eyewash station is accessible. A medical emergency response phone number should be nearby.
7. Install detectors and provide fire extinguishers. Conduct annual fire training and an annual fire inspection.
8. Conduct other disaster (eg, earthquake, flood, tornado, or bombing) training on a regular basis.
9. Conduct radiation safety training, if applicable.
10. Regularly schedule training in blood-borne pathogens and the transportation of infectious substances.
11. Provide trash or biological waste sanitation training.
12. Obtain, and make available, copies of the material safety data sheet and communications regarding hazardous agents.

risk of exposure to microorganisms that cannot be eliminated.

A facility must monitor staff and the environment to ensure that sterile technique is being followed. The procedure that each facility uses to monitor aseptic technique will be based on that facility's initial validation and subsequent validations after major shifts in monitored environmental sterility levels. Table 14-3 contains examples of contamination control measures.

Emergency Preparedness and Action Plans

In addition to basic biological safety, other types of safety survival skills must be addressed in a CT facility. The following questions represent some of the issues that should be considered:

- Are facility personnel prepared to handle accidents, emergencies, and other unexpected events such as hazardous material spills, toxic fumes, the release of ionizing radiation, exothermic reactions, medical emergencies, utility failures, bomb threats, and suspicious packages?
- How does a facility address fire drills during cellular manufacturing?
- Is the facility equipped to assist individuals with mobility or visual and hearing impairments?

- Is someone in the facility responsible for maintaining emergency supplies?

Manuals and procedures for emergency preparedness should be readily available to staff to minimize adverse effects from accidents and potential disasters. Staff should become aware of the location of emergency intercoms and panic buttons, if available. Emergency telephone numbers should be posted within all manufacturing spaces. See Table 14-4 for a suggested checklist for emergency preparedness implementation.

Contamination Control

High-efficiency particulate air (HEPA) filters facilitate the maintenance of air classifications in critical manufacturing areas. HEPA filters, however, are only part of the solution for maintaining sterility in labs performing open-system manufacturing of cellular products. Numerous standard *operational controls* help to limit contaminants in the manufacturing areas (see Table 14-3).

One effective practice for preventing the entry of unwanted microbes in the manufacturing area is the use of tack mats. These are sticky floor mats, usually 2 mm thick, lined with a polyethylene gluey pane that is engineered to remove soil and particulates from the bottom of footwear when stepped on. Each tack mat sheet is impregnated with a

Table 14-3. Contamination Control Measures

1. Follow personnel flow instructions and diagrams through the facility.
2. Promote one-time use materials and disposables.
3. Use powder-free gloves.
4. Use tack mats for shoe debris and for removing dirt on cart wheels.
5. Employ validated cleaning methods. Make disinfectant solutions according to the manufacturer's instructions.
6. Maintain and practice good autoclave procedures.
7. Prohibit particle-shedding paper, paper towels, boxes, or notebooks in the manufacturing areas unless they have been released by QA.
8. Place SOP pages in plastic liners or use a rolling read-only laptop computer.
9. Rewrap and re-autoclave materials that are past the sterilization period.
10. Use primary safety barriers such as the BSC and PPE.
11. Keep BSC sashes and centrifuge lids closed. Cover microscopes when they are not in use.
12. Use sharps containers to prevent needle sticks and cuts.
13. Dispose of biohazardous waste and chemical wastes in appropriately labeled containers.
14. Conveniently locate, use, and replenish spill control kits.

QA = quality assurance; SOP = standard operating procedure; BSC = biological safety cabinet; PPE = personal protective equipment.

Table 14-4. Emergency Preparedness Implementation Checklist

1. Appoint a person to coordinate facility emergency preparedness.
2. Develop emergency notification, reporting, and call-back procedures for staff.
3. Identify an area for facility staff to assemble during an emergency situation.
4. Encourage individuals with permanent or temporary disabilities who might require special assistance in an emergency to identify themselves. Assign a coworker "buddy" to provide assistance to them during an emergency.
5. Monitor and report any nonstructural earthquake and safety hazards to the appropriate facility engineers or campus environment and safety officer.
6. Procure and maintain adequate emergency supplies for facility staff (eg, bottled water, flashlights, extra batteries, first aid supplies, a transistor radio, a screw driver, and a wrench). Rotate the emergency supplies.
7. Annually review and familiarize staff with a standard plan of action for emergencies.
8. Orient new staff and students to emergency procedures.
9. Conduct practice drills for different types of emergency situations.
10. Post facility and campus emergency phone numbers in a visible place.
11. Routinely update the names of all employees on a list to provide to emergency personnel.
12. Become familiar with how to report suspicious activities to the proper authorities.

microbial agent that provides long-lasting protection against the growth of organisms, including mold, mildew, and bacteria. These mats are placed outside the entrance to a controlled area.

Large quantities of contaminants may be released into the air from cardboard boxes and paper brought into the facility. These contaminants should not be brought into cellular manufacturing areas. After supplies and materials are released by quality assurance (QA), they should be removed from their cardboard boxes and then transferred to plastic bins or placed on shelves that are protected with zippered, dust-proof covers. Secondary outer plastic bags should be wiped down with 70% isopropyl alcohol or with an effective decontamination agent before the bags are brought into a cleanroom.

Containment of infectious substances is achieved through use of BSCs. The BSC is the principal device that controls infectious splashes or aerosols generated by many open-system cellular-processing procedures. Proper operation of the BSC when it is used in conjunction with good aseptic technique affords an effective containment system for microorganisms. Class II BSCs have HEPA-filtered air flowing down across the work surface. When working in the BSC or vertical laminar flow hood, staff should follow procedures to prevent obstruction of downward airflow.

Ergonomic Safety

Ergonomic safety is the science of fitting jobs to the people who work in them. Many institutions and university medical centers have ergonomics programs through their environmental health and safety departments. The goal of an ergonomics program is to reduce work-related musculoskeletal disorders developed by workers when a major part of their jobs involves reaching, stooping, bending over to lift heavy objects, using continuous force with equipment and vibrating materials, or doing repetitive motions. Awkward posture while working with one's arms over the head or holding fixed positions often contributes toward musculoskeletal disorders. It is important for a manufacturing facility to understand ergonomic safety and to provide a procedure for staff to report any signs or symptoms. Managers should be aware of early warnings of cumulative trauma disorders such as back pain, neck and shoulder pain, and hand or wrist pain that may contribute to repetitive motion injuries.

Safety While Using Compressed Gas Cylinders

Some CT facilities may perform operations (eg, cell expansions, cryopreservation, and sterile autoclaving) that require the use of compressed gases con-

Table 14-5. Sections of the Material Safety Data Sheet

1. Product information: Identification of the substance, scientific name, common name, manufacturer and emergency phone numbers, and hazard rating.
2. Composition and information on ingredients.
3. Hazards identification: Data on flammability, reactivity, chronic hazardous exposure (eg, highly caustic or severely irritating to eyes and skin).
4. First aid measures: Description of recommended immediate first aid.
5. Firefighting measures: Flash point information, recommended firefighting apparatus, methods, and products to use.
6. Accidental release: Measures to be taken if a chemical is spilled on soil, spilled into waterways, or mixed into sources of drinking water.
7. Recommended handling and storage.
8. Exposure control and personal protection: Occupational exposure limits and specific PPE required (eg, respiratory protection; skin, eye, and face protection).
9. Physical and chemical properties: Unique characteristics such as weight, water solubility, appearance, odor, boiling point, pH, viscosity, evaporation rate, freezing point, vapor pressure, and vapor density.
10. Stability and reactivity: Incompatible materials, conditions to avoid, and dangerous by-products of decomposition.
11. Toxicological information: Possible data on known carcinogenic properties and information on the acute and chronic toxicity if swallowed, inhaled, or absorbed.
12. Ecological information: Information on the ecotoxicity of the chemical substance and its biodegradability in different environments (eg, "Do not release into the environment without proper government permits").
13. Disposal considerations: References to local requirements regarding disposal of the hazardous substance.
14. Transport information: Shipping name; hazard class; UN number; package group by ground, air, or sea; reference to DOT regulations.
15. Regulatory information: EPA and EU classifications, hazard symbols, safety phrases, and applicable state regulations.
16. Other information: Abbreviations used in the MSDS and references to EU directives or ISO standards.

PPE = personal protective equipment; DOT = Department of Transportation; EPA = Environmental Protection Agency; UN number = United Nations identification number; EU = European Union; MSDS = material safety data sheet; ISO = International Organization for Standardization.

tained in cylinders. These operations pose special risks because the cylinders contain gas under high pressure. Regardless of the properties of the gas, any gas under pressure can explode if the cylinder is improperly stored or handled. Likewise, inappropriately releasing the gas from a compressed gas cylinder may be extremely dangerous because a sudden release of gas can cause a cylinder to become a missile-like projectile.

To prevent dangerous situations, the following measures are suggested:

- Cylinders should be stored in a well-ventilated area, away from heat and ignition sources.
- Empty cylinders should not be stored with full cylinders.
- Cylinders that contain oxidizers must be stored at least 20 feet away from flammable gases.
- Cylinders must not be dropped, allowed to fall, or allowed to be struck by another object. They should be chained and racked in an upright position during use and storage. If the tanks are not securely held in racks, they should be double strapped to the wall.
- Before a cylinder is used, a proper pressure-reducing regulator should be installed on the valve. After installation, the user should verify that the regulator is working, all gauges are operational, and all connections are tight.
- All systems must be leak-tested at every connection after setup and after changing cylinders.
- When a cylinder is moved, even for a short distance, all valves must be closed, the regulator removed, and the valve cap installed.
- A properly designed cart with straps should be used to move a cylinder. Slings or magnets should never be used.
- Cylinders should never be permitted to contact live electrical equipment or grounding cables.

- Cylinders should be protected from the sun's direct rays, especially in high-temperature climates.
- Valves should be opened slowly by hand, not with a wrench.

Material Safety Data Sheets and Hazardous Materials

A comprehensive safety program or hazardous material (HAZMAT) program includes developing, maintaining, and training staff who handle hazardous materials used in the facility. The document that contains information about a given hazardous material is called the material safety data sheet (MSDS) and may be requested directly from the manufacturer or the distributor of the material. MSDS information must be up to date and should be available both to workers exposed to the materials and to emergency personnel.

The HAZMAT program should describe the safe handling, storage, and disposal of chemical agents and should delineate the potential health effects of exposure to dangerous chemicals.

MSDS formats may range from one page to numerous pages. The American National Standards Institute (ANSI) "Standard for Hazardous Industrial Chemicals—Material Safety Data Sheets—Preparation" (Z400.1-1998) requires that the MSDS contain 16 sections as shown in Table 14-5.

References/Resources

1. Padley D, ed. Standards for cellular therapy product services. 3rd ed. Bethesda, MD: AABB, 2008.
2. Code of federal regulations. Current good manufacturing practices: Applicability of current good manufacturing practice regulations. Title 21, CFR Part 210.2. Washington, DC: US Government Printing Office, 2008 (revised annually).
3. Code of federal regulations. Good manufacturing practices: Buildings and facilities. Title 21, CFR Part 211.42. Washington, DC: US Government Printing Office, 2008 (revised annually).
4. Code of federal regulations. Biologics regulations: Physical establishments, equipment, animals, and care. Title 21, CFR Part 600.11. Washington, DC: US Government Printing Office, 2008 (revised annually).
5. Code of federal regulations. Quality systems. Title 21, CFR Part 820. Washington, DC: US Government Printing Office, 2008 (revised annually).
6. Code of federal regulations. Human cells, tissues, and cellular and tissue-based products. Title 21, CFR Part 1271. Washington, DC: US Government Printing Office, 2008 (revised annually).
7. Code of federal regulations. Occupational safety and health standards: Hazard communications; guidelines for employer compliance. Title 29, CFR Part 1910.1200. Washington, DC: US Government Printing Office, 2008 (revised annually).
8. Code of federal regulations. Hazardous materials regulations. Title 49, CFR Part 171. Washington, DC: US Government Printing Office, 2008 (revised annually).
9. Food and Drug Administration. Guidance for industry: Sterile drug products produced by aseptic processing—current good manufacturing practice. (September 2004) Rockville, MD: CBER, CDER, and ORA, 2004.
10. Food and Drug Administration. Pharmaceutical cGMPs for the 21st century—a risk-based approach. Second progress report and implementation plan. (September 3, 2003) Rockville, MD: CDER, 2003.
11. American National Standards Institute. American national standard for hazardous industrial chemicals—material safety data sheets—preparation. ANSI Z400.1-1998. Washington, DC: ANSI, 1998.
12. International Organization for Standardization. Cleanrooms and associated controlled environments—Part 1: Classification of air cleanliness. ISO 14644-1, 1999. Geneva, Switzerland: ISO, 1999.
13. University of California at San Francisco, Office of Environmental Health and Safety. Safe use of compressed gas cylinders. Safety update newsletter (October/November/December) 2007;7:3.
14. State of California. Hazard communications regulation. 8 California Code of Regulations 5194. Sacramento, CA: State of California, 2008.
15. State of California. Repetitive motion injuries. 8 California Code of Regulations 5110. Sacramento, CA: State of California, 2001.
16. Centers for Disease Control and Prevention. General safety training manual. (December 1, 2004) Atlanta, GA: CDC Office of Health and Safety, 2004. [Available at http://www.cdc.gov/od/ohs/safety/safety.htm (accessed January 14, 2009).]

Facilities: General Procedures

THE CONDITIONS OF THE ENVIRONMENT within which cellular therapy (CT) products are manufactured, tested, and stored often have a direct impact on the potency, safety, and stability of those products. Besides the importance of the design of the facility, its operation and maintenance are critical factors in the suitability of the facility for its intended purpose. Among the key variables that must be considered when the design and operational controls of the facility are being developed are the following:

- The type and number of products intended to be processed.
- The open or closed nature of the processes.
- The number and type of staff required.
- The equipment, reagents, and supplies required.
- The stage of product development involved, from preclinical studies to commercial production.

The Food and Drug Administration (FDA) has divided ex-vivo processing of cellular products into two categories: *minimally manipulated* and *more-than-minimally manipulated.* The manufacture of minimally manipulated cellular products uses procedures that do not alter the basic characteristics and function of the cells. Some examples of minimal manipulation are cryopreservation, thawing, density gradient separation, the washing and diluting of cell products before reinfusion, and simple cell selection and depletion. The manufacture of more-than-minimally manipulated products involves procedures that may alter the biological characteristics of the cells in the cellular products and includes ex-vivo expansion and gene modification. The FDA regulates all CT products and CT manufacturing facilities in the United States, regardless of the type of manipulation performed. However, the agency uses a risk-based approach to

Section Editors: Robert A. Preti, PhD, President and Chief Scientific Officer, Progenitor Cell Therapy, LLC, Hackensack, New Jersey, and John R. Godshalk, MSE, MBA, Senior Consultant, Biologics Consulting Group, Inc, Alexandria, Virginia

The editors have disclosed no conflicts of interest.

the regulation of products in the two categories. Manufacturers that perform minimal manipulation are required to follow current good tissue practice (cGTP)—as defined in the Code of Federal Regulations (CFR) Title 21, CFR Part 1271—whereas manufacturers involved with more-than-minimally manipulated procedures must comply with current good manufacturing practice (cGMP), as defined in 21 CFR 211, as well as the core cGTPs. Manufacturers who perform both types of procedures must comply with the regulations applicable to the specific procedure being performed on a particular cellular product.

In: Areman EM, Loper K, eds
Cellular Therapy: Principles, Methods, and Regulations
Bethesda, MD: AABB, 2009

◆ ◆ ◆   **15**   ◆ ◆ ◆

Key Considerations and General Procedures for Facilities

Robert A. Preti, PhD, and John R. Godshalk, MSE, MBA

THE FOLLOWING SPECIFICATIONS ARE CRITical in the design and operation of cellular therapy (CT) manufacturing facilities, especially facilities subject to the drug and biologics regulations [current good manufacturing practice (cGMP)]. Many of these factors are described in more detail in the chapters that follow.

- Facility design should provide sufficient capacity for the products anticipated to be manufactured, tested, and stored within the facility.
- The facility should conform to all local, regional, and national codes and regulations appropriate to handling biological products and to aseptic manufacturing. This includes the requirement to obtain and maintain all necessary licenses to do business as a pharmaceutical or biological manufacturer in the location where the company will be operating.
- As an entity engaged in the manufacture of a product that is subject to licensure under Section 351 of the Public Health Service (PHS) Act (42 US Code 262) as amended by the Food and Drug Administration Modernization Act of 1997

(Public Law 105-115), a facility should be registered with the FDA in accordance with registration and listing provisions in 21 CFR 207, 607, or 807. The facility must comply with applicable provisions of the Food, Drug, and Cosmetic Act (FD&C Act), 21 CFR 207, 607, or 807. Facilities that manufacture cellular products regulated solely under Section 361 of the PHS Act must also register with the FDA as described in 21 CFR 1271.3. In the United States, certain states may also have requirements.

- The facility should contain the following key areas: administrative and office space; computer, networking, and telephone system space; warehousing and shipping and receiving areas; mechanical and utility areas; quality control (QC) and microbiology laboratory space; manufacturing support areas; and appropriate manufacturing space.
- The administrative and other manufacturing support functions (where products are not present) may be performed in locations separate from the manufacturing facility. Personnel break

Robert A. Preti, PhD, President and Chief Scientific Officer, Progenitor Cell Therapy, LLC, Hackensack, New Jersey, and John R. Godshalk, MSE, MBA, Senior Consultant, Biologics Consulting Group, Inc, Alexandria, Virginia

The authors have disclosed no conflicts of interest.

rooms and training rooms should be provided both in the manufacturing building and at support locations.

- The facility design should incorporate unidirectional raw material or component, product, operator, and waste flow to ensure maximum segregation and minimum crossovers.
- The facility design should consider the requirements for perimeter security and access restrictions to controlled areas within the facility.
- There should be sufficient parking available for staff and couriers and adequate lighting and safety features in the parking area to support the standard operating hours of the facility.
- The facility should meet Occupational Safety and Health Administration (OSHA) standards and other local, state, and federal codes for laboratory environments.
- The facility should have established appropriate design requirements for mechanical systems.
- A detailed construction design specification document should be issued to all contractors. This document sets standards and requirements for all mechanical, plumbing, piping, and electrical systems appropriate to the products being processed.
- Facility sanitization in GMP should use the appropriate grade of water [pharmaceutical grade water (water for injection, or WFI) or purified water grade systems that comply with USP standards] for cleaning. The appropriate quality of water (according to USP standards) should be used to formulate cleaning and sanitization solutions for the facility, either by on-site production or by purchase from outside ven-

dors. Sterile filtered water may be used to formulate solutions intended for cleaning and disinfecting aseptic processing areas.
- The facility should maintain an appropriate pest control and sanitation program according to approved procedures.

Manufacturing Area Requirements

The nature of the cellular products intended for manufacture in the facility should dictate the air classification of the manufacturing suites (see Table 15-1). In general, all products that are manufactured by the use of open systems should be manufactured in International Organization for Standardization (ISO) 5 (formerly Class 100) biological safety cabinets (BSCs) in rooms that are designed to control the environment to a degree commensurate with the products being processed. The manufacturer should consult with a qualified consultant and with the FDA before finalizing facility classifications. For most CT products subject to cGMP regulations, the aseptic processing guidance should be followed.[2] Manufacturing should be performed in ISO 7 manufacturing suites and all open steps performed in ISO 5 BSCs located within an ISO 7 area.

For products that are manufactured in systems that have been demonstrated to be closed through aseptic process validation, "unclassified but controlled" manufacturing suites are typically used. For design purposes, these areas are built with the same materials and systems as ISO 8, including high-efficiency particulate air (HEPA) filtered air,

Table 15-1. Air Classification Standards: US Federal and ISO Comparisons and Viable Count Action Levels[1]

Clean Area Classification (0.5 μm particles/ft³)	ISO Designation	>0.5 μm Particles/m³	Active Air Action Levels (Viable CFU/m³)	Passive Air Sampling Action Levels*
100	5	3,520	1	1
1,000	6	35,200	7	3
10,000	7	352,000	10	5
100,000	8	3,520,000	100	50

*Microbiological settling plates diameter of 90 mm; CFU/4 hours.
ISO = International Organization for Standardization; CFU = colony-forming unit.

but they are not controlled or monitored as ISO 8 systems. In Europe, these areas may be referred to as Class D or E, whereas in the United States the term most often used is "unclassified but controlled."

The facility should be designed and operated in compliance with appropriate FDA regulations, including 21 CFR 210, 211, 600, 610, and 1271.

The requirements for the provision of dedicated (cleanroom) areas that are adequately segregated from other products being manufactured in the facility should be considered on the basis of the nature of the products and the volume of processing.

The build-out plan should take into consideration such requirements as clean spaces with non-shedding materials, sealed seams, coved corners at walls and floor meeting junctions, and a monolithic construction design that will make the processing areas and room finishes (ceilings, floors, walls) easily cleanable. Requirements for the frequency and intensity of environmental monitoring should be considered.

The facility should be equipped with and monitored for appropriate air ventilation, HEPA filtration, air exchanges, and air pressure differentials. Positive pressure to the less clean environment should be maintained. Access should be limited to appropriately trained individuals and controlled to maintain pressurization differentials.

Consideration should be given to the level of design qualification (DQ), installation qualification (IQ), operational qualification (OQ), and performance qualification (PQ) of the facility and systems.

The conceptual facility plan should anticipate the appropriate flow of the product, materials, personnel, and waste through the facility. The plan should incorporate the principles of single-direction with minimal crossover, as feasible, and should allow for appropriate levels of segregation and isolation. All aseptic manufacturing areas, adjacent corridors, and associated gowning and de-gowning rooms should be at a minimum classification of ISO 8. Pressurization or airflow and classification or air handler diagrams should be part of the conceptual design plan.

Facility design should allow for multiple levels of gowning for the different ISO cleanroom classifications and should ideally provide for independent gowning and de-gowning areas. However, when closed systems are employed, one level of gowning may be adequate. Levels of gowning appropriate to each functional area within the manufacturing facility should be described and posted. Gowning and de-gowning rooms should be provided to facilitate unidirectional personnel flow, particularly when personnel are performing aseptic processing. Such gowning rooms should have the same classification as the area that they safeguard.

The design of the facility should take into account segregation through individual air-handling units and restrictions on personnel movement between "modules" to avoid mix-up or cross-contamination during manufacturing. This subject is discussed in detail later in this section.

Ideally, each cleanroom should have an independent heating, ventilation, and air conditioning (HVAC) unit with ceiling terminal HEPAs and side-wall- or low-wall-ducted returns for recycling and exhaust. The air-handling units should be accessible so that maintenance can be conducted from the outside without breaching the classified environment inside the modules. Air handlers for classified processing areas must be separate from those for unclassified and office areas.

Design and construction should allow for modular growth and expansion of facility space to meet the ramp-up of volume demand without affecting ongoing manufacturing processes. Use of the modular approach should be considered to permit expansion of the manufacturing areas in more than a single direction, if necessary. The plan should anticipate the need for the expansion of one or more modules at a time and connection to existing operational areas, after validation is completed and after any required regulatory approvals have been obtained.

Temperature and Humidity

The cleanroom processing area should be able to operate at a range of temperature and humidity levels determined by the product being manufactured and the comfort of the operators. Humidity must be controlled in classified areas. Typical relative humidity (RH) control limits are 20-80% RH or 30-70% RH. Ideally, in rooms where liquid nitrogen freezers are used, the humidity will be kept low to avoid excess frost buildup, whether or not these areas are classified. All controlled areas should be monitored and controlled by a validated HVAC system.

Space Requirements

The CT manufacturing area must be of adequate space to maintain the aseptic environment and the product segregation required for the specific operation, considering the equipment and the number of personnel. The facility should provide for secured storage of raw materials, components, and controlled documentation. Areas within the manufacturing space should be provided for accessioning of incoming cellular components and for quarantine and holding of finished products until their release.

Because the requirements for cleanliness are less stringent for QC and testing laboratories than for manufacturing areas, it may be practical to separate these sections from one another by using pass-through boxes or windows to transfer test samples. Accessioning and sampling areas may also be separate from processing areas, using the same pass-through design.

An additional or separate manufacturing area may be required to process samples from high-risk or seropositive patients or donors. Such areas should be designed as containment areas and should be segregated at the workstation level, including the installation of an independent HVAC system with 100% exhaust. Ideally, personnel entering these areas of the facility should not be allowed into other manufacturing areas on the same day, and the requirement for re-gowning should be considered.

Manufacturing Support Area Requirements

Considerations should be made for operating adjacent laboratories as controlled clean spaces. One way to accomplish this is to arrange for appropriate ISO 8 cleanroom areas (manufacturing support or laboratories) that surround or are adjacent to the ISO 7 manufacturing areas that have ISO 5 BSCs (for open processes) within the ISO 7 area.

Entry to the manufacturing support area should be restricted to personnel who are authorized to access the manufacturing space.

QC Laboratory and Microbiology Laboratory Requirements

Depending on the hazard level of the products tested, QC and microbiology laboratory spaces may be operated as controlled clean spaces and maintained at an appropriate positive or negative pressure differential to the surrounding laboratory and office space. The following factors should be considered in the design of the QC and microbiology laboratory components of the CT manufacturing facility:

* QC and microbiology labs should be designed to support current and future in-process and product release testing requirements at the projected load capacity.
* If mycoplasma testing is performed, QC labs should have an appropriate segregated space to accommodate mycoplasma testing by polymerase chain reaction (PCR).
* Microbiology labs should provide appropriate segregation for sterility analysis samples from other analytical or microbiological work spaces. This provision often includes having classified areas for sterility testing.
* QC labs should contain dedicated space for the accessioning of incoming cellular raw material and the release (hold and shipment) of the final manufactured products.
* QC labs should include controlled and monitored temperature and humidity storage.
* Appropriate provisions should be made for the QC and microbiology laboratories to conduct environmental-monitoring activities.
* The QC and microbiology laboratories should be sized to accommodate facility production and should be environmentally controlled according to the requirements of the products manufactured or tested in the facility.

Information Technology Infrastructure

Consideration should be given to the current or future computerization of the operations in the QC, materials, manufacturing, and microbiology areas. Validated instrumentation may be associated with each workstation and integrated with individual pieces of equipment when electronic interface capability is available for the instrument. In addition, each of these instruments may be equipped with bar-code-reading capability for identifying samples and matching them with their origin. Depending on the level of development of an electronic batch record, sample analytical data may be uploaded into a database, which will reduce the need for calculations and paperwork. Software used for any part of production must be validated or verified. Software and computer validation are discussed later in this section.

Mechanical and Utility Requirements

Facility and Equipment Monitoring, Maintenance, and Alarm Systems

Consideration should be given to selecting an automated building management system that will incorporate control, monitoring, and alarm functions. At a minimum, an appropriate alarm monitoring system with call-out capability should be installed for critical equipment. Facility, equipment, and environmental controls should be described in an equipment master plan. Equipment and HVAC should be subject to an appropriate level of IQ, OQ, or PQ to meet or exceed product manufacturing standards. Consideration should be given to each piece of equipment's IQ requirement for space, utilities, and monitoring. In the absence of a dedicated metrology department, the company must qualify and engage a subcontractor to manage the calibration and routine preventive maintenance needs of the facility. Equipment redundancy and support by an emergency backup generator ensure uninterrupted processing capability.

Compressed Gases

The facility may need medical grade CO_2, N_2, and compressed air, with appropriate backup systems. Sufficient space should be provided within mechanical areas of the manufacturing building for the storage and operation of a medical gas system, including automated tank changeover, monitoring, and alarm system, as required.

Liquid Nitrogen

The need for liquid nitrogen storage should be considered and should be provided for in a manner appropriate to the facility layout and requirements. Liquid nitrogen is often used for storage of cryopreserved CT products. Ideally, a central tank for the bulk storage of liquid nitrogen with an appropriate delivery system and monitoring should be employed.

Emergency Backup Power Systems

An emergency uninterruptible power supply (UPS) and electrical generation system should be considered to maintain the operation of appropriate systems in all manufacturing and support areas. The emergency generator should supply power automatically in the event of a power failure, and full power should be restored within an interval appropriate to the manufacturing tolerances and criticality of the products processed in the facility.

Warehouse Requirements

The warehouse should have appropriate attributes and environmental controls for the types of materials stored and should comply with appropriate cGMP requirements for quarantined and released inventory. It should be environmentally controlled to prevent the damage and deterioration of items that require storage at room temperature and should provide secured material storage areas off the floor. Restricted access to all quarantine and storage areas should be required. The warehouse should have clearly visible GMP signage for all material areas. Appropriate controlled and monitored temperature and humidity storage for both quarantined and released products should be provided. The shipping and receiving (S/R) area should contain an appropriate number and type of loading docks for receiving raw materials and gas tanks from commercial vehicles. S/R areas should provide adequate space for staging, shipping, and receiving materials that range from individual boxes to full pallets. Consideration should be given to the segregation and control of incoming cellular materials and final product pickup.

All of the factors described in this chapter are critical to the design and operation of a facility that manufactures GMP CT products, and many of these factors also apply to products that are minimally manipulated (GTP). The rest of this section describes systems and processes for developing and operating a quality CT facility.

References/Resources

1. International Organization for Standardization. Cleanrooms and associated controlled environments—Part 1: Classification of air cleanliness. ISO 14644-1, 1999. Geneva, Switzerland: ISO, 1999.

2. Food and Drug Administration. Guidance for industry: Sterile drug products produced by aseptic processing—current good manufacturing practice. (September 2004) Rockville, MD: CBER, CDER, and ORA, 2004.

In: Areman EM, Loper K, eds
Cellular Therapy: Principles, Methods, and Regulations
Bethesda, MD: AABB, 2009

◆◆◆   16   ◆◆◆

Aseptic Processing

Angela Ondo, MT(ASCP)

ASEPTIC PROCESSING IS THE STRICT CONtrol of a manufacturing process to minimize the risk of contamination or cross-contamination of the manufactured product. Because terminal sterilization, (the sterilization of the product in its final container), is not feasible for cell therapy (CT) products composed of living cells,[1] aseptic processing must be used during product manufacturing, especially when open manipulations are performed. Aseptic manipulations typically occur in an ISO 5 (formerly Class 100) environment under laminar airflow [in a biological safety cabinet (BSC)].

Aseptic processing is a complete approach to product manufacturing and is not limited to the manipulation of the product. The aseptic processing approach encompasses all activities that are performed, to reduce the risk of contamination of the product, including activities that concern the environment and its controls, personnel training and monitoring, and the validation of the aseptic process itself. An example of a procedure for performing aseptic technique in a cell-processing facility is shown in Method 16-1.

The Environment

The environment for aseptic processing is usually an ISO 5 (Class 100) BSC within an ISO 7 background. The facility in which the BSC is located, however, may range from a laboratory with controlled air quality to a cleanroom suite with classified air quality. Emphasis should be placed on performing all open manipulations under aseptic conditions in an ISO 5 BSC with at least a controlled (unclassified but controlled), and preferably an ISO 7, background. See Method 16-2 for an example of a procedure for operation and maintenance of the BSC.

The maintenance and cleaning of the manufacturing environment are critical components of aseptic processing, and standard operating procedures (SOPs) should be in place that specify cleaning methods and frequency of use. At the end of component processing, a documented changeover process often occurs. Depending on the type of facility, the type of products processed, and the risk to the process, this changeover may involve saniti-

Angela Ondo, MT(ASCP), Quality Assurance Officer, Cell Therapy Laboratory, Sidney Kimmel Cancer Center at Johns Hopkins, Baltimore, Maryland

The author has disclosed no conflicts of interest.

zation of the BSC and all equipment used during the process and may even include sanitization of the entire processing suite.

Laboratory controls should be established to monitor the environment of the processing area throughout the manufacturing process. An environmental monitoring program should provide information on the quality of the aseptic environment. At a minimum, the program should involve periodic use of a passive air sampler or settling plate in the BSC during open processing. When there are extensive open manipulations, it may also be useful to obtain sampling of the BSC surfaces with a touch plate or swab. The environment in which the BSC is located can affect the aseptic processing environment. Therefore, a procedure should be in place for determining the air quality of the manufacturing area. The extent and frequency of air quality monitoring outside the BSC will depend on the type and history of the environment. When the aseptic processing method requires the facility to maintain a high level of air quality, active air monitoring should be employed to assess the microbial content of the air. In an unclassified but controlled background outside the BSC, the air quality can be monitored, at a minimum, with routine particle monitoring to detect deviations in the normal air cleanliness.

Personnel

Personnel Training

Proper training in aseptic processing is necessary for all individuals who will be performing steps in the aseptic manufacturing process. Training should include the following[1]:
- Aseptic technique.
- Cleanroom behavior.
- Working in the BSC.
- Microbiologic techniques.
- Appropriate hygiene.
- Gowning.
- Cleanroom safety.
- Specific aseptic processing procedures.

Basic aseptic technique should be described in an SOP, which should include at least the following requirements:

- The workspace must be disinfected before aseptic processing.
- After the initial gowning, protective gloves should be regularly sanitized or changed, and sterile gloves should be used where appropriate.
- All items should be disinfected before they are placed in the BSC.
- Gloved hands should not be passed over an open container containing the product or media.
- After initial training, there should be a continuing education program for aseptic processing.
- Manufacturing operators should be regularly evaluated for adherence to aseptic processing procedures.

Personnel Monitoring

Personnel can significantly affect the quality of the environment and the CT product. A personnel monitoring program should be established to minimize potential contamination of the production environment.

The monitoring program should be developed to complement aseptic processing needs, considering the type of facility and the potential risk to the product. When an operator is working in a BSC that is located in an unclassified facility (for example, in Phase I production), sampled sites may include the operator's gloves and sterile sleeve covers. When an operator is working in a BSC that is located in a classified area where there is a higher demand for asepsis, additional sampling sites on the operator's gown may be included. The frequency and sites of monitoring will depend on the potential impact to the product. For processing with a high risk of personnel impact on product sterility, the sampling may be performed after critical steps or at the end of processing. When the risk to the product is lower, sampling may not be necessary with each batch but, rather, as part of an ongoing assessment of aseptic processing at regular intervals. Regardless of the sampling sites and frequency, the results of monitoring should be used to continuously assess the quality of aseptic processing and to determine if retraining is required.

Validation of Aseptic Processing

An aseptic processing operation should be validated through performance of the process with the substitution of microbiological growth media for the CT product. This technique is also known as a "media fill" and involves exposing microbiological growth media to product contact surfaces of equipment, container closures, critical environments, and process manipulations to closely simulate the exposure that the actual product will undergo.[1] Media fills can be used to assess the aseptic training of new personnel, to monitor aseptic competency, or to evaluate the aseptic processing of a new or revised manufacturing process such as a closed system. All closed systems that are expected to maintain asepsis must be validated for aseptic processing.

Reference/Resource

1. Food and Drug Administration. Guidance for industry: Sterile drug products produced by aseptic processing—current good manufacturing practice. (September 2004) Rockville, MD: CBER, CDER, and ORA, 2004.

Method 16-1. Aseptic Technique for Cell Processing

Purpose

Aseptic technique is performed to minimize the risk of contamination of a product.

Summary of Procedure

1. Infection control.
2. Gowning.
3. Working in the biological safety cabinet (BSC).
4. Working with sterile supplies.
5. Product sampling.
6. The addition of media and cells.
7. Environmental and personnel monitoring.
8. Changeover procedures.

Equipment

BSC.

Supplies and Reagents

70% isopropyl alcohol. Cleanroom wipers.

Safety

1. Refer to the material safety data sheets for all cleaning reagents.
2. Personnel must handle and dispose of human tissue and blood components according to facility standard operating procedure (SOP).

Policy

A. *Infection Control*
1. Personnel who exhibit chills or a fever are not permitted to enter the processing facility and must notify their supervisor.
2. Personnel who are exposed to a communicable disease to which they are susceptible (during or away from work) must notify the appropriate institutional departments.
3. Exposed, susceptible employees may be excluded from duty for the entire period of potential communicability.

B. *Gowning*
1. Disposable, fluid-resistant gowns must be worn by anyone who enters the processing area.
2. Hands should be washed according to the facility procedure for hand hygiene and skin antisepsis whenever anyone enters the laboratory to process products, between products, before and after eating or using the restroom, after touching any inanimate object likely to be contaminated, and when hands are soiled.
3. Clean nitrile gloves should be put on before products are handled. Gloves should be changed or disinfected often to avoid contamination of the product and must be changed immediately after completion of processing one product and before processing another.
4. When dictated by the process-specific procedure involving open manipulations, individuals involved in processing should gown and don sterile gloves and sleeves before working in the BSC.
5. The operator should don a pair of nitrile gloves and open the sleeve cover package carefully to avoid contamination. Sleeve covers should be removed from the package one at a time, handled by the turned back "inside" of the sleeve. The hand is placed inside the sleeve cover, which is then unrolled, with care being taken not to touch the outside of the sleeve.
6. The operator should sit directly in front of the BSC and open sterile gloves. The gloves should be handled by their turned back "inside." Gloves should be pulled on one at a time, with care taken not to contaminate the outside of the gloves. Hands should be placed in the BSC without touching contaminated surfaces outside the BSC.

7. When dictated by the SOP, hair covers must be used during open processing.

8. If it is necessary to obtain supplies outside the BSC during processing, gloves should be sprayed or wiped with 70% isopropyl alcohol before the person returns to the BSC.

Procedure

A. *Working in the BSC*

1. Before working in the BSC, the operator should ensure that it has been cleaned according to SOP and that the cleaning has been documented. The BSC blower should be allowed to run for 5 to 10 minutes before the start of processing.

2. All items must be sprayed with 70% isopropyl alcohol before placement in the BSC.

3. When possible, all items necessary for processing should be placed in the BSC before the start of processing. However, an excess number of items should be avoided because they could interfere with BSC airflow and the appropriate sterile technique.

4. Before processing, a clean area in the BSC should be established for unused supplies, and a waste area should be designated for the placement of used or contaminated supplies.

5. Movements should be slow and limited, and entering and exiting should be minimized.

6. All open processing should be closed whenever it is necessary to exit the BSC to obtain supplies or discard waste materials. When the person returns, gloves should be changed or sanitized according to gowning requirements.

7. In the event of a spill, a clean wiper should be placed over the spill. All open processing should be closed and the area disinfected as indicated by cleaning procedures.

B. *Working with Sterile Supplies*

1. All supplies must be disinfected with 70% isopropyl alcohol before they are placed in the BSC.

2. All sterile, wrapped supplies should be unwrapped inside the BSC, and the unwrapped item should not come in contact with the outer wrapping.

3. All items suspected to be contaminated should be discarded and segregated from the sterile supplies in the BSC.

4. Paper-wrapped supplies that have been sprayed with alcohol but have not been used should be discarded.

5. Sterile container tops intended for reuse throughout a procedure may be placed cap side up on a clean surface (such as an alcohol pad) free of other supplies and debris. Nothing should be passed over the cap (eg, pipette, sleeve, or gloved hand).

6. Waste containers for liquids must be sterile, and the aseptic technique must be maintained when liquids are transferred into the waste bottle.

7. During pipetting, the pipette package should be opened to expose the top end of the pipette. After the top end of the pipette is inserted into the pipettor, remaining packaging should be removed without touching the pipette. Liquids should be pipetted above the opening of the vessel, and the pipette should not come in contact with the vessel or its contents. If any contact occurs, a new pipette must be used to maintain sterility.

C. *Product Sampling*

1. Sterile bag spikes or sampling site couplers should be used whenever possible.

2. The outer wrap of the spike or coupler should be carefully removed.

3. The tabs of the protective covering of the bag port should be grasped and separated to expose the port. The exposed port should not come in contact with any other surface before the spike or coupler is inserted.

4. The cap may then be removed from the spike or coupler and the spike or coupler inserted in the port.

   a. A bag can be sampled through a spike using a syringe with a threaded or blunt cannula after the site is wiped carefully with alcohol. When multiple samples are to be removed, the sampling site should be wiped between samples.

   b. Samples can be removed with a syringe attached to a sampling site coupler that will be removed. Care must be taken to maintain the sterility of the coupler and cap.

5. Syringes used to remove cells from conical tubes must be sterile. Needles or cannulas should be carefully attached and removed without the barrel of the syringe being handled.

6. A syringe barrel may be used for transferring cell suspensions and other liquids to sterile bags. The syringe package must be opened carefully without its contents being touched. The outer packaging can be gripped to hold the syringe barrel in place while the plunger is removed from the barrel.

D. Addition of Media or Cells

1. One aseptic method for transferring media or cells from bottles or flasks to sterile culture bags makes use of a ring stand that has been disinfected, a Cobe 2991 coupler (CaridianBCT, Lakewood, CO), and a sterile transfer pack.

   a. After all of the required supplies are placed in the BSC, the Cobe coupler is used to spike the transfer pack.

   b. The barrel is removed from a 60-mL syringe and attached to the coupler, and the syringe cap is placed on an alcohol pad.

   c. The syringe barrel is clamped to the ring stand.

   d. The media or cell suspensions are transferred with a sterile pipette to the bag by dispensing them through the syringe barrel. The end of the pipette should not touch the barrel. Alternatively, media can be poured from the bottle into the bag through the syringe barrel. The bottle should not touch the barrel of the syringe.

   e. The cap is then securely replaced on the coupler.

2. When media or cells are transferred from bags to tubes, bottles, or flasks, the roller clamp on a spike-spike sterile transfer set should be closed, and one spike aseptically inserted through a sterile port into the bag.

   a. Caps should be removed from the tubes, flasks, or bottles and placed in an undisturbed area of the BSC.

   b. The bag should be elevated and the protective covering removed from the remaining spike. The spike is then positioned above the first receptacle and the roller clamp opened. The spike should not come into contact with any surface. When the appropriate volume has been transferred, the roller clamp is closed and the same procedure is performed with the next container.

   c. Spills that may occur should be covered with a clean wiper until the transfer of media or cells is complete.

E. Environmental and Personnel Monitoring

1. For all processing that involves open containers of cells or media, it may be advisable to place a settling plate in the BSC for monitoring aseptic processing.

2. The monitoring of personnel gloves with touch plates should be performed as part of the initial processing validation and as part of the annual competency evaluation.

F. Changeover Procedures

1. All items should be removed from the BSC before the BSC is disinfected, and the action should be documented according to established procedure.

2. All equipment used in the procedure should be disinfected according to the appropriate equipment procedure, and the action should be documented on the equipment log.

References/Resources

1. Operator's manual for BSC by the manufacturer.
2. Food and Drug Administration. Guidance for industry: Sterile drug products produced by aseptic processing—current good manufacturing practice. (September 2004) Rockville, MD: CDER Office of Training and Communication and CBER Office of Communication, Training, and Manufacturer's Assistance, 2004.

Method 16-2. Operating and Maintaining the Biological Safety Cabinet

Purpose

The biological safety cabinet (BSC) is the appropriate environment for all aseptic processing of cellular therapy products. Proper operation and maintenance of the BSC are important elements of aseptic processing.

Time for Procedure

1. Cleaning before and after processing takes approximately 10 minutes.
2. The scheduled cleaning every 6 months takes approximately 30 minutes.

Summary of Procedure

1. Cleaning of the BSC before and after each use.
2. Operation of the BSC.
3. Removal of the grill and bottom tray every 6 months for BSC cleaning.
4. BSC certification.

Equipment

BSC.

Supplies and Reagents

1. CaviCide spray (Metrex, Romulus, MI) or equivalent intermediate-level surface disinfectant effective against tuberculosis, viruses, bacteria, and fungi.
2. CaviWipes XL (Metrex, Romulus, MI) or equivalent.
3. 70% isopropyl alcohol.
4. Spor-Klenz or equivalent agent for use in the microbial control (including spores) and disinfection of hard surfaces.
5. Cleanroom wipers.

Safety

1. Material safety data sheets should be available for all cleaning reagents.
2. Personnel must handle and dispose of human tissue and blood components according to appropriate standard operating procedure (SOP).
3. Nothing should be stored in or on the BSC.
4. The BSC should never be operated while a warning light or alarm is on.
5. Open flames must not be used in the BSC.

Procedure

A. *Cleaning the BSC before and after Use*
   1. The BSC blower should be turned on for 5-10 minutes before use.
   2. When the BSC door is raised, CaviCide should be sprayed on the work surface of the BSC, including the walls, side, back, interior surface of the window, and front lip.
   3. The CaviCide must have wet contact with the surfaces for a minimum of 3 minutes, after which the surfaces may be wiped with a CaviCide-saturated wipe or CaviWipes XL. The person performing the wiping should work from side to side, moving from the back to the front.
   4. The surfaces should then be sprayed with 70% isopropyl alcohol.
   5. The BSC door should be left open 8 inches and the surfaces permitted to air dry.
   6. All BSC cleaning should be documented in the BSC cleaning log and on the batch production record, as appropriate.

B. *Operation of the BSC*
   1. The BSC should be cleaned before and after component processing.
   2. Only one sample or product should be permitted in the BSC at any given time.
   3. If multiple samples or components are being processed, the BSC must be cleaned between processes.

4. The operator should be seated so that his or her armpits are level with the bottom of the BSC sash.

5. All items should be sprayed with 70% isopropyl alcohol and wiped with a cleanroom wiper before being placed in the BSC.

6. Items should never be placed on the front or rear grills because of the creation of air turbulence that increases the risk of contamination to the user or the product.

7. When processing is complete, all items should be removed from the BSC.

8. The interior surfaces of the BSC should be cleaned according to the steps for cleaning before and after use, and the cleaning should be documented.

9. At the end of the day, the BSC should again be cleaned, the blower turned off, and the sash closed.

C. *Semiannual Maintenance of BSC*
1. The bottom tray and grill should be removed from the BSC.

2. The tray, grill, and all interior surfaces of the BSC should be cleaned with Spor-Klenz, followed by a rinse with sterile water.

3. All parts should be sprayed with 70% isopropyl alcohol and wiped dry.

4. The grill and bottom tray may be replaced in the BSC.

5. Environmental monitoring should be performed according to the institutional SOP.

D. *Annual Certification*
1. The BSC should be certified annually by an appropriately qualified individual.

2. The individual who performs the certification will verify the proper operation of the filter system and airflow and will prepare a report of the certification.

3. When reviewing the BSC certification report, the laboratory should verify that all parameters are within specification.

References/Resources

1. Operator's manual for BSC from the manufacturer.
2. Manufacturer's instructions for CaviCide.
3. Manufacturer's instructions for Spor-Klenz.

In: Areman EM, Loper K, eds
Cellular Therapy: Principles, Methods, and Regulations
Bethesda, MD: AABB, 2009

◆◆◆   **17**   ◆◆◆

Cross-Contamination Issues in the Manufacture of Cellular Therapy Products

John Finkbohner, PhD

ONE OF THE MAJOR CHALLENGES IN DESIGN-ing and implementing a process that consistently and reliably produces high-quality product is identifying the possible routes of contamination and implementing controls that minimize the risk to the product and, thereby, the risk to the patient. Controlling product quality and resultant risk to the patient can be especially complex when working with cell- and tissue-based products from human sources, which may vary with respect to the presence and level of adventitious agents. The risk management approach to identifying process weaknesses described in the International Conference for Harmonisation (ICH) Q9 document[1] can be a valuable tool in ensuring patient safety by providing a structured pathway for prospectively defining process risk so that the identified concerns can be controlled. Control of cross-contamination in the manufacture of cellular therapy (CT) products involves the identification, ranking, and mitigation of all process- and product-related risks.

Overall process control can be achieved through a combination of engineering and procedural controls. Engineering controls can include the use of single-use, presterilized, disposable processing materials to minimize potential batch-to-batch cross-contamination or the potential failure of in-house sterilization processes, and the use of controlled processing environments such as those afforded by biological safety cabinets (BSCs). For situations in which containment may be a special concern, the use of Class II BSCs (Type 2B or analogous unit) may be especially helpful. High-efficiency particulate air (HEPA) filtration of all exhaust air fully traps all airborne (aerosolized) adventitious agents within HEPA-filtered barriers. Procedural controls include adherence to documented processing directions (batch records), the supporting procedure documentation that provides directions for specific unit operations, and the establishment of a training and qualification program for operators who perform the processing operations to ensure continuous adherence to processing directions.

The critical quality attributes for CT products are often based on the maintenance of the viability of the CT product, the removal of routes that might introduce adventitious agents to the product while

John Finkbohner, PhD, Director, Regulatory Affairs, MedImmune, LLC, Gaithersburg, Maryland

The author has disclosed no conflicts of interest.

it is manipulated ex vivo, and the maintenance of the product in a state suitable for reintroduction to the patient. These requirements for critical quality attributes often dictate the nature of the product release criteria, which include confirmation of sterility, confirmation of freedom from adventitious agents, verification of viability, and assessment of the concentration of stabilizers or other excipients that are intended to prolong viability of the product before introduction or reintroduction to the patient. Critical quality attributes must be maintained while risks associated with cross-contamination are mitigated.

Identifying Process Risks: Process Mapping

One of the first steps in designing a robust CT manufacturing process is defining the process flows and optimizing each step to maintain the highest possible product quality while ensuring that the end product remains fit for use. The steps in the process may include harvesting cells or tissue, storing harvested material until processing is initiated, processing the material, and packaging or storing the product for use in a clinical setting. A number of transportation operations are likely to be involved, including movement within a medical center and intrastate, interstate, and international transport to processing locations, storage facilities, and end user clinical sites. One of the difficulties in controlling possible routes of cross-contamination in the manufacture of CT products is the potential occult and pre-existing adventitious agent burden introduced to equipment by the processing of materials derived from differing donors. This difficulty is minimized to a large extent through the use of disposable, presterilized, single-use processing equipment (eg, cell and tissue collection materials and surgical-grade instruments, bags, tube sets, reaction vessels, cell culture bags, and tissue expansion growth flasks). In situations in which it is impossible or infeasible to use disposable equipment, reusable equipment must be carefully controlled to ensure that materials that contact the product are returned to a state that is fit for reuse. Equipment processing for reusable equipment and instruments may include cleaning, sterilization, depyrogenation, and sterile packaging.

Once the process stream has been completely mapped and all unit operation criteria fully defined, the challenges are to identify possible means for the tissue or cellular preparation to become contaminated and to take steps to build in controls to provide robust process isolation from these routes of contamination. Tissue harvesting operations and associated routes of potential contamination provide a good example of areas in which methods for minimizing the risk to product quality are needed. In addition to routine sterile field precautions in surgical settings or during fluidic tissue collection and standard blood banking type controls, donor screening for known human pathogens will be required for nonautologous patients. For autologous CT product operations, donor screening may not be required, but it may be advisable if key processing equipment must be reused (eg, tissue macerators or sonicator probe assemblies). All reusable equipment should be assumed to have been exposed to the worst-case range of human adventitious agents when procedures for cleaning and preparation for reuse are designed. In many cases, the equipment should be considered to have been exposed to transmissible spongiform encephalopathies (TSEs).

Minimizing Process Risks: Optimizing Manufacturing Unit Operations and Validating Unit Operation Robustness

Individual unit operations will involve the definition of processing parameters to maintain the highest level of product quality and to minimize potential risk to the patient. Parameters that must be defined include operational limits for the processing time at each step and conditions for process hold steps (eg, maximum hold time, temperature conditions, media or buffers for use during hold steps, and types of containers that may be used). Hold steps allow samples that have been taken for testing to yield results before continued processing of in-process intermediates. For live cells and tissues, however, these hold steps may contribute to loss of viability. In situations in which cell viability is labile, hold steps may not be possible and processing needs to continue before test results become available ("processing at risk"). In these situations, it is important to understand what risks to the processing equipment may result from later receipt of test results that indicate that the material and associated processing equipment have been exposed to potential adventitious agents.

Continued processing of material at risk is not uncommon in CT processes because of the need to maintain product viability by minimizing the time that the product is manipulated ex vivo before it is returned to a patient or cryopreserved. Therefore, it is important to consider actions that will be required if unacceptable test results are received. These actions may include conducting extraordinary cleaning or decontamination, using quarantine barriers, and, if post-treatment patient testing reveals adventitious agents that were not present before treatment, employing "look-back" actions. Look-back actions notify patients who may have been affected by the contamination event, for example, if equipment cross-contamination involved the processing of multiple production lots of material used in multiple patients.

Maceration and dissolution to produce cellular suspensions may be important early operations in the preparation of CT products where source materials are collected from organs or solid tissues. Often, these operations will involve the use of nondisposable equipment, which must be rigorously controlled for reuse. Preparation for reuse will often involve a decontamination and cleaning operation, followed by sterilization or depyrogenation. In situations in which TSEs may be involved, preparation for reuse sometimes includes reconditioning the stainless steel process stream contact surfaces (eg, repassivation). Careful consideration must be applied to the design of procedures for operations after use because the worst-case exposure of the equipment to potential adventitious agents will need to be addressed. Once the procedures for return of reusable equipment to a state appropriate for use in production of another batch of material have been defined, a validation study for each process should be conducted. This study will ensure that the parameters defined in the reuse processing directions result in the equipment's being exposed to the appropriate conditions during every procedure. For cleaning, this validation may include defining the worst-case soiling agent and cleaning operations reflecting a worst-case procedure to ensure that the routine operation achieves the needed level of cleanliness with an additional

level of assurance built in. For sterilization operations, the validation of the selected cycle should ensure a high level of sterility. Guidance available from the Food and Drug Administration (FDA) and in technical reports available through the Parenteral Drug Association (PDA) explains the development of these validation protocols. Consulting with experts in the field can be a valuable resource in ensuring that the systems for processing reusable equipment meet regulatory expectations.

Processing Considerations

Additional ex-vivo processing of CT products may include the expansion of the cells or enrichment of cell preparation for cell subtypes through gradient centrifugation, cell selection, or cell sorting. The parameters for these operations also need to be carefully studied and optimized to maximize the viability and subsequent suitability of the product for use in the recipient. Some CT processes include cytokines or other cytoactive agents to modify cell function or activate cellular behaviors that are desirable for patient treatment. In these instances, operational parameters may require the monitoring of cell response to the ex-vivo agent and may challenge process consistency when cell treatment varies by cell source and donor characteristics. These types of process controls are discussed elsewhere in this book.

For contamination control, the critical factor to consider is the nature of the cytoactive agent and its source. If it is an animal-derived material, the verification of control over the source material is critical because it could be a significant source of adventitious agents. Wherever possible, the use of materials that are not of animal origin is highly advisable. When the cytoactive agent that is used to manipulate cell behavior is a biotechnology-derived material, animal-derived materials may still have been used in the preparation of the agent. In this situation, the CT manufacturer is required to have full knowledge of the sources of potential adventitious agents in the preparation of the cytoactive agent and to have an arrangement for notification by the vendor should a lot of released agent be found to be nonconforming after release for use. As in the case of implantable devices, the CT product manufacturer may be required to perform a look-back operation to notify patients who may have been exposed to adventitious agents through the ex-vivo agent. This risk can be minimized when the agent is a product licensed for use in treating human disease. When nonlicensed materials are used, due diligence is required in conducting vendor audits and determining the agent's fitness for use and is critical to minimizing risks to patients.

Aseptic Processing

With rare exceptions, CT products must be produced using aseptic technique from the initial harvest of the cellular material through final packaging for introduction to the patient. All process stream contact materials should be presterilized, and solutions that are used to support processing should be rendered sterile through physical means (eg, steam or radiation sterilization) or through sterile filtration, where feasible. Sterile filtration processes should be validated through the conduct of a microbial challenge study. Advice on the parameters to include in such a study can be gained through contact with the technical service departments of sterile filter manufacturers, who will often design and conduct a study of the processing conditions for the specific process for a fee.

All operations that involve aseptic processing should be qualified through a media challenge approach. This approach involves identifying the worst-case operational conditions that can be expected during routine operations and performing a mock operation using a microbial growth medium capable of supporting the growth of a wide range of microorganisms. For the modeling of aseptic processing operations for CT or tissue manipulations, it may be appropriate to conduct media challenges using a combination of solid agar and fluid growth media. Initial validation of aseptic processing capability should be achieved through the conduct of three consecutive successful media challenges. A single media challenge should be performed at least once per year to requalify the aseptic operations. In addition, operators who perform aseptic operations should be fully qualified through a worst-case mock process using growth media that follows the same rules outlined for the overall process. See Chapter 16 (Aseptic Processing) for a more detailed discussion of this topic.

Minimizing Process Risks: Controlling Routine Operation Variables

In addition to the substantial challenge of the initial definition of operational parameters, it is critical to maintain process capability by defining all variables that may affect the process over time. The identification of sources of potential process variability will allow the design of controls to minimize the impact to the process. For example, processes that use donor tissues from exogenous sources to treat patients may require donor screening questions to establish the background exposure of the donor to potential adventitious agent risks. The FDA provides guidance documents that describe donor screening approaches for differing types of cells and tissue, and early dialogue with the agency is wise when developing a CT process in which allogeneic donor materials will be used to manufacture the product.

During process development and optimization, the criteria for conducting individual unit operations are defined, validated, and documented. A well-designed process is still vulnerable to poor performance if sources of routine variation are not controlled. One significant source of variability in ongoing operations arises from the inconsistency of human operators in performing the processing steps. Other sources of variability are donor source materials, vendor-supplied materials, the performance of equipment systems, and process stream inputs.

The human factor is best managed through thoroughly documented processes and procedures and the implementation of a separate quality unit. The quality unit is responsible for maintaining controlled documents, verifying operations (including review of batch production records), leading investigations into processing deviations, and performing vendor qualification programs to ensure the ongoing quality of incoming raw materials. A quality unit can consist of a limited number of individuals, but it is important that they are knowledgeable and empowered to make decisions related to process performance and product disposition (eg, release or rejection of the production lot).

The master document in which process directions are defined and key processing data are captured is the batch record. The batch record provides the directions for conducting the entire process and should be maintained as a controlled document as part of the larger quality system. Safety-related controls for the process must be implemented during the investigational phase of product development, and full compliance with current good manufacturing practice (cGMP) must be in place for licensure of the product and process. Although other sections of this book provide greater detail on compliance with cGMP requirements, those requirements are mentioned briefly in this chapter in order to appropriately address the topic of contamination control.

Once a process is defined and optimized for product quality (including minimization of the risk of contamination), the challenge becomes the ability to continue producing a high-quality product. A number of variables need to be controlled to ensure the ongoing ability to manufacture products that conform to release criteria. These criteria include the quality of vendor-supplied materials and components, the quality and consistency of operations performed by humans, the ability of equipment to perform as intended, and the maintenance of the sterile barrier. The importance of vendor audits and the institution of a vendor qualification program has already been noted. The vendor qualification program should include verification that the materials used in processing routinely meet fitness-for-use criteria, and periodic monitoring must be performed to ensure that incoming raw materials continue to meet the predefined criteria for use in processing.

Qualification of equipment capability involves not only the initial assessment of processing capability and validation in regard to operational procedures performed using the equipment, but also the periodic reverification that equipment performs as intended. This reverification usually involves a combination of calibration and routine requalification of equipment performance to support manufacturing operations. For equipment with critical components or subsystems that may need periodic replacement, criteria must be defined for how to release the replacement component for use and to ensure that the replacement component functions as intended. In addition, if equipment performance is likely to vary according to a change in component performance over time, it may be necessary to

define system suitability measures to assess equipment performance before use as part of each manufacturing operation (eg, verification of light source intensity for photo-activated processes).

The greatest risks to the process in regard to contamination include the addition of adventitious agents through process stream inputs, previously noted in regard to the use of ex-vivo, cytoactive agents, and the introduction of microbial contamination during the conduct of unit operations that is due to equipment or procedural-control failure. Even though operators may be qualified for their ability to perform aseptic operations through media challenge studies, failure to maintain the sterile barrier can still lead to product contamination.

Materials

For presterilized, disposable, single-use systems, it may be difficult to verify the integrity of the sterile barrier before each use. A small percentage of these materials develops breaches that may allow exposure of the process stream to the external environment, especially when the physical barrier is compromised because of material stress from handling or manipulation at ultra-low temperatures. It is important to remember that disposable processing equipment is often composed of multilayer laminates of polymeric material that may undergo a glass transition to a brittle state at ultra-low temperatures. If processing will include disposable processing systems at ultra-low temperatures, the manufacturer must ensure that the vendor has certified the ability of the polymeric materials to perform under the conditions of use and must qualify this ability under the conditions of use for its own process by using a mock process model. If it is possible to perform a pressure hold or other verification of the integrity of the sterile barrier before use, it would be expected under cGMP. However, such a verification may be difficult or impossible for some disposable processing equipment systems.

Product Manipulation

Other than materials, the most likely route of introduction of adventitious agents to the process stream occurs at open manipulation steps such as open container operations that are conducted in BSCs and during use of equipment that may preclude the use of a closed system such as sonication or maceration. In situations where open operations must be performed, it is critical to maintain the cleanliness of the operational environment and to take all precautions to avoid the introduction of microorganisms into the aseptic field. Controlling the immediate environment where open operations occur is critical to minimize the potential routes for microbial contamination. The environment can be controlled through a combination of equipment maintenance and upkeep, including HEPA filter requalification in situ, routine monitoring of the air quality in the BSC relative to both viable and nonviable airborne particulates, the establishment of sterile gowning procedures including the qualification of operators, and rigorous maintenance of a cleaning and sanitization schedule for the operation areas. These control techniques are covered in more detail in other sections of this book.

When an aseptic operations area is established in a BSC, it is also important to control all exterior surfaces for materials introduced into the area through a wipe down with qualified disinfectants. Often, the most robust means of establishing an effective aseptic operations area includes the presence of two operators: one who performs the aseptic operations within a BSC and another who prepares supporting materials for introduction into the aseptic zone. The second operator can make entries into the batch record, freeing the primary operator from the need to cycle in and out of the aseptic operations area and allowing the primary operator to focus on the task at hand.

In addition to the immediate production environment, other sources of potential contamination should be considered, including operators with an active infection, potential cross-contamination from other patient materials, and air intakes from areas where infectious airborne particulates may be generated or otherwise present. Operators should be trained to recognize the criticality of maintaining an appropriate level of control over sources of contamination, including their own illnesses. Provisions should be made to allow operators who report to work with an active infection to perform duties unrelated to the processing of CT materials until they become noninfectious. During initial design of the production space, the location of air intakes should be considered relative to the exhaust from other areas of a building.

Conclusion

As noted previously in this chapter, the importance of documenting the process, including detailed operational parameters for each unit operation, is critical to maintaining a reliable and repeatable process. This chapter noted the importance of conducting validation and qualification activities to establish the capability of individual unit operations and supporting systems. Documentation of all initial validation and qualification activities is of key importance to establishing a cGMP-compliant process that may be licensed at a later time. These tasks and a number of additional activities under the responsibility of the quality unit drive the need to implement a quality organization and quality system early in the process development cycle.

Reference/Resource

1. Food and Drug Administration. Guidance for industry: Q9 quality risk management. (June 2006) Rockville, MD: CDER Office of Training and Communication, and CBER Office of Communication, Training, and Manufacturers Assistance, 2006. [Available at http://www.fda.gov/RegulatoryInformation/Guidances/ucm128050.htm (accessed June 19, 2009).]

In: Areman EM, Loper K, eds
Cellular Therapy: Principles, Methods, and Regulations
Bethesda, MD: AABB, 2009

◆◆◆   **18**   ◆◆◆

Computer Systems in the Cellular Therapy Facility

Paula L. Brown, MT(ASCP), JD

ALL COMPUTER SYSTEMS, WHETHER BUILT in-house or purchased and customized, that are used in the procurement, manufacturing, testing, or administration of cellular therapy (CT) products must be validated before being placed into service. They must also be routinely calibrated, inspected, and verified according to a written program that is designed to ensure proper performance.[1] Thus, before building or purchasing a computer system, the facility should develop and use a written plan approved by the quality management team for computer system selection and validation.[2]

Regulatory authorities and accrediting bodies provide regulations, standards, and guidance for the implementation and use of computer systems in CT facilities. Although these documents may differ in the level of detail, all stress that the facility must validate the performance of the computer system for its intended use. More information on software validation can be found in the next chapter of this section.

Computer System Selection

Before building or purchasing a computer system, the CT program should identify a knowledgeable individual or group of individuals within the facility to oversee the project. This individual or group should work with potential users of the system to identify the system functions and to draft and submit a written computer system selection plan. This plan should also be used in developing the computer validation plan.

The computer system selection plan should describe the mandatory functions and features of the system to ensure the preparation, storage, and release of safe and effective CT products and to meet regulatory and accreditation requirements.

Mandatory Computer Functions

The computer system selection plan should, at a minimum, mandate the following:

Paula L. Brown, MT(ASCP), JD, Quality Officer, Division of Cell Therapy/Transfusion Medicine, University of Arkansas for Medical Sciences, Little Rock, Arkansas

The author has disclosed no conflicts of interest.

- That the computer system be secure and limit access to authorized users.[1]
- That the computer system ensure the authenticity, integrity, and confidentiality of all records.[2]
- That computer records be ready for retrieval promptly.[2]
- That the computer system have a backup feature that will allow the records to be stored off site in a secure location.[1]
- That the computer system have appropriate controls to ensure that only authorized personnel can make changes to the main computer functions, hardware, and software.[1]
- That potential physical or environmental restrictions such as temperature and humidity be considered.
- That the facility have a specified number of licensed users.

Quality Assurance Computer Functions

Facility

In addition to the above, a CT facility computer system might require the following important quality assurance (QA) features and functions:

- A hard drive or other storage media that is large enough to store all relevant information for an extended period such as 10 years.
- A mechanism for tracking the cellular product from the time it is procured until its final disposition.
- A mechanism for tracking adverse reactions and deviations associated with a particular product.
- The ability to interface with other facility computers.
- The ability to read and print International Society of Blood Transfusion (ISBT) 128 labels.
- The ability to quarantine products until they are available for release and the ability to stop the release of nonconforming products.
- Truth tables and control records.
- Complete collection and processing records that identify the personnel, equipment, and materials involved in each lot.
- The ability to access information during downtime.

Vendor

The following items should be supplied by potential vendors:
- Validation templates.
- Vendor support for the life of the computer, including updates and patches to comply with new regulations.
- Vendor-supported training.
- A list of acceptable scanners, printers, and computer terminals needed to connect to and run the computer system.
- A list of other facilities that currently use the computer system.
- The ability to convert and transfer old computer files to the new computer system.

For an example of a computer system selection plan, see Appendix 18-1.

Completing the Evaluation and Selection Process

After the specifications are received from outside vendors or in-house developers and appropriate demonstrations have been performed, the information contained in the computer system selection plan should be evaluated by the designated individuals. A written recommendation should be prepared, including the rationale for the recommendation, and should be provided to upper management and the QA team for review and approval.

Computer Validation Plan

After the purchase contract is signed with the selected vendor, a validation plan must be developed that includes or addresses the following elements:

- A timetable (approximate times) for the installation of the computer system.
- The physical dimensions of the hardware and the version number of the software.[2]
- Validation of the hardware.[2]
- A description of system security.[3]
- A description of the process for authorizing and documenting modifications to the system and for system maintenance.[3]
- The training of all personnel.[3]
- Risk analysis and evaluation of post-implementation performance.[3]
- Data backup and downtime processes.[3]

• Validation approval from the quality management team.[2]

The vendor may be able to supply the facility with validation templates, which should be used with the facility's selection plan to write validation test scripts to test the limits of the computer. The validation test scripts should address 1) the objective of the validation test script, 2) the procedure to be performed to prove the objective, 3) the expected results, 4) the actual results obtained, 5) whether the validation passed or failed, and 6) quality management review. For an example of an installation plan, see Appendix 18-2.

Test scripts should be written for the following elements:

• Security and access that are limited to authorized users.[1]
• Backup and restoration procedures of the computer system in case of downtime.
• Interface with other computer systems in the facility.
• Product tracking.
• Each critical step or element identified in the selection plan.

• If the computer has a truth table that prevents inappropriate product release, testing of the truth table to verify that it is functioning properly.

Computer systems are critical elements of a quality system. The goal of computer validation is to prove that the computer system is operating within a state of control and is functioning properly in the preparation and release of safe and effective cellular products.

References/Resources

1. Code of federal regulations. Current good manufacturing practice for finished pharmaceuticals. Automatic, mechanical, and electronic equipment. Title 21, CFR Part 211.68. Washington, DC: US Government Printing Office, 2008 (revised annually).
2. FACT-JACIE international standards for cellular therapy product collection, processing, and administration. 3rd ed. Omaha, NE: Foundation for the Accreditation of Cellular Therapy and the Joint Accreditation Committee of ISCT and EBMT, 2006.
3. Padley D, ed. Standards for cellular therapy product services. 3rd ed. Bethesda, MD: AABB, 2008.

◆

Appendix 18-1. Computer System Selection Plan

Selection Process

	Name of Computer and Vendor	Address	Phone Number	Contact Person
Computer System 1				
Computer System 2				
Computer System 3				

Physical Requirements of the Computer System

To fill out the form, enter the facility's specifications or requirements for the computer in the column "Facility Physical Requirements for the Computer System." Under each computer system, enter the computer's specifications.

	Facility Physical Requirements for the Computer System	Computer System 1 Specifications	Computer System 2 Specifications	Computer System 3 Specifications
Facility-required RAM and GB capabilities				
Platform and operating system required by the facility				
Temperature and humidity requirements of the system				
Physical dimensions of the computer system				
Number of users for license				

RAM = random access memory; GB = gigabyte.

(Continued)

Appendix 18-1. Computer System Selection Plan (Continued)

Regulatory Requirements of the Computer System

To fill out the form, mark an "X" for "yes" and leave the cell blank for "no." If the answer is neither "yes" nor "no," leave the cell blank and record the reason in the comments section.

Computer or Vendor Functions	Computer System 1	Computer System 2	Computer System 3	Comments
Is the computer system secure, and does it limit access to authorized users?				
Does the computer system ensure the authenticity, integrity, and confidentiality of all records?				
Can computer records be easily and promptly retrieved?				
Does the computer system have a backup feature?				
Does the computer system have controls to ensure that only authorized personnel can make changes to the main computer functions, hardware, and software?				
Will information be accessible during downtime?				

Vendor Functions

To fill out the form, mark an "X" for "yes" and leave the cell blank for "no." If the answer is neither "yes" nor "no," leave the cell blank and record the reason in the comments section.

Computer or Vendor Functions	Computer System 1	Computer System 2	Computer System 3	Comments
Does the vendor supply templates for validation?				
Does the vendor offer support for the life of the computer system, including updates and patches?				
Does the vendor supply training?				
Can the vendor supply a list of acceptable scanners, printers, and computer terminals needed to run the system?				
Can the vendor convert the old computer data to the new system?				
Can the computer vendor supply the facility with a list of facilities currently using this version of the computer system? Document the names of the facilities and attach them to this form.				

(Continued)

Appendix 18-1. Computer System Selection Plan (Continued)

Quality Assurance Review

The quality assurance team should test functions. To fill out the form, mark an "X" for "yes" and leave the cell blank for "no." If the answer is neither "yes" nor "no," leave the cell blank and record the reason in the comments section.

Computer or Vendor Functions	Computer System 1	Computer System 2	Computer System 3	Comments
Can the system track an incoming HPC from the time of procurement until distribution?				
Can the system track adverse patient reactions, deviations, and engraftment data?				
Does the computer have written interfaces that will connect facility computers?				
Does the computer system have the ability to perform billing functions?				
Does the computer system have labeling capabilities?				
Can the computer system read and print ISBT 128 labels?				
Does the computer system have the ability to quarantine unacceptable products and the ability to stop the release of nonconforming products?				
Is the computer system FDA approved?				

HPC = hematopoietic progenitor cell; ISBT = International Society of Blood Transfusion; FDA = Food and Drug Administration.

Approval of the Computer System Selection Plan

Plan prepared by/date: _____

Evaluation of Computer Systems

Hematopoietic Progenitor Cell Department

Name of the computer system recommended:

_____

Reason for the recommendation of the above computer system:

_____

_____

_____

Upper Management

Name of the computer system approved for purchase by upper management and quality management:

_____

_____

Approval

Upper management signature/date: _____

Quality management signature/date: _____

Appendix 18-2. Sample Computer System Installation Plan

Objective

To confirm that the computer room environment is compliant with environmental and safety requirements as well as with computer system requirements.

Procedure

1. Confirm that the computer room is supplied with emergency power, which is tested weekly.
2. Confirm that the computer room will maintain a constant temperature within computer server limits.
3. Confirm that the size of the computer room is adequate for equipment and storage.
4. Confirm that fire extinguishers are mounted on the wall.
5. Establish computer facility security: access procedure and surveillance.

Expected Results

The computer room environment is adequate to maintain the facility information systems while remaining compliant with environmental and safety procedures:

1. The computer room is supplied with emergency power and is tested each Wednesday.
2. The computer room maintains a constant temperature.
3. The size of the room is adequate for storage.
4. Fire extinguishers are mounted on the wall
5. Everyone must sign in to enter the room, and security cameras are operational.

PASS ☐
FAIL ☐

Performed by/date: _____

Quality management review/date:_____

In: Areman EM, Loper K, eds
Cellular Therapy: Principles, Methods, and Regulations
Bethesda, MD: AABB, 2009

◆◆◆   **19**   ◆◆◆

Software Considerations for Cellular Therapy Products

John R. Godshalk, MSE, MBA

SOFTWARE IS USED IN MULTIPLE PROCESSES and systems for the production of cellular therapy (CT) products. Software is found in cell processing equipment, tracking databases, analytical equipment, recordkeeping systems, and many other systems. Software that is used in the production of CT products or for electronic records during such production must be validated or verified to meet the requirements of the Code of Federal Regulations (CFR), Title 21, Parts 11 and 1271.[1] Some systems that require validation are the following:

- Computer systems that match donors and recipients of CT products by using HLA matching, where the risk of mismatch or mix-up is high.
- Tracking software for a CT vaccine to ensure that autologous cells that are manipulated ex vivo are returned to the correct patient.
- Preparation and maintenance of an electronic batch record, where automated cell-processing or testing equipment supplies data directly to the batch record. All data flowing to the batch record must be checked for accuracy, and printouts of the batch record must match the electronic

form. In addition, the requirements of 21 CFR 11 must be fulfilled for the electronic batch record.

CT products that are considered biologic drug products are subject to the 21 CFR 1271 regulations, the good manufacturing practice (GMP) regulations of 21 CFR 210 and 211, and the production software regulations of 21 CFR 11. Most CT products are currently in the clinical trial stage, and companies will ideally be working toward, if not already meeting, these Food and Drug Administration (FDA) regulatory requirements.

If a computer system is relied on to meet core current good tissue practice (cGTP) requirements (for products regulated under 21 CFR 1271) such as donor screening and donor eligibility determination, the computer system must be validated.

Verification vs Validation

A short risk analysis for each computer system that is used for production is helpful in determining whether verification or validation is appropriate for

---

John R. Godshalk, MSE, MBA, Senior Consultant, Biologics Consulting Group, Inc, Alexandria, Virginia

The author has disclosed no conflicts of interest.

the system. Computer systems that are in the higher risk categories (which might result in injury or death to the patient) must be validated, while systems in lower risk categories can be verified. Table 19-1 provides a risk class ranking for a hypothetical CT product for cancer patients.

Software Validation Basics

Software validation consists of objective tests and evidence that the software is fit for use and is working the way it was designed to work. From the FDA perspective, software validation is "confirmation by examination and provision of objective evidence that software specifications conform to user needs and intended uses, and that the particular requirements implemented through software can be consistently fulfilled."[2] From a practical standpoint, validation activities include design control, testing as the software is being developed, inspections and analyses, user site testing, and functionality testing in a simulated environment. *Software verification* is used in this chapter as defined by the International Organization for Standardization (ISO) Standard 8402[3]: it is not as thorough as full validation and refers only to verification that design outputs meet the specified requirements. The objective

of verification is consistency, completeness, and correctness. Guidance for software validation that elucidates these points is available from the FDA.[2] One practical example is Microsoft Excel, whose spreadsheets are verified, not validated, because Excel is off-the-shelf software.

CT companies and organizations that use software in production must validate or verify the software for fitness in its intended use for Phase II and III studies or full licensure. For example, computer systems that are often used in the manufacture of CT products for the following functions must be validated: laboratory information management, building management, recording production information and electronic batch records, donor eligibility, patient HLA matching, release and/or release information, document management, and corrective and preventive action (CAPA) management.

Software used in the production of any CT product must be validated to demonstrate that it has the attributes of fitness for use and design controls. Most problems in software arise in the design phase. Therefore, careful design and documentation of the software lifecycle process[4] are paramount in software validation. Documentation is not an end unto itself or merely a regulatory burden. Rather, documentation encourages software engineers and developers to design, test, and build

Table 19-1. Software Risk Class Ranking for a Hypothetical Cellular Therapy Product

Computer System Function	Risk Class	Validation or Verification	Basis
e-Batch record	High	Validation	Critical GMP document
Release test record	High	Validation	Critical GMP document
Weighing of materials	Medium	Calibration or verification	Firmware
Cell sorter output for production	Medium	Validation for normal ranges of input and output	Critical process
System for label production	Medium	Validation	Critical nature of labeling (identity)
Sterility test record that is relayed to the e-batch record	High	Test validation combined with validation of data transfer	Critical release test
pH in-process test relayed to e-batch record	Medium	Calibration combined with verification of data transfer	In-process test has a medium risk because of the wide acceptance range
ERP system for storage and retrieval of matched stem cells	High	Validation	Retrieval of wrong unit is possible

GMP = good manufacturing practice; ERP = enterprise resource planning.

software in a way that minimizes potential risk and errors and allows for logical testing and deployment. The FDA and CT standards organizations such as AABB[5] and the Foundation for the Accreditation of Cellular Therapy (FACT)[6] are concerned that software used in the production of CT products work consistently in the way it was designed and that its design and function fit its use. Validation is simply the written proof for inspectors that the company has thought about the risks that may arise in using software and has mitigated those risks through validation.

Software Validation Performance

Software validation can be performed in many ways, at many different levels. Although it is not a good idea to forego software validation, it is not necessary to validate every line of code. The basic elements of software validation and compliance with 21 CFR 11 are enough to satisfy most FDA inspectors. The method of software validation is up to the company, and FDA has stated that manufacturers have latitude and flexibility in defining how the validation is done. Most validation protocols are based on the Good Automated Manufacturing Practice (GAMP) standard,[7] although other standards and methods can be used.

Following are the basic elements of software validation and documentation:
- Design input document, which provides software specifications and requirements (intended use and user needs).
- Design documents (architecture, detailed design, and traceability).

- Risk management defined by level of concern (if applicable).
- Integration testing [operational qualification (OQ)].
- Installation qualification (IQ).
- Testing under actual use conditions, which validates fitness-for-use criteria, including data integrity testing [performance qualification (PQ)].
- A description of the lifecycle, plans, and system and supporting documents.
- Documentation of system security, operation, training, and maintenance.
- Configuration change management and change control.

Software validation and documentation consist of writing and executing a protocol that is based on these basic elements and producing the supporting documentation. Validation includes the verification and documentation of design elements as well as the testing of the software and documentation of its installation and configuration. The heart of software validation is software testing for fitness for use, which is always necessary regardless of the extent to which the software is validated. Testing cannot be done without a design because the traceability matrix (linking the design elements with the functions) is part of the validation exercise.

Documenting the software validation and creating supporting documentation are just as important as performing the validation. Supporting documents such as lifecycle description, system description, and security overview are helpful additions to the validation package. There are other documents that are not required for validation but are nonetheless needed for GMP-related processes.

Table 19-2. An Example of Risk Analysis for Three Computer Systems

Computer System	Risk Level (1 = Highest)	Analysis Outcome
HPLC computer; HPLC used for release test	Level 3	Separate computer validation not necessary; part of the method validation
Preliminary HLA-matching system	Level 2	Validation required but not part of the production system; a person performs the final match
LIMS system	Level 1	Validation required; level 1 because this system stores release data

HPLC = high-performance liquid chromatography; LIMS = laboratory information management system.

Examples include system operation, training, and maintenance documents.

All software changes must be revalidated if significant changes are made after the initial validation protocol is completed.

Risk Analysis

A risk analysis should be performed for each computer system that is used. Table 19-2 shows the outcome and rationale for the risk analysis of three computer systems. The validation effort should reflect the criticalness of the computer system and its risk analysis level. Typically, risk analysis is conducted in teams; therefore, there may be variance in the outcome.

Regulations for Software Used in the Production of Cellular Therapy Products

Code of Federal Regulations, Title 21, Part 1271 Compliance

Software systems that are used in the production of CT products need to be validated according to Part 1271 regulations. Any software that is used for production, facilities, or equipment, or for quality functions must be validated to ensure its fitness for the intended use. The specific regulation and its application can be found in 21 CFR 1271.160(d):

You must validate the performance of computer software for the intended use, and the performance of any changes to that software for the intended use, if you rely upon the software to comply with core CGTP requirements and if the software either is custom software or is commercially available software that has been customized or programmed (including software programmed to perform a user defined calculation or table) to perform a function related to core CGTP requirements. You must verify the performance of all other software for the intended use if you rely upon it to comply with core CGTP requirements. You must approve and document these activities and results before implementation.

Table 19-3 shows the core cGTP requirements for which related software must be validated.

Code of Federal Regulations, Title 21, Part 11 Compliance

For higher-risk CT products that are regulated as drugs, 21 CFR 211.68 regarding automatic, mechanical, and electronic equipment also applies:

(a) Automatic, mechanical, or electronic equipment or other types of equipment, including computers, or related systems that will perform a function satisfactorily, may be used in the manufacture, processing, packing, and holding of a drug product. If such equipment is so used, it shall be routinely calibrated, inspected, or checked according to a written program designed to assure proper performance. Written records of those calibration checks and inspections shall be maintained.

(b) Appropriate controls shall be exercised over computer or related systems to assure that changes in master production and control records or other records are instituted only by authorized personnel. Input to and output from the computer or related system of formulas or other records or data shall be checked for accuracy. The degree and frequency of input/output verification shall be based on the complexity and reliability of the computer or related system. A backup file of data entered into the computer or related system shall be maintained except where certain data, such as calculations performed in connection with laboratory analysis, are eliminated by computerization or other automated processes. In such instances a written record of the program shall be maintained along with appropriate validation data. Hard copy or alternative systems, such as duplicates, tapes, or microfilm, designed to assure that backup data are exact and complete and that it is secure from alteration, inadvertent erasures, or loss shall be maintained.

For production systems and quality systems software, Part 11 requirements must be met. The Part 11 requirements are controls that ensure that computer systems work as intended and are equivalent to, or more reliable than, paper-based systems.

Production and quality computer systems should meet all of the following requirements:

Table 19-3. Core cGTP Requirements (21 CFR) That Pertain to Software

Core cGTP Requirement	Example
Requirements that relate to facilities in Parts 1271.190(a) and (b)	Building management system that monitors and controls the room pressure and temperature
Requirements that relate to environmental control in Part 1271.195(a)	Building management system that monitors and controls the room pressure and temperature; a system that logs particulate level in the air of an ISO 7 area
Requirements that relate to equipment in Part 1271.200(a)	Automated cell-processing equipment that is computer controlled
Requirements that relate to supplies and reagents in Parts 1271.210(a) and (b)	Laboratory information management system used to store quality tests for incoming raw materials
Requirements that relate to recovery in Part 1271.215	A system that gathers CT product data during recovery
Requirements that relate to processing and process controls in Part 1271.220	A system used to control and record controlled rate freezing of a CT product
Requirements that relate to labeling controls in Parts 1271.250(a) and (b)	A barcode label system for identification of the CT product for in-process controls and testing
Requirements that relate to storage in Parts 1271.260(a) through (d)	A system that monitors and records the level of liquid nitrogen in the CT product storage Dewar
Requirements that relate to receipt, predistribution shipment, and distribution of an HCT/P in Parts 1271.265(a) through (d)	A system that records receipt and acceptance of a CT starting material; a system that is used for release to inventory
Requirements that relate to donor eligibility determinations, donor screening, and donor testing in Parts 1271.50, 1271.75, 1271.80, and 1271.85	A system that is used to gather donor eligibility information
Requirements that relate to computer batch records in Part 211.180(c)	An electronic batch record

cGTP = current good tissue practice; CFR = Code of Federal Regulations; ISO = International Organization for Standardization; CT = cellular therapy; HCT/Ps = human cells, tissues, and cellular and tissue-based products.

- Validation: The validation extent (validation rigor) is at an appropriate level with respect to the risk to the product or patient.
- Record maintenance: The system has the ability to maintain copies of records, and these records can be maintained for a time that is consistent with the firm's record retention policy.
- Access: The system has limited and controlled access.
- Backup: The system automatically and consistently backs up data and records.
- Record retrieval: The system is able to retrieve records accurately and promptly.
- Electronic signatures: If the system has electronic signatures, they must include the name of the person signing, the date and time, and the meaning of the signature, and they must be permanent, secure, and unique. The identity of the

person signing must also be verified before the e-signature is assigned.

Summary

Computer systems that are used in the production of CT products, for CT quality control functions, or to meet any of the core requirements of 21 CFR 1271 must be validated for their intended use. Risk analysis for computer systems can be used to determine the extent of validation necessary and any compliance needs related to 21 CFR Part 11. Validation methods and protocols vary both in type and extent. Firms should have a rationale for the validation extent (rigor) chosen and should be able to refer to a method, guidance, or reference for development of the protocol. Validation involves documenting that the software is fit for its intended use, was designed with user requirements in mind, and is able to perform consistently.

References/Resources

1. Code of federal regulations. Food and drugs. Title 21, CFR Parts 11 and 1271. Washington, DC: US Government Printing Office, 2008 (revised annually).
2. Food and Drug Administration. General principles of software validation; final guidance for industry and FDA staff. (January 11, 2002) Rockville, MD: CDRH/FDA, 2002.
3. International Organization for Standardization. Quality management and quality assurance—vocabulary. ISO 8402:1994. Geneva, Switzerland: ISO, 1994.
4. American National Standards Institute. Medical device software—software life cycle processes. ANSI/AAMI SW68:2001. Arlington, VA: Association for the Advancement of Medical Instrumentation, 2001.
5. Padley D, ed. Standards for cellular therapy product services. 3rd ed. Bethesda, MD: AABB, 2008.
6. FACT-JACIE international standards for cellular therapy product collection, processing, and administration. 3rd ed. Omaha, NE: Foundation for the Accreditation of Cellular Therapy and the Joint Accreditation Committee of ISCT and EBMT, 2006.
7. Good automated manufacturing practice (GAMP) guide for validation of automated systems, GAMP 4. Tampa, FL: International Society for Pharmaceutical Engineering, 2001.

In: Areman EM, Loper K, eds
Cellular Therapy: Principles, Methods, and Regulations
Bethesda, MD: AABB, 2009

◆◆◆ **20** ◆◆◆

Approaches to Validation for Cellular Therapy Products

Gary C. du Moulin, PhD, MPH

QUALITY CANNOT BE TESTED INTO A PRODuct. This well-known adage underscores the need to mitigate variability by first understanding and then controlling the critical parameters of a process, which will lead to the safe and efficacious manufacture of a pharmaceutical product. The process by which variability is assessed and controlled is validation and is particularly relevant for cellular therapy (CT) products. Regulators have emphasized the need for validation with the increasing acceptance of the therapeutic potential and commercial realization for these products.[1-8] Moreover, the clarification by the US Food and Drug Administration (FDA) of "351" vs "361" products, the promulgation of the good tissue practice regulations [Code of Federal Regulations (CFR) Title 21, Part 1271], and the emergence of global regulatory paradigms for these products reinforce the importance of validation.[5,6] Historically, the application of the concepts of validation focused on aspects of the manufacturing process and assurance of a sterile product. However, since the creation of regulated CT products, specific vali-

dation guidance has been published, and validation programs are reviewed during preapproval inspections that encompass facility, equipment, raw materials, cleaning, and software aspects.[2] In fact, every aspect of a regulated process requires validation as an accepted means of defending the science and demonstrating the robustness of the manufacturing process.

The FDA has developed definitions for validation that have stood the test of time, such as "establishing *documented* evidence which provides a high degree of *assurance* that a specific process will *consistently* produce a product meeting its *predetermined* specification and quality attributes" (emphasis added).[8] Inherent in this definition is the demonstration that the process is understood and that it is controlled. Inspectors are given guidance before reviewing validation submissions and are taught that the requirement of process validation is implicit in the language of 21 CFR 211.100 of the current good manufacturing practice regulations, which states, "There shall be written procedures for production and process control to assure that drug

Gary C. du Moulin, PhD, MPH, Vice President, Quality Operations, and Senior Director, Quality Compliance, Genzyme Biosurgery, Cambridge, Massachusetts

The author has disclosed no conflicts of interest.

products have the identity, strength, quality, and purity they purport or are represented to possess."[4] This chapter reviews the elements of validation required for CT products and describes elements that should be incorporated into a robust validation program. FDA guidance documents are available and should be consulted to more fully appreciate the concepts and application principles for validation.

Unique Requirements for the Validation of Cellular Therapy Products

The inherent biological nature of CT products presents a series of issues that differs in complexity from traditional pharmaceutical and biopharmaceutical practice. CT product developers must be prepared to address challenging quality concerns in the quest to ensure product safety and efficacy.[9-12] For example, in products that are based on autologous therapeutic modalities, patient biopsies that are collected in various clinical surroundings under differing conditions may result in variances in size, condition, and site of harvest. These and other variables are outside the control of the cell-processing facility and can affect the growth and performance of the living cells. The issues are less problematic for allogeneic products. However, cell lines are still subject to change as a result of their culture environment and conditions of storage (eg, freezing). The control of cell propagation, maintenance, expansion, and purification must be monitored and the mechanism of action or potency must be demonstrated.

A number of CT products are characterized by a limited shelf life, resulting in a need to develop release assays that are rapid and also exhibit the appropriate specificity and ruggedness to assess compliance to release specifications. For autologous CT products, each patient lot receives the full complement of in-process and final release testing. Tissues and cellular materials transported to the cell-processing facility as well as the final cell product returned to the patient must be shipped in specially engineered packaging systems that ensure a controlled, protective environment for living cells. Shipping containers must maintain the integrity of cells within a defined temperature range over a period to allow transit to and from points of origin. Cell transit and processing activities are governed by the known limited shelf life of the living cells.

Cellular Therapy Processes That Should Be Validated

The number of validations that must be conducted will depend on the manufacturing process and the ancillary systems that support it. These processes and systems include any sterilization process, the establishment of the cleanroom condition and environmental controls (static and in operation), all aseptic filling and manipulation processes through process simulations and media fills, and cleaning processes. In addition, validation should be performed to assess the conditions of shipping, including the tissue procurement procedure and the controls engineered into the container for transporting the CT product. There are well-established protocols for validating these processes because they may be considered "devices" and would require assessment under International Organization for Standardization (ISO) Standard 13485 and the Medical Devices Directives.[13] All analytical procedures used for in-process and lot-release testing require validation before Phase III or pivotal clinical investigations commence. Finally, process validation should take into account the inherent variability of the ancillary materials and components and the potential for drift of the quality of the product if these materials are changed or modified by the manufacturer during scale-up of the process.[14] Because most CT manufacturing processes are not automated, the skill and ability of personnel to work in an aseptic processing environment must be assessed by process simulation and media fill studies.

Elements and Definition of Validation

Validation is a serious endeavor. Developers of CT products must understand the constituents of a validation program and learn the terminology that will ensure that regulatory reviews will be productive. Several elements comprise a validation program. Because manufacturing processes of most of these products require input regarding the facility, equipment, ancillary materials, and personnel qualification, these elements need to be considered early and incorporated into a well-documented validation master planning process that articulates the validation approach and the contribution of each of these elements into a product design. The qualification process of each of these elements is clearly defined within this living document throughout the early phases of a product life cycle. The validation master plan therefore becomes the blueprint for the project and provides information for document formatting, organization, and resource management. A complete list of standard operating procedures (SOPs), flow diagrams, and drawings should be included as they are developed. The validation master plan will be inspected later during the preapproval inspection process and should be one of the best maintained documents within the quality program. Reviews of inspection outcomes show that validation issues are one of the most frequently cited areas of concern.[15] The validation master plan should describe the goals and objectives of what must be validated and include procedures that define how validation protocols are constructed, validation experiments conducted, data collected and evaluated, and summary reports written, and it should give the process for approval of changes, amendments, and deviations.

Validation has its own vocabulary and terminology. A few definitions are germane to the discussion of validation:

- **Design qualification (DQ)** identifies and qualifies critical parameters and conditions of the product. If the product has features that will define it as a device, a well-described process and details can be found in the device quality system regulations (21 CFR 800) and ISO 13485.[13]
- **Installation qualification (IQ)** ensures that systems are installed in accordance with the approved design, specifications, and regulatory codes and that the manufacturer's installation recommendations have been taken into consideration.
- **Operational qualification (OQ)** verifies that the equipment can operate as designed and tested and is capable of repeatable operation throughout the entire operating range of process variables.

- **Process qualification (PQ)** documents that processes operate consistently and reliably at the normal operating limits of critical parameters, especially when appropriate challenges are applied. Critical parameters or attributes should normally be identified during the development stage, and the necessary ranges for the reproducible operation should be defined.

Three elements need to be considered when formulating a plan for validation:

1. The critical quality attributes of the product need to be defined.
2. The process parameters that could affect the critical quality attributes of the product must be identified.
3. The range for each critical process parameter to be used during routine manufacturing and process control should be determined.[7]

Once these determinations have been made, process validation can be performed by development, approval, and execution of a validation protocol. Validation can also be accomplished prospectively, retrospectively, or concurrently. However, prospective validation is considered the preferable approach when a product is being developed for regulatory approval. To ensure that a product is manufactured that meets approved specifications and standards, a number of lots of the product are prepared under normal conditions of scale. The number of conformance batches or lots that are prepared should be determined by considering the goal to demonstrate consistency and confidence in the manufacturing process. Acceptance criteria should be developed that provide quantitative measurements to demonstrate process understanding and consistency. For each validation element, a validation protocol should be generated that includes the methodology for testing acceptance criteria, the means of collecting and evaluating data, and expected conclusions. The protocol should also contain instructions for the investigation of failures and procedures for re-evaluating and retesting.

Creating Procedures and Constructing a Protocol

SOPs should be drafted that define uniform procedures for validation activities. The procedures should apply to all equipment, utilities, facilities, computerized systems, software, processes, subprocesses, and assays that may contribute to the variability of the finished product. Because validation projects include a mix of many disciplines, including representation from quality assurance, engineering, and manufacturing, responsibilities should be clearly defined. The procedure should have a section in which all terms used in validation are defined. Normally, a validation study director is appointed who oversees the project. This person is chosen on the basis of his or her expertise and the nature of the proposed validation. Clear guidance should be provided in this overarching procedure for defining the components of an IQ, OQ, or PQ of equipment or systems or the validation of an assay or process. The procedure should also define the structure of the protocol and the format of the final report. Finally, the procedure should describe steps to follow if any planned or unplanned digression from the approved validation protocol occurs. Depending on the size and complexity of the organization, additional procedures may be drafted that describe revalidation policies or specific guidance for highly intricate protocols, such as for assay validation.

The validation protocol should be developed in compliance with the procedures. Elements to consider in the development of validation protocols include the identification of the process, equipment, or system to be validated, and the determination of objective and measurable criteria concerning the length and duration of the validation, the personnel involved, special controls or conditions, and statistical methods for data collection and analysis. The protocol should clearly define what will be verified or measured, how it will be verified or measured, and how many repetitions or runs need to be measured. These elements, along with quantitative acceptance and rejection criteria, form the basis of a robust validation protocol.

Product development is a part of the product life cycle in which validation plays a crucial role, not only in making the process fully understandable and controlling its inherent variability, but also in providing a baseline and compendia of information for later improvements in the product or process. Moreover, successful validation provides the basis for the development of robust SOPs, appropriate training, and maintenance that ensure that

the manufacturing process will remain consistent over time.

Maintaining a State of Validation

Maintaining a process in a validated steady state requires continual evaluation of data derived from in-process testing and monitoring and analysis of trends observed over time. Statistical process control methodology is widely used in other manufacturing industries but is problematic if applied to CT product manufacturing. Because of the inherent variability in the biological nature of the product, it is difficult to identify and assess drift. Process evaluation is more difficult because of the inherent variability of the primary raw material (eg, patient tissue), operator-to-operator variability, and variability in the ancillary materials used in the process (eg, enzymes and media). It can be difficult to determine quickly when product variations are caused by a process variable that has undergone a change or when performance fluctuations represent uncontrollable and natural biological variations. The problem is exacerbated in early product development because large numbers of manufacturing procedures are not performed, which makes the determination of unacceptable variation difficult. However, the collection of process data such as cell growth, process yields, and product qualities such as morphology and viability can be useful for determining the typical operating range of the process. This data collection may help to establish the normal level of biological variability inherent within the process.

Process or Product Changes

Changes in process because of unanticipated modifications in ancillary materials or anticipated modifications as a result of process improvements require revalidation. FDA guidance instructs that validation protocols must be developed to "demonstrate the lack of an adverse effect for the specified types of change on the identity, strength, quality, purity, or potency of the product as it relates to the safety and effectiveness of the product."[16] For regulated products, process changes and protocol parameters are usually discussed with the FDA before execution of the validation. However, changes that occur in products under development or during clinical trials should undergo similar scrutiny by the developers and should be made only when one can reliably predict and assess the impact of the change on the product. A number of guidance documents are available, but in the end the protocol should be well defined, detailed, and scientifically sound.

Conclusion

Validation is an essential component in the development of CT products. It is a skill set that may appear arduous and time consuming. However, if the goal is to develop products that can exert a powerful biological repair function, then the investment of time to learn and apply the principles of validation are well worth it. Seminars and conferences on validation topics are sponsored throughout the year by a number of organizations (eg, the Parenteral Drug Association). A facility can ensure that CT products are prepared properly, exhibit the necessary therapeutic characteristics, and are safe for patient administration by applying the principles of validation.

References/Resources

1. Food and Drug Administration. Guidance for industry: Validation of procedures for processing of human tissues intended for transplantation; final guidance. (March 2002) Rockville, MD: CBER Office of Communication, Training, and Manufacturers Assistance, 2002.
2. Food and Drug Administration. Guidance for FDA reviewers and sponsors: Content and review of chemistry, manufacturing, and control (CMC) information for human somatic cell therapy investigational new drug applications (INDs). (April 2008) Rockville, MD: CBER Office of Communication, Training, and Manufacturers Assistance, 2008.
3. Food and Drug Administration. Draft guidance: Analytical procedures and methods validation. Chemistry, manufacturing, and controls documentation. (August 2000) Rockville, MD: CDER Office of Communication and Training and CBER Office of Communication, Training, and Manufacturers Assistance, 2000.
4. Food and Drug Administration. Guidance for industry: Sterile drug products produced by aseptic processing—current good manufacturing practice. (September 2004) Rockville, MD: CDER Office of Communication and Training and CBER Office of Communication, Training, and Manufacturers Assistance, 2004.
5. Food and Drug Administration. Compliance program inspection of human cells, tissues, and cellular and tissue-based products (HCT/Ps)—7341.002. Rockville, MD: CBER Office of Compliance and Biologics Quality, 2005.
6. Food and Drug Administration. Compliance program inspection of biological drug products—7345.848. Rockville, MD: CBER Office of Compliance and Biologics Quality, 2005.
7. Food and Drug Administration. ICH Guidance for industry—Q7A good manufacturing practice guidance for active pharmaceutical ingredients. (August 2001) Rockville, MD: CDER Office of Communication and Training and CBER Office of Communication, Training, and Manufacturers Assistance, 2001.
8. Food and Drug Administration. Guideline on general principles of process validation. (May 1987) Rockville, MD: CDER Office of Compliance, 1987.
9. Schaeffer S, Stone BB, Wolfrum JM, Du Moulin GC. Ex vivo autologous cell therapies. In: Sofer G, Zabriskie DW, eds. Biopharmaceutical process validation. New York: Marcel Dekker, 2000:361-72.
10. Ostrovski S, Du Moulin GC. Achieving compliance and validation and metrology in cell and gene therapy. Biopharm 1995;8:20-8.
11. Du Moulin GC, Pitkin Z, Shen YJ, et al. Overview of a quality assurance/quality control compliance program consistent with FDA regulations and policies for somatic cell and gene therapies: A four year experience. Cytotechnology 1994;15:365-72.
12. United States Pharmacopeia. Cell and Gene Therapy Expert Committee. <1046> Cell and gene therapy products. In: USP 31-NF 26. Rockville, MD: The United States Pharmacopeial Convention, 2007.
13. International Organization for Standardization. ISO 13485:2003: Medical devices—quality management systems. Requirements for regulatory purposes. Geneva, Switzerland: ISO, 2003.
14. United States Pharmacopeia. Cell and Gene Therapy Expert Committee. <1043> Ancillary materials for cell, gene, and tissue engineered products. In: USP 31-NF 26. Rockville, MD: The United States Pharmacopeial Convention, 2007.
15. Buchholz S, Gangi VJ, Johnson A, et al. Results of a survey of biological drug and devices industries inspected by FDA under the Team Biologics Program. PDA J Pharm Sci Technol 2007;61:211-22.
16. Code of federal regulations. Change to an approved application. Title 21, CFR Part 601.12. Washington, DC: US Government Printing Office, 2008 (revised annually).

Process and Product Development
for Cellular Therapeutics

PROCESS DEVELOPMENT AND PRODUCT development are terms that describe the series of steps to bring a new cellular therapy (CT) product from a research environment to a clinical one. These terms may also be applied to the transition of a process or product from early-phase safety studies to Phase III studies to demonstrate the product's safety, effectiveness, and readiness for commercialization. This section focuses on the use of a risk-based approach to process and product development for early-phase clinical studies. Steps in product development can include scale-up and optimization of manufacturing processes; supply, reagent, and equipment evaluation; technology transfer; and draft document preparation [eg, standard operating procedures (SOPs), batch production records, test sample lists, and procedure flowcharts]. Phase I clinical studies are designed to evaluate safety, but it is never too early to consider Phase III and commercialization issues such as potency assays. Even if the long-term plan is to transfer the process or product to another company or to outsource product manufacturing, decisions about the Phase I study may affect future clinical trials because process changes made during late-stage studies must ensure that the product that has been manufactured is the same as in Phase I.[1]

This section is written from the perspective of a university-based CT laboratory translational program. Other models of product and process development are used by nonacademic organizations. However, in all cases it is wise to include the clinical CT laboratory input early in development.

Section Editors: Janice M. Davis-Sproul, MAS, MT(ASCP)SBB, Manager, Cell Therapy and Development Laboratories, Sidney Kimmel Comprehensive Cancer Center at Johns Hopkins, Baltimore, Maryland, and Olive J. Sturtevant, MHP, MT(ASCP) SBB/SLS, Quality Assurance Manager, Connell & O'Reilly, Cell Manipulation Core Facility, Dana-Farber Cancer Institute, Boston, Massachusetts

The editors have disclosed no conflicts of interest.

In: Areman EM, Loper K, eds
Cellular Therapy: Principles, Methods, and Regulations
Bethesda, MD: AABB, 2009

♦♦♦ **21** ♦♦♦

Overview of Process Development

Jo Lynn Procter, MEd, MT(ASCP)SBB; Amy McDaniel, PhD;
Diane Kadidlo, MT(ASCP)SBB; Lizabeth Cardwell, MT(ASCP),
MBA, RAC; Michele W. Sugrue, MS, MT(ASCP)SBB;
and Douglas Padley, MT(ASCP)

IN THE SETTING OF INVESTIGATIONAL CEL-
lular therapies, process development often
begins with an investigator's having an idea and
some preclinical experimental data. The goal of
development, within the framework of the translation of basic research findings into clinical evaluation, is to create a process that generates a safe
product in a consistent fashion given the limitations of working with biological products and the
confines of government regulations. The plan
should be to build quality into the processes and
products from the beginning. An overview of the
product development process with steps or tasks
for each phase is shown in Fig 21-1. A flowchart
that depicts the steps that support the implementation of a new process is shown in Fig 21-2.

Another approach to development that incorporates the concepts described for a risk-based
approach but uses the language of the medical
device sector is design control. This approach relies
on a sequence of project design and development
steps to ensure that the design requirements for the
device are met. The Code of Federal Regulations
(CFR) Title 21, Part 820.30 of the Quality System
Regulation (QSR) provides specific steps for documenting the development and revision of medical
device manufacturing. It also requires that responsibility for change implementation be assigned for
all phases of development, even postimplementa-
tion changes that are made to meet changing market needs or to correct original design flaws. For
cellular therapy (CT) products, "input" is defined

*Jo Lynn Procter, MEd, MT(ASCP)SBB, Supervisor of Operations, Cell Processing Section, National Institutes of Health Clinical Center,
Bethesda, Maryland; Amy McDaniel, PhD, Associate Director, Microbial Science and Technology, Wyeth Biotech, Andover, Massachusetts;
Diane Kadidlo, MT(ASCP)SBB, Director, Molecular and Cellular Therapeutics, University of Minnesota, and Technical Supervisor, Cell
Therapy Clinical Laboratory, University of Minnesota Medical Center Fairview, St Paul, Minnesota; Lizabeth Cardwell, MT(ASCP), MBA,
RAC, Principal, Compliance Consulting, Seattle, Washington; Michele W. Sugrue, MS, MT(ASCP)SBB, Coordinator, Research Programs,
Division of Hematology/Oncology, Department of Medicine, University of Florida and Shands Hospital, Gainesville, Florida; and Douglas
Padley, MT(ASCP), Development Coordinator, Human Cellular Therapy Laboratory, Division of Transfusion Medicine, Mayo Clinic,
Rochester, Minnesota*

The authors have disclosed no conflicts of interest.

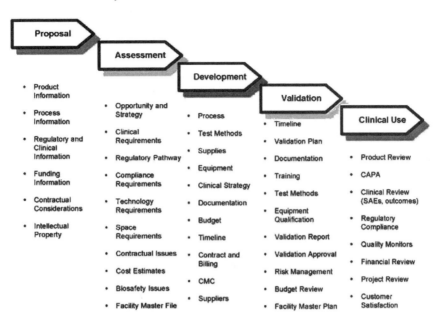

Figure 21-1. Product development process overview.
CMC = chemistry, manufacturing, and controls; CAPA = corrective and preventive action; SAE = serious adverse event.

as the user requirements, which are the technical specifications or acceptance criteria for the product. Development viewed in this fashion evaluates the interactions of inputs and processes as they relate to the manufacture of products with reproducible characteristics. A flowchart for design control for CT is shown in Fig 21-3.

Development Process Initiation

Product and process development should always begin with a meeting. The attendees should include, at a minimum, the principal investigator and a representative of the CT laboratory. The purpose of the meeting is to discuss the goals of the project. In this first step, some basic scientific and practical questions need to be addressed. The answers define a broad product concept and its intended use. What is the product? Are there unique product characteristics? What has the investigator done in the research setting to prove that the proposal has merit? Have animal or human studies been performed? If so, what are the results?

In the excitement of a new discovery and its translation to the clinic, the financial aspects of development may be overlooked. However, the cost of development is not trivial and should be discussed early in the process. The use of clinical-grade materials, the expense of product testing, and the cost of technologist time add up. Research grants may or may not be written with development studies in mind. Therefore, it is important to educate investigators on the need to include translational studies in their grants. Routine financial requirements need to cover labor, overhead, supplies, equipment, cellular source material, and quality control (QC) testing for development and validation studies. Other costs, which may add several hundred thousand dollars to the project's bottom line, may be incurred for additional qualification testing of raw materials, the purchase of additional equipment, or the development of new tests.

After the initial meetings, when possible, a representative of the CT laboratory should observe the research procedure to begin to understand the process and the expected outcomes. A flowchart of the

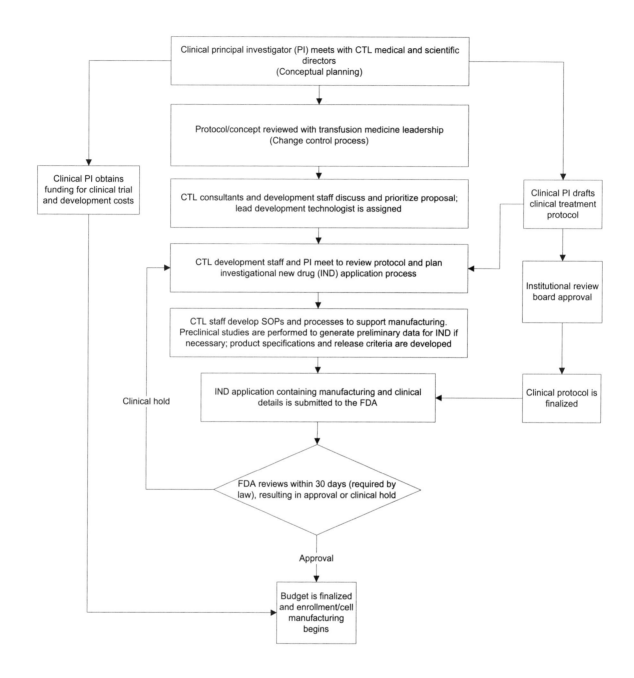

Figure 21-2. Flowchart for new process implementation.
CTL = cellular therapy laboratory; SOP = standard operating procedure.

research process that includes as many details as possible is helpful during this time. The representative should identify the goal of each processing step and ask the researcher the importance of certain parameters. For example, are cells centrifuged at a certain speed in the research laboratory because of routine practice or for a scientific or practical reason? It is important to prepare a list of equipment,

supplies, and materials used in the process. On the basis of the information gathered, a systematic and risk-based approach to the transition from research to clinical-scale production should be developed. Risk management methodologies are described at the end of this section, though risk assessment is referred to throughout. Safety considerations should focus on providing a safe product but also

Design Control for Cell Therapy

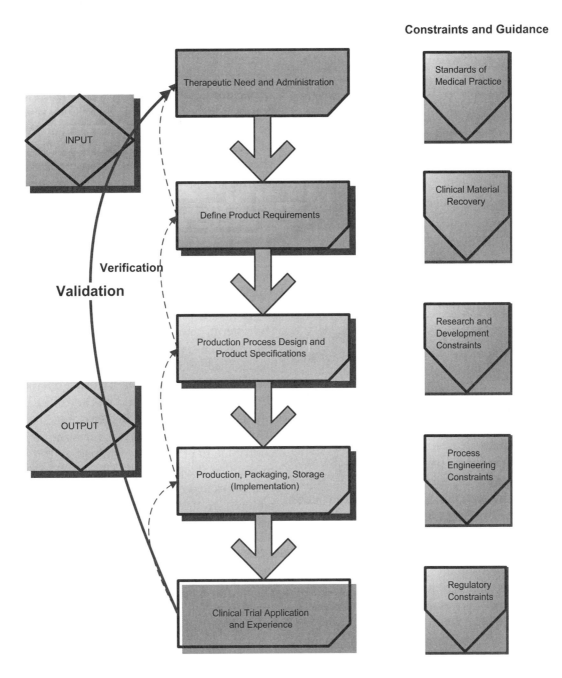

Figure 21-3. Design control flowchart for cellular therapy.

should address any safety considerations for the staff who are performing the procedure and for the environment. Throughout the development process, it is important to evaluate the changes made and how they affect the product that is manufactured. Have the development changes resulted in

the manufacture of the same product that was generated using the research protocol? Switching reagents from animal-based materials to those approved for human use may or may not affect the final product. Therefore, appropriate control materials should be included in these evaluations.

Depending on the product and process, assays may need to be developed to monitor the process and characterize the final product. A detailed discussion of considerations for assay development is presented later in this section.

This section presents an overview of considerations for process and product development for early-phase CT products. In brief, the keys to success during process and product development are 1) a clear understanding of the deliverables or goals, 2) the productive use of team members, and 3) a focus on risk and quality throughout the process. The topics within this section were divided for presentation, but in actual process and product development they are often addressed concurrently and should be linked.

Development Team and Communication

One key element for a successful development project is to bring the right people together for the planning, design, and implementation phases of the project. The number and scope of the necessary team members will depend on the project. If the project could affect areas other than the cell-processing laboratory, representative members from other groups should be on the team. Usually, the more complex the organization, the more team members are needed. Team members can include the investigator, the research technicians, clinical laboratory staff, quality assurance (QA) staff, the clinical investigator, and others as necessary. Having a diversified group review the project and analyze what needs to be accomplished helps to ensure success. Different perspectives enrich the process and reduce the risk of failure.

Team meetings are critical elements of development. It is important to prepare meeting minutes to provide a record of decisions and the reasons for the decisions. Process and product decisions are made for various reasons when using a risk-based approach to development, including scientific and financial considerations. Therefore, meeting minutes are a valuable communication tool as staff transition on or off the team. Minutes also may provide insights if there are failures during process validation. In addition to documenting decisions,

meeting minutes can include timelines and identify individuals who are responsible for action items.

As a project progresses through the development process, obtaining documentation of management approvals is necessary, and approaches will vary depending on the size of the organization. Examples for documentation include a study report (Appendix 21-1) and a design-phase transition approval form (Appendix 21-2). Study reports can be included in regulatory submissions. Appendix 21-3 is a template for a final pre-implementation checklist, which can be used after the development work is complete and before clinical implementation.

Facility Assessment

Before initiation of a new project, a facility risk assessment should be performed as part of the development process. If the process is simple and short term, and the cell manipulations occur in closed systems, then the facility can be a controlled, unclassified laboratory work space. If the processes include long-term cell culture using open systems, then the work space should be controlled and classified to help ensure that the environment does not adversely affect the product during processing or contribute to product contamination. If it is determined that the process does need to be performed in a controlled environment, the next questions to address are 1) What degree of classification is needed? and 2) Should the airflow in that environment be positive or negative in relation to the surrounding environment? Again, risk assessment of the product, process, and ancillary agents used in the process determines the degree of facility control that is required.

Table 21-1 lists the facility controls to consider on the basis of the type of process performed, and Table 21-2 lists the types of processes that can be performed in a classified area. It should be remembered that the risk might be to the product, the employees, or the environment. Another factor that should be considered is whether there is adequate space for the new process. If new equipment or supplies are needed, assessments can determine 1) if the items can be incorporated into the current workspace and 2) if current processes would be jeopardized by the new equipment or supplies.

Table 21-1. Facility Controls According to Processes Performed

Processing	Facility Controls	Classification	Airflow
Routine (minimal manipulation) closed procedures	Temperature Humidity Airflow Security	Unclassified	Positive
Routine (minimal manipulation) open procedures	Temperature Humidity Airflow Security	Classified BSC: Class 100 Level 2	Positive
Cell expansion with no viral vectors (open systems)	Temperature Humidity Airflow Security Viable and nonviable monitoring	Classified BSC: Class 100 Level 2	Positive
Cell expansion with viral vectors (open systems)	Temperature Humidity Airflow Security Changeover procedures Viable and nonviable monitoring	Classified BSC: Class 100 May need biological safety Level 3	Negative
Viral vectors (open systems)	Temperature Humidity Airflow Security Changeover procedures Viable and nonviable monitoring	Classified BSC: Class 100 May need biological safety Level 3	Negative

BSC = biological safety cabinet.

Table 21-2. Examples of Operations That May Be Performed in Classified Areas[1]

Class/ISO Equivalent	Example of Operation
Class 100/ISO 5	• Open manipulations • Aseptic processing
Class 1000/ISO 6 Class 10,000/ISO 7	• Surround Class 100 (bioburden control) • Centrifugation • Location of incubators and closed systems
Class 100,000/ISO 8*	• Surround Class 10,000 (areas requiring moderate control) • Centrifugation and labware storage • Placement of incubators and closed systems

ISO = International Organization for Standardization.
*If additional microbiological controls are required, the procedure should be performed in a Class 10,000 area.

Regardless of the facility classification, cell-processing laboratories need to have control of the temperature, humidity, access, and workflow to ensure adequate protection of the product during processing. Again, the extent of control is based on the processing that is performed in the facility. Temperature and humidity can be critical for the survival of cell cultures, proper chemical reactions for certain tests, and the safe operation of equipment. For example, equipment that has lasers is sensitive to humidity levels in the environment, as are sterile connecting devices.

The aseptic processing guidelines from USP General Chapter <797> suggest that any open procedure should occur in a controlled, classified space to minimize the risk of contamination.[2] Open procedures need to occur in at least a Class 2 biological safety cabinet (BSC). The space around the cabinet should be controlled and classified as appropriate. Figure 21-4 provides an example of the controlled space surrounding a BSC. Movement around the cabinet space needs to be limited to prevent contaminants from flowing into the BSC workspace. As the clinical trial moves along the pathway from Phase I to Phase III, the manufacturing environment may change. If the new procedure involves hazardous chemicals, then a chemical safety cabinet vented to the exterior of the building is needed to protect the employees from harm during the proce-

dures. Chemicals not used in routine cell processing can creep into the process, especially when the cell-processing laboratory is involved with translational preclinical process development. Solvents such as formaldehyde for fixing slides, acids for dissolving gels, or other hazardous materials are common in the preclinical setting. Risk assessment for a new process should consider any hazardous materials or waste that might be generated that would affect whether the facility and the employees can safely handle the new process.

Facilities that perform both open and closed processes as well as routine, preclinical, and investigational manufacturing need additional and appropriate space to maintain segregation of products and raw materials. Study materials need to be isolated from routine supplies and materials. This may mean having a dedicated piece of equipment or creating a separate storage area within a storage area (eg, refrigerator, freezer, room temperature) for routine use. What might be acceptable for one facility may not be possible for another. Facility needs are based on the size, scope, and complexity of operations. Most regulatory bodies will use a risk-based approach to assess facility requirements. The regulatory standards do not clearly define the differences in the size or the complexity of manufacturing facilities. The facility must assess product volume, complexity levels, the mixed uses of the

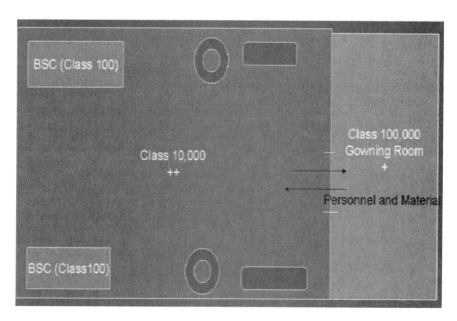

Figure 21-4. Example of the controlled space around a biological safety cabinet (BSC).[1]

facility (routine and complex), and safety risks before moving forward with a new process or procedure.

Cell-processing facilities that perform open processes in a BSC should determine which controls are appropriate to ensure that the cabinets are functioning properly. Viable and nonviable particle testing should be used as necessary. Table 21-3 is a USP <1116> chart[3] that provides suggested monitoring for sterile products. A modification of this chart can be developed according to the identified risks.

Equipment Assessment

Equipment evaluation is an integral part of development. Consideration should be given to the process-specific equipment that is required. Is it necessary for the clinical laboratory to purchase equipment? If so, is more than one piece of equipment needed and is the equipment manufactured by a single vendor? Depending on the situation, it may be necessary for the initial development studies to be performed in the investigator's research laboratory. If this decision is made, a study plan should be prepared to transition from the research to the clinical laboratory. Other risks to be evaluated include the cleaning requirements for the equipment, the risk of product cross-contamination during equipment use, any unique safety hazards associated with the equipment, facility issues

(special room temperatures, power sources, or airflow), and staff training. When a piece of equipment is selected for use, the risk of breakdown should be addressed as it relates to the manufacturing process and the final product. Depending on the type of product, whether the product is manufactured for a single patient or for multiple patients (an off-the-shelf product), and the cell production goals, equipment needs may change as the study advances from Phase I to Phase III. Therefore, additional development studies related to equipment may be anticipated over the course of the project. Additionally, any regulatory requirements related to the equipment should be identified.

Ancillary Reagents and Materials Assessment

The types of reagents and materials used in CT manufacturing include antibiotics, buffers, cell culture media, cytokines, chemokines, cryoprotectants, dyes, density gradient solutions, enzymes, lysing solutions, magnetic particles, membrane columns, monoclonal antibodies, peptides, plasma, plasmids, proteins, serum, starches, synthetic matrices, toxins, tumor antigens, and viruses. These agents are used during manufacturing to produce a desired effect and are not usually a primary constituent of the final product. These reagents and materials are used in the preparation

Table 21-3. Environmental Classifications and Limits*

	Classification	
	Class 100 **M3.5**	**Class 10,000** **M5.5**
Frequency	Each shift	Each shift
Total particle counts	100/ft³ (>0.5 μm)	10,000 ft³ (>0.5 μm)
Airborne viables	0.1 CFU/ft³	0.5 CFU/ft³
Surface viables (except floor)	3 CFU	5 CFU
Surface viables (floors)	3 CFU	10 CFU
Personnel gowns	5 CFU	20 CFU
Personnel gloves	3 CFU	10 CFU

*Reprinted with permission.[3]
ft³ = cubic foot; CFU = colony-forming unit.

of both "351" and "361" products as defined by the Food and Drug Administration (FDA).

When a product is submitted for an investigational new drug (IND) classification from the FDA, a chemistry, manufacturing, and controls (CMC) section is required as part of the submission. Providing comprehensive and detailed information on the use of ancillary reagents and materials is essential to assessing the risk to subjects who are enrolled in clinical trials under an IND classification. Developing a system for the selection and qualification of ancillary reagents and materials should be paramount to CT programs involved in Phase I and II clinical trials. Such a system is especially important when the reagent or material is being used "off label" and is neither approved nor licensed for the intended manufacturing use. A critical part of development, in addition to the qualification of materials, is the evaluation of alternate materials that may be more suited for clinical use. For example, if a cell line is expanded in a medium containing fetal bovine serum, will it expand in a serum-free medium? This type of development study is essential to reduce the risk of the unnecessary exposure of the product to materials not approved for human use. It may also indicate that there is no suitable substitute material.

One approach for the qualification of reagents and materials used in the preparation of CT products that do not have a clinical-grade formulation is a risk-based, tiered approach. The tiered approach to qualification allows the development team to focus more of its efforts on the materials that are the most risky. When there is greater risk to the patient, there are more stringent requirements for the qualification of the reagent or material. *USP 30—National Formulary 25*,[4] a combination of two official compendia of pharmaceutical standards, describes a comprehensive system for the qualification of ancillary reagents and materials for cell-, gene-, and tissue-engineered products that uses a risk-based classification system. In general, the degree of risk associated with a reagent or material depends on the answers to the following questions:

- Is the source material licensed or approved for therapeutic use?
- Is the manufacturing process for the material controlled and documented?
- How is the material used in the CT product manufacturing process?

- How much of the material is used?
- Is the material part of the final product formulation?

If the reagent or material is licensed or approved by the FDA for therapeutic use, then routine vendor qualification is the only requirement. However, if the reagent or material is not licensed or approved for therapeutic use, additional vendor information is needed. This information includes 1) material characterization and release test results, 2) toxicological profiles, and 3) manufacturing procedures. From the CT development perspective, risk is assessed according to 1) how the material is to be used in the manufacturing process, 2) whether the material comes in direct contact with the cells or tissue and, if so, whether the material can be washed out of the final product, and 3) whether there is a history of use of the material in previous clinical trials. The answers to these questions determine the risk associated with the use of the material.

Development of a risk-based approach for the qualification of reagents and materials is a way to systematize and manage the oversight of ancillary reagents and materials in a laboratory. The USP approach has four tiers. Table 21-4 contains examples of reagents that have been classified using this approach.

Tier I materials are described as low risk and highly qualified (ie, licensed or approved for therapeutic use). Qualification documentation would include a drug master file cross-reference, certificate of analysis, documentation of lot-to-lot performance, documentation of removal from the final product, and documentation of stability during the process.

Tier II materials are also described as low risk and are well characterized. However, the "FDA seal of approval" is not available in the form of a license or approval for therapeutic use. Therefore, in addition to the documentation listed for Tier I materials, it may be necessary to perform a functional assay or to further qualify a vendor by performing an audit.

Tier III materials are described as moderate risk and are produced for in-vitro diagnostic or reagent-grade use. In addition to the steps taken for Tier I and II materials, Tier III materials may require working with the manufacturer to have the manufacturing process upgraded to good manufac-

Table 21-4. Examples of a Risk-Based Approach for Material Classification

USP Risk Level	Materials
Tier I	Human serum albumin • FDA-approved for human use • Package insert
Tier II	Human AB serum • Manufactured internally for use as a reagent only • Source is a "pedigreed" (repeatedly tested) donor who meets FDA and AABB criteria for allogeneic whole blood donation • Procedure • Documentation of reagents and disposables used • Safety assays (sterility culture) • HLA antibody screening
Tier III	Cell and tissue culture media • Manufacturer certificate of analysis • Vendor qualification • Confirm certificate of analysis test results critical to product (could include functional assays) • Upgrade manufacturing process for material to GMP
Tier IV	Fetal bovine serum • Certificate of analysis • Assess lot-to-lot variability • Verify traceability to country of origin • Ensure that the country of origin is qualified as safe with respect to source-relevant animal diseases, including transmissible spongiform encephalopathy • Lot-to-lot biocompatibility, cytotoxicity, and adventitious agent testing

FDA = Food and Drug Administration; GMP = good manufacturing practice.

turing practice (GMP) status or to develop internal specifications, which may include lot-to-lot biocompatibility, cytotoxicity, or adventitious agent testing.

Tier IV materials are designated as high risk and should be avoided for manufacturing clinical products whenever possible. It may be necessary to take extra precautions such as verifying the country of origin and performing adventitious agent testing for animal-source materials.

The following are guidelines for establishing a comprehensive qualification program for ancillary materials:
- Qualify each vendor.
- Create a master list of materials that states the intended use and storage requirements for each.
- Qualify reagents for off-label use.
- Maintain records of receipt, qualification, review, and release for use in processing.

- Perform necessary quality control according to the manufacturer's recommendations and as required for the intended use.
- Perform stability studies if the expiration date is not known.
- Characterize the reagent or material for biologic properties that pertain to its function.
- Determine the quantities required to sustain the desired effect.
- Assess the toxicity level of the materials for human use.
- Develop assays to verify that the final product is safe.

Process Assessment

Process details vary with the project and are linked to the facility, equipment, and material decisions.

One challenge with many CT procedures is that the process needs to be adapted from an open system to a closed or functionally closed system process to reduce the risk of contamination. For example, rather than expanding cells in a flask, a development study could evaluate the use of cell culture bags or cell factories. Other considerations include optimization studies that focus on the optimal media volume in the culture vessels, the number of media changes during expansion, the cell concentration for culture initiation, and the length of the expansion process. During these types of development studies, it is important to evaluate the short-term stability of the product during in-process manipulations. Consideration should be given to possible delays in processing, and the study should determine the acceptable storage temperatures and times. Cryopreservation studies may also be included in process development. These studies may be used later as part of a stability program.

A challenge during development is to determine the appropriate starting material for the studies. What cells should be used for development? The starting material for the clinical study may not be available or may not be available in the appropriate volume or total cell dose. Are surrogate cells available? Are disease-specific products necessary for the process? If development studies are performed by using fewer cells or smaller volumes, holding steps should be included in the evaluation to simu-

late the expected processing times for full-scale production. Depending on the project, the starting material may be a cell line. Information about the cell line (for example, source and infectious disease test results) should be gathered early in the development process to determine whether the cell line is suitable for clinical use.

Assay Development

A cell-processing laboratory may need to develop a new test or, at the very least, adapt a clinical test method for use with specimen types that differ from those for which the assay was specifically designed. It is important to determine the validity of test methods for use on cellular products.

Appropriate method development and validation are critical for the use of a new analytical method. The International Conference on Harmonisation (ICH) has provided guidelines on the validation of analytical methods,[5] and numerous references are available on the subject.[6,7] Nevertheless, because of the variety of methods available, the need to allow for alternative acceptable approaches, and analyses during method development and validation, the terminology in these guidance documents is often vague, which creates difficulty for scientists in this area.

Method validation (see Fig 21-5) is the process of establishing documented evidence by laboratory

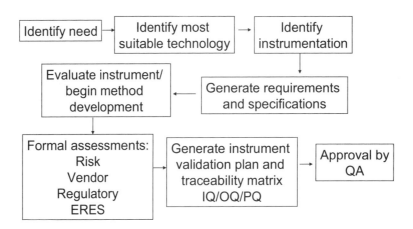

Figure 21-5. Example of validation process flow for a new method.
ERES = electronic records and electronic signatures; IQ = installation qualification; OQ = operational qualification; PQ = performance qualification; QA = quality assurance.

studies to provide assurance that a method is scientifically sound and will consistently produce results that meet predetermined acceptance criteria. The extent of the validation generally depends on the stage of product development. During early stages of development or the clinical trial, analytical methods may be qualified. Qualification is an activity that precedes validation, whereby key attributes are evaluated and documented in order to support the intended use of the method. Method validation must be completed before application for a license for a CT product.

The first stage of assay method development is to categorize the method according to its role in assessing the identity, potency, purity, concentration, safety, and quality parameters of a product. Methods may be classified according to the following three major categories, as defined by the ICH guidelines:

1. Analytical methods for quantitation of major components or excipients of bulk drug substances or active ingredients in finished pharmaceutical products.

2. Analytical methods for testing for impurities, product-related species, and degradation compounds in bulk drug substances or in finished pharmaceutical products. Methods included in this category may be further classified as either a quantitative test or a limit test.

3. Analytical methods for the identification of an analyte in a sample, which usually involves the comparison of a property of a sample (eg, spectrum, chromatographic behavior, or chemical reactivity) to that of a reference material.

When the method pertains to either quantitation or testing, the expected content or concentration range and the desired accuracy and precision of the determination should be considered and assessed as part of the method development. The accuracy and precision of the developed method must be adequate to make appropriate decisions that are based on the final results. During development of assays that test for impurities, the limit of detection should also be considered and assessed, as well as the potential for interference from other components. For identity tests, method development must address the ability of the method to distinguish the test article from other potential substances. Additional consideration during method development should be given to the

amount of the available sample, which might limit the choice of the analytical method, depending on the volume needed for the test. Furthermore, if large numbers of samples are expected, or if the results of the analysis are required before processing can continue, consideration should be given to the analysis time (per sample) and the sample throughput. Sample stability during the analysis procedure, as well as during storage before analysis, should be assessed. Automation should be considered if large numbers of samples are expected regularly. On the other hand, if only a few samples are expected, a manual method might produce results more quickly. Finally, if the method is intended to be employed at multiple locations, consideration should be given to the ease of transferring the method, the availability of equipment and reagents, and the ability to recruit or train staff with the required expertise to perform the method.

As part of the method validation, a protocol should be written to describe the test method, the recording of critical assay control parameters, and the collection of data for the method. In addition, the protocol should describe safety measures, as applicable. The written protocol should be complete, unambiguous, and easy to follow, and it should contain sufficient detail to permit a trained analyst to perform the test method. The data reduction instruments that are used to collect assay data or to perform data and statistical analysis for validation and routine testing (eg, statistical package and system-specific software) should be documented in the protocol. Furthermore, the validation protocol must detail where data will be captured during the execution of the validation.

Any method-specific requirements that must be achieved to accept the assay as valid (ie, assay acceptance guidelines) should be documented. Documentation should be referenced such that information is traceable to the original source. Any specific system suitability, sample acceptance criteria, or sample stability issues (such as data to demonstrate the stability of all sample preparations throughout the time required to complete the analysis) should be described, and guidance should be provided for assay performance within these constraints. If this information is not available before the validation studies, it should be considered within the design of the test method validation. Although system suitability is not part of method validation, it is an integral part of the test method. Therefore, the appropriate criteria should be built into the test method to show that the equipment, electronics, and analytical operations are accurately performed.

The validation parameters that will be evaluated for the test method should be listed in the protocol. The typical validation parameters for each analytical method (using the ICH guidelines as a model) are listed in Table 21-5. Additional or alternative validation parameters may be defined for the test method, when applicable. The method validation protocol should describe the parameters tested and should include a rationale for their selection. Wherever possible, a combined approach that uses one data set for multiple parameters is recommended.

Risk Assessment Methodology

Many tools can be used to assess risk and prevent errors, accidents, and unacceptable outcomes.[3] The following paragraphs review flowcharting, risk assessment, and failure mode effects analysis (FMEA). As stated previously, risk assessment should begin when the project is in the initial phases of development. This early assessment allows quality to be built into the design from the beginning. When a facility is developing a new product or process, it should assess, rework, educate, and evaluate before trying to validate and implement.

During development, laboratory staff may be working with multiple new elements: products, reagents, methods, equipment, or clinical peers (people). Each brings unique challenges and risks—opportunities for things to go wrong or to have an undesired outcome. Quality improvement or risk assessment is about mitigating or preventing negative outcomes.

Basic risk assessment should be addressed at the start of a new process or product evaluation. Most individuals do this instinctively but, by following a defined process or using formal tools such as a fault tree analysis or FMEA, one may uncover potential risks that otherwise might not have been expected. Once identified, risks or negative outcomes may be objectively measured over time.

As previously stated, selecting appropriate team members and preparing a process flowchart are the first steps in the development process. The next

Table 21-5. Parameters for the Validation of Analytical Methods*

| | Type of Analytical Method | | | |
| | | Testing for Impurities | | |
Validation Parameter	Quantitation of Major Components or Excipients	Quantitation	Limit Test	Identification
Accuracy	+	+	−	−
Precision	+	+	−	−
Specificity	+	+	+	+
Detection limit	−	−	+	−
Quantitation limit	−	+	−	−
Linearity	+	+	−	−
Range	+	+	−	−
Robustness	+	+	+	+

*The requirements for the validation of biological activity methods are not specified in International Conference on Harmonisation guidance. Therefore, these are recommended minimum parameters for validation. Some complex biological assays may require validation of additional parameters.
+ = the validation parameter is normally evaluated; − = the validation parameter is not normally evaluated.

steps are to 1) identify as many risks and potential risks as possible, and 2) rate the risks by using a system that is based on the likelihood of occurrence and the severity of the deviation or event if it occurs. Using that information, the laboratory can identify critical control points in the process, which can detect a failure. The facility should consider different perspectives when assessing and weighing risks, including patient safety, regulatory approval, contamination of clinical laboratory space, safety of staff, cost, time, the loss of irretrievable material, and feasibility.

FMEA is a systematic, proactive method for evaluating a process to identify where and how it might fail to assess the relative impact of different failures and, ultimately, to identify the parts of the process that are most in need of change or monitoring. FMEA is particularly useful for evaluating a new process before implementation and for assessing the impact of a proposed change to an existing process.

FMEA includes the following steps:
1. Flowchart the process and identify the critical testing steps. (An example for a hypothetical product is shown in Fig 21-6.)
2. Identify the areas in which failure might occur and classify them according to the following criteria:
   a. List the failure causes. (Why would the failure happen?)
   b. List the failure effects. (What would be the consequences of each failure?)
   c. Assign a numeric value to each failure mode. This is known as the risk priority number (RPN). For each failure mode, assign an RPN for likelihood of occurrence, likelihood of detection, and severity (see Table 21-6).
3. Calculate the RPN. For each failure mode, multiply the three scores obtained (the 1-to-10 scores for the likelihood of occurrence, detection, and severity). In Table 21-7, the failure

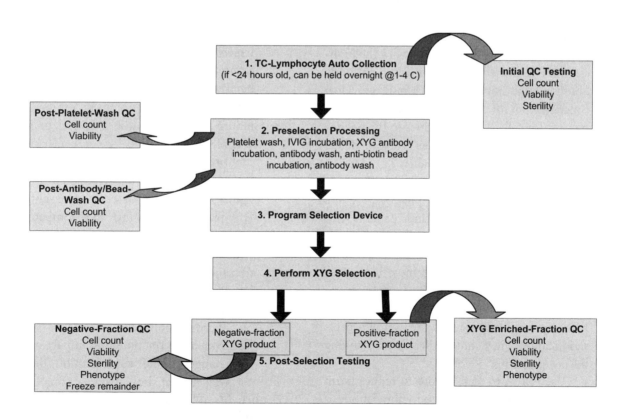

Figure 21-6. Process flowchart for hypothetical product cell (XYG) selection.
QC = quality control; TC = therapeutic cells; IVIG = intravenous immunoglobulin.

Table 21-6. Risk Priority Numbers for Failure Modes*

Likelihood of...	Score of 1	Score of 10
Occurrence	Very unlikely to occur	Very likely to occur
Detection	Very likely to be detected	Very unlikely to be detected
Severity	Very unlikely that harm will occur	Very likely that severe harm will occur

*In patient care examples, a score of 10 for harm often denotes death.

mode "final product purity <80%" may be due to several failure causes. If the cell count of the starting product is too high, the selection process may be compromised. This failure cause has the following profile: a "3" for likelihood of occurrence, a "1" for likelihood of detection, and a "4" for severity, for an overall RPN of "12." Although failure to adjust the starting cell count before selection would result in a poor yield for the final product, the product is salvageable. The negative fraction of the final product could be reselected. The lowest possible score will be 1, and the highest, 1000. Identify the failure modes with the top 10 highest RPNs. These are the causes of failure that should be considered first as improvement opportunities. The failure cause with the highest RPN is caused by a nonspecific antibody binding with tumor cells, which results in a low concentration of the desired cell population plus tumor cells. The similarities in the phenotypes will determine whether one can detect the tumor cells by flow cytometry. The inability to detect tumor cells may lead to a contaminated product. Aside from phenotyping the product, one may need to exclude patients with this tumor type from the selection protocol.

4. Plan improvement efforts. Failure modes with high RPNs are probably the most important parts of the process on which to focus improvement efforts. Failure modes with very low RPNs are not likely to affect the overall process significantly. They should therefore be among the last priorities.
   a. Use FMEA to plan actions to reduce harm from failure modes if the failure mode is likely to occur.
   b. Evaluate the causes and see if any or all of them can be eliminated.

   c. Consider adding a forcing function or change that makes committing an error impossible.
   d. Add a verification step, such as action or alert QC checks.
   e. Modify other processes that contribute to the causes.

5. Identify failures that are unlikely to be detected:
   a. Identify other events that may occur before the failure mode that can serve as flags that the failure mode might happen.
   b. Add a step to the process that intervenes at the earlier event to prevent the failure from occurring (eg, prepare a Gram's stain of a sample from each individual culture before pooling or harvesting if this is a critical or irreversible point).
   c. Consider technological alerts such as devices with alarms to warn users when values are approaching unsafe limits if the failure is likely to cause a critical or irreversible situation.
   d. Identify early warning signs that a failure mode has occurred, and train staff to recognize these signs for early intervention. Use proficiency testing and competency assessment to ensure that staff can detect a situation. For example, use validation runs to train staff through the following:
      i. Providing information and resources, such as reversal agents and antibiotics at critical points.
      ii. Evaluating the potential impact of the changes under consideration during trial runs or simulated trial runs.

The benefits of FMEA include the following:
- The collective knowledge of a team.
- Improvement of the quality, reliability, and safety of the process.

Table 21-7. Example of Failure Analysis

Steps in Process	Failure Mode	Failure Causes	Failure Effects	Likelihood of Occurrence (1-10)	Likelihood of Detection (1-10)	Severity (1-10)	Risk Profile Number	Action to Reduce Failure
5	Final product purity <80%	Selected cell count >10 × 10^9	Cell loss if count exceeds antibody dose	3	1	4	12	Cell count before selection
		Antibody specificity	Marker occasionally found on tumor cells	3	8	8	192	Phenotyping of selected product
		Instrument failure	Failure to run instrument in a timely manner may overexpose cells to antibody	4	1	8	32	Monitor start and end times
		Incubation times	Cells/antibody bond is time dependent	3	1	8	24	Try different incubation times
							260	

- A logical, structured process for identifying areas of concern.
- Reduction of process development time and cost.
- Documentation and tracking of risk-reduction activities.
- Less time spent on considering the potential problems of a design concept.
- Continual awareness of the crucial elements of the project.

Additional Points to Consider

Variation is a constant, and it may diminish a facility's ability to consistently produce quality results. How many trial runs are enough to gain confidence in the new process? In theory, once processes, methods, and documents are prepared, the process should produce the same outcomes consistently. However, what is the minimum number of trial runs necessary to be confident in the process? The answer is "it depends." Many factors need to be considered: limited resources, starting raw material, staff, space, dollars, and time. What is the probability of detecting a systematic error? What is the acceptable risk allowed with the process? Is failure an option? Again, the answer is based on risk assessment.

By planning, identifying possible failure points, and assigning probability of occurrence or detection, a laboratory can assess how well the process is working. How much variation was seen during the development? What variation can be expected during validation? Data from the development studies should be used to determine the acceptance criteria and release specifications of the process and product for validation. Standardizing and controlling the process will minimize some variation, but it will not eliminate random variation or control for biological variation. The initial starting material (cells or tissue) is the most variable factor in the cell-processing laboratory, and creating acceptance criteria that do not account for biological variations is unwise. The best approach is to create systems that control the variation in the process, the equipment, and the materials (supplies and reagents). During process development, more than one starting material should be used to determine the biological variation with the process after hav-ing used only one starting material to assess the inherent variability of the process.

Information Systems and Databases

Most cell-processing laboratories use a combination of commercial software systems and self-created databases to capture data and endpoints. If the new processes or procedures create new or additional data requirements, it is important to include the data capture system in the development process. Often the vendor or information services group needs substantial lead time to create new tests or product groups, or meet other connectivity requirements. As ISBT product codes become the standard, one must also factor in the time needed to request such codes.

Summary

The success of clinical trials using cellular therapies hinges on many variables. One factor that should remain consistent is the manufacture of a safe product. A risk-based approach to process and product development improves the odds of manufacturing success. Risk should be assessed as it relates to the starting material (cells or tissues); reagents, materials, and formulation agents; facility; equipment; release assays; and staff. Not all hazards can be eliminated. However, efforts should be made to identify and control manufacturing risks using the methods described in this section.

References/Resources

1. Crim J. Facility design and cGMP considerations for cell therapy products. Presented at the International Society for Cellular Therapy 6th Annual Symposium, September 25-27, 2006.
2. General chapter <797>. Pharmaceutical compounding—sterile preparations. In: USP Pharmacists' Pharmacopeia. 2nd ed. Rockville, MD: USP, 2008.
3. General chapter <1116>. Microbiological controls and monitoring environments used for the manufacture of healthcare products. In: USP Pharmacists' Pharmacopeia. 2nd ed. Rockville, MD: USP, 2008.
4. USP 30—National formulary 25. (November 2006) Rockville, MD: United States Pharmacopeial Convention, 2006.

5. International Conference on Harmonisation. Validation of analytical procedures: Text and methodology: Q2(R1). (November 2005) Geneva, Switzerland: ICH, 2005.

6. Walfish S. A statistical perspective on the ICH Q2A and Q2B guidelines for validation of analytical methods. BioPharm Int 2006;19:28-36.

7. Krause S. Analytical method validation for biopharmaceuticals: A practical guide. Guide to validation. BioPharm Int 2005;3(Suppl 1):26-34.

8. International Conference on Harmonisation. Quality risk management: Q9. (June 2006) Geneva, Switzerland: ICH, 2006.

Appendix 21-1. Example of a Development Study Report

Development Laboratory	Control Number: D-S-0095
	Revision: Final
	Page: 1 of __
Study Report	
Evaluation of Post-Thaw Stability for Ex-Vivo Expanded CT Cells	

CONFIDENTIAL

STUDY REPORT:

Evaluation of Post-Thaw Stability for a Hypothetical Ex-Vivo Expanded CT Cell Product

Control Number:	D-S-0095	
Revision:	Final	
Author (responsible):	Author	Signature and Date
Read and Approved by:	Laboratory Director Operations	
	Technical Director Manufacturing	
	Quality Assurance	
Department:	Development	
Date:	May 14, 2007	
Study Performed:	July 2006 and May 2007	
Key Words:	Post-thaw stability, room temperature, CT cells	

TABLE OF CONTENTS

List of Tables

1. **Summary**

This study was performed to examine 1) the post-thaw viability of cellular therapy (CT) cells cryopreserved in XYZ cryoprotectant in ABC cryobags, and 2) the post-thaw stability of CT cells stored at room temperature. On the basis of this study, the following conclusions can be made:

- CT cells can be effectively cryopreserved and stored using XYZ cryoprotectant and ABC cryobags.

- After thawing, CT cells can be stored at room temperature in ABC cryobags for 2 hours.

2. **Introduction**

This study was designed to support the clinical trial "Use of CT Cells in Transplant." The autologous cellular therapy products that will be used to support this study are CT cells. After expansion, the cells will be concentrated and washed according to standard operating procedure. The washed cells will be cryopreserved in XYZ cryoprotectant. Before infusion, the ABC cryobag will be thawed in a 37 C water bath, and the cells will be infused without manipulation.

In anticipation of possible bedside delays before infusion, a short-term stability "hold" study was performed and measured cell viability at 0, 15, 30, 45, 60, and 120 minutes after the thaw.

The purpose of this study was to examine 1) the post-thaw viability of CT cells cryopreserved in XYZ cryoprotectant in ABC cryobags, and 2) the post-thaw stability of CT cells stored at room temperature.

3. **Materials and Reagents: Starting Cells**

CT cells derived from bone marrow aspirates obtained from three patients, expanded and cryopreserved in the development laboratory.

Material	Manufacturer	Lot Number	Expiration Date
XYZ cryoprotectant			
ABC cryobags			

XYZ and ABC are hypothetical products.

4. **Equipment**
   4.1 Biological safety cabinet (BSC).
   4.2 Microscope.
   4.3 Water bath.

5. **Methods**
   5.1 Thaw the CT product using the 37 C water bath.
   5.2 After the cells are thawed, place the ABC cryobag in the BSC.

5.3 Use a syringe to determine the total volume.

5.4 Mix the suspension in the bag, and remove a sample for a cell count and viability determination.

5.5 At 15, 30, 45, 60, and 120 minutes after thawing, mix the suspension in the cryobag, and remove a sample for a cell count and viability determination.

6. Acceptance Criteria

For acceptable post-thaw storage at room temperature, CT cells should have a viability of ≥70%.

7. Results

The tables that follow show the viability and viable cell recovery results. At no time during the 2-hour room-temperature storage period did cell viability decrease below 78%. The difference between the viabilities at 0 and 120 minutes after thawing were –8%, +2%, and –6%. The average viable cell recovery immediately after thawing was 83%, and after 1 hour of storage, it was also 83%. After the second hour of storage, the average viable cell recovery dropped 5% to 78%. The acceptance criterion for room-temperature storage of thawed CT cells was met at up to 2 hours of storage.

Cell Viability (%) Results

	Experiment 1: CT Cell Sample 27	Experiment 2: CT Cell Sample 26	Experiment 3: CT Cell Sample 31
Prefreeze	90	90	83
Time after Thawing			
0 minutes	90	79	84
15 minutes	Not done	78	86
30 minutes	83	82	85
45 minutes	84	78	82
60 minutes	81	81	82
120 minutes	82	81	78

Viable Cell Recovery (%) Results

	Experiment 1: CT Cell Sample 27	Experiment 2: CT Cell Sample 26	Experiment 3: CT Cell Sample 31
Prefreeze	100	100	100
Time after Thawing			
0 minutes	81	84	84
15 minutes	Not done	92	75
30 minutes	80	99	72
45 minutes	85	92	75
60 minutes	77	96	75
120 minutes	86	80	67

8. **Discussion**

In this study, CT cells were stored after having been thawed at room temperature without manipulation in a cryobag. During this period for the three products evaluated, cell viability did not decrease below 78%. Immediate post-thaw average viable cell recovery was 83%. This was unchanged after 1 hour of room-temperature storage. There was no evidence of cell clumping over the course of the study.

9. **Conclusions**

The study was successfully completed and the acceptance criteria were met for the storage of CT cells at room temperature for up to 2 hours after thawing. The intention of the clinical trial is to infuse CT cells immediately after thawing. However, there may be circumstances whereby infusion is delayed. This study demonstrated that thawed CT cells may be held at room temperature for as long as 2 hours in XYZ cryoprotectant without the loss of viability.

10. **Data Documentation**

Data for this study are documented in worksheets stored in the CT laboratory.

11. **References**

Standard operating procedures for references:
Determination of cell number and viability.
Operation of the BSC.
Operation of the microscope.
Operation of the water bath.

12. **Appendix**

None

Appendix 21-2. Template for a Design-Phase Transition Approval Form

---

Design Phase I (Input)

Describe product selection and concept for therapeutic application (include disease assessment, biological hypothesis, therapeutic hypothesis, preliminary draft clinical development plan). This should be a 5-10 page attachment generated by the advocate for the human cells, tissues, and cellular and tissue-based product (HCT/P) therapy. It may also include any market analysis if other cellular therapy (CT) laboratories are also generating a similar HCT/P.

Approval Signatures for Phase II

Chief Medical Advisor

_____
Signature and Date

Chief Development Advisor

_____
Signature and Date

Quality or Regulatory Advisor

_____
Signature and Date

Design Phase II (Input)

Prepare product requirements by working with clinical raw material recovery and therapeutic administration staff for realistic expectations and needs. Work with cell laboratory development staff to determine process and product characterization requirements and feasibility. Generate and attach a 5-to-10-page report on the requirements and feasibility of the proposal from Design Phase I. Attach the data, and generate a conclusion and action plan for HCT/P product development to the next phase. Verify that Phase I therapeutic and HCT/P product hypotheses have been met or adequately modified.

Approval Signatures for Phase III

Chief Medical Advisor

_____
Signature and Date

Chief Development Advisor

_____
Signature and Date

Quality or Regulatory Advisor

_____
Signature and Date

Design Phase III (Output)

Attach the report on the development of the HCT/P production process specifications and developed product characterization. Data presentations will include healthy donor process development, component and raw material availability, draft records for all production requirements, and identification and optimization of critical process parameters. Propose conclusions and project the plan for Phase IV. Verify that Phase II product requirement inputs from the clinical staff and development staff have been adequately satisfied.

Approval Signatures for Phase IV

Chief Medical Advisor

_____
Signature and Date

Chief Development Advisor

_____
Signature and Date

Quality or Regulatory Advisor

_____
Signature and Date

Design Phase IV (Output): Investigational New Drug (IND) Application Preparation and/or Investigational Review Board (IRB) Application

Design and follow the project plan for further product and process characterization and data collection for chemistry, manufacturing, and controls (CMC); animal models; stability; residual disease; or impurities. Prepare clinical trial documentation. Generate clinical protocol, investigator brochure, informed consent forms, case report forms, etc. Establish an adequate quality structure in compliance with current good manufacturing practice (cGMP), good tissue practice (GTP), and good clinical practice (GCP). Have a pre-IND meeting with the Food and Drug Administration (FDA) and file an IND application. Verify that the clinical product and development process requirements continue to be met or are adequately modified to reflect the current objectives of all team members.

Approval Signatures for Clinical Trial

Chief Medical Advisor

_____
Signature and Date

Chief Development Advisor

_____
Signature and Date

Quality or Regulatory Advisor

_____
Signature and Date

Clinical Trial Phase V (Output): Clinical Hypothesis Validation

Follow the clinical trial plan for cGMP or GTP product manufacturing and data collection.
Determine the structure for reporting routine clinical trial updates to involved parties. At each planned update, collect signatures from decision-makers to continue on the clinical trial plan.

Approval Signatures for Clinical Trial

Chief Medical Advisor

_____
Signature and Date

Chief Development Advisor

_____
Signature and Date

Quality or Regulatory Advisor

_____
Signature and Date

Clinical Trial Phase VI (Output): Clinical Trial Reporting

Follow the clinical trial plan for cGMP or GTP product manufacturing and data collection.
Determine the structure for reporting routine clinical trial updates to involved parties. At each planned update, collect signatures from decision-makers to continue on the clinical trial plan.

Approval Signatures for Clinical Trial

Chief Medical Advisor

_____
Signature and Date

Chief Development Advisor

_____
Signature and Date

Quality or Regulatory Advisor

_____
Signature and Date

3 of 3

Appendix 21-3. Example of a Preimplementation Review Checklist

Cellular Therapy Clinical Trial Summary and Preimplementation Review Human Cellular Therapy Development Laboratory

Clinical Trial Name:

Brief Description:

IND#   IRB #   Change Control #

Date Open for Enrollment:

Roles and Responsibilities

Title or Role	Name	Contact Information
IND Principal Investigator		
Clinical Principal Investigator		
Lead Development Technologist		
Clinical Coordinator		
Manufacturing Technologist		
Product Release		
Additional Roles or Responsibilities		

Systems Review Checklist

Comments

Organization

Is there a document that defines the key personnel and their roles in the trial?	Yes No	
Has the project team within the CTL development group been identified?	Yes No	
Has the project been through the change control process?	Yes No	
Has the test-tracking database been updated to reflect the current status of the trial?	Yes No	

Comments

Facilities and Safety

Does this product need a containment clean-room?   Yes No

Will this product be manufactured in one of the cleanroom suites?   Yes No

Is there sufficient cleanroom capacity for this trial?   Yes No NA

Are there any special room changeover procedures to be followed once the facility has finished manufacturing this product?   Yes No

Does this project require any special safety or personal protective equipment?   Yes No

Documents and Data Management

Are process-specific SOPs and forms finalized or in provisional mode?   Yes No

Are there any data collection forms for internal or external collaborators?   Yes No

Has the scheduled due date for the IND annual report been forwarded to the CTL IND or regulatory coordinator?   Yes No NA

Is the IND file in the CTL complete and up to date?   Yes No NA

Have the current versions of the relevant manufacturing SOPs and forms been submitted to the FDA?   Yes No NA

Are training documents, modules, and profiles complete?   Yes No

Personnel

Have adequate numbers of technical personnel been trained in manufacturing and final product preparation and administration?   Yes No

Are those trained personnel listed in the roles and responsibility log or as members of the development team?   Yes No

Is an adequate number of QA staff trained in product release?   Yes No NA

Critical Materials and Services

Are critical materials and supplies listed in the appropriate SOPs or forms?   Yes No

Comments

Are specifications for the critical materials and supplies defined in the lot number database?	Yes No NA	
Is there a template or profile in the lot number database to record the lot numbers of supplies used in manufacturing?	Yes No NA	
Are certificates of analysis or package inserts for the critical materials and supplies available in the laboratory?	Yes No	
Are there any reagents or supplies for this trial that are lot-number specific or require a lot be set aside?	Yes No	
If yes, is there a sufficient quantity of those supplies to complete the trial?	Yes No	
Did any of the critical materials or supplies require validation or qualification testing?	Yes No	
If yes, are those records available?	Yes No	

Equipment

Is critical equipment listed in the appropriate SOPs or forms?	Yes No	
Was any equipment validated for use specifically for this trial?	Yes No	
Are those records available?	Yes No	
Was any new equipment purchased specifically for this trial?	Yes No	
Are there records for the required specifications, vendor qualification, IQ, and OQ for the new equipment?	Yes No	
Are there any special cleaning requirements for the equipment used in this trial?	Yes No	
Is there a schedule for QC and maintenance for the critical equipment used in this trial?	Yes No NA	
Has the equipment undergone maintenance and QC according to the schedule?	Yes No	

Process Control

Are there supporting data (eg, laboratory notebook) or validation documents for key steps in the manufacturing process?	Yes No NA	
Have pilot production runs been completed?	Yes No NA	

		Comments
Are the records for those pilots available?	Yes No NA	
Is there a plan for the collection, tracking, and trend analysis of manufacturing data such as phenotype and recoveries?	Yes No NA	
Are there additional CAP proficiency programs (or the equivalent) in which to participate?	Yes No NA	

Process Improvement

Are there plans to meet with the clinical coordinator shortly after the first patient is enrolled?	Yes No	
Has an audit or review of the preclinical data been performed by anyone outside the CTL development group?	Yes No	
Are the results of that audit available?	Yes No NA	

Events and Assessments

Are there any trial-specific event-reporting requirements for this trial (ie, other than the departmental event report form)?	Yes No	
Are there plans for a postimplementation audit to be performed by facility personnel?	Yes No	
Are there plans for an audit to be performed by external personnel such as a study sponsor or an outside agency? Please specify:	Yes No	

Sponsor Reimbursement

Is a mechanism to ensure reimbursement from the sponsor in place?	Yes No NA	

IND = investigational new drug (application/status); IRB = institutional review board; CTL = cellular therapy laboratory; NA = not applicable; SOP = standard operating procedure; FDA = Food and Drug Administration; QA = quality assurance; IQ = installation qualification; OQ = operational qualification; QC = quality control; CAP = College of American Pathologists.

Collection of Cells for Transplantation

HEMATOPOIETIC PROGENITOR CELL (HPC) grafts are generally obtained from human bone marrow (marrow), peripheral blood (PB), or umbilical cord blood (UCB), although new and potential sources are continuously being identified. Collection of marrow from cadaveric human donors is also feasible, and cadaveric donor marrow has been reported to engraft in the related recipient. In addition, it is possible to derive a graft from fetal liver or through tissue culture expansion of a minimal cell dose obtained from marrow, PB, or UCB.

Many facilities obtain grafts primarily by leukocytapheresis (apheresis) of PB rather than from marrow harvesting because apheresis generally provides larger yields and is more comfortable and convenient for the donor. However, traditional marrow transplantation may have several advantages over transplantation of HPCs from apheresis (HPC-A), including a decreased incidence of chronic graft-vs-host disease and potentially better long-term marrow function because of the presence of mesenchymal stromal cells (MSCs) that appear to be exclusive to the marrow niche. Some cell populations that are of interest for blood and marrow transplant or regenerative medicine are exclusive to, or more prevalent in, marrow than in PB. These populations include macrophages, reticular endothelial cells, endothelial progenitor cells, fibroblasts, adipocytes, and osteogenic progenitor cells. The extent to which any of these other cell populations exist in CB remains to be determined.

Section Editors: Michele Cottler-Fox, MD, Director, Division of Cell Therapy and Transfusion Medicine, Department of Pathology, University of Arkansas for Medical Sciences, Little Rock, Arkansas; Edward Snyder, MD, Professor of Laboratory Medicine, Yale University School of Medicine, and Director, Blood Bank and Apheresis/Transfusion Center, Yale-New Haven Hospital, New Haven, Connecticut; and Zbigniew M. Szczepiorkowski, MD, PhD, FCAP, Associate Professor of Pathology and Medicine, Dartmouth Medical School, Medical Director, Transfusion Medicine Service, Dartmouth-Hitchcock Medical Center, and Director, Cellular Therapy Center, Dartmouth-Hitchcock Medical Center, Lebanon, New Hampshire

The editors have disclosed no conflicts of interest.

Background and Historical Perspective

The technique described for marrow collection by Thomas and Storb in 1970 has undergone few major changes. Surgically resected ribs, cadaveric vertebral bodies, and complete ilia are potential sources of marrow that have been investigated but are rarely used. HPC mobilization into and collection from the PB is currently the most common source of cells for transplantation in adults, although the use of UCB for transplantation in adults as well as in children is increasing rapidly. Until recently, most comparisons of HPC collection and marrow harvesting have looked at mobilized peripheral progenitors vs steady-state, ie, unmobilized, marrow. To address this discrepancy, some groups have begun to compare both marrow and apheresis techniques for stem cell collection after mobilization for all patient groups. Their findings, paired with basic research into the nature and function of the marrow niche, suggest a definite role for traditional marrow harvesting.[1]

Current State of the Field

Many factors have been shown to influence the ability to mobilize HPCs from the marrow into the blood. Poor mobilization is currently defined as the inability to collect >2.0 × 10^6 CD34+ cells/kg of recipient body weight from an autologous or allogeneic donor. Mobilization using a combination of chemotherapy and growth factors has been shown to be significantly more effective than either type by itself in the autologous setting. Many chemotherapeutic agents have been used, followed closely by one or more growth factors (colony-stimulating factors, or CSFs).

Granulocyte colony-stimulating factor (G-CSF) and granulocyte-macrophage colony-stimulating factor (GM-CSF) are the agents that have been used most frequently since the late 1980s for mobilization. Both factors have been shown to increase the release of proteolytic enzymes from mature neutrophils in the marrow, which serve to disrupt the anchoring of the more immature HPCs, thus allowing their egress into the periphery. Both agents can cause bone pain, nausea, vomiting, diar-

rhea, insomnia, chills, fevers, and night sweats. In patients who mobilize poorly, GM-CSF combined with G-CSF has been demonstrated to increase CD34+ yields.

Overview of Section V

This section contains information on the acquisition of cells involved in hematopoiesis from a number of sources available for clinical use, including marrow, adult PB, and UCB. It also includes methods for assessing collection quality from the different cell sources. These methods cover the measurement of volume (which can help to assess collector competency as well as collection quality), the enumeration of cells in the product (a measure of purity that helps to assess collector competency, the collection quality, and possibly the quality of the donor), the measurement of viability (which measures potential efficacy and potency), the evaluation of the functionality of the cells in the product (which relates to potency), and the measurement of microbial contamination (a measure of safety). More extensive information pertaining to CT product evaluation and characterization is provided in Section VIII.

Future Directions

After many years of using the same growth factors, new agents for mobilization of adult HPCs are being developed. AMD-3100 (Mozobil, Genzyme, Cambridge, MA) is a new agent that may soon become available for clinical use. It acts as a reversible inhibitor of the CD34+ cell cytokine receptor, CXCR4. The CXCR4 receptor associates with its ligand, stromal-derived factor 1α (SDF-1α/CXCL-12), to mediate stem cell homing, trafficking, and retention. Once CXCR4 has been bound by AMD-3100, the ability of HPCs to migrate toward and adhere to the marrow niche is impaired, which increases the number of these cells that move into the circulation. When AMD-3100 is used in conjunction with G-CSF mobilization, the results are synergistic, with no increase in toxicity.

The GROβ chemokines are in early clinical development. They interact with receptors on neutrophils to cause the release of matrix metallo-proteinase-9 (MMP-9), one of the three primary enzymes involved in the bone marrow matrix degradation that is necessary for HPC egress. The effects of GROβ chemokines are noticeable within 15 to 30 minutes of administration, and they can increase yields of HPCs by more than 200-fold. The addition of GROβ chemokines, particularly in poor mobilizers, could decrease potential toxicity from higher G-CSF doses and significantly augment collection.

Although UCB has the disadvantage of limited cell numbers, unrelated recipients appear to be able to tolerate less-stringent HLA matches better than with marrow or HPC-A. Studies are under way that indicate that adult patients can safely receive 2 partially mismatched UCB units, a process that seems to provide more rapid engraftment than a single UCB transplant and compensates somewhat for the low cell numbers in one unit. But the primary advantage of this cell source over other HPC products is its immediate availability. Because UCB units are processed, cryopreserved, HLA-typed, and thoroughly tested before they are released to inventory, there is no waiting period for an identi-

fied donor to be screened, tested, and scheduled for donation. With these benefits and with recent and developing improvements such as simplified collection techniques, automated processing methods, and better methods of enumerating and evaluating the number and type of cells in the product, it is not surprising that UCB has quickly become an established source of cells for HPC transplantation.

As more is learned about the qualities of the different sources of cells for transplantation and other therapies, distinct advantages of particular types for different indications and applications will probably become evident. Meanwhile, it is important that the collection of all types of cellular products be performed in ways that will provide the highest possible yields and the best possible quality.

Reference/Resource

1. Weisdorf D, Miller J, Verfaillie C, et al. Cytokine-primed bone marrow stem cells vs peripheral blood stem cells for autologous transplantation: A randomized comparison of GM-CSF vs G-CSF. Biol Blood Marrow Transplant 1997;3:217-23.

In: Areman EM, Loper K, eds
Cellular Therapy: Principles, Methods, and Regulations
Bethesda, MD: AABB, 2009

◆◆◆ **22** ◆◆◆

Bone Marrow Collection

Thomas R. Spitzer, MD

MARROW TRANSPLANTATION FOR THE treatment of numerous life-threatening neoplastic and nonneoplastic hematologic and congenital disorders has greatly increased in scope and magnitude during the past 3 decades. Even though tens of thousands of transplants have been performed worldwide, there is little published information on a standardized methodology for marrow collection for transplantation. Moreover, there is considerable controversy about the optimal method of collection and little outcome data to support one technique over another.

Sources of marrow can be either autologous (self donor), allogeneic (nonself donor), or syngeneic (identical twin donor). Although the technique of marrow collection is similar regardless of the donor source, there may be individual considerations about the type of anesthesia or the desired dose of nucleated cells (NCs) that are relevant (see Table 22-1). Autologous donors who have received bleomycin, for example, may be prone to the development of oxygen-related acute lung injury. Regional anesthesia in these circumstances may be preferable. The source of allogeneic marrow may influence the desired NC yield. Requested cell numbers from the transplant center for unrelated donor trans-

plants often exceed those for related donor transplants. These increased cell numbers are the result of the increased risk of engraftment failure of an unrelated donor transplant, concerns about cell loss during transport, and an increased likelihood of performing ex-vivo T-cell depletion to prevent graft-vs-host disease (GVHD).

Recently, hematopoietic progenitor cells from apheresis (HPC-A) have become the preferred source for both autologous and allogeneic progenitor cell transplantation.[1-4] Faster recovery of neutrophil and platelet counts following HPC-A transplantation than following marrow transplantation has been documented in a number of randomized, controlled clinical trials.[1-3] Several randomized and nonrandomized trials have also shown faster resolution of donor symptoms related to stem cell collection, including fatigue and pain (secondary to growth factor administration in the case of HPC-A or the harvest procedure in marrow collection).[5-7] Despite the growing use of HPC-A for transplantation, marrow collection for transplantation is still an important option when it is the donor's preference and to avoid the increased risk of chronic GVHD following HPC-A transplantation for conditions where there is no beneficial

Thomas R. Spitzer, MD, Director, Bone Marrow Transplant Program, Massachusetts General Hospital, Boston, Massachusetts

The author has disclosed no conflicts of interest.

Table 22-1. Factors for Consideration before Marrow Harvesting

Donor Source	Factors Influencing Anesthesia and Collection
Autologous	• Previous therapy (eg, bleomycin) • Tumor cell contamination • Postoperative infusion with recovered red cells
Allogeneic	• Use of irradiated homologous blood components intraoperatively • Transfusion with predonated autologous red cells • Related vs unrelated donors • ABO status of donor or recipient
Syngeneic	• Transfusion with predonated autologous red cells • Confirmation of identity

effect of GVHD, such as aplastic anemia. This chapter discusses the most widely accepted methods of marrow collection, reviews the existing evidence in support of these techniques, and describes the complications associated with these procedures.

Development of Human Marrow Collection Technique

In 1939, Osgood and colleagues published the first description of marrow transplantation, in which 15 mL of sternal marrow aspirate was procured from multiple sternal punctures.[8] In the 1950s, numerous marrow transplants were performed for a variety of malignant conditions. The posterior ilium, sternum, and spines of the lumbar vertebrae were described by Wilson as potential sites of marrow collection.[9] Although a limited number of sternal punctures is possible (10-15 punctures, yielding 50-70 ml of marrow), the technique is not without risk, and the yield, at least in terms of the usual total volume needed, is small. Aspiration of sternal marrow is no longer commonly employed.

Wilson described the procurement of marrow from the posterior ilium in detail.[9] General anesthesia was said to be preferred, particularly for debilitated patients. The patients were placed on their side with their knees sharply flexed, similar to the preparation for a lumbar puncture. The first point of aspiration was the posterior iliac crest; the second was the posterior superior iliac spine. It was

recommended that the operator form a mental image of the marrow cavity, dividing it into the posterior iliac crest, cephalad and caudad portions of the posterior ilium, and finally the region of the postero-superior iliac spine. Each of these divisions was then partitioned into at least three planes from medial to lateral, extending from the sacroiliac joint laterally to the free edge of the posterior ilium. Wilson's technique involved advancing the needle through the marrow cavity with 180-degree clockwise turns. Marrow was aspirated each time the needle was advanced until the opposite cortex was reached or the needle was obstructed by bone spicules. With this technique, 15 to 20 different positions on each side were said to suffice, and 50 to 150 mL of marrow and blood were aspirated from the two sides.

The field of marrow transplantation was revolutionized by E. Donnall Thomas in the 1960s and 1970s. Thomas described both the techniques and the clinical outcomes of marrow transplantation by using elegant animal models and subsequent clinical trials of transplantation in patients with refractory hematologic malignancies. In a review of marrow transplantation in 1975, Thomas et al described a technique of marrow collection.[10] Spinal anesthesia was said to be preferred. Following insertion of the marrow aspiration needle into the marrow cavity, vigorous suction was applied. Thomas et al suggested that the volume aspirated from each site should be limited to 1 to 3 mL to minimize dilution by peripheral blood (PB). They described the placement of marrow into a beaker containing tissue culture medium and preservative-free heparin, followed by filtration of the marrow through stainless steel screens of 0.3 mm, then through screens of 0.2 mm.

The author previously described a technique for marrow collection as part of a comparative analysis that evaluated the impact of the collection center on the quality of marrow harvested from volunteer unrelated donors.[11] This technique is detailed in the procedure for marrow harvesting in Method 22-1 and is described below.

Anesthesia

All marrow harvests are performed in the operating room under sterile conditions using either general, regional (epidural or spinal), or local anesthesia (see Table 22-2). The choice of anesthetic varies considerably from center to center (and from patient to patient). Regional anesthesia may be associated with fewer postoperative complications, particularly in autologous donors with comorbid conditions, and is the choice of donors who prefer to be awake. Severe or life-threatening complications associated with anesthesia are very rare among healthy allogeneic or syngeneic donors and are as likely to occur with regional anesthesia as with general anesthesia. The risks of the different anesthetic methods are described in the "Donor Complications" section of this chapter.

Marrow harvests with reportedly adequate pain control have also been performed by using local anesthesia, with sedation or patient-controlled analgesia.[12,13] Although postoperative morbidity may be slightly lessened, achieving a degree of operative anesthesia equivalent to the other methods is unlikely, especially when the discomfort associated with aspiration is considered.

Collection Technique

The collection of marrow requires at least two individuals, usually an attending physician with a fellow, a medical resident, or a nurse practitioner. The method of collection at one facility is described in Method 22-1.

Following the induction of anesthesia, donors are placed in the prone position. The posterior iliac crest areas are antiseptically prepared and draped in a sterile fashion. Ball-top aspiration needles, such as those used at the University of Washington, Seattle, WA (or other 11-14-gauge aspiration needles with similar comfort features), are inserted through the skin overlying each posterior iliac crest. Marrow is then vigorously aspirated into 30-ml plastic syringes, which have been flushed with a heparinized solution. The marrow volume from each aspiration site should be limited to 5 mL to minimize contamination with PB. The needles are rotated approximately 180 degrees following each aspiration to maximize the cellular yield of each aspirate. The needles, with syringes attached, are removed from the bone after each aspiration. After the aspirated marrow is placed in a heparin-containing receptacle, the syringes are serially flushed with normal saline and heparinized normal saline. Needles are repeatedly reinserted through the same skin puncture site into different bone sites until approximately 20% to 33% of the intended marrow volume is collected. Given the wide area of accessible bone beneath each skin puncture site, it is usually not necessary to use more than 3 to 5 skin puncture sites on each side. Subsequent skin sites should be superolateral to the initial puncture sites. These puncture locations follow the contour of the posterior iliac crest and ensure that areas inferior to the posterior superior iliac spine, where, for example, the sciatic nerve exits, are not approached. Through each subsequent skin puncture site, mul-

Table 22-2. Types of Anesthesia Used in Marrow Harvesting

- General
- Epidural
- Spinal
- Local with sedation
- Local with patient-controlled analgesia
- Local infiltration of harvest sites following general or regional anesthesia

tiple aspirations are again performed. Ultimately, the entire marrow volume can be collected from 3 to 5 different skin puncture sites overlying each iliac crest. Of 133 allogeneic-related donor marrow harvests performed at the author's facility, an adequate NC yield was obtained from the posterior iliac crest areas in all cases (Spitzer, unpublished observations).

Collected marrow is placed in a receptacle containing heparin and medium. The most commonly employed apparatus for marrow collection is a disposable collection bag (eg, manufactured by Fenwal, Lake Zurich, IL), to which plastic filters of 500 and 200 microns are attached. This design allows for easy and uninterrupted filtration of the marrow following completion of the collection. The marrow can then pass directly into a sterile transfer container.

The optimal medium for the collection and type (and amounts) of anticoagulant have not been fully defined. Earlier collections often used RPMI tissue culture medium, Hanks solution, or a similar balanced salt solution. These media are not, however, approved by the Food and Drug Administration (FDA) for human use. Plasma-Lyte A (Baxter Healthcare, Deerfield, IL), an FDA-licensed electrolyte solution, was previously evaluated as a substitute solution for marrow collection.[14] The data showed excellent cell viability, and Plasma-Lyte A is now commonly employed in collection practices. Heparin is used to prevent clotting of the marrow. Ten to 15 units of heparin per mL of collected marrow are sufficient in most cases to prevent clotting. However, given the potential for "clumping" (likely due to platelet aggregation) of the marrow during more extended storage (as might be the case when the marrow is transferred to another center for transplantation), additional anticoagulation may be used. Acid (or anticoagulant)-citrate-dextrose formula A (ACD-A) at a 10% concentration appears to lessen the chance of clotting and clumping of the marrow.

Following the marrow collection, the skin puncture sites along the posterior iliac crest area are cleansed with a sterile saline solution, and a pressure dressing is applied. Upon completion of the procedure, the donor is transferred to the recovery room.

Postoperative Care

Adequate hydration and pain control are essential components of postoperative management. Infusion of autologous predonated red cells either intra- or postoperatively is often prescribed. Additionally, recovered red cells obtained during the postharvest processing of the autologous marrow can also be reinfused. With these practices, an allogeneic red cell transfusion is rarely required. Furthermore, replacement of known or anticipated blood volume loss with sufficient intravenous crystalloid hydration (usually 2.5 to 3 times the blood loss volume) is essential.

Pain control can initially be achieved either by oral or parenteral narcotic administration or via an indwelling epidural catheter for patients who received epidural anesthesia. A reduction in postoperative harvest-site pain may also be achieved by using local infiltration with a long-acting local anesthetic (eg, bupivacaine).[15] Donors are often hospitalized overnight for pain control, as well as for monitoring of vital signs and hydration. Recently, however, the feasibility and safety of outpatient harvesting have been established.[16,17]

Narcotic analgesia (eg, oral acetaminophen with codeine or oxycodone) is required for an average of 3 days after the harvest but, on occasion, may be required for several weeks.[12] Oral iron supplements are generally recommended for 2 to 4 weeks after the harvest. Donors should be advised to avoid heavy lifting or strenuous exertion affecting the pelvis for 2 to 3 weeks following the harvest. Medical attention should be sought for the increasing intensity (or a change in the quality, such as to suggest nerve root irritation) of pain, fever, or signs of local infection.[18]

Nucleated Cell Yield and Quality Control

Historically, a yield of greater than or equal to 3×10^8 NCs/kg of recipient bodyweight has been a goal of both autologous and allogeneic marrow harvests. This desired yield was derived by an extrapolation from animal data that suggested improved engraftment with this cell dose.[19] In a study by Storb and colleagues, which evaluated the impact of cell dose on engraftment, patients with aplastic anemia who received $<3 \times 10^8$ NCs/kg had a higher rate of graft rejection than patients who received a dose higher than 3×10^8 NCs/kg.[20] However, engraftment has also been shown to be reliably achieved following marrow transplantation by using lesser numbers of NCs. In the situation of a major ABO incompatibility, for example, processing of the marrow on a cell separator instrument to prepare a mononuclear-cell-enriched fraction may reduce the number of NCs in the product by almost 1 log. Stable trilineage engraftment has been reliably achieved in these situations as well.[21]

Maximizing the NC yield, while keeping marrow collection volume to a minimum, is an essential goal of marrow harvesting. Three studies have addressed the impact of the aspirate volume on NC, T-cell, and cellular subset yield. Because T-cells are not produced in the marrow, they serve as an indicator of the level of PB contamination in a marrow collection. These studies are summarized in Table 22-3.

Bacigalupo and colleagues evaluated 11 marrow donors who donated 1000 mL of marrow.[22] In six donors, the first 500 mL were harvested in 2-ml aliquots and the second 500 mL in 20-mL aspirates.

In the other five cases, the first 500 mL were obtained in 20-mL aliquots, whereas the final 500 mL were obtained in 2-mL aspirates. Significantly more NCs and colony-forming units—granulocyte-macrophage (CFUs-GM) concentrations and fewer CD3-positive T-cells were seen in the small-volume aspirates, consistent with the notion that larger-volume aspirations are associated with increased PB contamination.

A detailed immunophenotypic analysis of the cellular composition of the first 1.0 mL of marrow aspirate compared with that of an aliquot taken from the marrow harvest at the end of the procedure was evaluated in 17 allogeneic marrow donors.[23] Considerably more PB contamination was seen in the end marrow product, and CFU-GM concentrations were significantly higher in the initial marrow aliquot samples. The marrow was collected from approximately six skin and 200 bone puncture sites. The average volume per aspiration was 4 to 5 mL. The study did not address the impact of individual aspirate volumes on cell yield, but it did suggest that small-volume aspirates at the beginning of a harvest procedure were enriched for hematopoietic progenitors.

Table 22-3. Summary of Trials That Evaluated Different Approaches to Marrow Harvesting

Investigator and Marrow Source/Harvest Site	Patient (n)	Design	Outcome
Bacigalupo[22] Allo/PIC	11	Prospective comparison of 2-mL and 20-mL aspirations	2-mL aspirate: ↑ NCs (p = 0.02) ↑ CFU-GM (p = 0.03) ↓ CD34+ cells (p = 0.01)
Batinic[23] Allo/AIC and PIC	17	Comparison of first 1.0-mL and end-product aliquots	First 1.0-mL aspirate: ↑ NCs (threefold) ↑ CFU-GM (10-fold) ↑ T cells (twofold) No difference in CD56+, CD13+, CD33+, and CD34+ cells
Spitzer[11] Allo/PIC*	20	Retrospective comparison of GUMC (5-mL aspirations) and outside harvest center (10 aspirations at GUMC vs 10 aspirations at outside center)	GUMC (5-mL aspirate): ↑ NCs (p = 0.0014) ↑ CD34+ cells (p = 0.001) ↓ CD3+ cells (p = 0.0008) ↓ CD4+ cells (p = 0.0006) ↑ CD19+ cells (p = 0.0032) No difference in CD8+ cells

*Harvest for aspirates performed at Georgetown University Medical Center.
Allo = healthy allogeneic donors; PIC = posterior iliac crest; NC = nucleated cell; CFU-GM = colony-forming unit—granulocyte-macrophage; AIC = anterior iliac crest; GUMC = Georgetown University Medical Center.

The author compared the quality of marrow collected at his institution with marrow collected at outside harvest centers.[11] This study was prompted by a perceived difference in NC concentrations that were perhaps affected by differences in marrow harvesting techniques. There were significantly higher NC concentrations and CD34 antigen-positive cell content and correspondingly lower CD3 and CD4 antigen-positive T-cell numbers in the marrow harvested in this study. These data confirmed the existence of significant variability in marrow collection practices between institutions. Although the marrow collection practices of individual outside harvest centers could not be determined in this study, the results did show that strict adherence to a collection procedure in which small-volume marrow aspirations from multiple skin puncture sites were performed resulted in a product with a high number of HPCs and minimal PB contamination.

A fundamental question is whether NCs or cell subset yields affect donor risks or recipient clinical outcomes following marrow transplantation. Because target numbers of NCs (according to the previously discussed considerations) are similar among marrow transplant programs, it is likely that the major difference in achieving the target number is the blood volume loss during the harvest procedure. Thus, large-volume harvests might be associated with increased transfusion (autologous or allogeneic) needs. If in fact large-volume harvests are associated with the collection of significantly fewer CD34+ progenitor cells, engraftment could also be affected. There are no available clinical data, however, to support this conclusion. A higher number of T cells in an allogeneic marrow graft probably does not influence the incidence of acute GVHD but may increase its severity.[24] The recent experience with allogeneic HPC-A transplants, in which a number of T cells that has been increased by approximately 1 log are infused without an apparent increased risk of acute GVHD, further calls into question whether an association between T-cell numbers and GVHD risk exists.[2]

The HLA-matched unrelated-donor transplant experience has underscored the importance of developing standardized practices of marrow collection to optimize the quality of the harvested marrow. Transplants from unrelated donors are associated with higher engraftment failure risks than transplants from HLA-matched related donors.[25] Stem cell loss during transport or processing emphasizes the need for optimizing the number of harvested HPCs. These harvests must be performed in the context of an acceptable blood loss volume (<20 mL/kg donor bodyweight). An analysis of recipient clinical outcomes according to the NC and cell subset content of the marrow product will ultimately be necessary to define the optimal practice of marrow collection.

Donor Complications

Related Marrow Donors

Several large-series studies have described a range of related-donor complications following marrow harvesting. Whereas certain complications (such as local soreness and bruising) are common, others (for example, fat embolism) are the subject of only individual case reports. Overall, a less-than-1% risk of life-threatening complications has been reported. Complications according to their frequency are described in Table 22-4.

The largest of these published series was an analysis of 2027 transplants reported to the Interna-

Table 22-4. Complications of Marrow Harvesting

Common (>50%)

- Local discomfort lasting <3 weeks
- Bruising

Uncommon (1%-10%)

- Pressure neuropathies
- Fever
- Pain lasting >3 weeks
- Postoperative nausea, vomiting, urinary retention, and spinal headache

Rare (<1%)

- Infection
- Arrhythmias
- Pulmonary embolism
- Fat embolism syndrome
- Acute pancreatitis
- Mechanical ileus
- Cardiopulmonary arrest

tional Bone Marrow Transplant Registry and 1263 transplants performed at the Fred Hutchinson Cancer Research Center in Seattle.[26] Most of these aspirations were performed from the posterior iliac crest, although the anterior iliac crest and, occasionally, the sternum were used in some cases. An overall 0.27% of life-threatening complications were reported. These complications included septicemia, a femoral vein thrombosis at the site of an indwelling femoral vein catheter, pulmonary embolism, aspiration pneumonia, cerebral infarction, arrhythmia (ventricular tachycardia), and cardiopulmonary arrest.

In a separate and more detailed account of donor complications by Buckner and colleagues from Seattle, 1270 procedures performed on 1160 donors were analyzed.[27] Most (72%) of these harvests were performed under general anesthesia. In the majority of instances (69%), both the anterior and posterior crests were aspirated. In 9% of harvests, the sternum was also aspirated.

As expected, all donors experienced transient aspiration site discomfort. In only 10 (0.8%) of the procedures did greater-than-expected operative site morbidity occur. In six of these instances, pressure neuropathy that was likely caused by hematomas was reported. In one case, sciatic pain was still present at 18 months after harvest. The most common complication other than local discomfort was postoperative fever, which occurred in 10% of donors. In only two cases were bacterial infections documented. Eight of 328 donors who received a spinal anesthetic reported "postspinal headaches," and one donor required an epidural blood patch procedure. Nine donors required catheterization for urinary retention.

Other rarely reported complications include fat embolism, fracture of the ilium, acute pancreatitis, and mechanical ileus.[28-31] There are also four known deaths that occurred during or following a related-donor marrow harvest. These deaths were a result of cardiac complications, adult respiratory distress syndrome following anaphylaxis during anesthesia, fatal neurologic injury precipitated by cardiac arrest, and a fatal pulmonary embolism.[32]

In addition, apprehension about the procedure before the marrow harvest and anxiety related to the procedure are experienced by the majority of marrow donors. According to an analysis of predonation and postdonation self-report question-naires, related marrow donors were found to have significantly more pain than unrelated donors, which raised a question about the possible psychosocial factors that influence the incidence and severity of postharvesting complications.[33]

Unrelated Donor Complications: The National Marrow Donor Program Experience

Because only 25% to 30% of patients will have an HLA-identical sibling, there has been an increasing use of volunteer unrelated-donor marrow transplants for a variety of hematologic malignancies and other conditions that can potentially be cured by marrow transplantation. Data from the harvests of healthy volunteer unrelated donors provides a unique perspective on the experience of marrow donation. The National Marrow Donor Program (NMDP) has prospectively analyzed the experiences of thousands of volunteer unrelated donors. Other studies have examined a number of psychosocial factors that influence both willingness to donate and perceptions of the harvest experience.[33-35] Volunteer unrelated donors are a highly motivated, altruistic group of individuals. As discussed above, differences in perception of the harvest experience (less pain when compared with related marrow donors) have been documented.

A prospective analysis of the experiences of the first 493 unrelated marrow donors in the NMDP was performed by Stroncek and colleagues.[36] Marrow donors were surveyed within 3 days following the donation, then 1 week after marrow collection, and weekly thereafter. Of the original surveys, 97.8% were completed. Marrow from the 493 donors was collected at 42 different centers. General anesthesia was used in 77.8% of collections, spinal anesthesia in 7.5%, and epidural anesthesia in 14.6%. The median duration of anesthesia was 110 minutes, and the median time to collect the marrow was 60 minutes (range = 8-196). A wide range of marrow volumes was also documented. The median volume was 1050 mL (range = 180-2983). Most donors (89.8%) received at least 1 unit of autologous Red Blood Cells. Three donors received allogeneic blood.

Twenty-nine donors (5.9%) experienced an acute complication. Six donors experienced hypotension, and two of these donors had a syncopal episode.

Four donors had a fever that required an extension of their hospital stay or treatment with antibiotics. Hospitalization was prolonged in four other donors because of local pain or a postdural puncture headache. The most serious complication was an apneic episode, which occurred during the administration of spinal anesthesia. The complication resolved, and the marrow collection proceeded uneventfully.

In the majority of cases, donors fully recovered from the procedure within 19 days of the donation procedure. However, 54 donors (12.6%) reported that they had not recovered completely by 30 days. In most of these cases, donors described pain or soreness at their site of marrow collection. Three donors had temporary numbness in the leg or foot, and one had loss of bladder sensation. Twenty-two donors reported that they had not resumed all normal physical activities, and eight reported that they had not resumed normal work-related activities. One year following the collection procedure, individuals were asked if they had suffered a side effect or complication related to donating marrow. Forty donors (11.1%) indicated that they had suffered a side effect or complication.

In a multivariate analysis, a statistically significant correlation was seen between donor pain or fatigue following the collection and the duration of the marrow collection procedure. There was also a statistically significant correlation between the number of donors who experienced a complication or side effect 1 year after the marrow collection and the volume of marrow collected. These data further support the recommendation that marrow harvest volumes (and, correspondingly, the length of the marrow collection procedure) be kept to a minimum.

Additional Issues

Increasing the Yield of Hematopoietic Progenitors

A combination of chemotherapy and recombinant-growth-factor-mobilized HPC-A has become the preferred source for autologous and allogeneic transplantation, as previously discussed. Larger numbers of CD34+ progenitor cells are reliably procured by these methods, and transplantation of

these products is associated with considerably faster engraftment. Corresponding to this increasing use of HPC-A for transplantation has been a decrease in the number of marrow harvests performed. Although an increased incidence of acute GVHD following allogeneic stem cell transplantation is not apparent, there is a significantly increased risk of chronic GVHD.[4] The long-term safety of recombinant growth factor use in healthy allogeneic donors remains to be established.

Recently, several investigators have shown that the administration of recombinant myeloid growth factors before a marrow harvest procedure can increase the yield of HPCs. Increased yields of CD34+ progenitor cells and the expansion of myeloid progenitors in short-term liquid cultures have been demonstrated in healthy donors who have received Interleukin-3 or granulocyte colony-stimulating factor (G-CSF) and granulocyte-macrophage colony-stimulating factor (GM-CSF) before marrow harvesting.[37,38] There is also preliminary clinical evidence that hematologic recovery following transplantation with growth-factor (G-CSF)-mobilized marrow is faster (and comparable to hematologic recovery following mobilized HPC-A transplants) than with unmobilized marrow.[39,40] In normal donors, the administration of growth factors could result in a reduced harvest volume, which may be a relevant issue for donors of small size.[41] The overall value of this strategy, however, remains to be determined. A major advantage of using HPC-A is the avoidance of an operative procedure. Even if increased numbers of HPCs can be procured and comparable engraftment kinetics compared with PB stem cell transplants can be achieved with growth-factor-mobilized marrow, this approach would involve both the donor safety concerns of recombinant growth factor administration (at least in healthy allogeneic donors) and an operative procedure.

Cadaveric Bone Marrow Harvesting

In light of recent experimental and preliminary clinical evidence suggesting that donor-specific allotolerance can be induced by using donor marrow to induce mixed lymphohematopoietic chimerism,[42,43] the harvesting of cadaveric marrow has gained considerable interest. Rapid marrow recovery from vertebral bodies following donor multiorgan procurement has been described.[44,45] Adult vertebral bodies provide a rich source of marrow with minimal T-cell contamination. Placement of bone fragments in a medium with gentle agitation until free cell suspensions are created, followed by filtration through mesh screens, has been described. Excellent cell viability and in-vitro immunological function have been demonstrated.[45] Significant yields, although lower than those obtained from the vertebra, can also be obtained from the ilia. However, the number of NCs procured from a single ilium is substantially lower than the number of cells obtained from a conventional marrow harvest using multiple iliac crest aspirations, which confirms that significant PB contamination of the products occurs with conventional marrow harvesting.

Conclusions

Despite the widespread practice of marrow harvesting for human transplantation, the methodology for this procedure remains poorly standardized. Large-volume marrow harvests are still frequently performed, often with poor cellular yields. Although a strong correlation exists between the number of HPCs (usually measured by CD34+ cell content) infused and engraftment following HPC-A transplantation, similar data for NC (or CD34+ cell) yields of marrow harvests and engraftment are not readily available. Individual small-volume aspirations have clearly been shown to be associated with higher cell yields, and, in one study, with significantly higher CD34+ cell numbers. Because donor complications are related to the length of the harvest procedure (and likely the number of aspirations during the procedure), efforts should be made to define whether a correlation between marrow harvest cell yields and clinical outcomes exists. If engraftment can then be reliably achieved with either fewer cell numbers than previously believed to be necessary or higher percentages of early progenitor cells, less invasive (ie, fewer) aspirations and more efficient (ie, small-volume, high-progenitor-cell-yield) aspirations should be encouraged. Efforts should also continue to evaluate safe ways of increasing the progenitor cell yield of marrow harvests.

Acknowledgments

The author thanks Joseph H. Antin, MD, from the Dana-Farber Cancer Institute, and Zbigniew M. Szczepiorkowski, MD, PhD, FCAP, from Dartmouth-Hitchcock Medical Center, for sharing their marrow harvest SOPs, and Christine Colby for assistance in the preparation and review of the manuscript.

References/Resources

1. Brunvand MW, Bensinger WI, Soll E, et al. High-dose fractionated total-body irradiation, etoposide, and cyclophosphamide for treatment of malignant lymphoma: Comparison of autologous bone marrow and peripheral blood stem cells. Bone Marrow Transplant 1996;18:131-41.
2. Bensinger WI, Martin PJ, Storer B, et al. Transplantation of bone marrow as compared with peripheral-blood cells from HLA-identical relatives in patients with hematologic cancers. N Engl J Med 2001;344:175-81.
3. Schmitz N, Beksac M, Bacigalupo A, et al. Filgrastim-mobilized peripheral blood progenitor cells versus bone marrow transplantation for treating leukemia: 3-year results from the EBMT randomized trial. Haematologica 2005;90:643-8.
4. Stem Cell Trialists' Collaborative Group. Allogeneic peripheral blood stem-cell compared with bone marrow transplantation in the management of hematologic malignancies: An individual patient data meta-analysis of nine randomized trials. J Clin Oncol 2005;23:5074-87.
5. Rowley SD, Donaldson G, Lilleby K, et al. Experiences of donors enrolled in a randomized study of allogeneic bone marrow or peripheral blood stem cell transplantation. Blood 2001;97:2541-8 [erratum appears in Blood 2001;98:1301].
6. Favre G, Beksac M, Bacigalupo A, et al. Differences between graft product and donor side effects following bone marrow or stem cell donation. Bone Marrow Transplant 2003;32:873-80.
7. Karlsson L, Quinlan D, Guo D, et al. Mobilized blood cells vs bone marrow harvest: Experience compared in 171 donors with particular reference to pain and fatigue. Bone Marrow Transplant 2004;33:709-13.
8. Osgood EE, Riddle MC, Mathews TJ. Aplastic anemia treated with daily transfusions and intravenous marrow; case report. Ann Intern Med 1939;13:357-61.
9. Wilson RE. Techniques of human-bone-marrow procurement by aspiration from living donors. N Engl J Med 1959;261:781-5.
10. Thomas E, Storb R, Clift RA, et al. Bone-marrow transplantation (first of two parts). N Engl J Med 1975;292:832-43.

11. Spitzer TR, Areman EM, Cirenza E, et al. The impact of harvest center on quality of marrows collected from unrelated donors. J Hematother 1994;3:65-70.

12. Hill HF, Chapman CR, Jackson TL, Sullivan KM. Assessment and management of donor pain following marrow harvest for allogeneic bone marrow transplantation. Bone Marrow Transplant 1989;4:157-61.

13. Sim KM, Boey SK, Wong LT. Bone marrow harvesting using local anaesthesia and PCA-alfentanil: A feasible alternative to general or regional anaesthesia. Bone Marrow Transplant 1996;18:787-90.

14. Areman EM, Dickerson SA, Kotula PL, et al. Use of a licensed electrolyte solution as an alternative to tissue culture medium for bone marrow collection. Transfusion 1993;33:562-6.

15. Chern B, McCarthy N, Hutchins C, Durrant ST. Analgesic infiltration at the site of bone marrow harvest significantly reduces donor morbidity. Bone Marrow Transplant 1999;23:947-9.

16. Bolwell BJ, Maurer W, Anderson J, et al. Outpatient bone marrow harvest: The Cleveland Clinic experience. Bone Marrow Transplant 1995;16:703-5.

17. Thorne AC, Stewart M, Gulati SC. Harvesting bone marrow in an outpatient setting using newer anesthetic agents. J Clin Oncol 1993;11:320-3.

18. Aleem A, Lovell R, Holder K, et al. Performing bone marrow harvest on an outpatient basis: A single center UK experience. Acta Haematol 2004;112:200-2.

19. Vriesendorp HM, van Bekkum DW. Role of total body irradiation in conditioning for bone marrow transplantation. Haematol Blood Transfus 1980;25:349-64.

20. Storb R, Prentice RL, Thomas ED. Marrow transplantation for treatment of aplastic anemia. An analysis of factors associated with graft rejection. N Engl J Med 1977; 296:61-6.

21. Spitzer TR. Bone marrow and stem cell processing. In: Areman EM, Deeg HJ, Sacher RA, eds. Bone marrow and stem cell processing: A manual of current techniques. Philadelphia: FA Davis, 1991:95-9.

22. Bacigalupo A, Tong J, Podesta M, et al. Bone marrow harvest for marrow transplantation: Effect of multiple small (2 mL) or large (20 mL) aspirates. Bone Marrow Transplant 1992;9:467-70.

23. Batinic D, Marusic M, Pavletic Z, et al. Relationship between differing volumes of bone marrow aspirates and their cellular composition. Bone Marrow Transplant 1990; 6:103-7.

24. Atkinson K, Farrelly H, Cooley M, et al. Human marrow T cell dose correlates with severity of subsequent acute graft-versus-host disease. Bone Marrow Transplant 1987; 2:51-7.

25. Kernan NA, Bartsch G, Ash RC, et al. Analysis of 462 transplantations from unrelated donors facilitated by the National Marrow Donor Program. N Engl J Med 1993; 328:593-602.

26. Bortin MM, Buckner CD. Major complications of marrow harvesting for transplantation. Exp Hematol 1983; 11:916-21.

27. Buckner CD, Clift RA, Sanders JE, et al. Marrow harvesting from normal donors. Blood 1984;64:630-4.

28. Beamish N, Schwarer AP, Watson AM, et al. Acute pancreatitis complicating a bone marrow harvest. Bone Marrow Transplant 1997;19:525-6.

29. Klumpp TR, Mangan KF, MacDonald JS, Mesgarzadeh M. Fracture of the ilium: An unusual complication of bone marrow harvesting. Bone Marrow Transplant 1992; 9:503-4.

30. Baselga J, Reich L, Doherty M, Gulati S. Fat embolism syndrome following bone marrow harvesting. Bone Marrow Transplant 1991;7:485-6.

31. Wolf HH, Heyll A, Hesterberg R, et al. Mechanical ileus following bone marrow harvesting: An unusual complication (letter). Bone Marrow Transplant 1994;14:179-80.

32. Confer DL, Stroncek DF. Bone marrow and peripheral blood stem cell donors. In: Thomas ED, Blume SJ, Forman KG, eds. Hematopoietic cell transplantation. Malden, MA: Blackwell Science, 1999:421-30.

33. Chang G, McGarigle C, Spitzer TR, et al. A comparison of related and unrelated marrow donors. Psychol Med 1998;60:163-7.

34. Switzer GE, Dew MA, Butterworth VA, et al. Understanding donors' motivations: A study of unrelated bone marrow donors. Soc Sci Med 1997;45:137-47.

35. Butterworth VA, Simmons RG, Bartsch G, et al. Psychosocial effects of unrelated bone marrow donation: Experiences of the National Marrow Donor Program. Blood 1993;81:1947-59.

36. Stroncek DF, Holland PV, Bartch G, et al. Experiences of the first 493 unrelated marrow donors in the National Marrow Donor Program. Blood 1993;81:1940-6.

37. Sosman JA, Stiff PJ, Bayer RA, et al. A Phase I trial of interleukin 3 (IL-3) pre-bone marrow harvest with granulocyte-macrophage colony-stimulating factor (GM-CSF) post-stem cell infusion in patients with solid tumors receiving high-dose combination chemotherapy. Bone Marrow Transplant 1995;16:655-61.

38. Solomon SR, Mielke S, Savani BN, et al. Selective depletion of alloreactive donor lymphocytes: A novel method to reduce the severity of graft-versus-host disease in older patients undergoing matched sibling donor stem cell transplantation. Blood 2005;106:1123-9.

39. Couban S, Messner HA, Andreou P, et al. Bone marrow mobilized with granulocyte colony-stimulating factor in related allogeneic transplant recipients: A study of 29 patients. Biol Blood Marrow Transplant 2000;6:422-7.

40. Ostronoff M, Ostronoff F, Souto Maior P, et al. Pilot study of allogeneic G-CSF-stimulated bone marrow transplantation: Harvest, engraftment, and graft-versus-host disease. Biol Blood Marrow Transplant 2006;12: 729-33.

41. Pession A, Locatelli F, Prete A, et al. G-CSF in an infant donor: A method of reducing harvest volume in bone marrow transplantation. Bone Marrow Transplant 1996; 17:431-2.

42. Sharabi Y, Sachs DH. Mixed chimerism and permanent specific transplantation tolerance induced by a nonlethal preparative regimen. J Exp Med 1989;169:493-502.

43. Fudaba Y, Spitzer TR, Shaffer J, et al. Myeloma responses and tolerance following combined kidney and nonmyeloablative marrow transplantation: In vivo and in vitro analyses. Am J Transplant 2006;6:2121-33.

44. Bottino R, Linetsky E, Selvaggi G, et al. Human vertebral body bone marrow harvest: Comparison between manual and automated methods. Transplant Proc 1995;27:3340.

45. Olson LC, Ricordi C, Karatzas T, et al. Vertebral body procurement from multiorgan donors for bone marrow harvest. Transplant Proc 1997;29:2243-5.

Method 22-1. Harvesting Bone Marrow

Purpose

Human bone marrow contains mature red and white blood cells, platelets, committed hematopoietic progenitor cells (HPCs), mast cells, fat cells, plasma cells, and pluripotent hematopoietic cells. Some of these cells are capable of reconstituting the marrow of an autologous or allogeneic recipient after myeloablative or nonmyeloablative conditioning. This treatment may be indicated for certain malignancies, immune deficiencies, hematologic diseases, and congenital disorders.

Description

This procedure details the marrow harvesting procedure performed in the operating room (OR), including the preparation of required instruments and reagents; filtration after collection; labeling; and transport of the marrow.

Note: This standard operating procedure (SOP) requires that a laboratory staff member assist the harvesting physician and OR nursing staff with the collection procedure. Individual staffing and facility practices may vary.

Summary of Procedure

Marrow cells are obtained from the posterior iliac crests and occasionally from the anterior crests or, rarely, the sternum of the donor through multiple needle aspirations. The marrow is placed in a labeled sterile collection container with an electrolyte solution and an anticoagulant. The volume collected is determined by the weight of the recipient and is usually in the range of 500 to 1500 mL or approximately 10 mL/kg of the recipient's weight. The volume collected may also be limited by the donor size. After the marrow is collected, it is filtered in the OR to remove fat, bone particles, and cellular debris. Once the marrow has been filtered and the label is complete, it is transported to the processing laboratory.

Time for Procedure

Varies according to the volume collected.

Equipment

(Autoclaved and usually kept in the OR area)
1. Marrow harvesting needles
2. Marrow collection stand consisting of the following:
   a. Round base.
   b. Support rod.
   c. Collection container retainer.
   d. Collection container support with thumbscrew.
3. 600-mL stainless steel beaker.
4. 250-mL stainless steel beaker.
5. Hemostat.

Reagents

1. Plasma-Lyte A (Baxter, Deerfield, IL) injection.
2. Preservative-free heparin (1000 units/mL).
3. Acid (or anticoagulant)-citrate-dextrose formula A (ACD-A).
4. Sterile water.
5. Sterile 0.9% sodium chloride injection.

Supplies

1. Validated product transport cooler.
2. Marrow collection kit [eg, 4R2104, Fenwal, Lake Zurich, IL].
3. 35-mL disposable luer-lock syringes.

Safety (Personal Protective Equipment)

1. Sterile surgical gown.
2. Shoe covers.
3. Surgical head cover.
4. Face shield.
5. Sterile gloves.

Procedure

A. *Day before Harvest—Preparation of Transport Cooler*
   1. A completed and signed prescription or collection order is obtained:

a. For local donors, a prescription for collection and processing is obtained.

b. For National Marrow Donor Program (NMDP) donors, a copy of the prescription and prescription verification forms is obtained from the marrow transplant coordinator or the NMDP donor center and placed in the cooler.

- Any special requests from the transplant program (eg, other-than-usual media or a different anticoagulant ratio) are noted and verified.

- If a request has been made for marrow sample tubes to be sent with the product, this should be noted.

2. Labels are prepared and placed in the cooler.

3. A laboratory requisition form for requesting a white cell count is completed.

a. The form should be completed with the appropriate donor information, laboratory name and phone number, and instructions for delivery of the sample to the laboratory.

b. The completed form is placed into the cooler with the marrow harvest record.

4. Also placed into the cooler are at least 3 large zipper-seal bags that will be used for transporting the collected and filtered marrow to the laboratory.

B. Day of Harvest in the OR—Preparation

Note: Sterile technique must be observed throughout the procedure.

1. Upon arrival in the OR, a staff member retrieves the marrow harvest record form from the cooler and records the lot numbers and expiration dates of all reagents to be used for the harvest.

2. The telephone number of the OR in which the procedure is taking place is filled in on the miscellaneous laboratory requisition. The requisition will be sent to the laboratory with the midharvest sample for a nucleated cell (NC) count.

3. The harvest medium, prepared by the pharmacy, is obtained.

a. For local autologous and allogeneic donors, the usual medium consists of 2 100-mL aliquots of Plasma-Lyte A,

each containing 15,000 units of preservative-free heparin.

Note: More of the medium will be needed if the volume collected is anticipated to be >1000 mL.

Note: For small-volume collections, that is, <500 mL (eg, for pediatric recipients), the amount of Plasma-Lyte A and heparin should be adjusted: usually 50 mL of Plasma-Lyte A and 7500 units of preservative-free heparin.

b. Occasionally, the transplant center requests a different medium for NMDP unrelated donors. This medium should be provided in advance so that it will be available for the harvest.

4. Staff who are participating in the harvest procedure perform the proper hand-scrubbing technique and don appropriate surgical scrub clothing (mask, head and foot covers, face protection).

5. The sterilized unassembled marrow collection stand and aspiration set are opened and inspected by the OR staff.

6. The collection stand is assembled according to the manufacturer's instructions.

7. The disposable collection container is assembled according to the manufacturer's instructions.

8. 100 mL of Plasma-Lyte A (50 mL for small collection) and 15 mL of preservative-free heparin (7.5 mL for small collection) are placed aseptically in the collection bag.

9. A 250-mL labeled stainless steel beaker is filled with sterile saline for initial rinsing of the syringes.

10. 100 mL of Plasma-Lyte A and 15 mL of preservative-free heparin are aseptically placed in a 600-mL labeled stainless steel beaker for a second rinsing of the syringes.

11. Six 35-mL plastic luer lock syringes are rinsed with heparinized Plasma-Lyte A and placed on the instrument stand along with the appropriate ball-top aspiration needles.

Note: Needle and trocar sets must be of identical length. The trocar should snap firmly into the needle. The sets are color-coded for ease of matching the two parts.

C. *Harvest Procedure*

1. After suitable (regional or general) anesthesia is administered, the donor is placed in the prone position. The posterior iliac crest areas are then cleaned with an antiseptic solution and draped in a sterile fashion.

2. The clinicians, one on each side of the patient, procure marrow by inserting the ball-top needles through the skin overlying each posterior iliac crest and into the bone, aspirating marrow into the heparinized syringes. A maximum amount of marrow, ranging from 5 to 10 mL, should be obtained with each aspiration.

3. Needles with attached syringes are then removed from the donor and placed on the instrument stand for transfer of the marrow to the collection bag.

4. Repeated aspirations are performed by reinserting the needle through the same skin puncture site into different bone sites until approximately 20% to 33% of the intended volume is collected. Skin puncture sites are then changed and the aspirations are repeated.

   Note: Because of the speed of the harvest, a laboratory staff member and scrub nurse usually share the duties of transferring the marrow to the collection bag and cleaning and rinsing the needles and syringes.

5. After the clinician has placed a syringe containing marrow on the stand, the assistant retrieves the syringe, pulls back on the syringe plunger to aspirate any residual marrow that may be in the needle, and removes the needle. The needle is placed in the water basin for rinsing. After expelling the marrow into the collection bag, the assistant gently squeezes it to mix the marrow with the anticoagulant and medium.

   Note: If it is necessary to collect >1000 mL of marrow, an additional collection bag should be used containing an appropriate volume of heparinized Plasma-Lyte A.

6. The scrub nurse or laboratory staff member rinses each syringe with saline from the small beaker before adding heparinized Plasma-Lyte A from the large beaker and

replacing the syringe on the stand for reuse.

7. Midway through the harvest, approximately 2 mL of marrow is drawn into a syringe from the sampling site at the bottom of the collection bag.

   a. The sample is given to the circulating nurse to send to the laboratory with the completed miscellaneous laboratory requisition.

   b. The technologist in the laboratory retrieves the sample, performs the NC count, and reports the results to the OR.

D. *Completion of Harvest*

1. For marrow that will be further processed, 10% ACD-A (10 mL of ACD-A per 100 mL of marrow) is added to the collection bag at the end of the procedure. For unrelated donors, if the transplant center requests ACD-A, it is added in the concentration requested.

2. After the desired volume of marrow has been collected and the ACD-A has been added, if applicable, the cap is closed and the collection bag is hung from an intravenous pole. The bag is mixed carefully.

3. The marrow is filtered to remove bone particles, fat, and clots, and it is collected into a 600- or 2000-mL transfer pack. Filters and transfer bags are provided with the collection kit. The 500-micron filter (red) is connected to the collection bag first, followed by the 200-micron filter (blue).

   Note: If a filter becomes blocked, it is replaced with another of the same size and color (supplied with the kit). The tubing should be closed with hemostats and roller clamps before the filters are removed.

4. The marrow bags are labeled with the labels provided in the cooler.

5. The marrow is placed in a zipper-seal bag and the seal is closed to prevent leakage. The sealed bag is placed into the product transport cooler and taken to the processing laboratory.

6. When the marrow arrives in the laboratory, it is usually stored at room temperature (22

±2 C) until it is infused or further processed, unless other arrangements have been made.

7. The data from the marrow harvest record and the NC count that was obtained after the completion of the harvest are recorded in the laboratory database.

References/Resources

1. Thomas E, Storb R. Technique for human marrow grafting. Blood 1970;36:507.
2. Herzig RH, Meagher RC. Bone marrow harvest: Disposable collection kit. In: Areman EM, Deeg HJ, Sacher RA, eds. Bone marrow and stem cell processing: A manual of current techniques. Philadelphia: FA Davis, 1992:53-5.
3. Fenwal Bone Marrow Collection Kit. Package insert. Version 07-19-55-841 REV:C. Lake Zurich, IL: Fenwal, 2008.
4. Areman EM, Dickerson SA, Kotula PL, et al. Use of a licensed electrolyte solution as an alternative to tissue culture medium for bone marrow collection. Transfusion 1993;33:562-6.
5. Padley D, ed. Standards for cellular therapy product services. 3rd ed. Bethesda, MD: AABB, 2008.
6. FACT-JACIE international standards for cellular therapy product collection, processing, and administration. 4th ed. Omaha, NE: Foundation for the Accreditation of Cellular Therapy and the Joint Accreditation Committee of ISCT and EBMT, 2008.

In: Areman EM, Loper K, eds
Cellular Therapy: Principles, Methods, and Regulations
Bethesda, MD: AABB, 2009

◆◆◆   **23**   ◆◆◆

Collection of Cellular Therapy Products by Apheresis

Michael L. Linenberger, MD, FACP

DURING STEADY-STATE HEMATOPOIESIS, the concentrations of pluripotent stem cells and committed progenitors circulating in the peripheral blood are low. These cells, collectively referred to as hematopoietic progenitor cells (HPCs), tend to reside within the marrow because of cytoadhesive interactions between membrane receptors and ligands expressed on microenvironmental stromal cells and within the extracellular matrix.[1] Two important progenitor-associated surface molecules are the integrin very late antigen 4 (VLA-4), which binds to vascular cell adhesion molecule 1 (VCAM-1), and the chemokine CXCR4, which binds to stromal-cell-derived factor 1 (SDF-1). Marrow HPCs emigrate into the blood when these (and other) cell:cell and cell:matrix cytoadhesive interactions are disrupted.[1]

HPCs transiently leave the marrow and enter the circulation during normal recovery after myelosuppressive chemotherapy. HPCs can also be induced into the bloodstream by certain exogenously administered cytokines, such as granulocyte col-

ony-stimulating factor (G-CSF), granulocyte-macrophage colony-stimulating factor (GM-CSF), and stem cell factor (SCF). The molecular and biological mechanisms involved in chemotherapy- and cytokine-induced mobilization are incompletely understood but appear to involve chemokine activation of proteases within the microenvironment that, in turn, hydrolyze cytoadhesive bonds and liberate HPCs.[1-3] Because of the growing interest in clinical applications of adult HPCs, pharmacologic agents are being developed that selectively interfere with receptor: ligand interactions (such as AMD3100, a reversible inhibitor of CXCR4 and SDF-1 binding) as a means to rapidly mobilize HPCs into the blood for collection and use.[3]

The CD34 antigen is another clinically important molecule expressed on the surface of primitive and committed HPCs. Although its exact function is undefined, CD34 has been extremely useful for identifying, quantitating, and purifying marrow and blood progenitors. Early trials in humans confirmed that CD34+ cells mobilized into the

---

Michael L. Linenberger, MD, FACP, Medical Director, Apheresis and Cellular Therapy, Seattle Cancer Care Alliance; Professor, Division of Hematology, Department of Medicine, University of Washington; and Associate Member, Clinical Research Division, Fred Hutchinson Cancer Research Center, Seattle, Washington

The author has disclosed no conflicts of interest.

peripheral blood (PB) and, when collected for transplantation, were similar to marrow-derived cells in their ability to fully reconstitute hematopoiesis after myeloablative conditioning. The numbers of transplanted CD34+ cells correlated with engraftment kinetics.[4,5] Since the mid-1990s, mobilization of HPCs with chemotherapy and cytokines and collection by mononuclear cell (MNC) leukocytapheresis (apheresis) became the preferred method for procuring large numbers of CD34+ cells for autologous and allogeneic transplantation.

Although the proliferative and regenerative potentials of marrow and mobilized blood CD34+ HPCs are similar, biological differences exist. Compared to steady-state CD34+ marrow cells, mobilized CD34+ cells are less frequently in the active cell cycle, and their RNA profiles show relatively decreased levels of the expression of genes involved in DNA synthesis, cell cycle initiation, and cell cycle progression.[6,7] Mobilized CD34+ cells also express greater transcript levels of genes that direct apoptosis.[7]

The cellular composition of products containing mobilized HPCs collected by apheresis differs from HPC products procured from steady-state marrow. Compared to marrow harvest products, HPCs from apheresis (HPC-A) generally contain twofold to fivefold more CD34+ cells, roughly fivefold more type-2 dendritic cells, 10-fold more T lymphocytes and natural killer (NK) cells, and 20-fold more monocytes and B lymphocytes.[8] In turn, HPC-A products lack the significant numbers of mesenchymal stromal cells, endothelial progenitors, osteogenic progenitors, and other microenvironmental cells found in aspirated marrow.

The relatively higher CD34+ cell content of HPC-A products offers advantages over marrow products for progenitor cell transplantation. After myeloablative conditioning, neutrophil and platelet engraftment occurs roughly 4 to 7 days sooner, and immune function recovers earlier for recipients of HPC-A compared to recipients of marrow.[8] The more rapid engraftment with HPC-A translates into lower early transplant-related morbidity and mortality, particularly for autologous recipients, along with fewer hospital days and lower costs.

Transplantation with HPC-A may be associated with disadvantages in the allogeneic recipient. Some retrospective analyses and nonrandomized

trials of myeloablative transplants for hematologic malignancies have observed significantly higher rates of chronic (but not acute) graft-vs-host disease (GVHD) among recipients of sibling donor HPC-A compared to marrow.[9-11] Moreover, the severity, duration, and infectious complications associated with chronic GVHD appear to be worse in HPC-A recipients than in patients who received marrow.[12,13] An increased risk of chronic GVHD in this setting has been linked to high CD34+ cell doses.[14]

In contrast to the early retrospective studies, some prospective randomized trials observed no differences in the incidence rates of chronic GVHD among recipients of either HPC-A or marrow.[15,16] To address these discordant data, a meta-analysis was performed on nine prospective randomized trials that had compared blood and marrow stem cell sources and outcomes of transplantation after myeloablative conditioning.[17] That analysis identified a significant association between HPC-A and a higher rate of chronic GVHD; however, individuals who had received HPC-A for treatment of aggressive and late-stage hematologic malignancies also developed significantly fewer relapses and had lower relapse-related mortality. Thus, those observations support the findings by others[18] that chronic GVHD related to HPC-A can be associated with a more potent graft-vs-tumor effect. Retrospective data suggest that these positive effects of donor alloreactivity in adults are not recapitulated in pediatric patients who have higher rates of chronic GVHD and mortality after transplantation with HPC-A.[19]

Since the mid-1990s, HPC-A transplants have been increasingly substituted for marrow as the preferred stem cell source for transplantation for hematologic malignancies. Currently, HPC-A products are used for more than 75% of adult and 30% of pediatric (mostly unrelated donors) allogeneic transplants and for 85% to 90% of autologous transplants.[20,21] Nonmyeloablative (also called reduced-intensity) conditioning regimens have also recently driven the preference for allogeneic HPC-A products because the higher CD34+ cell content optimizes engraftment and minimizes the risk of rejection. Despite the benefits of HPC-A and the growing use of these products, the optimal graft source for most allogeneic transplantation indications has not been systematically evaluated in prospective, randomized clinical trials. Some studies suggest that a marrow product with a high nucleated cell (NC) dose may be superior to HPC-A for some diseases.[22] For these reasons, the Blood and Marrow Transplant Clinical Trials Network has initiated a multicenter, prospective, randomized trial to assess engraftment, GVHD rates, and survival among patients who are undergoing myeloablative transplantation for hematologic malignancies using either unrelated donor marrow or HPC-A procured through the National Marrow Donor Program (NMDP).

HPC Mobilization Regimens and Kinetics

HPC-A products are collected by apheresis after CD34+ cells are mobilized with myelosuppressive chemotherapy alone, chemotherapy with cytokine stimulation, or cytokine stimulation alone.[2,3] For patients with malignancy who require cytoreductive treatment, chemotherapy is given and HPC-A collection is performed during spontaneous hematopoietic recovery or, more commonly, when CD34+ cell mobilization is enhanced by posttreatment administration of a recombinant cytokine. The agents approved for this indication by the Food and Drug Administration (FDA) include recombinant human GM-CSF (sargramostim) and recombinant human G-CSF (filgrastim, a nonglycosylated molecule). A glycosylated form of recombinant G-CSF (lenograstim) is not available in the United States but is used for HPC mobilization in Europe. A pegylated form of recombinant G-CSF (pegfilgrastim) is approved by the FDA for febrile neutropenia but not for HPC mobilization. Single-dose pegfilgrastim has been successfully and safely used for mobilization of patients and healthy donors.[23,24]

Not all myelosuppressive chemotherapeutic drugs and regimens are effective for mobilization.[2] Cyclophosphamide, used alone or in combination regimens, is one of the most reliable mobilizing agents for patients with non-Hodgkin lymphoma and myeloma. By comparison, nucleoside analogues and alkylating agents that are progenitor cell toxins are less-effective mobilizers and can reduce the marrow reserve of CD34+ cells available for mobilization.[25]

For patients who do not require chemotherapy and for healthy allogeneic donors, peripheral blood progenitor cells (PBPCs) are procured by apheresis when the circulating CD34+ cell counts are maximal after subcutaneous injections of GM-CSF or, more commonly, G-CSF. Daily doses of G-CSF or a single dose of pegfilgrastim mobilize CD34+ PBPCs from steady-state hematopoiesis (ie, without recent prior chemotherapy) with predictable and reproducible kinetics. From a baseline concentration of $<5 \times 10^6$/L, blood CD34+ cell counts increase by 10- to 30-fold at 96 to 144 hours after the first daily dose of G-CSF or after a single injection of pegfilgrastim.[24,26] Peak blood CD34+ cell counts usually occur at 120 hours (ie, day 5) of mobilization with G-CSF alone.

Because the kinetics of cytokine-induced HPC mobilization from steady-state hematopoiesis and the resultant CD34+ cell yield by leukocytapheresis are predictable and reproducible, precollection monitoring of blood CD34+ cell counts is not routinely required. However, precollection measurement of peripheral CD34+ cells is used as an indicator of adequate circulating PBPCs by many programs. Apheresis is usually initiated at 96 to 120 hours after the start of G-CSF administration if an appropriate level of peripheral CD34+ cells is achieved. By comparison, the pace of hematopoietic recovery and the day of maximal CD34+ cell mobilization after myelosuppressive chemotherapy are generally not predictable. Therefore, blood cell count parameters must be followed to determine the optimal time to start apheresis.

The most reliable predictor of HPC-A product yield is the PB CD34+ cell count, which is usually determined by cytofluorometric methods.[27,28] A blood CD34+ cell concentration ≥8 to 10×10^6/L correlates closely with the number of product CD34+ cells that are collected either by standard blood volume processing or large-volume leukocytapheresis (LVL).[29,30] When a blood CD34+ cell count is not available, alternative parameters that roughly estimate HPC mobilization and apheresis CD34+ cell yield can be used. These may include the number of circulating immature cells, as determined by a manual differential count of a stained blood smear,[31] or the number of circulating progenitor cells, determined by using an automated instrument that assesses cell size, density, and resistance to osmotic lysis.[32] Blood measurements that are sometimes used, but are less indicative of circulating progenitor cell content, are the white cell (WBC) and MNC count.

A number of variables negatively affect the success of chemo-mobilization in patients and, in turn, the ability to procure adequate numbers of PBPCs for autologous transplantation. These variables include current or prior use of stem cell toxic chemotherapeutic agents, extensive prior myelosuppressive chemotherapy exposure, irradiation of marrow-bearing bones, exclusion of adjunctive cytokine stimulation after mobilization chemotherapy, heavy marrow involvement with malignancy, older age, and baseline thrombocytopenia (reflecting compromised steady-state hematopoiesis).[2,33,34]

Roughly 5% to 30% of patients are "poor mobilizers" and fail to generate at least 2×10^6 CD34+ cells/kg. Although lower CD34+ cell doses can reconstitute hematopoiesis after myeloablative conditioning,[35] 2×10^6 CD34+ cells/kg is usually considered the minimum acceptable cell dose to ensure timely engraftment of neutrophils and platelets. Salvage approaches for remobilization and collection can, in many cases, yield sufficient additional PBPCs for transplantation.[36] These approaches include the use of different mobilization chemotherapy regimens; higher-dose G-CSF, either alone or following chemotherapy; and large-volume leukapheresis (LVL).[2] For selected patients, combinations of mobilization agents can be considered to augment the effect of chemotherapy or G-CSF alone. These agents include adjunctive GM-CSF, SCF (ancestim, which is available in Europe and Canada but not in the United States), and AMD3100 (currently in investigational status).[37-39]

Healthy related and unrelated volunteer donors mobilized with standard doses and schedules of G-CSF may also occasionally fail to produce the expected numbers of CD34+ cells for allogeneic HPC-A transplantation. In a number of studies, donor ages of ≥38, 45, 50, and 55 years have been identified as independent predictors of significantly lower CD34+ cell yields on the first day of apheresis compared to yields from younger donors.[40-44] Additional factors associated with significantly lower CD34+ yields in multivariate analyses include female sex[42] and lower body weight.[44]

Instruments and Methodologies for HPC-A Collection

Continuous- or intermittent-flow blood cell separators that efficiently collect MNCs are suitable for HPC-A procurement. The use of these instruments is based on the principle that the CD34+ HPCs have the same relative density as lymphocytes. Therefore, they can be collected along with the buffy coat cells from a centrifuge bowl or drawn from a separation chamber that isolates the MNC population. The apheresis instruments that are used for MNC collections differ somewhat in their hardware specifications, separation technologies, disposable collection kits, extracorporeal volume (ECV) requirements, and levels of automated vs semiautomated (ie, computerized) operational capabilities.[45-47]

The relative performance characteristics of apheresis instruments for HPC-A collections are summarized in Table 23-1. The COM.TEC cell separator and software applications (Fresenius HemoCare, Bad Homburg, Germany) are used most commonly in Europe. This instrument incorporates a continuous-flow, automated system with single- or dual-stage separation chambers and cyclic MNC collections that optimize HPC collection efficiency (CE).[48-50] An additional feature is a software application that allows individualized blood volume processing according to the predicted product yield of CD34+ cells.

A number of retrospective and prospective, randomized studies have compared cell yield, CE, process volume, runtime, and PB cell effects (particularly on the platelet count) of HPC-A collections using different instruments and systems. Equivalent CD34+ cell product cell yields are achieved with either the COBE Spectra V4.7 semiautomated system (CaridianBCT, formerly Gambro BCT, Lakewood, CO) or the Spectra automated V6.0 system,[51-53] although some trials report lower-mean CD34+ cell CE with the V6.0 system,[51] and others report a higher CE.[53] All of the comparative studies observed shorter procedure times with the V4.7 system and higher product platelet contamination that, in turn, translated into greater blood platelet count decrements after the procedure.

The Haemonetics MCS+ cell separator (Haemonetics Corp, Braintree, MA), which uses discon-

Table 23-1. Instruments Used for HPC-A Collection and Their Relative Performance Characteristics

Instrument	References	Process	Inlet Flow Rate (mL/min)	ECV (mL)	Red Cell ECV (mL)	Blood Plt Count Decrease (range of mean %)*	MNC Collection Efficiency (range of mean %)*	CD34+ Collection Efficiency (range of mean %)*
Baxter CS 3000 Plus[†]	53-56, 58, 59	Continuous blood flow; continuous MNC collection	50-75	460	100	8	82	29-87
Baxter Amicus[†]	58-60, 62, 63	Continuous blood flow; cyclic MNC collection	35-75	210	60	18-22	107-113	46-121
COBE Spectra Manual (V4.7)[‡]	48-50, 51, 53-55, 61, 63	Continuous blood flow; continuous MNC collection	40-150	285	114	33-46	33-108	45-93
Gambro Spectra Auto (V6.0 and V6.1)[‡]	48, 50-52, 56, 62	Intermittent blood flow; cyclic MNC collection	35-75	165	66	15-34	15-91	38-77
Haemonetics MCS+[§]	51, 52	Intermittent blood flow; cyclic buffy coat collection	20-30	480	180	39-46	NR	NR
Fresenius COM.TEC (Auto MNC)[‖]	45-47	Continuous blood flow; cyclic MNC collection	NR	NR	NR	37-49	NR	67-95

*Mean percentages with the processing of 2 to 3 blood volumes.
[†]Baxter Healthcare, Deerfield, IL.
[‡]CaridianBCT, Lakewood, CO.
[§]Haemonetics Corp, Braintree, MA.
[‖]Fresenius USA, Walnut Creek, CA.
HPC-A = hematopoietic progenitor cells from apheresis; ECV = extracorporeal volume; MNC = mononuclear cell; Plt = platelet; NR = not reported.

tinuous blood flow and intermittent MNC collection methodologies, requires 30% more time and processes roughly one-third less blood than comparable apheresis procedures that use the Spectra V4.7 and V6 systems.[54,55] As a result, HPC-A products collected with the MCS+ instrument contain significantly fewer MNC and CD34+ cells. In addition, the product volume is significantly less, and platelet contamination is similar to products collected with the Spectra V6 system.[54,55] The major advantage of the MCS+ system is that single-needle access is adequate to collect HPC-A.

Small randomized trials and larger retrospective studies have compared HPC-A collections using the Spectra systems with the Baxter CS 3000 Plus system (Baxter, Deerfield, IL).[56-60] When similar blood volumes are processed, the relative yields of product progenitors and CD34+ cells are equivalent, regardless of the instrument or the system. One study, which included many patients with high preapheresis WBC and CD34+ cell counts, reported a lower mean CD34+ cell CE with the CS 3000 Plus (when compared with the Spectra V4.7), primarily because of a significant drop in the CE when the WBC count was $>50 \times 10^9$/L and the CD34+ cell count was $>50 \times 10^6$/L.[58] Other trials using the CS 3000 Plus system observed either similar mean CD34+ cell CEs to the Spectra V4.7,[56,57] or a mean CE that was superior to that obtained with the Spectra V6.0 system.[59] The latter study noted that a low preapheresis WBC count was associated with a high CD34+ cell CE when the CS 3000 Plus is used.[59]

A newer automated cell separator, the Baxter Amicus (Baxter Healthcare, Deerfield, IL), incorporates a two-stage separation module with intermittent MNC collection cycles to maximize CD34+ cell CE. Comparative studies that collected HPC-A from patients using both the Amicus and the CS 3000 Plus (ie, the day 1 apheresis using one instrument, and the day 2 apheresis using the other)[61] or by randomizing patients to either instrument[62] observed significantly higher mean CD34+ cell CEs for the Amicus. Mean CD34+ CE was 65% for the Amicus vs 43% for the CS 3000 when alternating instruments, and 54.9% for the Amicus vs 46.4% for the CS 3000 when patients were randomized to either instrument. However, the CE with the Amicus instrument, like the CS 3000 Plus, decreases significantly when the precollection WBC

count is >40 to 50×10^9/L. For patients and donors with high WBC counts, modifications to the cycle volumes and whole blood flow rates can improve the performance of the Amicus system.[62,63]

Studies that compared the Amicus instrument and the automated Spectra systems have observed either no difference in HPC-A product CD34+ cell CEs (Amicus vs Spectra V6.0 system)[64] or a superior CE for Amicus (compared to the Spectra V6.1 system).[65] Platelet contamination is significantly greater in HPC-A products collected with the Spectra automated systems. Standard-volume collections with the Amicus result in a decrease of approximately 20% in postprocedure blood platelet count compared to a 30% decrease with the Spectra. Similarly, the semiautomated Spectra V4.7 system collects greater numbers of platelets during HPC-A collection,[66] resulting in a 30% to 50% decrease in postprocedure platelet count. However, the mean CEs for MNC and CD34+ cells are not different between the Amicus and Spectra V4.7 system.[66] Other collection systems by various manufacturers are in development.

Standard Procedures for HPC-A Collections

Mobilization regimens are used to optimize the concentration of circulating CD34+ cells that are available for collection by MNC apheresis. Standard operating procedures (SOPs) for HPC-A collections are designed to maximize the yield of CD34+ cells with each procedure. An example of an SOP for HPC-A collection using the MNC protocol for the COBE Spectra instrument can be found in Method 23-1. Standard treatment plans that accompany the MNC protocol and outline modifications of the procedure for LVL or alternative anticoagulant usage are found in Appendices 23-1 through 23-3.

Peripheral venous access, using antecubital and forearm veins, is usually adequate for HPC-A collections from healthy adult donors who require only one to three procedures. However, 7% to 10% of healthy donors, and up to 20% of female donors, will require a temporary central venous catheter (CVC).[67,68] For these adult donors and most pediatric sibling donors under 12 years of age,[69] temporary access is achieved with a short-term, dual-lumen apheresis/dialysis-type CVC placed in the jugular vein or, particularly in children, the femoral vein. Patients who undergo HPC-A collection for autologous transplantation commonly undergo placement of a semipermanent, tunneled apheresis/dialysis-type CVC that will be adequate for both the apheresis procedures and for long-term intravenous management throughout the posttransplant period.

The choice of an anticoagulant for HPC-A collection is frequently based on local institutional practices. Standard options include citrate-containing solutions alone [eg, acid (or anticoagulant)-citrate-dextrose formula A (ACD-A) used at an inlet blood:anticoagulant ratio of 1:7 to 1:15] or a combination of a citrate solution with unfractionated heparin (eg, 10 units heparin/mL ACD-A used at an inlet blood:anticoagulant ratio of 1:15 to 1:35) (see Method 23-1). Regardless of the solution, extra anticoagulant is often added to the product collection bag either before or immediately after HPC-A procurement to prevent clot formation. The advantage of combining heparin with citrate is minimization of the cumulative exposure to citrate during the procedure, thereby reducing the likelihood of hypocalcemic side effects and the need for calcium replacement. The concern with using heparin is its ability to induce temporary physiological anticoagulation, possibly increasing the risk of bleeding in patients with more severe thrombocytopenia or coagulopathy. In addition, heparin-induced thrombocytopenia (HIT) and associated thrombotic complications could develop in a newly exposed patient or donor, or rapid-onset complications might occur in a patient with a recent prior history of HIT.

Procurement of HPC-A from a patient or donor typically involves processing two to three times the total blood volume, or 10 to 12 L for an adult, by MNC apheresis. However, LVL, which involves processing between three and six times the total blood volume (24-36 L in an adult), is frequently performed to collect higher numbers of autologous HPC-A from pediatric and adult patients.[70,71] These procedures must take into account the logistical and clinical risks associated with a longer process time, a greater loss of platelets, and the side effects related to increased exposure to heparin or citrate anticoagulant.[72-74] Over the past few years, LVL has been more commonly used for HPC-A collections

from healthy related[73-74] and unrelated adult volunteer donors. Requirements include good venous access (to support procedures that last for up to 5 hours) and, especially when ACD-A is used alone for anticoagulation, routine supplementation with intravenous calcium chloride or calcium gluconate.

The intraprocedure concentration of CD34+ cells within the PB during either a standard-volume MNC apheresis or LVL appears to remain relatively constant or even to increase.[75-81] By comparison, concentrations of blood platelets and granulocytes decrease appreciably during collection.[75] This phenomenon of "recruitment" of CD34+ cells into the PB, although variable and not observed in all studies,[82] appears to correlate directly with the patient's total blood volume and the amount of blood processed (ie, recruitment is greater during LVL). The mechanisms responsible for HPC recruitment are undefined but may relate to the mobilization kinetics of the G-CSF that is administered before the procedure, the effects of heparin or ACD-A on cytoadhesive interactions within the marrow microenvironment, and the perturbation of feedback signals within the marrow that sense the concentration of circulating CD34+ cells.

Observations with standard-volume HPC-A collections and LVL have shown a direct correlation between the yield of CD34+ cells and the pre-apheresis blood CD34+ cell count when that count was ≥ 10 to 20×10^6/L.[29,70,71,73,74,81] More accurate methods to predict the effect of HPC recruitment during LVL and to thereby individualize the duration of apheresis to achieve the desired CD34+ cell goal have included midcollection assessments of circulating CD34+ cell concentrations and product CD34+ cell counts.[77,79] The circulating leukocyte count at the time of LVL must also be considered because the CD34+ cell CE of some cell separators is compromised at WBC counts of $>35 \times 10^9$/L, whereas the effect with other instruments may be variable or negligible.[83-86]

Whether high precollection blood CD34+ cell counts affect the CD34+ cell CE during MNC apheresis is unclear. Significantly lower CE has been reported with some instruments when the circulating CD34+ cell count was ≥ 40 to 50×10^6/L,[87] whereas no effect was seen with other instruments,[53,58,60] or the effects were attributable to a concurrent high WBC count rather than to the CD34+ count.[62]

Variations in instrument collection methodologies or donor characteristics may also affect the relative numbers and types of non-CD34+ cells within the apheresis product. These collection-related differences in product cellular composition might, in turn, affect transplant outcomes.[88,89] The potential roles of technical, donor, and patient variables on HPC-A product content have not yet been systematically investigated or characterized.

Collecting HPC-A from Pediatric Donors

Pediatric HPC-A collections, including LVL and procedures in extremely low-weight infants, can be safely carried out when autologous transplantation is indicated for solid tumors and hematologic malignancies.[71,90-93] Healthy pediatric sibling donors can also safely undergo G-CSF mobilization and successful HPC-A collection as an alternative to marrow harvest, although HPC-A collection is not a standard practice in all transplant centers.[69,94,95] Special procedural considerations in these patients and donors include the following[69,90,91,93,96]:

- The ethical, legal, and regulatory aspects of informed consent for a minor.
- The selection and use of a CVC for access.
- Indications for sedation or anesthesia.
- Emotional complications.
- The potential need for homologous red cells to prime the instrument (according to the patient or donor's total blood volume and the extracorporeal red cell volume required for the apheresis circuit and cell separation set).
- Proper adjustments of flow rates during the procedure and rinseback at completion to achieve the planned fluid balance at the end.
- The choice of an anticoagulant and the associated risks, including requirements for calcium supplementation.
- Expected postprocedure changes in blood platelet count and hematocrit.

The CD34+ cell CE for procedures in pediatric patients is equivalent to that for procedures in adults that use similar cell separation instruments.[97] If available, midprocedure product CD34+ cell measurements can help to predict the final blood process volume necessary to achieve the desired goal.[98]

Adverse Effects and Complications of CD34+ Cell Mobilization and HPC-A Collection

Side effects of G-CSF that is used to mobilize blood CD34+ cells occur frequently, but they are usually mild, transient, and dependent on dose and schedule.[67,99-106] Notably, however, adult donors of HPC-A do not experience significantly less overall pain, discomfort, and emotional distress than marrow donors.[67,100-102,107] Roughly 40% to 85% of HPC-A donors experience bone and musculoskeletal pain, and up to 40% require some analgesic medication.[67,99-104,106] Fatigue is reported by 30% to 70% and headache by 12% to 55%, whereas nausea occurs in 3% to 29%, insomnia in 5% to 30%, and fever in 3% to 13%.[67,99-103,106] Mild, transient splenomegaly occurs after 5 days of G-CSF in most donors[108] and may be responsible in part for a decrease in blood platelet count. Rare complications include marked splenomegaly and splenic rupture, severe thrombocytopenia, acute lung injury, and exacerbation of inflammatory conditions such as gout and iritis.[94,106]

Laboratory abnormalities attributable to G-CSF, in addition to neutrophilia, include mild, transient thrombocytopenia and elevations in liver enzymes, lactate dehydrogenase (LDH), and uric acid.[67,104-106] One prospective, long-term, follow-up study of 94 sibling donors observed mild lymphopenia at 14 days after collection in 25 individuals and neutropenia at 14 days after collection in 26 individuals.[106] Mild lymphopenia and neutropenia were still present in 5 and 4, respectively, out of 38 otherwise-healthy donors evaluated 3 years after collection.

The long-term safety of brief G-CSF exposure for HPC-A procurement remains an open question. Some investigators have reported that mobilization doses of G-CSF induce transient genetic and epigenetic changes in circulating lymphocytes and myeloid cells from healthy donors, which raises the concern that even short-term exposure may lead to an increased risk of hematologic malignancies.[109-111] By comparison, a study using different methodologies to assess blood MNC from donors after 4 days of G-CSF stimulation found only rapidly resolving, "nonpathological" alterations in gene expression.[112]

Single-institution, retrospective, and prospective follow-up studies of donors have observed no cases of hematological malignancy or myelodysplasia at 3 to 6 years after HPC-A collection.[106,113,114] However, a survey of adverse drug reactions identified two cases of acute myelogenous leukemia (AML) among 200 sibling HPC-A donors who had undergone collection on clinical trials 4 and 5 years previously.[115] The recipients in each case had AML, and the mother of one sibling pair also had secondary AML, suggesting that familial leukemia risk factors might be involved. The publication of this study prompted a review by the NMDP of the experiences of unrelated HPC-A donors whose PBPCs had been mobilized and collected, and no cases of leukemia or lymphoma were identified among 4015 donors at 1 year or 897 donors at 4 years beyond collection.[116] Similarly, no increased rates of hematologic malignancies have been observed among donors who have participated in HPC-A collections through international registries.[94] Ongoing prospective studies of unrelated HPC-A donors are being carried out by the NMDP and other registries to obtain sufficient long-term follow-up information to define the relative risks and safety of limited G-CSF treatment.

Primarily, adverse events related to the apheresis procedure include pain and complications from venous access, hypotension, hypocalcemia symptoms because of citrate toxicity, and thrombocytopenia secondary to platelet loss into the product. A CVC is required for 7% to 10% of all healthy adult donors and up to 20% of women.[67,68] Catheter or needle-site pain is reported by 1% to 50% of donors.[67,100,101] Venous access flow problems or alarms occur during roughly 7% of procedures.[117]

Citrate-related symptoms, including paresthesias, headache, and nausea, are more common in women and with LVL procedures, particularly if ACD-A alone is used as an anticoagulant.[72,74,118] With intravenous calcium prophylaxis during LVL using citrate only, mild paresthesias occur in roughly 15% of all donors and up to 28% of women, and nausea occurs in 3%.[74,118] By comparison, a citrate reaction occurs in 20% of donors who undergo standard-volume (12 L) apheresis with ACD-A plus heparin.[101] Retrospective survey data of HPC-A donations at European centers revealed

that citrate toxicity was reported in 13% to 20% of collections.[117,119] Hypocalcemia and citrate reactions are treated by slowing the infusion rate of citrate and infusing supplemental calcium chloride or calcium gluconate.

Unexpected acute adverse events occur in 0.06% to 1.5% of donors who undergo HPC-A collection.[68,119,120] These include severe pain, nausea, headache, hypotension or syncope, arrhythmias, citrate reactions, angina, thrombosis, bleeding (sometimes due to thrombocytopenia), splenic rupture, and pneumonitis.

Donors whose HPC-A are mobilized with G-CSF and collected by apheresis do not experience the acute procedure-related pain felt by donors who undergo marrow harvesting. However, cumulative daily G-CSF side effects translate into an extended duration of discomfort, and the overall pain and symptom burden felt by HPC-A donors is similar to that of marrow donors.[67,100-102,107] In addition, although symptoms resolve more rapidly after HPC-A collection, the short- and long-term recovery times are, with a few exceptions, equivalent to the recovery times for marrow donors.[67,101,107] In comparison to marrow harvest, the HPC-A collection process requires less time away from work and incurs a low risk of hospitalization. However, the levels of anxiety and psychological stress associated with these procedures are not appreciably different.[67,100-103,107]

Adverse events during pediatric HPC-A collections are similar to those encountered with adult patients and donors.[90] Additional concerns include the risks related to sedation or anesthesia, emotional and behavioral consequences, and exposure to red cell blood components.[69,91,94] In general, pediatric procedures are safe and well tolerated. Young and small-bodyweight children must be monitored closely for hypovolemia, fluid overload, and citrate reactions, particularly when donors cannot verbalize symptoms because they are too young or are sedated.[92,93] Children experience milder G-CSF-associated musculoskeletal pain symptoms than adult donors.[69] However, the same concerns regarding the potential long-term adverse effects of G-CSF apply to pediatric donors, and these must be weighed against the risks and complications of marrow harvest.[95]

References/Resources

1. Papayannopoulou T. Current mechanistic scenarios in hematopoietic stem/progenitor cell mobilization. Blood 2004;103:1580-5.

2. Kessinger A, Sharp JG. The whys and hows of hematopoietic progenitor and stem cell mobilization. Bone Marrow Transplant 2003;31:319-29.

3. Cashen AF, Lazarus HM, Devine SM. Mobilizing stem cells from normal donors: Is it possible to improve upon G-CSF? Bone Marrow Transplant 2007;39:577-88.

4. Schwartzberg L, Birch R, Blanco R, et al. Rapid and sustained hematopoietic reconstitution by peripheral blood stem cell infusion alone following high-dose chemotherapy. Bone Marrow Transplant 1993;11:369-74.

5. Weaver C, Hazelton B, Birch R, et al. An analysis of engraftment kinetics as a function of the CD34 content of peripheral blood progenitor cell collections in 692 patients after the administration of myeloablative chemotherapy. Blood 1995;86:3961-9.

6. Graf L, Heimfeld S, Torok-Storb B. Comparison of gene expression in CD34+ cells from bone marrow and G-CSF-mobilized peripheral blood by high density oligonucleotide array analysis. Biol Blood Marrow Transplant 2001;7:486-94.

7. Steidl U, Kronenwett R, Ulrich-Rohr P, et al. Gene expression profiling identifies significant differences between the molecular phenotypes of bone marrow-derived and circulating human CD34+ hematopoietic stem cells. Blood 2002;99:2037-44.

8. Körbling M, Anderlini P. Peripheral blood stem cell versus bone marrow allotransplantation: Does the source of hematopoietic stem cells matter? Blood 2001;98:2900-8.

9. Ringdén O, Labopin M, Bacigalupo A, et al. Transplantation of peripheral blood stem cells as compared with bone marrow from HLA-identical siblings in adult patients with acute myeloid leukemia and acute lymphoblastic leukemia. Am J Clin Oncol 2002;20:4655-64.

10. Guardiola P, Runde V, Bacigalupo A, et al. Retrospective comparison of bone marrow and granulocyte colony-stimulating factor-mobilized peripheral blood progenitor cells for allogeneic stem cell transplantation using HLA identical sibling donors in myelodysplastic syndromes. Blood 2002;99:4370-8.

11. Schmitz N, Eapen M, Horowitz MM, et al. Long-term outcome patients given transplants of mobilized blood or bone marrow: A report from the International Bone Marrow Transplant Registry and the European Group for Blood and Marrow Transplantation. Blood 2006;108:4288-90.

12. Flowers M, Parker PM, Johnston LJ, et al. Comparison of chronic graft-versus-host disease after transplantation of peripheral blood stem cells versus bone marrow in allogeneic recipients: Long-term follow-up of a randomized trial. Blood 2002;100:415-20.

13. Anderson D, DeFor T, Burns L, et al. A comparison of related donor peripheral blood and bone marrow transplants: Importance of late-onset chronic graft-versus-host disease and infections. Biol Blood Marrow Transplant 2003;9:52-9.

14. Heimfeld S. HLA-identical stem cell transplantation: Is there an optimal CD34 cell dose? Bone Marrow Transplant 2003;31:839-45.

15. Bensinger WI, Martin PJ, Storer B, et al. Transplantation of bone marrow as compared with peripheral-blood cells from HLA-identical relatives in patients with hematologic cancers. N Engl J Med 2001;344:175-81.

16. Couban S, Simpson DR, Barnett MJ, et al. A randomized multicenter comparison of bone marrow and peripheral blood in recipients of matched sibling allogeneic transplants for myeloid malignancies. Blood 2002;100:1525-32.

17. Stem Cell Trialists' Collaborative Group. Allogeneic peripheral blood stem cell compared with bone marrow transplantation in the management of hematologic malignancies: An individual patient data meta-analysis of nine randomized trials. J Clin Oncol 2005;23:5074-87.

18. Sohn SK, Kim JG, Kim DH, et al. Impact of transplanted CD34+ cell dose in allogeneic unmanipulated peripheral blood stem cell transplantation. Bone Marrow Transplant 2003;31:967-72.

19. Eapen M, Horowitz MM, Klein JP, et al. Higher mortality after allogeneic peripheral blood transplantation compared with bone marrow in children and adolescents: The Histocompatibility and Alternate Stem Cell Source Working Committee of the International Bone Marrow Transplant Registry. J Clin Oncol 2004;22:4872-80.

20. Miano M, Labopin M, Hartmann O, et al. Haematopoietic stem cell transplantation trends in children over the last three decades: A survey by the paediatric diseases working party of the European Group for Blood and Marrow Transplantation. Bone Marrow Transplant 2007;39:89-99.

21. Gratwohl A, Baldomero H, Frauendorfer K, et al. Results of the EBMT activity survey 2005 on haematopoietic stem cell transplantation: Focus on increasing use of unrelated donors. Bone Marrow Transplant 2007;39:71-87.

22. Gorin NC, Labopin M, Rocha V, et al. Marrow versus peripheral blood for geno-identical allogeneic cell transplantation in acute myelocytic leukemia: Influence of dose and stem cell source shows better outcome with rich marrow. Blood 2003;102:3034-51.

23. Kroschinsky F, Hölig K, Platzbecker U, et al. Efficacy of single-dose pegfilgrastim after chemotherapy for the mobilization of autologous peripheral blood stem cells in patients with malignant lymphoma or multiple myeloma. Transfusion 2006;46:1417-22.

24. Kroschinsky F, Hölig K, Poppe-Thiede K, et al. Single-dose pegfilgrastim for the mobilization of allogeneic CD34+ peripheral blood progenitor cells in healthy family and unrelated donors. Haematologica 2005;90:1665-71.

25. Tournilhac O, Cazin B, Lepretre S, et al. Impact of front-line fludarabine and cyclophosphamide combined treatment on peripheral blood stem cell mobilization in B-

cell chronic lymphocytic leukemia. Blood 2004;103:363-6.

26. Stroncek DF, Clay ME, Herr G, et al. The kinetics of G-CSF mobilization of CD34⁺ cells in healthy people. Transfus Med 1997;7:19-24.

27. Sutherland DR, Anderson L, Keeney M, et al. The ISHAGE guidelines for CD34+ cell determination by flow cytometry. J Hematother 1996;5:213-26.

28. Venditti A, Battaglia A, Del Poeta G, et al. Enumeration of CD34+ hematopoietic progenitor cells for clinical transplantation: Comparison of three different methods. Bone Marrow Transplant 1999;24:1019-27.

29. Yu J, Leisenring W, Fritschle W, et al. Enumeration of HPC in mobilized peripheral blood with the Sysmex SE9500 predicts final CD34⁺ cell yield in the apheresis collection. Bone Marrow Transplant 2005;25:1157-64.

30. Moncada V, Bolan C, Ying Yau Y, et al. Analysis of PBPC cell yields during large-volume leukapheresis of subjects with a poor mobilization response to filgrastim. Transfusion 2003;43:495-502.

31. Kozuka T, Ikeda K, Teshima T, et al. Predictive value of circulating immature cell counts in peripheral blood for timing of peripheral blood progenitor cell collection after G-CSF plus chemotherapy induced mobilization. Transfusion 2002;42:1514-22.

32. Lefrere F, Zohar S, Beaudier S, et al. Evaluation of an algorithm based on peripheral blood hematopoietic progenitor cell and CD34+ cell concentrations to optimize peripheral blood progenitor cell collection by apheresis. Transfusion 2007;47:1851-7.

33. Kuittinen T, Nousiainen T, Halonen P, et al. Prediction of mobilization failure in patients with non-Hodgkin's lymphoma. Bone Marrow Transplant 2004;34:907-12.

34. Ford CD, Green W, Warenski S, et al. Effect of prior chemotherapy on hematopoietic stem cell mobilization. Bone Marrow Transplant 2004;33:901-5.

35. Weaver CH, Potz J, Redmond J, et al. Engraftment and outcomes of patients receiving myeloablative therapy followed by autologous peripheral blood stem cells with a low CD34⁺ cell content. Bone Marrow Transplant 1997;19:1103-10.

36. Bensinger W, Appelbaum F, Rowley S, et al. Factors that influence collection and engraftment of autologous peripheral-blood stem cells. J Clin Oncol 1995;13:2547-55.

37. Boeve S, Strupeck J, Creech S, et al. Analysis of remobilization success in patients undergoing autologous stem cell transplants who fail an initial mobilization: Risk factors, cytokine use and cost. Bone Marrow Transplant 2004;33:997-1003.

38. Dawson MA, Schwarer AP, Muirhead JL, et al. Successful mobilization of peripheral blood stem cells using recombinant human stem cell factor in heavily pretreated patients who have failed a previous attempt with a granulocyte colony-stimulating factor-based regimen. Bone Marrow Transplant 2005;36:389-96.

39. Flomenberg N, Devine SM, Diperso JF, et al. The use of AMD3100 plus G-CSF for autologous hematopoietic progenitor cell mobilization is superior to G-CSF alone. Blood 2005;106:1867-74.

40. Rubia J, Arbona C, de Arriba F, et al. Analysis of factors associated with low peripheral blood progenitor cell collection in normal doors. Transfusion 2002;42:4-10.

41. Shimizu N, Asai T, Hashimoto S, et al. Mobilization factors of peripheral blood stem cells in healthy donors. Ther Apher 2002;6:413-18.

42. Martino M, Callea I, Condemi A, et al. Predictive factors that affect the mobilization of CD34+ cells in healthy donors treated with recombinant granulocyte colony-stimulating factor (G-CSF). J Clin Apher 2006;21:169-75.

43. Anderlini P, Przepiorka D, Seong TL, et al. Factors affecting mobilization of CD34+ cells in normal donors treated with filgrastim. Transfusion 1997;37:507-12.

44. Ings S, Balsa C, Leverett D, et al. Peripheral blood stem cell yield in 400 normal donors mobilized with granulocyte colony-stimulating factor (G-CSF): Impact of age, sex, donor weight and type of G-CSF used. Br J Haematol 2006;134:517-25.

45. Burgstaler EA. Current instrumentation for apheresis. In: McLeod BC, Price TH, Weinstein R, eds. Apheresis: Principles and practice. 2nd ed. Bethesda, MD: AABB Press, 2003.

46. Mechanic SA, Krause D, Proytcheva MA, et al. Mobilization and collection of peripheral blood progenitor cells. In: McLeod BC, Price TH, Weinstein R, eds. Apheresis: Principles and practice. 2nd ed. Bethesda, MD: AABB Press, 2003.

47. Moog R. Apheresis techniques for collection of peripheral blood progenitor cells. Transfus Apher Sci 2004;31:207-20.

48. Movassaghi K, Jaques G, Schmitt-Thomssen A, et al. Evaluation of the COM.TEC cell separator in predicting the yield of harvested CD34+ cells. Transfusion 2007;47:824-30.

49. Dal Fante C, Perotti C, Viarengo G, et al. Clinical impact of a new automated system employed for peripheral blood stem cell collection. J Clin Apher 2006;21:227-32.

50. Schwella N, Movassaghi K, Scheding S, et al. Comparison of two leukapheresis programs for computerized collection of blood progenitor cells on a new cell separator. Transfusion 2003;43:58-64.

51. Rowley SD, Prather K, Bui KT, et al. Collection of peripheral blood progenitor cells with an automated leukapheresis system. Transfusion 1999;39:1200-6.

52. Wilke R, Brettell M, Prince HM, et al. Comparison of COBE Spectra software version 4.7 PBSC and version 6.0 auto PBSC program. J Clin Apheresis 1999;14:23-30.

53. Ravagnani F, Siena S, De Reys S, et al. Improved collection of mobilized CD34+ hematopoietic progenitor cells by a novel automated leukapheresis system. Transfusion 1999;30:48-55.

54. Morrison AE, Watson D, Buchanan S, et al. Prospective randomized concurrent comparison of the COBE Spectra Version 4.7, COBE Spectra version 6 (Auto PBSC™) and Haemonetics MCS+ cell separators for leucapheresis

in patients with haematological and non haematological malignancies. J Clin Apher 2000;15:224-9.

55. Abdelkefi A, Maamar M, Torjman L, et al. Prospective randomized comparison of the COBE Spectra version 6 and haemonetics MCS+ cell separators for hematopoietic progenitor cells leucapheresis in patients with multiple myeloma. J Clin Apher 2006;21:111-15.

56. Stroncek DF, Clay ME, Smith J, et al. Comparison of two blood cell separators in collecting peripheral blood stem cell components. Tranfus Med 1997;7:95-9.

57. Hitzler WE, Wolf S, Runkel S, Kunz-Kostomanolakis M. Comparison of intermittent- and continuous-flow cell separators for the collection of autologous peripheral blood progenitor cells in patients with hematologic malignancies. Transfusion 2001;41:1562-6.

58. Mehta J, Singhal S, Gordon L, et al. COBE Spectra is superior to Fenwal CS 3000 Plus for collection of hematopoietic stem cells. Bone Marrow Transplant 2002;29:563-7.

59. Ford CD, Lehman C, Strupp A, et al. Comparison of CD34+ cell collection efficiency on the COBE Spectra and Fenwal CS-3000 Plus. J Clin Apher 2002;17:17-20.

60. Padley D, Strauss RG, Wieland M, et al. Concurrent comparison of the COBE Spectra and Fenwal CS3000 for the collection of peripheral blood mononuclear cells for autologous peripheral stem cell transplantation. J Clin Apher 1991;6:77-80.

61. Snyder EL, Baril L, Cooper DL, et al. In vitro and post-transfusion engraftment characteristics of MNCs obtained by using a new separator for autologous PBPC transplantation. Transfusion 2000;40:961-7.

62. Jeanne M, Bouzgarrou R, Lafarge X, et al. Comparison of CD34+ cell collection on the CS-3000+ and Amicus blood cell separators. Transfusion 2003;43:1423-7.

63. Hartwig D, Dorn I, Kirchner H, et al. Recommendations for optimized settings of the Amicus Crescendo cell separator for the collection of CD34+ progenitor cells. Transfusion 2004;44:758-63.

64. Adorno G, Del Proposto G, Palombi F, et al. Collection of peripheral progenitor cells: A comparison between Amicus and COBE-Spectra blood cell separators. Transfus Apher Sci 2004;30:131-6.

65. Ikeda K, Ohto H, Kanno T, et al. Automated programs for collection of mononuclear cells and progenitor cells by two separators for peripheral blood progenitor cell transplantation: Comparison by a randomized crossover study. Transfusion 2007;47:1234-40.

66. Ikeda K, Ohto H, Nemoto K, et al. Collection of MNCs and progenitor cells by two separators for PBPC transplantation: A randomized crossover trial. Transfusion 2003;43:814-19.

67. Favre G, Beksac M, Bacigalupo A, et al. Differences between graft product and donor side effects following bone marrow or stem cell donation. Bone Marrow Transplant 2003;32:873-80.

68. Pulsipher M, Kurian S, Leitman SF, et al. Unrelated-donor PBSC collection facilitated by the NMDP, 1999-2005: Efficacy and toxicities, serious unexpected events,

and outcomes of standard vs. large volume collections (abstract). Blood 2005;106:556a.

69. Pulsipher MA, Levine JE, Hayashi RJ, et al. Safety and efficacy of allogeneic PBSC collection in normal pediatric donors: The pediatric blood and marrow transplant consortium experience (PBMTC). Bone Marrow Transplant 2005;35:361-7.

70. Abrahamsen JF, Stamnesfet S, Liseth K, et al. Large-volume leukapheresis yields more viable CD34+ cells and colony-forming units than normal-volume leukapheresis, especially in patients who mobilize low numbers of CD34+ cells. Transfusion 2005;45:248-53.

71. Bolan CD, Yau YY, Cullis HC, et al. Pediatric large-volume leukapheresis: A single institution experience with heparin versus citrate-based anticoagulant regimens. Transfusion 2004;44:229-38.

72. Humpe A, Riggert J, Munzel U, et al. A prospective, randomized, sequential crossover trial of large-volume versus normal-volume leukapheresis procedures: Effects on serum electrolytes, platelet counts, and other coagulation measures. Transfusion 2000;40:368-74.

73. Gašová Z, Marinov I, Vodvárková Š, et al. PBPC collection techniques: Standard versus large volume leukapheresis (LVL) in donors and in patients. Transfus Apher Sci 2005;32:167-76.

74. Bolan C, Carter C, Wesley R, et al. Prospective evaluation of cell kinetics, yields and donor experiences during a single large-volume apheresis versus two smaller volume consecutive day collections of allogeneic peripheral blood stem cells. Br J Haematol 2003;120:801-7.

75. Humpe A, Riggert J, Munzel U, et al. A prospective, randomized, sequential, crossover trial of large-volume leukapheresis procedures: Effect on progenitor cells and engraftment. Transfusion 1999;39:1120-7.

76. Knudsen LM, Nikolaisen K, Gaarsdal E, et al. Kinetic studies during peripheral blood stem cell collection show CD34+ cell recruitment intra-apheresis. J Clin Apher 2001;16:114-19.

77. Humpe A, Riggert J, Koch S, et al. Prospective, randomized, sequential crossover trial of large-volume vs. normal-volume leukapheresis procedures: Effects on subpopulations of CD34+ cells. J Clin Apher 2001;16:109-13.

78. Rowley SD, Yu J, Gooley T, et al. Trafficking of CD 34+ cells into the peripheral circulation during collection of peripheral blood stem cells by apheresis. Bone Marrow Transplant 2001;28:649-56.

79. Ford CD, Greenwood J, Strupp A, et al. Change in CD34+ cell concentration during peripheral blood progenitor cell collection: Effects on collection efficiency and efficacy. Transfusion 2002;42:904-10.

80. Cull G, Ivey J, Chase P, et al. Collection and recruitment of CD34+ cells during large-volume leukapheresis. J Hematother 1997;6:309-14.

81. Fontana S, Groebli R, Leibundgut K, et al. Progenitor cell recruitment during individualized high-flow, very-large-volume apheresis for autologous transplantation improves collection efficiency. Transfusion 2006;46:1408-16.

82. Cassens U, Momkvist PH, Zuelsdorf M, et al. Kinetics of standardized large volume leukapheresis (LVL) in

patients do not show a recruitment phenomenon of peripheral blood progenitor cells (PBPC). Bone Marrow Transplant 2001;28:13-20.

83. Burgstaler E, Pineda A, Winters J. Hematopoietic progenitor cell large volume leukapheresis (LVL) on the Fenwal Amicus blood separator. J Clin Apher 2004;19: 103-11.

84. Sarkodee-Ardoo C, Taran I, Guo C, et al. Influence of preapheresis clinical factors on the efficiency of CD34+ cell collection by large-volume apheresis. Bone Marrow Transplant 2003;31:851-5.

85. Ford CD, Pace N, Lehman C. Factors affecting the efficiency of collection of CD34-positive peripheral blood cells by a blood cell separator. Transfusion 1998;38:1046-50.

86. Gidron A, Verma A, Doyle M, et al. Can the stem cell mobilization technique influence CD34+ cell collection efficiency of leukapheresis procedures in patients with hematologic malignancies? Bone Marrow Transplant 2005;35:243-6.

87. Heuft H, Dubiel M, Rick O, et al. Inverse relationship between patient peripheral blood CD34+ cell counts and collection efficiency for CD34+ cells in two automated leukapheresis systems. Transfusion 2001;41:1008-13.

88. Katipamula R, Porrata LF, Gastineau DA, et al. Apheresis instrument settings influence absolute lymphocyte count affecting survival following autologous peripheral hematopoietic stem cell transplantation in non-Hodgkin's lymphoma: The need to optimize instrument setting and define a lymphocyte collection target. Bone Marrow Transplant 2006;37:811-17.

89. Panse JP, Heimfeld S, Guthrie KA, et al. Allogeneic peripheral blood stem cell graft composition affects early T-cell chimaerism and later clinical outcomes after non-myeloablative conditioning. Br J Haematol 2005;128: 659-67.

90. Kim HC. Therapeutic pediatric apheresis. J Clin Apher 2000;15:129-57.

91. Sevilla J, Díaz MA, Fernández-Plaza S, et al. Risks and methods for peripheral blood progenitor cell collection in small children. Transfus Apher Sci 2004;31:221-31.

92. Cecyn KZ, Seber A, Ginani VC, et al. Large-volume leukapheresis for peripheral blood progenitor cell collection in low body weight pediatric patients: A single center experience. Transfus Apher Sci 2005;32:269-74.

93. Sevilla J, Fernández Plaza S, González-Vicent M, et al. PBSC collection in extremely low weight infants: A single-center experience. Cytotherapy 2007;9:356-61.

94. Pulsipher MA, Nalger A, Iannone R, et al. Weighing the risks of G-CSF administration, leukopheresis, and standard marrow harvest: Ethical and safety considerations for normal pediatric hematopoietic cell donors. Pediatr Blood Cancer 2006;46:422-33.

95. Grupp SA, Frangoul H, Wall D, et al. Use of G-CSF in matched sibling donor pediatric allogeneic transplantation: A consensus statement from the Children's Oncology Group (COG) Transplant Discipline Committee and Pediatric Blood and Marrow Transplant Consortium

(PBMTC) Executive Committee. Pediatr Blood Cancer 2006;46:414-21.

96. Ravagnani F, Coluccia P, Notti P, et al. Peripheral blood stem cell collection in pediatric patients: Feasibility of leukapheresis under anesthesia in uncompliant small children with solid tumors. J Clin Apher 2006;21:85-91.

97. Witt V, Fischmeister G, Scharner D, et al. Collection efficiencies of MNC subpopulations during autologous CD34+ peripheral blood progenitor cell (PBPC) harvests in small children and adolescents. J Clin Apher 2001;16: 161-8.

98. Sidhu RS, Orsini E, Giller R, et al. Midpoint CD34 measurement as a predictor of PBPC product yield in pediatric patients undergoing high-dose chemotherapy. J Clin Apher 2006;21:165-8.

99. Anderlini P, Donato M, Chan K-W, et al. Allogeneic blood progenitor cell collection in normal donors after mobilization with filgrastim: The MD Anderson Cancer Center experience. Transfusion 1999;39:555-60.

100. Switzer GE, Goycoolea JM, Dew MA, et al. Donating stimulated peripheral blood stem cells versus bone marrow: Do donors experience the procedures differently? Bone Marrow Tranplant 2001;27:917-23.

101. Rowley S, Donaldson G, Lilleby K, et al. Experiences of donors enrolled in a randomized study of allogeneic bone marrow or peripheral blood stem cell transplantation. Blood 2001;97:2541-8.

102. Heldal D, Brinch L, Tjønnfjord G, et al. Donation of stem cells from blood or bone marrow: Results of a randomised study of safety and complaints. Bone Marrow Transplant 2002;29:479-86.

103. Fortanier C, Kuentz M, Sutton L, et al. Healthy sibling donor anxiety and pain during bone marrow or peripheral blood stem cell harvesting for allogeneic transplantation: Results of a randomized study. Bone Marrow Transplant 2002;29:145-9.

104. Beelen DW, Ottinger H, Kolbe K, et al. Filgrastim mobilization and collection of allogeneic blood progenitor cells from adult family donors: First interim report of a prospective German multi-center study. Ann Hematol 2002;81:701-9.

105. Gutierrez-Delgado F, Bensinger W. Safety of granulocyte colony-stimulating factor in normal donors. Curr Opin Hematol 2001;8:155-60.

106. Tassi C, Tazzari PL, Bonifazi F, et al. Short- and long-term haematological surveillance of healthy donors of allogeneic peripheral haematopoietic progenitors mobilized with G-CSF: A single institution prospective study. Bone Marrow Transplant 2005;36:289-94.

107. Kennedy GA, Morton J, Western R, et al. Impact of stem cell donation modality on normal donor quality of life: A prospective randomized study. Bone Marrow Transplant 2003;31:1033-5.

108. Stroncek D, Shawker T, Follmann D, et al. G-CSF induced spleen size changes in peripheral blood progenitor cell donors. Transfusion 2003;43:609-13.

109. Kaplinsky C, Trakhtenbrot L, Hardan I, et al. Tetraploid myeloid cells in donors of peripheral blood stem cells

treated with rhG-CSF. Bone Marrow Transplant 2003;32: 31-4.

110. Nagler A, Korenstein-Ilan A, Amiel A, et al. Granulocyte colony-stimulating factor generates epigenetic and genetic alterations in lymphocytes of normal volunteer donors of stem cells. Exp Hematol 2004;32:122-30.

111. Shapira MY, Kaspler P, Samuel S, et al. Granulocyte colony stimulating factor does not induce long-term DNA instability in healthy peripheral blood stem cell donors. Am J Hematol 2003;73:33-6.

112. Hernández JM, Castilla C, Guitiérrez NC, et al. Mobilization with G-CSF in healthy donors promotes a high but temporal deregulation of genes. Leukemia 2005;19: 1088-91.

113. Cavallaro AM, Lilleby K, Majolino I, et al. Three to six year follow-up of normal donors who received recombinant human granulocyte colony-stimulating factor. Bone Marrow Transplant 2000;25:85-9.

114. Anderlini P, Chan FA, Champlin RE, et al. Long-term follow up of normal peripheral blood progenitor cell donors treated with filgrastim: No evidence of increased risk of leukemia development. Bone Marrow Transplant 2002;30:661-3.

115. Bennett C, Evens AM, Andritsos L, et al. Haematological malignancies developing in previously healthy individuals who received haematopoietic growth factors: Report from the Research on Adverse Drug Events and Reports (RADAR) project. Br J Haematol 2006;135:642-50.

116. Confer DL, Miller JP. Long-term safety of filgratim (rhG-CSF) administration. Br J Haematol 2007;137:76-8.

117. Moog R. Adverse events in peripheral progenitor cell collection: A 7-year experience. J Hematother Stem Cell Res 2001;10:675-80.

118. Bolan C, Cecca SA, Wesley R, et al. Controlled study of citrate effects and response to IV calcium administration during allogeneic peripheral blood progenitor cell donation. Transfusion 2002;42:935-46.

119. De Silvestro GD, Marson P, Russo GE, et al. National survey of apheresis activity in Italy (2000). Transfus Apher Sci 2004;30:61-71.

120. Yoshihisa K, Shunichi K, Harada M, et al. Severe adverse events of allogeneic related peripheral blood stem cell donors—results of nation-wide 3,262 consecutively and prospectively registered case-survey in Japan and of its comparison to the outcome of retrospective survey shared with EBMT for stem cell donors (abstract). Blood 2005;106:326a.

Appendix 23-1. Examples of Treatment Plans from Three Institutions for Adult Mononuclear Cell Collection by Leukocytapheresis

Physician Notification

- Notify the apheresis center medical director or designee of severe adverse reactions during the procedure.
- Notify the referring provider of collection results daily.

Procedure

	Institution A	Institution B	Institution C
Standard operating procedure (SOP)	Institutional SOP for mononuclear cell (MNC) collection on a specific instrument	Institutional SOP for MNC collection on a specific instrument	Institutional SOP
Target inlet volume processed	12 L or according to doctor's order	12 L or according to doctor's order	30 L or according to doctor's order
Anticoagulant (AC) solution	500 mL of ACD-A + 5000 units of heparin (or according to doctor's order)	500 mL of ACD-A	1000 mL of ACD-A + 5000 units of heparin
Inlet:AC ratio	15:1 to 35:1	12:1 to 15:1	31:1
Inlet flow rate	Not to exceed 100 mL/ minute	60-75 mL/minute	150 mL/minute
AC infusion rate	Not to exceed 0.8 mL/ minute/L of patient total blood volume (TBV)	Not to exceed 0.8 mL/ minute/L of patient TBV	0.8 mL/minute
Collect flow rate	1.5 mL/minute	1.0 mL/minute	1.5 mL/minute
AC added to component	40 mL of ACD-A + 400 units of heparin solution (or according to doctor's order)	None or 25 mL of ACD-A	10 mL of ACD-A at 10 L, 20 L, and 30 L
Ending fluid balance	Not to exceed ±15% donor TBV	Not to exceed ±15% donor TBV	Not specified
Plasma collection for overnight storage	100 mL of plasma collected	100 mL of plasma collected if product <200 mL	No plasma collected
Restrictions	No infusions other than calcium during procedure	No infusions other than calcium during procedure	No infusions other than calcium during procedure

ACD-A = acid (or anticoagulant)-citrate-dextrose formula A.

Laboratory Sample Testing

	Institution A	Institution B	Institution C
Pre-apheresis	• Complete blood count (CBC), ABO/Rh • Infectious disease testing (if not performed within 30 days)	• CD34, CBC, ABO/Rh • Infectious disease testing	• CBC, basic metabolic panel (BMP), ionized calcium (iCa), ABO/Rh • Infectious disease testing (if not performed within 30 days) • Pregnancy test
PRN	iCa	As dictated by clinical status	PRN
Postapheresis (drawn at the start of the rinseback)	CBC	CBC	Platelet count

PRN = as needed; iCa = ionized calcium; CBC = complete blood count.

Patient Care

Measure	Institution A	Institution B	Institution C
Vital signs (temperature, heart rate, and blood pressure)	Pre- and postprocedure and PRN	Pre- and postprocedure and every 15 to 30 minutes (according to doctor's order)	Preprocedure, at the halfway mark, and postprocedure; daily weight in kg
Additional	Repeat above every 30 minutes	None	PRN pulse oximetry

Medications

	Institution A	Institution B	Institution C
iCa levels	Reference ranges = 1.12 to 1.32 mmol/L	Not usually performed	Normal: 1.17 to 1.3 mmol/L
Hypocalcemia prophylaxis	Not applicable	Calcium gluconate (1 g in 60 mL): 60 to 180 mL/hour	1 to 2 g CaCl in 250 mL normal saline over 200 minutes
Prophylaxis/PRN for citrate-related grade 1 hypocalcemia	Calcium carbonate (500 mg tabs): • Two tabs PO q 30 minutes • Not to exceed 15 tabs/day	Increase rate of infusion up to 180 mL/hour	1 to 2 g calcium gluconate IV slow push plus oral calcium carbonate PRN
PRN for grade 2 to 4 symptomatic hypocalcemia	If iCa <1.10, give 1 g calcium gluconate IV push/bolus over 10 minutes; repeat × 1 PRN. Initiate calcium gluconate, 1 g/hr IV drip. Repeat iCa in 1 hr; if <1.10, increase calcium gluconate IV drip to 2 g/hr	Rarely observed; give 1 g of calcium gluconate over 10 minutes	1 to 2 g calcium gluconate IV slow push

Medications (continued)

	Institution A	Institution B	Institution C
PRN for hypotension	Normal saline IV bolus: • Up to 10 mL/kg of patient weight	Normal saline IV bolus: • Up to 10 mL/kg of patient weight	Rarely observed
PRN for allergic reactions: give medication, then notify provider	Diphenhydramine: • 25 to 50 mg IV q 30 minutes • Maximum dosage: 100 mg	Diphenhydramine: • 25 to 50 mg IV q 30 minutes • Maximum dosage: 100 mg	Diphenhydramine: • 25 to 50 mg intravenous push (IVP) • Methylprednisolone IVP
PRN for discomfort from line placement or cytokine therapy	Acetaminophen: • 650 mg PO q 3 to 4 hours	Acetaminophen: • 650 mg PO q 3 to 4 hours	Contact provider. Acetaminophen, oxycodone, fentanyl, propoxyphene
For anaphylaxis, give medication, then notify provider	• Epinephrine, 1:1000: give 0.3 to 0.5 mL SQ • Hydrocortisone, 100 to 250 mg IV • Diphenhydramine, 50 mg IV	• Epinephrine, 1:1,000: give 0.3 to 0.5 mL SQ • Hydrocortisone 100 to 250 mg IV • Diphenhydramine 50 mg IV	• Discontinue collection • Epinepherine, 1:1000: 0.3 to 0.5 mL SQ; may repeat × 1 • Diphenhydramine, 50 mg IV • Hydrocortisone, 100 mg IV

Tabs = tablets; PO = by mouth; q = every; IV = intravenous(ly); SQ = subcutaneous(ly).

Appendix 23-2. Examples of Treatment Plans from Three Institutions for Adult Large-Volume Mononuclear Cell Collection by Leukocytapheresis

Physician Notification

- Notify the apheresis center medical director or designee of severe adverse reactions during the procedure.
- Notify the referring provider of the collection results daily or when finished, according to institutional protocol.

Procedure

	Institution A	Institution B	Institution C
Standard operating procedure (SOP)	Institutional SOP for mononuclear cell (MNC) collection on a specific instrument	Institutional SOP for MNC collection on a specific instrument	Institutional SOP for MNC collection on a specific instrument
Target inlet volume processed	6 times the total blood volume (TBV), not to exceed 36 L or 6 hours of run time	300 to 360 minutes or according to doctor's order	According to doctor's order, not to exceed 40 L or 240 minutes
Anticoagulant (AC) solution	1000 mL ACD-A + 10,000 units heparin (or according to doctor's order)	1000 mL ACD-A	1000 mL ACD-A + 5000 units of heparin
Inlet:AC ratio	15:1 to 35:1	12:1 to 15:1	31:1
Inlet flow rate	Not to exceed 150 mL/minute	60-75 mL/minute	150 mL/minute
AC infusion rate	Not to exceed 0.8 mL/minute/L of patient TBV	Not to exceed 0.8 mL/minute/L of patient TBV	Not to exceed 0.8 mL/minute
Collect flow rate	1.5 mL/minute	1.0 mL/minute	1.5 mL/minute
AC added to component	40 mL ACD-A + 400 units heparin solution (or according to doctor's order)	None or 25 mL ACD-A	10 mL ACD-A at 10 L, 20 L, and 30 L
Ending fluid balance	Not to exceed ±20% of donor TBV	Not to exceed ±20% of donor TBV	Not specified
Plasma collection for overnight storage	Collect 100 mL of plasma to be added to the component bag	No modification	No modification
Restrictions	No infusions other than calcium during the procedure	No infusions other than calcium during the procedure	No infusions other than calcium during the procedure

ACD-A = acid (or anticoagulant)-citrate-dextrose formula A.   1 of 2

Laboratory Sample Testing

	Institution A	Institution B	Institution C
Pre-apheresis	• Complete blood count (CBC), ABO/Rh • Infectious disease testing (if not performed within 30 days) • Ionized calcium (iCa)	• CBC, ABO/Rh • Infectious disease testing	• CBC, basic metabolic panel (BMP), iCa, ABO/Rh • Infectious disease testing (if not performed within 30 days) • Pregnancy test, if appropriate
Midcollection	iCa	Laboratory tests*	Laboratory tests*
PRN	iCa	Laboratory tests*	Laboratory tests*
Postapheresis (drawn at the start of rinseback)	• CBC • ICa	CBC	Platelet count

*Speific tests not reported.
PRN = as needed; iCa = ionized calcium; CBC = complete blood count.

Patient Care

Measure	Institution A	Institution B	Institution C
Vital signs (temperature, heart rate, and blood pressure)	Pre- and postprocedure, every 30 minutes, and PRN	Pre- and postprocedure and every 15 to 30 minutes (according to doctor's order)	Preprocedure, midway, postprocedure, and PRN. Also, daily weight.

Appendix 23-3. Example of a Treatment Plan for Modified Anticoagulation for Apheresis

Physician Notification

- Discuss the patient or donor clinical condition with the apheresis unit medical director or designee before the procedure.
- Call the apheresis unit medical director or designee for severe allergic, febrile, or citrate reactions.

Indications for Heparin-Only Anticoagulation

- Patient or donor history of hypersensitivity to citrate anticoagulation.
- Patient or donor severe liver or renal dysfunction.

Procedure

Preprocedure bolus	40 units of heparin/kg bodyweight intravenously
Anticoagulant (AC) solution	500 mL normal saline + 7000 units heparin
Heparin infusion rate	40 units/minute
AC pump flow rate	2.9 mL/minute
Inlet:AC ratio	(desired inlet flow rate ÷ 2.9):1
Product bag additive	Call medical director or designee for orders

Laboratory Sample Testing

Pre- and postprocedure	Prothrombin time test (PT), activated partial thromboplastin time (aPTT), international normalized ratio (INR)
At 60 minutes, at midprocedure, and PRN thereafter (Call results to medical director or designee)	PT, aPTT (goal: 2 to 2.5 × control), INR

PRN = as needed.

Indications for Citrate-Only Anticoagulation if Heparin Is Routinely Used [Institution A (See Appendices 23-1 and 23-2)]

- Patient preprocedure platelet count >350,000.
- Patient with coagulopathy.
- Heparin allergy.
- Known or suspected heparin-induced thrombocytopenia (HIT).

Procedure

AC solution	ACD-A
Inlet:AC ratio	7:1 to 15:1
AC infusion rate	Not to exceed 0.8 mL/minute/L of patient TBV
Product bag additive	Add 40 mL ACD-A

ACD-A = acid (or anticoagulant)-citrate-dextrose formula A; TBV = total blood volume.

Laboratory Sample Testing

Preprocedure	Ionized calcium (iCa)
PRN and according to the standard treatment plan for each procedure	iCa

Patient Care

Monitor the patient closely for citrate-related symptomatic hypocalcemia	
Vital signs (heart rate and blood pressure)	Pre- and postprocedure and PRN
Additional	Repeat above every 30 minutes

Appendix 23-4. Example of an Apheresis Flow Sheet

CELL THERAPY
HPC Apheresis Flow Sheet

Procedure Type: _____ Product: _____ Date: _____

Procedure Number: _____ Directed Recipient: _____

Expiration Date: _____ _____

Allergy History: [ ] No known drug allergies   Other: _____

[ ] PCN   [ ] Codeine   [ ] GM CSF   [ ] Sulfa   [ ] Contrast   [ ] Adhesive   Assessed by: _____

CVL Assessment:	Time	Initials	CVL-Dressing change	Time	Initials
Site: L R			Stitches intact: [ ] yes [ ] no		
Dressing: [ ] clean [ ] dry [ ] intact			Signs of infection: [ ] yes [ ] no		
[ ] loose [ ] soiled [ ] bloody			CVL-restore patency		

CVL LAB	Time	Initials			
Infusaport: [ ]			CVL-resuture		
CVL lumen: [ ] blue [ ] brown [ ] red			CVL-remove		
[ ] white [ ] yellow			Peripheral LAB Draw	Time	Initials

CVL-Blood Cultures	Time	Initials	Site: # of attempts		
Infusaport: [ ]			Peripheral Blood Cultures	Time	Initials
CVL lumen: [ ] blue [ ] brown [ ] red			Site: # of attempts		
[ ] white [ ] yellow					

Pain Assessment		
Pre-Procedure: 0 1 2 3 4 5 6 7 8 9 10	Post-Procedure: 0 1 2 3 4 5 6 7 8 9 10	
Location:	Location:	
Intensity:	Intensity:	
Treatment:	Treatment:	

Product Results	Sex: Male Female	
Volume collected:	Ht: Wt:	
Cell yield X 10E8:	Vital Signs:	

CD 34%:	Time	Temp	Pulse	Respiration	Blood Pressure
Daily CD34 yield X 10E6:	pre				
Total CD34 yield:					
	post				

Comments: _____
_____
_____
_____
_____

CELL THERAPY
HPC Apheresis Flow Sheet

Procedure MEDS	Manufacturer	Lot #	Exp. Date	Accept √	Procedure Equipment	
ACDA:					Procedure machine:	
Heparin:					Fluid Warmer machine:	
1 L Saline:					VS machine:	
250 ml Saline:					IV Pump:	
Ca Chloride:					Alarm Checks	Nurse's Initials
IV Pump Tubing:					Yes or No	
Sampling Coupler:						
Stop Cock:						
Ca Gluconate:						
Procedure Kit						
Fluid Warmer Set						

PROCEDURE PARAMETERS:

Run Time:_____   ACD/WB Ratio:_____

Volume Processed:_____   Q Collected: _____

Volume ACD: _____   Vol Collect:_____

Time Proc	Vol.	RPM	Inlet Plasma/W.B.	QACD ADDED	ACDA	Comments

MEDICATION ADMINISTRATION

DISCHARGE STATUS:

Time	Medication	Dose	Route	Fluid	Device	Vol.Inf.	Initials
	CaCl		IV				
	GCSF		SQ				
	GMCSF		SQ				
	ASA	81	mg				
	NaCl 0.9%	10ml	IVP	to apheresis catheter x 2 lumens			
	Heparin 1000 units/ml	2ml	IVP	to apheresis catheter x 2 lumens			
	Heparin 100 units	___ml	IVP				

To: _____

Time: _____   Initials: _____

Mobility Status: [ ] ambulatory   [ ] wheelchair
                       [ ] stretcher

Accompanied by: _____

[ ] Unaccompanied

Condition: [ ] stable   or symptomatic with:

[ ] pain   [ ] fever   [ ] nausea

[ ] other:_____

Comments: _____

_____

Report to: _____   Given by: _____

Method 23-1. Mononuclear Cell Apheresis Collection Using COBE Spectra

Purpose

To ensure the safe collection of a peripheral blood (PB) mononuclear cell (MNC)-rich blood product by leukocytapheresis (apheresis).

Description

A specific fraction of the PB white blood cells [WBCs, including lymphocytes, monocytes, or hematopoietic progenitor cells (HPCs)] is targeted for collection by apheresis.

Time for Procedure

Varies from 120 to 300 minutes, and rarely more than 300 minutes.

Summary of Procedure

1. Donor is determined to be eligible to donate, and the eligibility is documented.
2. Appropriate pre-apheresis laboratory tests and donor examination are performed and documented.
3. The apheresis device is prepared for the procedure with all appropriate documentation.
4. Apheresis is performed, and the product is determined to be properly labeled before removal from the device.
5. The product is sent to the processing facility with the appropriate documentation.

Equipment

1. System: COBE Spectra Apheresis (Caridian BCT, Lakewood, CO).
2. Channel: COBE Spectra single–stage (Caridian BCT, Lakewood, CO).
3. Warmer: DataChem FloTem blood/fluid tubing (DataChem, Salt Lake City, UT) or Gambro SpectraTHERM blood/fluid tubing (Caridian BCT, Lakewood, CO).
4. Sealer: tubing (handheld or table model).

Reagents and Supplies

1. Normal saline: 1000- mL and 250-mLbags.
2. Acid (or anticoagulant)-citrate-dextrose formula A (ACD-A): 500- or 1000-mL bags.
3. Heparin: 5-10 mL (1000 units/mL).
4. Calcium chloride in normal saline: 10% (1g/10 mL × 2-3 vials) or according to institutional policy.
5. Gloves: clean.
6. Set: COBE WBC.
7. Set: blood warmer tubing.
8. Coupler: sampling site.
9. Syringes: sterile, 5 mL, 10 mL, 30 mL, 60 mL, according to institutional policy.
10. Container: biohazard sharps.
11. Spikes: intravenous (IV) bags (2).
12. Needles: 18 gauge (2).
13. Stopcocks: three-way (optional) (2).
14. Tubing clamps (2).
15. Venous access supplies.
16. Central venous catheter access supplies.
17. Wipes: alcohol.
18. Apheresis flow sheet (see Appendix 23-4 for an example)
19. Apheresis disclosure or consent form.

Safety (Personal Protective Equipment)

1. Each collection procedure is performed in a separate bay or patient room to maintain product integrity. The bay or work area and the COBE Spectra Apheresis System are cleaned after each procedure. Cleaning of bays or rooms is performed according to the hospital policy.
2. Standard precautions must be used at all times when employees are working with any biological specimens. All employees must complete training in bloodborne pathogens before performing this procedure.

3. Staff must don gloves and PPE, including scrubs or lab coats and eye protection, during the collection procedure.
4. Each procedure is performed using a sterile, disposable COBE WBC set.

Procedure

A. *Preprocedure Steps*
   1. Obtain physician orders for the procedures.
   2. Preprocedure samples:
      a. Label the appropriate Vacutainer tubes with a donor identification sticker, and add the date, the time, the indication "Pre," and the registered nurse's (RN's) initials.
      b. Collect samples of blood for pre-apheresis laboratory tests as ordered.
      c. Send samples with the corresponding laboratory request to the appropriate laboratories.
      d. Prepare component labels for the collection bag.
   3. Prepare the apheresis donor or patient chart, including a checklist on the first page, which includes the following:
      a. Physician order.
      b. Procedure cover sheet.
      c. Communication sheet.
      d. Laboratory results.
      e. Daily assessment sheet.
      f. Other documents as required.
   4. Prepare the anticoagulant specified by the physician orders or protocol.
   5. Label the anticoagulant container with the date, lot number, amount of heparin used, if applicable, expiration date, patient or donor label, and the RN's initials. Agitate the container gently.

B. *Machine Preparation*
   1. Load the COBE Spectra with single-stage channel and WBC set according to the COBE Spectra Apheresis System operator's manual.
   2. Load the blood warmer tubing onto the blood warmer, and then connect it to the return line of the WBC set.

3. Prime the Spectra with a normal saline and anticoagulant solution according to the COBE Spectra operator's manual.
4. Select SET #3 (WBC).
5. Select WBC PROCEDURE #1 (MNC).
6. At the automatic prime prompt, prime the blood warmer line, removing all air. Once it is primed, switch the blood warmer "on."
7. Add a three-way stopcock to both the access and return lines, and prime with saline.
8. Resume the prime procedure. When the prime procedure is complete, perform the alarm tests. Document the successful completion on the apheresis procedure flow sheet.
9. If ordered, add anticoagulant to the component collection bag using aseptic technique, and label the component bag with the amount and type of anticoagulant added.

C. *Donor Qualification*
   1. Each donor must undergo screening before each procedure, including vital signs, height, weight, and pain assessment, to document his or her qualification to undergo the procedure.
   2. Identify the donor by verifying the complete donor name, including the spelling; the date of birth; and the identifier number. Appropriately document this verification.
   3. Sign and present the "Apheresis Instructions and Follow-Up Care" form, and obtain the signature from the patient or donor.
   4. Review the leukocytapheresis procedure with the patient or donor and answer any questions.
   5. Check that the procedure consent is signed and filed with the medical records.
   6. If the donor does not meet the qualifying criteria (for both laboratory values and vital signs), hold the procedure. The procedure may not begin until the apheresis medical director or designee is notified and medical orders are given to proceed. A planned or unplanned variance form may be needed.

7. Apply the product label to the product collection bag.

D. *MNC Collection Procedure*

1. If ordered, perform a secondary blood priming of the cell separator.
2. Connect the COBE Spectra draw and return lines to the donor access lines. Check the access and return lines for air, and if air is present, run saline through the lines to clear them.
3. Begin apheresis and set the run parameters according to protocol or physician orders. Throughout the procedure, monitor and document the patient's vital signs.
4. If an adverse event occurs (eg, hypotension, chest pain, anaphylaxis, or severe citrate reaction), notify the apheresis medical director. Administer medication or treatment as ordered.
5. Observe the collect line closely throughout the procedure and adjust it to collect optimal MNCs.
6. Observe and document the machine parameters, which may include time, revolutions per minute (RPM), volume processed, blood flow rates, plasma flow rates, ACD-A volume, etc.
7. The run mode continues until the target values are reached.
8. Calcium supplementation according to institutional protocol may include continuous calcium chloride infusion, intermittent calcium gluconate IV as prophylaxis or treatment, and pro re nata (PRN) oral calcium carbonate.

E. *Postprocedure Steps*

1. Terminate the procedure as follows:
   a. When the target "inlet volume" is reached, select and initiate rinseback.
   b. Clamp the donor access line. Disconnect the COBE Spectra inlet line from the donor access line.
   c. Label postsample tubes with the patient or donor sticker and add the date, the time, the indication "Post," and the RN's initials.
   d. Draw postapheresis samples from the access line.
   e. Send the samples with the request form and corresponding paperwork to the appropriate laboratory.
   f. Remove the access line needle or flush the central venous catheter. Apply pressure to the venipuncture site.
   g. Obtain and record the postprocedure vital signs and patient status on the apheresis procedure flow sheet.
   h. Using input and output fluid balances, calculate the ending fluid balance and the percentage of total blood volume (TBV) using the following formulas:

      Input − Output = Ending Fluid Balance
      Ending Fluid Balance/TBV = % TBV

      If the ending percentage of TBV exceeds the balance in the procedure treatment plan (ie, ±15% for a standard-volume or ±20% for a large-volume procedure, if an applicable policy exists at the institution), complete the planned or unplanned variance form.
   i. Remove disposables and fluids according to the applicable COBE Spectra maintenance standard operating procedure.
   j. Clean the COBE Spectra and work surfaces.
2. Handle disposition of the patient or donor as follows:
   a. Transfer or discharge the patient from the care of the apheresis staff.
   b. Inpatient procedure: Give a report of the patient's status and procedure information to the patient's nurse.
   c. Outpatient procedure: Review postprocedure precautions with the patient or donor. The RN releases the patient from the apheresis center when the patient is stable.
3. Document by recording the medications given and place the apheresis procedure flow sheet in the patient/donor's medical record and in the apheresis patient/donor chart.
4. Complete the blood component and HPC transfusion records and place them in the patient's medical record chart and apheresis patient chart, if applicable.

References/Resources

1. Padley D, ed. Standards for cellular therapy product services. 3rd ed. Bethesda, MD: AABB, 2008.

2. FACT-JACIE international standards for cellular therapy product collection, processing, and administration. 4th ed. Omaha, NE: Foundation for the Accreditation of Cellular Therapy and the Joint Accreditation Committee of ISCT and EBMT, 2008.

In: Areman EM, Loper K, eds
Cellular Therapy: Principles, Methods, and Regulations
Bethesda, MD: AABB, 2009

◆◆◆ **24** ◆◆◆

Umbilical Cord Blood Collection

Julie G. Allickson, PhD, MS, MT(ASCP)

UMBILICAL CORD BLOOD (UCB) HAS BEEN collected for hematopoietic reconstitution since the mid-1980s. The first UCB transplant was performed in Paris in 1988.[1] The New York Blood Center, one of the first cord blood banks (CBBs) in the United States, began to store UCB for public use in 1991. Subsequently, private CBBs were established to store UCB for autologous and family use. At the time of this writing, more than 8000 UCB transplants have been performed, mostly in recipients not related to the donor. Transplants of UCB can provide hematopoietic reconstitution comparable to other sources of hematopoietic progenitor cells (HPCs) in pediatric patients, but with a delay in immunological reconstitution. However, UCB appears to lower the risk of graft-vs-host disease (GVHD), perhaps because of greater tolerance for HLA mismatching.[2] Since the first CBBs began operating in the 1990s, many have followed. There are now more than 50 CBBs in the United States alone.

UCB can be collected either in utero or ex utero. In the in-utero method, the UCB is harvested while the placenta is still in the uterus, and harvesting is typically performed by an obstetrician or midwife in the delivery suite. In the ex-utero method, the UCB is harvested after the placenta is expelled from the uterus, and the collection procedure is generally performed outside the delivery suite. Trained staff, often employed by the CBB, usually perform the ex-utero collection in a room close to the delivery suite. The placenta is elevated and placed on a stand, the cord is cleaned, the umbilical vein is punctured, and the UCB is collected with the help of gravity. Both collection techniques have been used successfully and are discussed in greater detail later in this section.

The first publications about UCB collection appeared in the 1950s and described the collection of cord blood samples for diagnostic purposes. CB in these studies was assessed for amino acid content, hematological characteristics, heparin activity, and fibrinogen levels and to explore diphtheria immunity.[3-6] A paper published in 1979 discussed the procurement of UCB from the umbilical vein into heparinized syringes.[7] The collected blood was cultured and coagulation studies performed to demonstrate the safety of UCB for treating iatrogenic blood loss. In 1981, UCB was used for the detection and diagnosis of neonatal bacteremia.[8] At

---

Julie G. Allickson, PhD, MS, MT(ASCP), Vice President, Laboratory Operations, Research and Development, Cryo-Cell International Inc, Oldsmar, Florida

The author has disclosed no conflicts of interest.

about the same time, Molloy described the collection of UCB at the time of delivery, and, in 1990, Brossard et al discussed the collection of UCB for possible hematopoietic reconstitution.[9,10] In the latter study, 158 donors were assessed to determine that cord blood could be collected safely with no adverse effects for the baby or mother.

Collection Methods Refined

A number of technical improvements have been attempted in the collection process over the years. For example, a closed collection system was developed to replace the original open collection system. The benefits of a closed system include less risk of microbial contamination and improved recovery of nucleated cells (NCs), especially HPCs.

In the early 1990s, several groups attempted to modify the existing collection techniques by performing a two-phase collection to optimize the volume and cell recovery of UCB. After the in-utero collection, multiple needle aspirations from the umbilical cord were performed to supplement the UCB volume.[11] Another modification combined in-utero with subsequent ex-utero collection following placental perfusion with an isotonic solution. This perfusion rinsed the residual UCB from the placental vessels and increased the total cell yield.[12] Both of these procedures were labor intensive compared to a one-step UCB collection. Similar modified techniques of UCB collection were assessed by other groups, but none were adopted for routine UCB collection. Although these protocols often demonstrated an increase in the total nucleated cell (TNC) content, they also increased the risk of bacterial contamination from the additional manipulations.

In 2007, Skoric and colleagues evaluated two in-utero collection methods.[13] The first was a syringe and flush ("syringe") method, and the second used the standard collection bag ("standard"). The syringe method resulted in a significantly higher volume, TNC number, and mononuclear cell (MNC) count, as shown in Table 24-1.[13]

In another report, the Madrid Cord Blood Bank, when using the standard method, reported a mean NC count of 1.00×10^9, with only 25% of the units reaching the target goal of 20×10^6 cells per kg of bodyweight in patients who weighed 50 to 70 kg.[14] To improve the yield, the authors performed a second collection after placental perfusion with 50 mL of heparinized 0.9% saline. The collections were combined, with the second fraction representing 32% of the total volume and 15% of the TNC count. The combined collections contained a mean volume of 123.7 ±50.1 mL and a TNC of 1.26 ±0.52 $\times 10^9$, with the composition of both fractions being similar. The microbial contamination rate of 2.8% was considered acceptable by the authors.

In another study, three different collection methods were analyzed. Participants in this study included 75 women who gave birth by vaginal delivery. One method used a standard blood collection bag (method 1), whereas the other two methods aspirated the UCB with syringes. The first syringe collection (method 2) was followed by a saline flush through the umbilical arteries in an open system. The second syringe method (method 3) collected UCB into a standard donation bag. Method 1 resulted in an average collection of 76.4 mL and a mean TNC count of 0.835×10^9. Method 2 yielded 174.4 mL and a TNC count of 1.62×10^9, and Method 3 yielded 173.7 mL and a TNC count of 1.69×10^9. The collection volume correlated with placental weight but not with the baby's weight or gestational age or the age of the mother. Because microbial contamination was significantly higher in method 2, the authors concluded that method 3 was optimal. These studies demonstrated that with increased collection efficiency it is possible to harvest sufficient UCB doses for adult transplantation.[15]

Table 24-1. Umbilical Cord Blood in-Utero Collection Methods

Method	N	Volume (mL)	TNCs ($\times 10^9$)	MNCs ($\times 10^8$)	Discard Rate (%)
Syringe	49	103 ±35.4	1.23 ±5.27	5.95 ±3.47	14
Standard	50	86 ±29.3	0.99 ±4.47	4.24 ±2.82	36

TNCs = total nucleated cells; MNCs = mononuclear cells.

Comparing Cord Blood Collection Methods

In-Utero Collection

A study by Surbek et al that assessed the characteristics of in-utero vs ex-utero UCB collections demonstrated significant superiority of products collected by the in-utero method in a number of categories, as shown in Tables 24-2 and 24-3. The study results agreed with other reports of the advantages of in-utero collection.[16]

Solves et al studied differences between in-utero and ex-utero UCB collections obtained from 569 vaginal deliveries and 70 cesarean section births. Rates of discard were 33% for vaginal ex-utero, 25% for vaginal in-utero, and 46% for cesarean deliveries. Volume, NC count, percentage of CD34+ cells, and colony-forming units (CFUs) were higher for vaginal deliveries where UCB was harvested in utero. There were no differences between ex-utero collections from cesarean and vaginal deliveries.[17]

In a study of 848 vaginal collections, 484 in utero and 364 ex utero, there was a significant difference in volume, TNCs, CD34+ stem cells, and CFUs.[18] The lower yields from the ex-utero collections resulted in a higher exclusion rate of 33%, compared to 25% from in-utero collections, which led to the authors' conclusion that in-utero collections were more efficient.

Wall et al assessed the feasibility of in-utero cord blood collections performed by the obstetrician after birth.[19] The study of 200 cord blood collections in about 40 different facilities demonstrated that collections performed in utero by a health-care professional compared favorably with those collected ex utero by trained staff.

In 1998, Surbek et al analyzed methods of optimizing the collection yield and were able to demonstrate that UCB collection is affected by the birth weight of the baby, the placental weight, the timing of collection after the birth of the baby, and the location of the cord clamping.[20] The study evaluated UCB collection before and after placental delivery in a prospective randomized study of vaginal births. The study variables were standardized to include double clamping of the cord and the transection of the cord within 30 seconds. For the ex-utero collection, the placenta was held, and the same decontamination and venipuncture were performed as for the in-utero collection. As shown in Table 24-2, in-utero collection yielded a greater mean volume and total MNC count than the ex-vivo method, even when the product volume and cell count were normalized for the weight of the baby.

In 2001, Wong and colleagues compared in-utero and ex-utero UCB collection and determined

Table 24-2. Comparisons of In-Utero and Ex-Utero Umbilical Cord Blood Collections for Volume and Total Nucleated Cell Content

Author	N (in utero or ex utero)	Volume (mL)			TNCs ($\times 10^8$)		
		In Utero	Ex Utero	p Value	In Utero	Ex Utero	p Value
Surbek[16]	21/19*	93 ±7.5	66 ±6.6	0.013	11.1 ±1.2	7.4 ±0.8	0.026
Solves[17]	264/309	108.8 ±28.6	98 ±28.5	<0.05	10.5 ±4.2	8.6 ±3.5	<0.05
Solves[17]	70*	NA	102.5 ±21.6	NA	NA	8.3 ±2.9	NA
Solves[18]	484/364	107.21 ±51.47	98.5 ±28.5	<0.05	10.34 ±3.83	8.56 ±3.54	<0.05
Wall[19]	293/41	81 (40-170)	75 (41-140)	NS	11.7 ±4.8	10.4 ±5.0	NS
Surbek[20]	23/19	83.3 ±7.9	48.4 ±4	0.0007	3.13 ±0.55	1.81 ±0.3	0.04
Pafumi[22]	21/26*	90.7 ±6	60.9 ±13.7	<0.05	10.1 ±1.2	7.1 ±0.8	<0.05

*Cesarean delivery.
TNCs = total nucleated cells; NA = not applicable; NS = not statistically significant.

Table 24-3. Comparisons of In-Utero and Ex-Utero Umbilical Cord Blood Collections for CD34 Content, CFU Capacity, and the Discard Rate

Author	N (in utero or ex utero)	CD34+ Cells (×10⁵)			CFUs (per 10,000 cells)			Discard Rate (%)		
		In Utero	Ex Utero	p Value	In Utero	Ex Utero	p Value	In Utero	Ex Utero	p Value
Surbek[16]	21/19*	30 ±6	17.4 ±2.4	NS	NR	NR	NA	NR	NR	NA
Solves[17]	264/309	36.5 ±33.8	29.6 ±22.5	NS	154 ±142	121 ±114	<0.05	25	33	<0.05
Solves[17]	70*	NA	30.8 ±19.7	NA	NA	153 ±153	NA	NA	46	NA
Solves[18]	484/364	35.3 ±29	30 ±22.4	<0.05	168 ±158	123 ±114	<0.05	25	33	<0.05
Wall[19]	293/41	NR	NR	NA	9.8 ±5.2	16.6 ±13	0.001	50	NR	NA
Pafumi[22]	21/26*	20 ±6.0	16.4 ±2.4	NR	NR	NR	NA	NR	NR	NA

*Cesarean delivery.
CFU = colony-forming unit; NS = not statistically significant; NR = not reported; NA = not applicable.

that TNCs and CFUs were significantly lower when the UCB was harvested ex utero.[21] Their cell analysis revealed a reduction in granulocytes, monocytes, and B cells in the ex-utero collections. There was also a significantly higher incidence of macroscopic clots in UCB collected ex utero (31% vs 1%).

Pafumi and others studied collections before and after placental uterine detachment in 47 women delivered by cesarean section.[22] This group also demonstrated higher collection numbers with the in-utero method than with the ex-utero technique, as shown in Table 24-2.

Collection Methods in Vaginal and Cesarean Section Deliveries

Sparrow et al investigated the role of the mode of birth on the yield of in-utero vs ex-utero UCB collection.[23] The UCB volume collected after 61 cesarean section procedures (76 mL) was significantly higher than the median volume from 157 vaginal deliveries (63 mL). However, the UCB from the vaginal deliveries had a significantly higher median TNC count (17.9×10^8) than cesarean section deliveries, which had a median TNC count of 13.6×10^8. Two other studies of in-utero and ex-utero collections from cesarean section deliveries did not show any significant differences in UCB collected by either method.[24,25]

A study was performed to compare UCB recovered from cesarean delivery with UCB collected after vaginal birth.[26] The mean volume from the cesarean deliveries (n = 29) was 103.9 ±33.6 mL, compared to 84.2 ±25.3 mL from the vaginal deliveries (n = 126). The percentage of CD34+ cells was similar, but, because of the higher volume collected, absolute numbers of CD34+ and nucleated cells were higher in the UCB obtained after cesarean section.

The Effect of Newborn Positioning

UCB collected after 51 vaginal deliveries was analyzed to determine whether the positioning of the newborn during the collection affected some properties of the UCB.[27] Upper and lower positions were assessed in 51 vaginal deliveries. Neonates were placed either on the maternal abdomen ("upper" position) or on the table ("lower" position) immediately after birth. Cord blood volume and total CD34+ cells collected from the babies in the upper position were significantly higher than those from the babies in the lower position. The neonatal hemoglobin levels and white cell (WBC) counts were monitored to confirm that the infants suffered no side effects from either position. The data demonstrated that placement of the newborn on the abdomen of the mother directly after birth appears to yield a larger UCB collection.

Standardization of UCB Collection

In 1996, the National Heart, Lung, and Institute (NHLBI) commissioned the Cord Blood Transplantation (COBLT) study to develop and perform standardized procedures for donor recruitment, UCB banking, and UCB transplantation as well as to build an ethnically diverse UCB product inventory.[28] From a total of 34,799 potential donors screened, 17,207 UCB units were collected, and 11,077 (64%) of the collected units were processed and stored. Of the processed units, 79% (approximately 50% of the total collections) met all eligibility requirements, were HLA typed, and were placed in the search registry. Collections were all performed ex utero, and those from cesarean sections yielded a higher volume and TNC count than those from vaginal deliveries. Products collected from African American donors contained fewer TNCs than UCB from other ethnicities. UCB volume and cell content correlated with birth weight. The study demonstrated that standardized procedures and data collection could be successfully implemented in a group of CBBs.

Microbial Contamination: In Utero vs Ex Utero

Although it is critically important to collect UCB units with the greatest possible volume and cell numbers, it is also important that the collected products be free of microbial contamination. A study that compared contamination rates of in-utero and ex-utero UCB collections showed that, although there was no difference between the methods in volume, TNC count, colony-forming units—granulocyte-macrophage (CFUs-GM), and CD34+ cells collected, the rate of bacterial contamination was higher for the in-utero collections.[29]

The introduction of a closed collection system significantly decreased the rate of microbial contamination from 12.5% to 3.3% in one report.[30]

Armitage et al analyzed the first 1000 ex-utero collections for the London Cord Blood Bank and found that, over time, the level of microbial contamination was reduced from 28% to 4% by using a bag collection method in which the cord was decontaminated with alcohol and chlorhexidine before puncture.[31]

Other Factors That Affect UCB Collection Quality

Many studies have demonstrated that certain variables have an effect on the number and type of cells collected from the umbilical cord at birth. For example, in a study of the collection and isolation of HPCs from UCB, Thierry et al were able to demonstrate that the number of HPCs in a UCB collection was inversely proportional to the time between conception and delivery (32 to 42 weeks).[32] Furthermore, HPCs derived from UCB appear to have higher proliferative potential than those derived from adult marrow, as demonstrated by a higher CFU-to-cell ratio in the UCB product.[33]

Cord blood bankers have evaluated variables in the collection process and have not always agreed on whether, or to what degree, different collection factors can affect the quality of the UCB product. In one study, UCB volume and MNC count correlated well with the delivery type, placental weight, neonatal bodyweight, and duration of pregnancy.[34] In addition, the UCB CD34+ cell count correlated with the MNC, while the tumor necrosis factor alpha (TNF-α) concentration demonstrated a negative correlation with the MNC, CFU-GM, and interleukin-1 beta (IL-1β) concentrations. Another group assessed cord blood variables in 190 UCB units that were harvested in utero from vaginal and cesarean deliveries and found that the TNC count was significantly increased in vaginal deliveries, in women over 25 years of age, in women with one or two parities, and from babies heavier than 3100 g.[35]

In a study of variables that affect ex-utero UCB collections, 2084 units were analyzed for placental weight and the presence of meconium in the amniotic fluid.[36] The mean volume of the units was 85.2 mL, with a TNC count of 1.19×10^9 and a CD34+ cell count of 5.2×10^6. In an assessment of collection variables, a placental weight of more than 500 g and meconium noted in the amniotic fluid correlated with a higher volume and a greater TNC and CD34+ cell count. This group noted that specimens collected after 40 weeks of gestation contained a greater volume and a higher TNC count. Other variables that were noted to produce higher collection yields were cesarean section, two trained collectors, and completion of the collection within 5 minutes. Another analysis of 300 UCB collections determined that larger babies produced a larger volume of UCB, resulting in a higher TNC count, higher CFU capacity, and higher CD34+ cell counts.[37] Some data even show that HPC and CFU concentrations correlate with the sex of the baby, with UCB from male infants containing significantly higher CD34+ cell counts than UCB from females.[38]

It seems intuitive that infant weight would have an effect on the amount of UCB available for harvest, and indeed this was shown to be true in a study of 304 UCB collections.[39] The authors showed by multivariate analysis that infant weight was a significant factor associated with UCB volume, TNC count, CD34+ cell count, and CFU-GM content. They also showed a relationship between higher collection parameters and such obstetric factors as placental weight, gestational age, cesarean delivery, and cord length.

Techniques to Improve Cord Blood Collection

Public CBBs assess the efficiency of their collection process by measuring the rates at which collected units do not meet acceptance criteria and are therefore excluded from banking. One method used by some European CBBs to reduce the number of unacceptable collections is to perform a precollection assessment of the placenta. This practice has lowered discard rates to 18% in one public CBB and to 29% in another.[40,41]

In a 1999 study similar to the study by Pafumi et al, neonates were assessed for their position after birth in relation to the cell content of the cord blood. Again it was clear that volume and cell numbers obtained with the baby placed on the mother's abdomen after delivery and before the cord was clamped were significantly higher than from UCB obtained from the baby in the lower position, with no significant difference in hemoglobin levels.[42] Another factor that can reduce the number of unacceptable units collected is the recording and evaluation of a maternal health history before delivery. In one study, more than 20% of collected UCB units were discarded largely because of the maternal health history.[43]

Summary

A great deal has been learned about UCB collection since the first collections and assessments were performed. Collection methods have evolved over time toward a safer product and a higher yield. Although two-phase collection methods were attempted and frequently demonstrated higher cell recoveries, the processes were complicated and labor intensive and often resulted in an increased level of bacterial contamination. The many reports of superior yields with in-utero UCB collection were countered with reports of increased microbial contamination and labeling errors. Comparisons may be difficult because of differences in standard operating procedures, levels of compliance, training models, and the environment in which the product is collected. The use of syringes for UCB collection has certain advantages but adds another step to the collection process because the UCB must be transferred to a receptacle. The introduction of closed collection systems along with rigorous training have probably had the greatest effect in reducing UCB contamination during collection.

Because parameters such as viability and TNC, MNC, CD34+, and CFU content can be analyzed by using different techniques and protocols, products from different CBBs may seem less similar than they really are. Results of a TNC count might be different when performed by an automated hematology analyzer rather than manually with a microscope and hemacytometer. The CD34+ cell analysis may be performed by single- or dual-platform flow cytometry and may evaluate only viable cells or include nonviable cells. The MNC count may depend on the judgment of the technologist who is performing the manual differential. On the other hand, an automated instrument may perform an inaccurate differential because the algorithm being used is based on normal peripheral blood (PB) morphology. Viability may appear higher when evaluated by a manual trypan blue assay than by flow cytometry and a fluorescent stain. Therefore, it is important to validate a new process or assay before making changes to a method.

Regulatory agencies and accrediting organizations have issued regulations and standards to guide cord blood banks in collecting safe and effective UCB products. Part 1271 of Title 21 of the US

Code of Federal Regulations (CFR) contains requirements for all manufacturers of human cells, tissues, and cellular and tissue-based products to register with the Food and Drug Administration, to determine donor eligibility, and to develop good tissue practices to prevent the introduction, transmission, and spread of communicable diseases. Public CBBs are also subject to current good manufacturing practices, as described in 21 CFR, Parts 210 and 211, and to the General Biological Products Standards (21 CFR, Part 610). Groups such as AABB and the Foundation for the Accreditation of Cellular Therapy/NetCord have published standards and perform assessments for organizations that wish to apply for accreditation by these bodies.

Cord blood collection plays an important role in providing a valuable cell source from a material that was once considered a biological waste product. The uses for these UCB cells beyond hematopoietic reconstitution are just now starting to be recognized, especially in the field of regenerative medicine. Optimizing the process for harvesting the most and best cells during the collection process continues to be the goal of many innovators in the UCB field.

References/Resources

1. Gluckman E, Broxmeyer HA, Auerbach AD, et al. Hematopoietic reconstitution in a patient with Fanconi's anemia by means of umbilical-cord blood from an HLA-identical sibling. N Engl J Med 1989;321:1174-8.
2. Rocha V, Wagner JE Jr, Sobocinski KA, et al. Graft-versus-host disease in children who have received a cord-blood or bone marrow transplant from an HLA-identical sibling. Eurocord and International Bone Marrow Transplant Registry Working Committee on Alternative Donor and Stem Cell Sources. N Engl J Med 2000;342:1846-54.
3. Schreier K, Stieg H. Amino acid content of umbilical cord blood. Z Kinderheilkd 1950;68:563-6.
4. Gaehtgens G. Hematology of the umbilical cord blood. Arch Gynakol 1950;178:211-2.
5. Halbrecht I, Brzoza H. Evaluation of hepatic function in newborn infants by means of chemical study of cord blood. Am J Dis Child 1950;79:988-95.
6. Barr M. A cord-blood survey of diphtheria immunity; comparison of 2 populations. Lancet 1950;24:1110-12.
7. Paxson CL. Collection and use of autologous fetal blood. Am J Obstet Gynecol 1979;134:708-10.
8. Polin JI, Knox I, Baumgart S, et al. Use of umbilical cord blood culture for detection of neonatal bacteremia. Obstet Gynecol 1981;57:233-7.
9. Molloy P. Collection of umbilical cord blood specimens at the time of delivery. Midwives Chron 1982;95:205.
10. Brossard Y, Van Nifterik J, De Lachaux V, et al. Collection of placental blood with a view to hemopoietic reconstitution. Nouv Rev Fr Hematol 1990;32:427-9.
11. Broxmeyer HE, Kurtzberg J, Gluckman E, et al. Umbilical cord blood hematopoietic stem and repopulating cells in human clinical transplantation. Blood Cells 1991;17:313-29.
12. Turner CW, Luzins J, Hutcheson C. A modified harvest technique for cord blood hematopoietic stem cells. Bone Marrow Transplant 1992;10:89-91.
13. Skoric D, Balint B, Petakov M, et al. Collection strategies and cryopreservation of umbilical cord blood. Transfus Med 2007;17:107-13.
14. Bornstein R, Flores AI, Montalban MA, et al. A modified cord blood collection method achieves sufficient cell levels for transplantation in most adult patients. Stem Cells 2005;23:324-34.
15. Elchalal U, Fasouliotis SJ, Shtockheim D, et al. Postpartum umbilical cord blood collection for transplantation: A comparison of three methods. Am J Obstet Gynecol 2000;182:227-32.
16. Surbek DV, Visca E, Steinmann C, et al. Umbilical cord blood collection before placental delivery during cesarean delivery increases cord blood volume and nucleated cell number available for transplantation. Am J Obstet Gynecol 2000;183:218-21.
17. Solves P, Moraga R, Saucedo E, et al. Comparison between two strategies for umbilical cord blood collection. Bone Marrow Transplant 2003;31:269-73.
18. Solves P, Mirabet V, Larrea L, et al. Comparison between two cord blood collection strategies. Acta Obstet Gynecol Scand 2003;82:439-42.
19. Wall DA, Noffsinger JM, Muecki KA, et al. Feasibility of an obstetrician-based cord blood collection network for unrelated donor umbilical cord blood banking. J Matern Fetal Med 1997;6:320-3.
20. Surbek DV, Schonfeld B, Tichelli A, et al. Optimizing cord blood mononuclear cell yield: A randomized comparison of collection before vs. after placenta delivery. Bone Marrow Transplant 1998;22:311-12.
21. Wong A, Yuen PM, Li K, et al. Cord blood collection before and after placental delivery: Levels of nucleated cells, haematopoietic progenitor cells, leukocyte subpopulations, and macroscopic clots. Bone Marrow Transplant 2001;27:133-8.
22. Pafumi C, Farina M, Bandiera S, et al. Differences in umbilical cord blood units collected during cesarean section, before or after the delivery of the placenta. Gynecol Obstet Invest 2002;54:73-7.
23. Sparrow RL, Cauchi JA, Ramadi LT, et al. Influence of mode of birth and collection on WBC yields of umbilical cord blood units. Transfusion 2002;42:210-15.
24. Solves P, Fillol M, Lopez M, et al. Mode of collection does not influence haematopoietic content of umbilical cord blood units from caesarean deliveries. Gynecol Obstet Invest 2006;61:34-9.

25. Tamburini A, Malerba C, Mancinelli F, et al. Evaluation of biological features of cord blood units collected with different methods after cesarean section. Transplant Proc 2006;38:1171-3.

26. Yamada T, Okamoto Y, Kasamatsu H, et al. Factors affecting the volume of umbilical cord blood collections. Acta Obstet Gynecol Sand 2000;79:830-3.

27. Pafumi C, Zizza G, Russo A, et al. Placing the newborn on the maternal abdomen increases the volume of umbilical cord blood collected. Clin Lab Haematol 2001; 23:397-9.

28. Kurtzberg J, Cairo MS, Fraser JK, et al. Results of the cord blood transplantation (COBLT) study unrelated donor banking program. Transfusion 2005;45:842-55.

29. Lasky LC, Lane TA, Miller JP, et al. In utero or ex utero cord blood collection: Which is better? Transfusion 2002; 42:1261-7.

30. Bertolini F, Lazzari L, Lauri E, et al. Comparative study of different procedures for the collection and banking of umbilical cord blood. J Hematother 1995;4:29-36.

31. Armitage S, Warwick R, Fehily D, et al. Cord blood banking in London: The first 1000 collections. Bone Marrow Transplant 1999;24:139-45.

32. Thierry D, Hervatin F, Traineau R, et al. Hematopoietic progenitor cells in cord blood. Bone Marrow Transplant 1992;9(Suppl 1):101-4.

33. Hows JM, Marsh JC, Bradley BA, et al. Human cord blood: A source of transplantable stem cells? Bone Marrow Transplant 1992;9(Suppl):105-8.

34. Szotomicka-Kurzawa P. Improved method for delivery room collection and storage of human cord blood cells for grafting. Ann Acad Med Stetin 2001;47:107-24.

35. Mohyeddin Bonab MA, Alimoghaddam KA, Goliaei ZA, et al. Which factors can affect cord blood variables? Transfusion 2004;44:690-3.

36. Askari S, Miller J, Chrysler G, McCullough J. Impact of donor- and collection-related variables on product quality in ex utero cord blood banking. Transfusion 2005;45: 189-94.

37. Solves P, Perales A, Moraga R, et al. Maternal, neonatal and collection factors influencing the haematopoietic content of cord blood units. Acta Haematol 2005;113: 241-6.

38. Aroviita P, Teramo K, Hiilesmaa V, Kekomaki R. Cord blood hematopoietic progenitor cell concentration and infant sex. Transfusion 2005;45:613-21.

39. Mancinelli F, Tamburini A, Spagnoli A, et al. Optimizing umbilical cord blood collection: Impact of obstetric factors versus quality of cord blood units. Transplant Proc 2006;38:1174-6.

40. Richter E, Eichler H, Leveringhaus A, et al. The Mannheim cord blood projection (abstract). Bone Marrow Transplant 1998;21(Suppl):522.

41. Bries G, Uttebroek A, Spitz B, et al. The Leuven cord blood banking project: Logistics and results (abstract). 3rd Eurocord Transplant Concerted Action Workshop, Annecy, France, 1998.

42. Grisaru D, Deutsch V, Pick M, et al. Placing the newborn on the maternal abdomen after delivery increases the volume and CD34 cell content in the umbilical cord blood collected: An old maneuver with new applications. Am J Obstet Gynecol 1999;180:1240-3.

43. Tamburini A, Malerba C, Picardi A, et al. Placental/ umbilical cord blood: Experience of St. Eugenio Hospital collection center. Transplant Proc 2005;37:2670-2.

Method 24-1. Collecting Cord Blood In Utero

Description

This standard operating procedure describes the in-utero collection of umbilical cord blood (UCB) and is applicable to both vaginal and cesarean section (C-section) delivery. UCB can be used as a source of hematopoietic stem cells and progenitor cells as well as other nonhematopoietic cells. The UCB is collected after the umbilical cord is clamped immediately after birth. The UCB is derived from the placenta as well as from the umbilical cord and is drawn from the umbilical vein. The collection volume generally ranges from 40 to 150 mL. UCB is harvested into an anticoagulant, usually citrate-phosphate-dextrose (CPD), but occasionally another anticoagulant such as heparin may be used.

Note: Maternal blood for infectious disease marker testing is collected within 7 days of the UCB harvest. The mother is tested as a surrogate for the UCB donor. Tests include those for human immunodeficiency virus (HIV), hepatitis B virus (HBV), hepatitis C virus (HCV), human T-cell lymphotropic virus (HTLV), syphilis, and cytomegalovirus (CMV). Labels in the collection kit are included for the tubes of maternal blood and require the date and time of collection as well as the collector's identification. The maternal and family health history is usually collected before the harvest at the time that consent is obtained for the collection, laboratory testing, and product storage. Labeling of all tubes and bags must comply with applicable regulations and standards.

Time for the Procedure

After supplies are set up, the actual collection of blood usually takes less than 15 minutes.

Summary of the Procedure

1. The umbilical cord is clamped.

2. After delivery of the baby, the umbilical cord is decontaminated with a combination of alcohol and iodine.
3. The needle, connected to a collection bag, is inserted into the umbilical vein, and the blood is drained from the vessel by gravity.
4. Once the collection is complete, the bag of cells is sealed and inverted gently with the anticoagulant to prevent clots.
5. After appropriate labeling and packaging, the UCB product is transported to the processing facility for cell processing and cryopreservation.

Equipment

Not applicable.

Supplies and Reagents

1. 250-mL sterile blood collection set with a 16-gauge, 1.5-inch sterile needle and 35 mL of CPD anticoagulant.
2. Sterile C-section adapter kit (for C-section collections only).
3. Iodine swabs.
4. Alcohol wipes.
5. Needle guard.
6. Plastic protective biohazard bag.
7. Absorbent towels.
8. Blue plastic placental basin.
9. Donor labels with barcodes.
10. Cord blood collection form.

Safety

Use the appropriate barrier and personal protective measures when handling UCB products. Handle all blood and tissue products as if they are capable of transmitting an infectious disease.

Procedure

A. *Vaginal Birth Procedure*

1. Confirm that all items needed for the collection are at the site for use.
2. Don gloves and appropriate attire before the UCB collection.
3. After delivery of the baby and before expulsion of the placenta, cleanse approximately 4 to 6 inches of the umbilical cord with the alcohol wipe and then with a tincture of iodine on a swab.
   a. Use a circular motion, starting at the center of the needle insertion site and moving to the periphery of the area.
   b. Wait 30 seconds to allow the area to dry after each alcohol and iodine wipe.
   c. For maximum volume, the needle insertion site should be directly above the clamp that remains on the cord.
   d. If the area is touched after it has been cleaned, it must be cleaned again with new alcohol and iodine swabs.
4. Remove the protective needle cap and cannulate the umbilical vein with the needle at the prepared site (bevel side facing away). Hold the needle in place until the collection is complete.
5. Allow as much UCB as possible to flow into the bag.
6. Check the bag and tubing periodically to confirm that the UCB is flowing.
7. If the umbilical vein collapses, an additional insertion site should be located further up the cord. Cleanse each site with alcohol and tincture of iodine, waiting 30 seconds for each application to dry.
8. When the collection is completed, strip the UCB in the tubing into the bag to mix with the anticoagulant.
9. Withdraw the needle from the cord and slide the needle guard over the exposed needle until it locks in place to safely discard it after removal.
10. At this point, the tubing may be clamped with a hemostat directly below the needle.
11. Seal or tie a tight knot in the tubing near the needle and directly below the hemostat.
12. Cut off the protected needle and discard it in the appropriate container.
13. Leaving at least 6 inches between the bag and the first seal or knot, seal the collection tubing twice more or tie at least two more secure knots in the tubing to prevent leakage during shipping.
14. Gently invert the bag several times to thoroughly mix the UCB and anticoagulant.
15. Confirm that all the needles are removed before shipment.
16. The bar-coded label must be completed with the appropriate donor identification as well as the date and time of the collection and the collector's identification.
    Note: Donor information will vary with the type of donation, public or private.
17. Confirm the identity of the UCB product with the collection form in the kit.
18. To prepare the product for shipment, wrap the UCB in the absorbent towels included in the kit and place it in the large zipper-top biohazard bag. Place the packaged UCB in the blue bin and seal and secure the bin with tape in the shipment box.
19. The product must be transported at room temperature to the processing facility so that processing can be performed within 48 hours of collection.

B. *C-Section Birth Procedure*

1. Confirm that all items needed for collection are at the site for use.
2. Don gloves and appropriate attire before the UCB collection.
3. Using sterile technique, allow only the C-section adapter kit with extension to be opened and placed on a sterile field, allowing the tubing to drape off the sterile field.
4. Insert the collection bag needle into the female adapter of the extension set.
5. With the needle guard in place, connect the UCB collection bag to the sterile C-section extension tubing outside the sterile field. This can be accomplished with assistance from the operating room circulator or by keeping the collection bag lower or off the sterile field.
6. Deliver the infant according to standard practice, double-clamping the cord after delivery.

7. After delivery of the baby and before expulsion of the placenta, cleanse approximately 4 to 6 inches of the umbilical cord with the alcohol wipe and then with a tincture of iodine on a swab.

   a. Use a circular motion starting at the center of the needle insertion site and moving to the periphery of the area.

   b. Wait 30 seconds to the allow area to dry after each alcohol and iodine wipe.

   c. For maximum volume, the needle insertion site should be directly above the clamp that remains on the cord.

   d. If the area is touched after it has been cleaned, it must be cleaned again with new alcohol and iodine swabs.

8. Remove the protective needle cap, and cannulate the umbilical vein by using the C-section extension set needle to initiate the collection (bevel side facing away). For maximum volume, the needle insertion site should be just above the clamp that remains on the cord.

9. Continue with steps 6-19 of the vaginal birth procedure.

Method 24-2. Collecting Cord Blood Ex Utero

Description

This standard operating procedure describes the ex-utero collection of umbilical cord blood (UCB) and is applicable to both vaginal and cesarean section (C-section) delivery. UCB can be used as a source of hematopoietic stem cells and progenitor cells as well as other nonhematopoietic cells. The UCB is collected after the umbilical cord is clamped immediately after birth. The UCB is derived from the placenta as well as from the umbilical cord and is drawn from the umbilical vein. The collection volume generally ranges from 40 to 150 mL. UCB is harvested into an anticoagulant, usually citrate-phosphate-dextrose (CPD), but occasionally another anticoagulant such as heparin may be used.

Note: Maternal blood for infectious disease marker testing is collected within 7 days of the UCB harvest. The mother is tested as a surrogate for the UCB donor. Tests include those for human immunodeficiency virus (HIV), hepatitis B virus (HBV), hepatitis C virus (HCV), human T-cell lymphotropic virus (HTLV), syphilis, and cytomegalovirus (CMV). Labels in the collection kit are included for the tubes of maternal blood and require the date and time of the collection as well as the collector's identification. The maternal and family health history is usually completed before the collection, at the time consent is obtained for the collection, laboratory testing, and product storage. Labeling of all tubes and bags must comply with applicable regulations and standards.

Time for Procedure

After supplies are set up, the actual collection of blood usually takes less than 15 minutes.

Summary of Procedure

1. The umbilical cord is clamped, and after placental delivery the organ is moved to an area outside the delivery suite for collection.

2. After the placenta is detached, it is elevated to facilitate the collection.
3. The umbilical cord is decontaminated with a combination of alcohol and iodine.
4. The needle, connected to a collection bag, is inserted into the umbilical vein, and the blood is drained from the vessel by gravity.
5. Once the collection is complete, the bag of cells is sealed and inverted gently to mix with the anticoagulant.
6. After appropriate labeling and packaging, the UCB product is transported to the processing facility for cell processing and cryopreservation.

Equipment

Collection stand or other elevated surface.

Supplies and Reagents

1. 250-mL blood collection bag containing 35 mL CPD anticoagulant and a 16-gauge, 1.5-inch sterile needle.
2. Iodine swabs.
3. Alcohol wipes.
4. Needle guard
5. Plastic protective biohazard bag.
6. Absorbent towels.
7. Blue plastic placental basin.
8. Donor labels with barcodes.
9. Cord blood collection form.
10. Sterile absorbent underpads.

Safety

Use the appropriate barrier and personal protective measures when handling UCB products. Handle all blood and tissue products as if they are capable of transmitting an infectious disease.

Procedure (Vaginal or C-Section Birth Procedure)

1. Confirm that all items for collection are at the site for use.
2. Don gloves and appropriate attire before the UCB collection.
3. After delivery of the baby and expulsion of the placenta, quickly transport the organ to the collection area.
4. The placenta must be elevated above the insertion site in the vein to facilitate the collection. This may be accomplished by using a sterile underpad (Chux) and stand or by placing the placenta on a high table with the fetal side facing down. If using a Chux, a hole or an opening is required for the cord.
5. Once the placenta is in place, cleanse approximately 4 to 6 inches of the umbilical cord with the alcohol wipe and then with a tincture of iodine on a swab.
   a. Use a circular motion, starting at the center of the needle insertion site and moving to the periphery of the area.
   b. Wait 30 seconds to allow the area to dry after each alcohol and iodine wipe.
   c. For maximum volume, the needle insertion site should be directly above the clamp that remains on the cord.
   d. If the area is touched after it has been cleaned, it must be cleaned again with new alcohol and iodine swabs.
6. Remove the protective needle cap, and cannulate the umbilical vein with the needle at the prepared site (bevel side facing away). Hold the needle in place until the collection is complete.
7. Allow as much UCB as possible to flow into the bag.
8. Check the bag and tubing periodically to confirm that the UCB is flowing.
9. If the umbilical vein collapses, an additional insertion site should be located further up the cord. Cleanse each site with alcohol and tincture of iodine, waiting 30 seconds for each application to dry.
10. If required to improve the collection, rotate the placenta, especially if the cord is particularly long. If the flow is extremely slow, another site may be used proximal to the placenta surface to increase the volume yield.
11. When the collection is completed, strip the UCB in the tubing into the bag to mix with the anticoagulant.
12. Withdraw the needle from the cord and slide the needle guard over the exposed needle until it locks in place to safely discard it after removal.
13. At this point, the tubing may be clamped with a hemostat directly below the needle.
14. Seal or tie a tight knot in the tubing near the needle and directly below the hemostat.
15. Cut off the protected needle and discard it in the appropriate container.
16. Leaving at least 6 inches between the bag and the first seal or knot, seal the collection tubing twice more or tie at least two more secure knots in the tubing to prevent leakage during shipping.
17. Gently invert the bag several times to thoroughly mix the UCB and anticoagulant.
18. Confirm that all needles are removed before shipment.
19. The bar-coded label must be completed with the appropriate donor identification as well as the date and time of collection and the collector's identification.

    Note: Donor information will vary with the type of donation, public or private.
20. Confirm the identity of the UCB product with the collection form in the kit.
21. To prepare the product for shipment, wrap the UCB in the absorbent towels included in the kit and place it in the large zipper-top biohazard bag. Place the packaged UCB in the blue bin and seal and secure the bin with tape in the shipment box.
22. The product is transported at room temperature and must arrive at the processing facility so that processing can be performed within 48 hours of collection.

In: Areman EM, Loper K, eds
Cellular Therapy: Principles, Methods, and Regulations
Bethesda, MD: AABB, 2009

♦♦♦   25   ♦♦♦

Assessment of Collection Quality

Grace S. Kao, MD

BECAUSE THERE IS THOUGHT TO BE A threshold dose for hematopoietic progenitor cells (HPCs) above which rapid hematopoietic reconstitution occurs, it is important to appropriately assess the quality and projected effectiveness of an HPC graft as early in the manufacturing process as possible. Hematopoietic grafts were originally evaluated solely on the basis of the total nucleated cells (TNCs) collected and infused per kg of recipient bodyweight, and it was believed that fewer cells were needed per kg in autologous transplantation than in allogeneic. However, the TNC count is only a surrogate for counting those cells that actually reconstitute hematopoiesis, and much effort has been expended to define a more appropriate measure of graft potential. Until recently, the most commonly used assay for the reconstituting ability of an HPC graft was the growth of the day-14 colony-forming unit—granulocyte macrophage (CFU-GM) in a semisolid culture. Estimates of threshold effective doses of CFU-GM differ widely but have been reported to be in the range of 0.1 to 1×10^4/kg for marrow. Because the colonies have not developed enough to be counted until 10 to 14

days after a harvest, real-time evaluation of a graft using this technique is not possible.

With the discovery of monoclonal antibodies specific for antigens on HPCs, many centers now enumerate and evaluate cellular therapy (CT) products by flow cytometry that uses antibodies against CD34 and other HPC cell-surface markers. Although technical problems with rare event analysis by flow cytometry originally made it difficult to compare results among centers, a standardized method for CD34 analysis was recently developed and is now commercially available. Because of this standardization, it has been possible for the field to agree on a dose of approximately 2.0×10^6 CD34+ cells/kg as clinically acceptable for the transplantation of HPCs from apheresis (HPC-A), with engraftment reliably occurring within 14 to 21 days of infusion without growth factor support.

Finally, microbiological evaluation of a graft for contamination resulting from the collection or processing procedures may be performed. Although grafts with positive microbial cultures have been infused without apparent adverse effects in the recipients, the US Food and Drug Administration

Grace S. Kao, MD, Assistant Medical Director, Cell Manipulation, Dana-Farber Cancer Center, and Instructor, Department of Pathology, Harvard Medical School, Boston, Massachusetts

The author has disclosed no conflicts of interest.

(FDA) does not permit distribution of these products [Code of Federal Regulations (CFR) Title 21, Part 1271.265(c)(2)] and requires that all cell- and tissue-based products be screened in a way that prevents the transmission of communicable diseases.

This chapter briefly discusses the evaluation of cellular products immediately after collection. Detailed methods for assessing products at all stages of production are described in Section VII.

Donor Issues

Cellular Therapy Sources

During the past decade, HPC transplants have become the standard of care for patients with certain hematological malignancies. The use of HPC sources for transplantation has evolved from marrow to cytokine-mobilized HPC-A and umbilical cord blood (UCB) cells. Moreover, there is growing evidence to support the use of lymphocytes or blood-derived cellular vaccines for the treatment of viral diseases and malignancies.[1] However, marrow, HPC-A, and UCB continue to dominate the CT field, even with the surge of interest in tissue engineering and regenerative medicine. Cell collection or procurement is the first step in CT product manufacturing. The quality of the starting product can greatly affect the subsequent cell-processing procedures and, likely, the clinical outcome of patients who receive the final CT product.

Because of their heterogeneous sources, the standardization of starting materials for CT products is difficult to achieve. The quality of the initial cell product is affected by the characteristics of the donor as well as by the quality of the collection technique. Initial donor assessment and donor testing can provide information to assist physicians in choosing the most appropriate donor and time for CT product collection. Therefore, quality control of the collection procedure and quality assessment of the collected product should be designed to reduce donor and recipient complications as well as to improve donor satisfaction and recipient clinical outcome.

Prevention of Infectious Disease Transmission

Proper donor evaluation by a careful review of donor health history and physical examination is critical for ensuring appropriate clinical care of the donor during the collection process and for preventing the transmission of infectious disease to the recipient and cell processing personnel. Since 2005, allogeneic donors and their cellular products have been evaluated, tested, and labeled according to the FDA current good tissue practice (cGTP) regulations (21 CFR 1271).[2] The primary concerns addressed by these regulations are the prevention of communicable-disease transmission and the assurance of safe processing and handling.

The first step in minimizing the opportunity for microbial contamination during the collection procedure is adherence to proper aseptic collection technique. For whole blood phlebotomy and apheresis collection, techniques described by the standards of professional organizations such as the AABB, the American Society for Apheresis (ASFA), the Foundation for the Accreditation of Cellular Therapy (FACT), and the College of American Pathologists (CAP), or by the National Marrow Donor Program (NMDP), should be followed.[3-5] For tissue or cellular samples taken from surgical sites, guidelines set forth by the American Association of Tissue Banks (AATB) for zone recovery and sequencing techniques are recommended.[6,7] The primary objective of zone recovery is to reduce the potential spread of microorganisms from one region of the body to another by employing isolation techniques and by documenting actions to facilitate suitability determinations from preprocessing culture results. Most important, all collected products should undergo microbial testing.

Quality Assessment of Cellular Products Intended for Hematopoietic Progenitor Cell Transplantation

Minimally manipulated marrow, HPC-A, and UCB are sources of cells that are routinely used to support HPC transplantation. Not surprisingly, the collection volume and cellular content of the products vary greatly depending on the cell source. Optimal products should be free of microbial contamination and contain high numbers of viable HPCs with minimal erythrocyte and granulocyte contamination.

The initial assessment of a CT collection is visual inspection of the product and product labels.

Clumping or noncellular debris observed in the product are early indicators of suboptimal collection or poor product quality. Labels and accompanying documents should be carefully reviewed, and problems should be resolved before the product is accepted for processing or infusion.

As previously noted, numerous studies have indicated that infusion of at least 2×10^6 CD34+ cells/kg recipient weight of allogeneic HPC-A will ensure early hematopoietic recovery after myeloablative therapy.[8-11] Enumeration of CD34+ cells by flow cytometric analysis is now routinely performed as a measure of HPC content because of its rapid turnaround time and proven correlation with posttransplant hematologic recovery.[12] Functional assays such as colony-forming unit (CFU) and long-term, culture-initiating cell (LTC-IC) assays can also measure the proliferative potential of collected cells. Although the results of these assays often correlate with posttransplantation hematopoietic recovery, their usefulness is limited by significant intra- and interlaboratory variability.

New tests have been developed to assess the content and quality of HPCs in CT products. For example, assays that measure intracellular aldehyde dehydrogenase (ALDH) activity and adenosine triphosphate (ATP) bioluminescence can be used to assess both the viability and the presence of early progenitor cells in the product.

Cell viability is essential to the integrity of the CT product, although viability assays can present both technical and scientific challenges. Trypan blue, a vital dye, is used routinely to distinguish dead from living cells. The trypan blue chromophore is negatively charged and does not enter the cell unless the membrane is damaged. Therefore, cells that exclude the dye are considered viable. Unfortunately, this method cannot distinguish the viability of subpopulations of cell types. Flow cytometry, an assay method required by some accrediting organizations, uses a fluorescent compound such as 7-amino-actinomycin D (7-AAD) for cell viability assessment.[12,13] The compound is excluded by viable cells but can penetrate the cell membrane of dying or dead cells and intercalates with double-stranded DNA. In flow-cytometry-based CT product analysis, this compound can be used in conjunction with other fluorescent cell markers to facilitate accurate documentation of cell viability within specific cell populations such as CD34+ cells.

Marrow

Large volumes of marrow are routinely harvested from autologous and allogeneic donors to support transplantation, as discussed previously in this section. The aspiration procedure uses sterile technique and multiple needle punctures through the posterior iliac crests, but contamination of the product by microbial skin flora can occur.

It has been estimated that the collection of approximately 10 to 15 mL of marrow/kg of recipient bodyweight should be adequate to support transplantation, provided that the donor has adequate marrow reserve.[14] The peripheral blood (PB) cell counts of the donor are highly predictive of the cellular yield of the product. The hematocrit of marrow products typically ranges from 20% to 35%, which is 10% to 20% below the donors' predonation PB hematocrit. The leukocyte concentration of the harvested marrow usually ranges from twofold to sixfold higher than the PB leukocyte concentration, and granulocytes and lymphocytes are the predominant cell types. However, the leukocyte yields tend to be lower for autologous donors with hematologic malignancies. Similarly, the CD34+ HPC yields are higher in healthy donor marrow products. Up to 2% of leukocytes collected in marrow products are CD34+ cells, a percentage that is approximately 1 log lower than the percentage in apheresis products from cytokine-stimulated (mobilized) allogeneic donors.

HPCs from Apheresis

At this time, mobilized HPC-A is the most commonly used HPC product for both autologous and allogeneic transplantation in adult patients because of the ease of collection and the ample number of CD34+ cells obtained.

Published reports that describe the correlation of the precollection, PB, circulating CD34+ cell count with the HPC yield have encouraged many centers to use this parameter to predict the collection efficiency of the HPC-A procedure.[15-17] Physicians may choose to postpone the procedure of a donor who does not demonstrate circulating CD34+ cells on the day of collection because the yield is expected to be poor. Furthermore, there is evidence to support the use of the PB CD34+ cell count before initiation of apheresis to optimize the planning and quality control of the collection.[18]

The measurement of collection efficiency is probably the most important quality indicator of the apheresis procedure. The apheresis collection efficiency for any cell type is calculated by dividing the number of cells in the apheresis component by the number of cells processed during the apheresis procedure. This latter number is estimated by multiplying the volume of PB processed by the average of the PB cell counts at the start and at the completion of the procedure. This formula, however, implies a steady-state presence of cells of interest in circulation. It has been noted that the concentration of some cell populations (eg, CD34) may vary at different times during the collection.[19] Documentation of collection efficiency should be part of the quality assurance program of any apheresis center to improve collection protocols and to identify substandard equipment and operators.

Optimizing the CD34+ cell collection efficiency of each apheresis procedure is especially important for patients who do not have high circulating PB CD34+ cell counts or for donors who may need to undergo multiple days of collection. Some studies have suggested that the apheresis procedure itself may mobilize CD34+ cells from marrow to blood circulation, and large-blood volume apheresis may be beneficial because it reduces the total number of collections needed to achieve a transplantable cell dose.[20-22] Midcollection PB CD34+ cell counts have also been used to predict the appropriate length of a collection procedure, minimizing unnecessarily extended collections.[23]

The leukocyte content of HPC-A is about two-fold higher than the leukocyte content of unstimulated blood and tenfold higher than that of marrow products. These white cells are primarily lymphocytes (40%-50%) and granulocytes (30%-50%), with a significant left shift and high concentration of immature cells. Therefore, a manual differential count may be more reliable than an automated differential count for HPC-A characterization. The CD34+ cell concentration of an HPC-A product stimulated by granulocyte colony-stimulating factor (G-CSF) is usually ten- to twenty-fold higher than that of a marrow product and forty- to fifty-fold higher than that of an unstimulated PB apheresis product. The erythrocyte contamination as measured by hematocrit is typically <5%, and products with higher hematocrit are generally considered to be of poorer quality. When a higher concentration of red cells occurs, the collection procedure, equipment, and venous access should be evaluated.

Umbilical Cord Blood

The use of UCB for transplantation has increased greatly in recent years because it has been shown to be a safe and effective alternative source of transplantable HPCs. The major limitation for its use in adult patients is the comparatively low cell dose. In unrelated UCB transplants, a dose greater than 3.7 $\times 10^7$/kg of infused cells usually predicts a higher probability of myeloid engraftment.[24] Therefore, optimizing collection methods to achieve a high cell dose for banking is essential.

As discussed in Chapter 24, the collection strategy is the first step in improving the quality of UCB units. Two main techniques are currently used for collecting UCB from the umbilical vein: 1) in the delivery room while the placenta is still in the uterus, by midwives and obstetricians, and 2) outside the delivery room after placental delivery, by trained technicians. Both methods produce comparable TNC and CD34+ cell counts, and CFU-GM numbers, but bacterial contamination, low volume, and clotting may be higher with in-utero collection.[25,26]

An estimate from a study in the United States suggests that approximately 30% of collected UCB products are finally accepted into inventory. The major reasons for discarding collected products are low volume, donor deferrals, and low cell counts.[27] Many banks use a minimum volume limit as the first-level selection criterion for processing because of the positive correlation between volume and cell yield. Discarding low-volume products before processing reduces the number of processed units that are disqualified for use, which results in reduced costs and improved efficiency. Maternal and neonatal factors appear to affect CB cell yield. Full-term pregnancies, primigravida, and mothers of European ethnicity who have placental weights of >500 g appear to be the donor characteristics most likely to provide large-volume products with high cell yield.[28,29] Nonetheless, strong consideration is given to HLA diversity, which is more likely to be found among ethnic and racial minorities.

Quality Assessment of Cellular Products Intended for Other Uses

Cell-Based Therapeutic Vaccines and Adoptive Immunotherapy

With advances in molecular technology, better understanding of human immunology, and increased interest in regenerative medicine, the use of CT products is no longer limited to transplantation. Applications of CT have expanded to include adoptive immunotherapy and therapeutic cancer vaccines. The most common cell sources for these therapies are PB cells collected by apheresis or simple phlebotomy. Concentrated PB mononuclear cells (PBMC) collected by apheresis are currently the preferred source for adoptive immunotherapy. Cell-based adoptive im-munotherapy involves the use of allogeneic donor or autologous recipient lymphocytes (T cells) to mount an immune reaction against malignant or virally infected cells. Allogeneic T cells from the original HPC donor are sometimes administered as a donor lymphocyte infusion (DLI) to treat patients with relapsed hematologic disease after transplantation. Patients with cancer and human immunodeficiency virus (HIV) who have damaged cellular immunity can donate their own blood for the generation of cancer or viral-antigen-specific, cytotoxic T lymphocytes (CTLs) to help the immune system fight the disease. PB has also been used to generate potent antigen-presenting cells (APCs) or dendritic cells (DCs) to stimulate in-vivo T cells in a disease-specific manner.[30]

The quality assessment of apheresis products intended for immunotherapy focuses on the collection efficiency of target cells. As a result, flow cytometry is often used to characterize subsets of immune cells in addition to routine cell counts and cell viability. For products intended for adoptive immunotherapy, lymphocytes such as CD3+, CD4+, CD8+, and CD20+ cells are routinely analyzed. Depending on the type of DCs to be generated from PB, monocytes (CD14+ cells) or CD34+ cells in the collection may also be assessed.[31,32] PB apheresis products are less cellular than cytokine-mobilized HPC-A but, like those products, should have a hematocrit of <5%. High granulocyte, erythrocyte, and platelet contamination in an apheresis product may indicate a problem with the collection procedure.

Tissue-Based Cellular Therapies

When tissue or a tumor is recovered for extraction of tumor-infiltrating lymphocytes, tissue engineering, or tumor vaccine production, procedures to prevent contamination and cross-contamination of tissue samples at recovery are crucial. Preprocessing microbial culture results should be available for review within a reasonable amount of time after recovery. Knowledge of a donor's preprocessing culture results could affect the suitability determination for the product. Statistical trends of contaminated collections should be tracked to modify tissue recovery procedures and to identify common sources of infection.

Nonhematopoietic Stem Cell Therapies

Interest in the application of CT for tissue regeneration has surged in the past few years because of encouraging preclinical data and human studies that have used autologous marrow cells to treat patients with myocardial infarction.[33] Nonhematopoietic tissue-committed stem cells (TCSCs) are believed to be present in the marrow and can potentially facilitate tissue regeneration. These nonhematopoietic TCSCs may be enriched within CD34+ and CD133+ cell populations, and it is thought that the clinical effect seen in some myocardial infarction studies may be the result of the promotion of angiogenesis by TCSCs present in the marrow.[34] Therefore, HPC-A and UCB, both enriched in CD34+ cells, are also good sources of TCSCs. Experiments have shown that mesenchymal stromal cells (MSCs) can be generated and expanded from marrow cells and that these MSCs can give rise to mesodermal tissue types, including bone, cartilage, tendon, muscle, and fat. With expanded use of cell-based therapy, quality assessment of procurement procedures and collected products will play an important role in supporting the future of CT.

References/Resources

1. June CH. Adoptive T cell therapy for cancer in the clinic. J Clin Invest 2007;117:1466-76.

2. Food and Drug Administration. Current good tissue practice for human cell, tissue, and cellular and tissue-based product establishments; inspection and enforcement; final rule. (November 24, 2004) Fed Regist 2004; 69:68611-88.

3. Goldman M, Roy G, Frechette N, et al. Evaluation of donor skin disinfection methods. Transfusion 1997;37: 309-12.

4. Sataro P. Blood collection. In: Kasprisin CA, Laird-Fryer B, eds. Blood donor collection practices. Bethesda, MD: AABB, 1993:83-104.

5. Smith L. Blood collection. In: Green TS, Steckler D, eds. Donor room policies and procedures. Arlington, VA: AABB, 1985:25-46.

6. Standards for tissue banking. 12th ed. McLean, VA: American Association of Tissue Banks, 2008.

7. Prevention of contamination and cross-contamination at recovery: Practices and culture results. (AATB guidance document). Version 2 (May 29, 2007). McLean, VA: American Association of Tissue Banks, 2007.

8. Mavroudis D, Read E, Cottler-Fox M, et al. CD34+ cell dose predicts survival, posttransplant morbidity, and rate of hematologic recovery after allogeneic marrow transplants for hematologic malignancies. Blood 1996; 88:3223-9.

9. Haas R, Witt B, Mohle R, et al. Sustained long-term hematopoiesis after myeloablative therapy with peripheral blood progenitor cell support. Blood 1995;85:3754-61.

10. Ketterer N, Salles G, Raba M, et al. High CD34(+) cell counts decrease hematologic toxicity of autologous peripheral blood progenitor cell transplantation. Blood 1998;91:3148-55.

11. Kiss JE, Rybka WB, Winkelstein A, et al. Relationship of CD34+ cell dose to early and late hematopoiesis following autologous peripheral blood stem cell transplantation. Bone Marrow Transplant 1997;19:303-10.

12. Allan DS, Keeney M, Howson-Jan K, et al. Number of viable CD34(+) cells reinfused predicts engraftment in autologous hematopoietic stem cell transplantation. Bone Marrow Transplant 2002;29:967-72.

13. Xiao M, Dooley DC. Assessment of cell viability and apoptosis in human umbilical cord blood following storage. J Hematother Stem Cell Res 2003;12:115-22.

14. Buckner CD, Clift RA, Sanders JE, et al. Marrow harvesting from normal donors. Blood 1984;64:630-4.

15. Rowley SD, Prather K, Bui KT, et al. Collection of peripheral blood progenitor cells with an automated leukapheresis system. Transfusion 1999;39:1200-6.

16. Benjamin RJ, Linsley L, Fountain D, et al. Preapheresis peripheral blood CD34+ mononuclear cell counts as predictors of progenitor cell yield. Transfusion 1997;37: 79-85.

17. Diaz MA, Garcia-Sanchez F, Lillo R, et al. Large-volume leukapheresis in pediatric patients: Pre-apheresis peripheral blood CD34+ cell count predicts progenitor cell yield. Haematologica 1999;84:32-5.

18. Yu J, Leisenring W, Bensinger WI, et al. The predictive value of white cell or CD34+ cell count in the peripheral blood for timing apheresis and maximizing yield. Transfusion 1999;39:442-50.

19. Ford CD, Greenwood J, Strupp A, Lehman CM. Change in CD34+ cell concentration during peripheral blood progenitor cell collection: Effects on collection efficiency and efficacy. Transfusion 2002;42:904-11.

20. Humpe A, Riggert J, Munzel U, et al. A prospective, randomized, sequential, crossover trial of large-volume versus normal-volume leukapheresis procedures: Effect on progenitor cells and engraftment. Transfusion 1999;39: 1120-7.

21. Abrahamsen JF, Stamnesfet S, Liseth K, et al. Large-volume leukapheresis yields more viable CD34+ cells and colony-forming units than normal-volume leukapheresis, especially in patients who mobilize low numbers of CD34+ cells. Transfusion 2005;45:248-53.

22. Fontana S, Groebli R, Leibundgut K, et al. Progenitor cell recruitment during individualized high-flow, very-large-volume apheresis for autologous transplantation improves collection efficiency. Transfusion 2006;46:1408-16.

23. Sidhu RS, Orsini E Jr, Giller R, et al. Midpoint CD34 measurement as a predictor of PBPC product yield in pediatric patients undergoing high-dose chemotherapy. J Clin Apher 2006;21:165-8.

24. Locatelli F, Rocha V, Chastang C, et al. Factors associated with outcome after cord blood transplantation in children with acute leukemia. Blood 1999;93:3662-71.

25. Askari S, Miller J, Chrysler G, McCullough J. Impact of donor- and collection-related variables on product quality in ex utero cord blood banking. Transfusion 2005;45: 189-94.

26. Solves P, Moraga R, Saucedo E, et al. Comparison between two strategies for umbilical cord blood collection. Bone Marrow Transplant 2003;31:269-73.

27. Lecchi L, Ratti I, Lazzari L, et al. Reasons for discard of umbilical cord blood units before cryopreservation. Transfusion 2000;40:122-3.

28. Mancinelli F, Tamburini A, Spagnoli A, et al. Optimizing umbilical cord blood collection: Impact of obstetric factors versus quality of cord blood units. Transplantation Proc 2006;38:1174-6.

29. Nakagawa R, Watanabe T, Kawano Y, et al. Analysis of maternal and neonatal factors that influence the nucleated and CD34+ cell yield for cord blood banking. Transfusion 2004;44:262-7.

30. Gilboa E. DC-based cancer vaccines. J Clin Invest 2007; 117:1195-203.

31. Glaser A, Zingsem J, Zimmermann R, et al. Collection of mononuclear cells in the Spectra for the generation of dendritic cells. Transfusion 1999;39:661-2.

32. Strasser EF, Berger TG, Weisbach V, et al. Comparison of two apheresis systems for the collection of CD14+ cells intended to be used in dendritic cell culture. Transfusion 2003;43:1309-16.

33. Orlic D, Kajstura J, Chimenti S, et al. Bone marrow cells regenerate infarcted myocardium. Nature 2001;410:701-5.

34. Stamm C, Westphal B, Kleine HD, et al. Autologous bone-marrow stem-cell transplantation for myocardial regeneration. Lancet 2003;361:45-6.

Appendix 25-1. Examples of Quality Characteristics (ie, Acceptance Criteria) of Cellular Therapy Products after Collection*

Characteristic	HPC-M	HPC-A	HPC-C	TC-A
TNC	See comment[†]	See comment[†]	>60 to 100 × 10⁷	See comment[†]
MNC content (%)	As measured	>60	As measured	>80
Viability (%)	>70	>90	>70	>90
Expiration time	24 hours	48 hours	48 hours	48 hours
Bacterial cultures[‡]	No growth	No growth	No growth	No growth
Fungal cultures[‡]	No growth	No growth	No growth	No growth
Potency assays				
Cellular content	Yes	No	Yes	Yes
CD34	No	Yes	Yes	No
CD3	No	No/Yes	No	Yes
CD14	No	No	No	Yes (TC-DC)
CD56	No	No	No	Yes (TC-NK)
CFU-GM	Yes/No	No	Yes	No

*The acceptable content of cells will vary widely according to the weight of the recipient and the expected level of postcollection manipulation.
[†]The acceptance criteria for this product depend on the desired function of the final CT product.
[‡]Microbial contamination needs to be assessed. The culture results are usually not available at the time of distribution from the collection facility to the processing facility.
HPC = hematopoietic progenitor cell; HPC-M = HPCs from marrow; HPC-A = HPCs from apheresis; HPC-C = HPCs from cord blood; TC-A = therapeutic cells from apheresis; TNC = total nucleated cell(s); MNC = mononuclear cell; DC = dendritic cell; NK = natural killer; CFU-GM = colony-forming unit—granulocyte-macrophage.

Production: Basic Processing

THIS SECTION FOCUSES ON THE BASIC procedures and applications involved in manufacturing clinical scale cellular therapy (CT) products for administration to human recipients. It begins with a brief discussion of issues to consider when working with CT products and describes some of the basic procedures performed in CT facilities. These procedures represent the more common applications in CT processing and manufacturing. All methods are presented as examples only, and they are not intended to substitute for appropriate procedure development and validation, as described in previous sections.

For the sake of brevity and consistency, details of aseptic processing steps (such as sanitizing work surfaces and cleaning injection sites) have been omitted from the methods presented in Sections VI and VII. It is expected that CT manufacturing facility personnel are trained in and adhere to strict aseptic processes and procedures at all times. Proper protective attire should always be worn and equipment manufacturers' instructions followed.

Lot numbers of critical supplies, reagents, and equipment, as well as identification of personnel performing the procedures, should be documented and the results recorded concurrently with the activities. These issues are discussed extensively in other sections.

Although the responsibility of the CT manufacturing facility for the CT product does not begin until after the source material is collected or recovered, effective communication between the collection facility and the clinical program can help identify mutual goals and resolve specific issues facing the processing facility. The final manufactured products should be available in a volume that is tolerable to the recipient and should contain concentrations of anticoagulant, cryoprotectant, or other additives that are also tolerable. The goal of the manufacturer or processing facility should be to provide a product of the highest possible quality. At a minimum, such a product must meet all specifications for safety, purity, and potency.

Section Editors: Melissa Croskell, MT(ASCP), Manager of Regulatory Compliance, Department of Pathology and Laboratory Services, and BMT Program Quality Manager, The Children's Hospital–Aurora, Aurora, Colorado; Kathy Loper, MHS, MT(ASCP), Director, Cellular Therapies, AABB, Bethesda, Maryland; and David H. McKenna, Jr, MD, Scientific and Medical Director, Molecular and Cellular Therapeutics, University of Minnesota, St Paul, Minnesota

M. Croskell and K. Loper have disclosed no conflicts of interest. D. McKenna has disclosed a financial relationship with BioE, Inc.

Product Handling

As discussed in an earlier section, best practices [eg, current good manufacturing practice (cGMP) and/or current good tissue practice (cGTP)] should be followed during CT product manufacturing. A controlled environment is essential for compliance with applicable regulations and standards. Work surfaces should be clean and uncluttered, allowing for safe and efficient manufacturing operations. Products should be handled individually to prevent contamination or mix-up. When available, closed systems should be employed. However, if use of an open system is necessary, care should be taken when sampling or introducing materials into the product. All supplies should be sterile and appropriate for their intended uses, and a system should be in place for tracking supplies. Reagents used during processing should be qualified and released for use. Ideally, a sterile connection device is used for attaching transfer bags during processing. If a sterile connection device is not available, care should be taken during the spiking procedure to reduce the potential for contamination. All ports or other sampling devices in use should be cleaned. To the extent possible, open manipulation should occur in a classified environment, such as a biological safety cabinet (BSC).

Collection Issues

Each CT source material presents a unique processing profile. Marrow collections are generally of a large volume, often over 1000 mL, and contain bone spicules, fat, clots, and anticoagulant(s). In-line serial filtration (larger pore to smaller pore) during marrow harvest keeps most bone spicules and other debris out of the CT product. If intraharvest filtration is not performed or if additional filtration is necessary before the product can be issued or processed, the marrow can be passed through a standard blood filter (170-260 micron). Fat content can be reduced by sedimentation, plasma removal, or washing of the marrow product. Washing may also be performed to reduce the anticoagulant concentration if the level is considered unacceptably high for infusion, as may be the case in some pediatric settings. A significant presence of red cells may pose a challenge in the setting of major ABO incompatibility.

The red cell and plasma content of CT products collected by apheresis may be altered to some degree by adjusting apheresis parameters during collection. Additional plasma may be collected during the procedure for use in subsequent manufacturing or storage procedures. If there is a major ABO incompatibility between donor and recipient, maintaining a low hematocrit during collection is desirable.

For umbilical cord blood (UCB) products, the issue of major or minor ABO incompatibility is of less consequence than it is with marrow because most UCB products are depleted of both plasma and red cells during processing. UCB units are unique among hematopoietic progenitor cell (HPC) transplant products because they are not collected and processed for a particular recipient, but they are "banked" and, therefore, may be identified and secured in a shorter time than other sources of HPCs.

Variables Affecting Product Manufacturing

When selecting basic processing methods, various parameters such as volume, cellular content, and ABO compatibility must be considered by the clinical program and the processing facility. Collection additives or cryoprotectants may need to be removed or diluted before infusion, depending on the clinical condition of the recipient. Such factors as patient age, weight, and renal function should be evaluated to determine the criteria and manufacturing procedures for the final product.

Processing Endpoints

For HPC products, cell dose is critical to engraftment and patient outcome.[1-3] Therefore, processing decisions should be made on the basis of factors such as cell dose [nucleated cell (NC) and/or CD34+ cell dose] in the starting material, expected cell loss from processing, and expected final NC and/or CD34+ cell dose. Sometimes these factors may dictate an alternate course of action or a modification of plans for processing.

Blood Group Compatibility

Incompatibility of ABO blood groups between donor and recipient may affect the type of processing required for an HPC product. In the case of a minor ABO incompatibility, the CT facility must consider the presence of donor alloantibodies (agglutinins) in the administered CT product against red cells in the recipient's circulation. For example, plasma contained in a CT product from a group O donor contains A, B, and A,B antibodies able to react with antigens on the red cells of a recipient who is either group A, B, or AB.[4] Plasma depletion techniques can significantly reduce the level of donor alloantibodies in the product at the time of infusion. Some laboratories determine the antibody titer when evaluating this potential reactivity—a step that gives them additional information for their decision process. With a major ABO incompatibility, where the recipient has circulating alloantibodies to antigens on the donor's red cells, a red cell depletion procedure is generally performed. Red cell depletion can be accomplished by several methods, discussed in detail later in this section, that do not significantly reduce the progenitor cell dose in the product.

In addition to ABO blood groups, there are other red cell antigens against which a donor or recipient may possess circulating alloantibodies. These antibodies are quite rare because they are almost always generated as an immune response, whereas the ABO agglutinins are naturally occurring. Although the blunted immune system of a transplant patient may reduce the potential for a significant antibody/antigen interaction, the possibility of a serious reaction should be weighed, especially in the setting of a preformed antibody with a current positive antibody screen.

Product Volume

When preparing a product for immediate infusion, the total amount of anticoagulant and product volume can be easily decreased by reducing the amount of plasma in the product. Reducing the overall volume may result in a product more easily tolerated by a pediatric or small adult patient and will decrease infusion time. As described in other sections of this text, the collection process for marrow, and occasionally apheresis, may result in a level of anticoagulant that could alter the coagulation status of the patient (particularly, smaller patients) upon infusion. Basic processing steps, such as plasma depletion and/or product washing, address some of these patient safety concerns.

Manipulation for Cryopreservation

The final product volume may be manipulated to achieve a specific cell dose in each cryopreservation container, if desired. Discussion of the primary manipulations, red cell and plasma depletion and nucleated cell enrichment, follows. The total volume of dimethyl sulfoxide (DMSO) and/or anticoagulant concentration should be taken into consideration, along with patient and treatment protocols, before freezing the cells. No standard expiration dating period has been established for cryopreserved HPC products, and each program should establish its own stability program and expiration dates. The principles and processes of cryopreservation are discussed later in this section.

DMSO

For products cryopreserved with DMSO, some transplantation programs limit the total DMSO infusion volume to 10 mL/kg/day.[5] When a treatment requires a large volume of frozen products, this limitation may require infusions to be split over several hours to limit DMSO toxicity. This is often the case for those patients treated with autologous HPCs from apheresis (HPC-A) who mobilize poorly and require a greater number of apheresis collections than do adequate mobilizers. When infusing cryopreserved cells, many pediatric programs have found that limiting the DMSO dose to <1g/24 hours reduces adverse reactions associated with DMSO infusion. Pharmacokinetic studies of DMSO have been described as linear in various animal studies, but such studies are limited in humans. Reactions possibly caused by DMSO include hypo- or hypertension, anaphylactic reactions, heart and respiratory failure, and, most commonly, nausea. DMSO can also be reduced by washing or diluting the thawed product before infusion. Reports of varied recovery endpoints illuminate the need for a comprehensive validation before implementing a wash procedure in the laboratory.[6,7]

References/Resources

1. Mavroudis D, Read E, Cottler-Fox M, et al. CD34+ cell dose predicts survival, post transplant morbidity, and rate of hematologic recovery after allogeneic marrow transplants for hematologic malignancies. Blood 1996; 88:3223-9.
2. Bittencourt H, Rocha V, Chevret S, et al. Association of CD34 cell dose with hematopoietic recovery, infections, and other outcomes after HLA-identical sibling bone marrow transplantation. Blood 2002;99:2726-33.
3. Dragani A, Angelini A, Iacone A, et al. Comparison of five methods for concentrating progenitor cells in human marrow transplantation. Blut 1990;60:278-81.
4. Roback JD, Combs MR, Grossman BJ, Hillyer CD, eds. Technical manual. 16th ed. Bethesda, MD: AABB, 2008.
5. Johns Hopkins Hospital, Custer JW, Rau RE, Lee CK. The Harriet Lane handbook. 18th ed. Philadelphia: Elsevier Mosby, 2008.
6. Laroche V, McKenna DH, Moroff G, et al. Cell loss and recovery in umbilical cord blood processing: A comparison of postthaw and postwash samples. Transfusion 2005;45:1909-16.
7. Porter DL, Collins RH Jr, Shpilberg O, et al. Long term follow-up of patients who achieved complete remission after donor leukocyte infusions. Biol Blood Marrow Transplant 1999;5:253-61.

In: Areman EM, Loper K, eds
Cellular Therapy: Principles, Methods, and Regulations
Bethesda, MD: AABB, 2009

♦♦♦   26   ♦♦♦

Basic Cellular Therapy Manufacturing Procedures

Melissa Croskell, MT(ASCP); Kathy Loper, MHS, MT(ASCP); and David H. McKenna, Jr, MD

WHEN EVALUATING AND PERFORMING any procedure, maintenance of a therapeutic dose (eg, nucleated cell and/or CD34+ cell dose) must always be the primary consideration. This and the following chapters describe some of the more common processing approaches in the manufacture of cellular therapy (CT) products. These methods are described as basic because of their more common use rather than because of their technical difficulty.

Basic Procedures

Unmanipulated Products

Processing of a fresh product may not be necessary, and aside from removal of samples for quality control testing, the product may be immediately sent to the patient care unit for infusion. The flow chart in Fig 26-1 outlines one possible thought process for an approach to hematopoietic progenitor cell (HPC) processing options.

Plasma Depletion

Some HPC products require plasma depletion to reduce total product volume or to reduce the level of plasma antibodies. This process is frequently required for products for pediatric recipients and/ or products with minor ABO incompatibility. Marrow and HPCs from apheresis (HPC-A) have characteristics similar to whole blood products, so techniques used in blood banking have been adapted for plasma depletion of HPC products. Plasma depletion can be performed using simple centrifugation and plasma expression or by more automated means such as with the COBE 2991 (CaridianBCT, Lakewood, CO; see Fig 26-2).

Melissa Croskell, MT(ASCP), Manager of Regulatory Compliance, Department of Pathology and Laboratory Services, and BMT Program Quality Manager, The Children's Hospital–Aurora, Aurora, Colorado; Kathy Loper, MHS, MT(ASCP), Director, Cellular Therapies, AABB, Bethesda, Maryland; and David H. McKenna, Jr, MD, Scientific and Medical Director, Molecular and Cellular Therapeutics, University of Minnesota, St Paul, Minnesota

M. Croskell and K. Loper have disclosed no conflicts of interest. D. McKenna has disclosed a financial relationship with BioE, Inc.

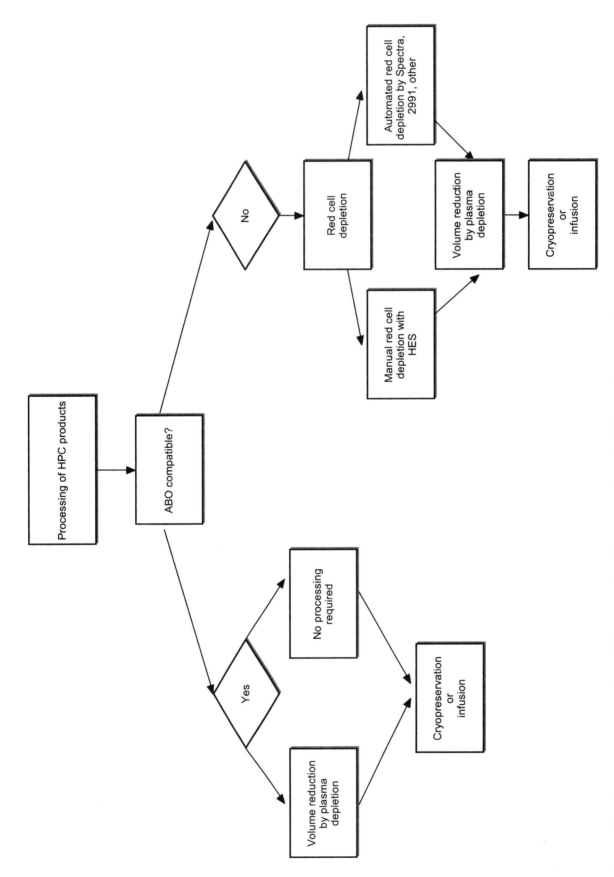

Figure 26-1. Sample processing tree. HPC = hematopoietic progenitor cell; HES = hydroxyethyl starch.

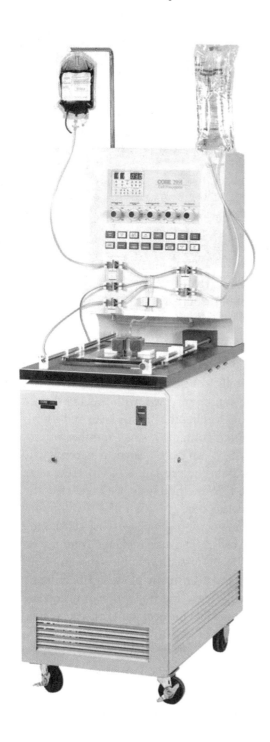

Figure 26-2. COBE 2991 Cell Processor. (Courtesy of CaridianBCT, Lakewood, CO.)

The manual procedure consists of centrifugation of the product, followed by expression of the plasma layer without disturbing the buffy coat or red cell layers, while preferably maintaining a closed system. Although centrifugation using an open system of conical tubes is possible, it is not recommended because of the potential for contamination. Centrifugation rates from 400 to 4000 *g* relative centrifugal force have been reported with similar success.[1]

An automated plasma depletion procedure can be performed with the COBE 2991 as well as with other similar instruments. These systems incorporate centrifugation with or without the addition of an isotonic solution. The volume of plasma removed varies and is often dictated by clinical needs. Some facilities add saline or other validated solutions [eg, Plasma-Lyte A (Baxter Healthcare, Deerfield, IL), human serum albumin] to the final product to adjust the cell concentration as needed. Sample methods for manual and automated plasma depletion are provided at the end of this chapter.

Red Cell Depletion

Centrifugation may also be used to remove mature red cells. In major ABO incompatibilities, recipient antibodies can hemolyze donor red cells in the graft. Therefore, the laboratory may be asked to reduce the red cell volume before transplantation. Unfortunately, the desirable progenitor and stem cell layer sediments very near the undesirable red cell layer when simple centrifugation is performed. If the available cell dose is generous, manual manipulation may be performed using a standard laboratory centrifuge. Basically, stem cell products are centrifuged port side down or inverted (with or without hydroxyethyl starch (HES) to facilitate sedimentation). The bottom red cell layer (closest to the ports) is manually expressed into a syringe or into an attached transfer bag. Because the HPC loss associated with the reduction of red cells in this procedure may be unacceptable, other techniques for reducing the red cell content are often preferred.

Semiautomated Red Cell Depletion

Commercial cell washing devices such as the COBE 2991 may be used for automated or semiautomated red cell depletion. The buffy coat is collected by manipulating a series of clamps and tubing into a collection bag. These procedures are relatively quick to perform and result in recovery of most of the nucleated cells in the product. Unfortunately, the product also contains a high level of red cells and granulocytes. These reduction procedures are most often used as a preparative debulking step for other procedures or in cases where the cell dose is such that no other suitable options exist.

Centrifugation with Hydroxyethyl Starch

The reduction of red cells using sedimentation with HES or sodium carboxymethyl starch has been used in marrow processing and, more recently, by the cord blood community with good nucleated cell recovery. However, when used for larger volume products with the intent of reducing red cells, the procedure becomes more challenging. A realistic and acceptable total nucleated cell (TNC) recovery should be established when validating this procedure in the laboratory. Although many institutions use this process for red cell depletion, there are numerous variations in concentration, timing, centrifugation, and temperature among different facilities.

Basically, HES or a similar compound is added to the CT product at a specific ratio (1:6, 1:8) or at 20% of product volume. The mature red cells will sediment over time (15-120 minutes), leaving a buffy coat layer and a small number of red cells in the plasma suspension. (See Figs 26-3 and 26-4.) Some facilities couple the HES incubation with gentle centrifugation to facilitate the sedimentation. The resulting clear plasma layer can be

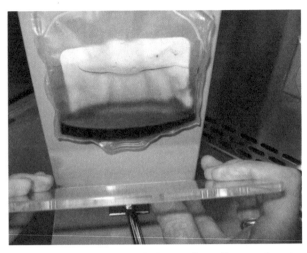

Figure 26-4. Hydroxyethyl starch sedimentation in bag. (Photo courtesy of David Matzilevich, New England Cord Blood Bank.)

expressed, as can the upper buffy coat layer, leaving the red cells to be discarded. Alternatively, the orientation can be reversed, withdrawing the red cells slowly and leaving the plasma layer and a buffy coat layer, which contains a small number of red cells. This process can be repeated, if necessary, to further separate the cell layers. UCB HPC recoveries with the HES method have been reported at 87.5% mononuclear cells (MNCs), 88.4% colony-forming units–granulocyte-macrophage (CFU-GM), and 87.4% CD34+ cells.[2] The use of large volumes of HES should be discussed with the laboratory medical director and transplant physician because it does not rapidly leave the body after infusion and has been responsible for occasional allergic reactions.

Red Cell Depletion by Automated Methods

Red cell depletion for CT products has been automated using devices usually employed for apheresis procedures. Designed for cell separation in a closed system, these instruments use sterile collection kits and a centrifuge to collect, separate, and return cells to the donor. When modified for cellular processing, the devices, programs, and/or processing kits can be used to perform these steps with a CT product, rather than a donor.[3] Instruments from several manufacturers are marketed in the United States, and others are in development.

One such instrument, the COBE Spectra (CaridianBCT; see Fig 26-5), uses a disposable kit to

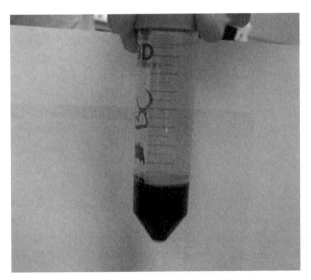

Figure 26-3. Hydroxyethyl starch sedimentation in conical tube. (Photo courtesy of David Matzilevich, New England Cord Blood Bank.)

recoveries are comparable to those of the Spectra, with 87% MNC recovery and 98% red cell reduction.[5] See Method 26-5 for Fenwal CS3000 red cell depletion.

There are some points to consider beyond red cell content when evaluating red cell removal from stem cell products. These platforms are designed to recover primarily an MNC fraction from the nucleated cell population. Because the target cell (ie, CD34+ cell) is in the MNC population, a differential of both the starting and final product is needed to calculate MNC recovery; this parameter is often used as a measure of quality control. Likewise, flow cytometry (CD34+ cell enumeration) may be used to evaluate process efficiency. These assay methods are further discussed in Section VIII.

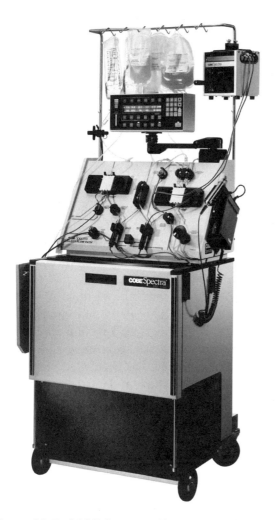

Figure 26-5. COBE Spectra. (Courtesy of Caridian-BCT.)

remove red cells from the marrow product. The disposable kit incorporates a white cell channel through which the HPC product enters and is separated into three layers: the red cells on the outside, the buffy coat of desirable white cells in the middle, and the platelet-rich plasma on the inside. While holding the red cell/plasma interface constant, the white cells are drawn from the channel through the white cell collection tube and transferred to a collection bag. Recoveries of 79% of MNCs and 77% of CD34+ cells have been reported using the Spectra.[4] Marrow grafts of less than 125 mL of red cell volume have reduced separation efficiency. (See Method 26-6.)

Another widely used platform is the Fenwal CS3000 Plus (Fenwal, Lake Zurich, IL; see Fig 26-6), which is a self-contained blood cell separator that uses continuous-flow centrifugation. Cell

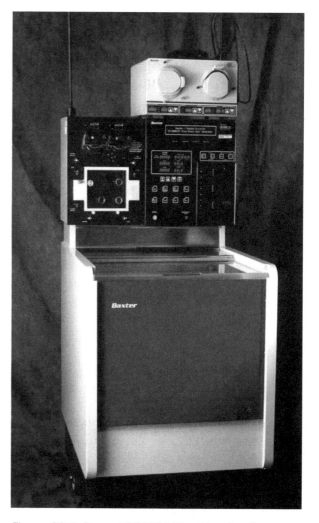

Figure 26-6. Fenwal CS3000 Plus blood cell separator. (Courtesy of Fenwal, Lake Zurich, IL.)

Mononuclear Cell Enrichment

As discussed in Section V (Collection of Cells for Transplantation), collection of a concentrated MNC product may be accomplished with several of the currently available apheresis devices. As previously noted, these devices yield relatively pure MNC products with good CD34 collection efficiency. The procedure is similar to the application for red cell removal; however, the cells are collected directly from the patient/donor. When the operator controls the product collection parameters, one can collect "lighter" when red cell presence is a concern, or "darker" when cell recovery targets are more critical than red cell content. With manual collections, collection efficiency greatly depends on the operator's skill and experience. MNC collections may be mobilized [eg, with granulocyte colony-stimulating factor (G-CSF)] or nonmobilized for production of HPC grafts or for other cellular therapies [eg, donor leukocyte infusion, natural killer (NK) cells, etc].

Cell Enrichment by Density Gradient

For years, cell biologists have used density gradient methods of cell separation and enrichment. Cells separate according to their density, which is relative to that of the density gradient medium. This process is expedited with the addition of centrifugation. A variety of density gradient media can be obtained with various densities or diluted and mixed in the laboratory to obtain the desired density or specific gravity, the most common of which are Ficoll-Hypaque (Ficoll or F/H, GE Healthcare, Chalfont St Giles, United Kingdom; often 1.077 specific gravity) and Percoll (GE Healthcare, Chalfont St Giles, United Kingdom; often 1.130 specific gravity). Ficoll is a high-molecular-weight polymer of sucrose and epichlorohydrin, often combined with Histopaque (Sigma-Aldrich, St Louis MO; a mixture of sodium diatrizoate) to form a discontinuous density gradient. Percoll is a silica colloid solution. However, because none of these media are approved by the FDA for human infusion, the cell isolation step is generally followed with sufficient washing steps to remove any residual density gradient medium. Studies have demonstrated the efficiency of the F/H gradient on a COBE 2991, yielding a highly purified MNC fraction with minimal red cells and neutrophils.[5] Cell recoveries can vary widely, and acceptance criteria should be established and methods validated by each laboratory. None of these media should alter the target cell population during separation. The benefits and risks, including cell loss, should be weighed. (See Method 26-7 for density gradient separation.)

Additional Platforms for Manipulations

Several instruments—such as the COBE 2991, Haemonetics V50 (Haemonetics, Braintree, MA), Fresenius AS104 cell separator (Bad Homburg, Germany), and Baxter Cytomate—have been developed that function well as platforms for plasma depletion and cell washing. Reportedly, these devices have also been used for the processing of products with major ABO incompatibility, volume reduction, and high-volume washing. Additionally, the Cytomate has been used for washing large-volume cell cultures and in regenerative medicine applications.[6] Because some of these devices were designed for other functions, there may be limitations on their efficiencies for CT product manipulations. In the case of procedures that use instruments for applications other than those for which they were developed or approved, it is imperative that the procedures be validated and that acceptable recovery levels be established for each method used.

Donor Lymphocytes for Infusion

Donor lymphocyte infusions (DLIs) are often used as posttransplant immunotherapy for allogeneic HPC transplantations. To induce remission after relapse of leukemia or to prevent recurrence of disease for those patients at high risk for relapse, DLIs are collected from the original stem cell donor, usually by apheresis. Dosage is generally based on lymphocyte content, and CD3+ T cells may be enumerated by flow cytometry. The desired dose (CD3+ cells/kg) is then calculated and aliquotted for infusion after initial testing is performed. Other than occasional volume reduction for smaller recipients, additional processing is not routinely performed. Some centers cryopreserve the leftover material in defined CD3+ doses for subsequent infusion. Another method of recovering donor lymphocytes is to freeze the unselected cells that are left after a CD34+ selection procedure, because most of the residual cells are T lymphocytes. From a processing perspective, it is important to ascertain whether the flow cytometry results are determined based on the total white cell (gate) or total lymphocyte population, because this factor is significant for the calculations and may result in incorrect dosing if the wrong variable is used. Some protocols also involve selecting certain target cell populations and employing novel applications such as CD8+ depletion.

Acknowledgments

Method 26-3 was submitted by Leigh Ann Stamps, MT(AMT), Cell Processing Technologist, Sarah Cannon Blood and Marrow Transplant Program at Centennial Medical Center, Nashville, Tennessee. Method 26-5 was submitted by Lizette Caballero, MT(ASCP), Manager, FHCI Cellular Therapy Laboratory, Florida Hospital, Orlando, Florida. Method 26-7 was submitted by Joy Cruz, CLS, MT(ASCP)SBB, Supervisor, Blood and Marrow Transplant Laboratory, Departments of Pathology and Laboratory Medicine, University of California-San Francisco, San Francisco, California.

References/Resources

1. Rowley SD, Bensinger WI, Gooley TA, et al. Effects of cell concentration on bone marrow and peripheral blood stem cell cryopreservation. Blood 1994;83:2731-6.
2. Regidor C, Posada M, Monteagudo D, et al. Umbilical cord blood banking for unrelated transplantation: Evaluation of cell separation and storage methods. Exp Hematol 1999;27:380-5.
3. Rodriguez JM, Carmona M, Noguerol P, et al. A fully automated method for mononuclear bone marrow cell collection. J Clin Apher 1992;7:101-9.
4. Koristek Z, Mayer J. Bone marrow processing for transplantation using the COBE Spectra cell separator. J Hematother Stem Cell Res 1999;8:443-8.
5. Davis JM, Schepers KF, Eby LL, et al. Comparison of progenitor cell concentration techniques: Continuous flow separation versus density-gradient isolation. J Hematother 1993;2:314-20.
6. Wirk B, Klumpp T, Ulicny J, et al. Lack of effect of donor-recipient Rh mismatch on outcomes after allogeneic hematopoietic stem cell transplantation. Transfusion 2008;48:163-8.

Method 26-1. Reducing Plasma in Marrow and Hematopoietic Progenitor Cells from Apheresis

Description

Hematopoietic progenitor cells (HPCs) are collected by leukapheresis or marrow harvest. The product is centrifuged, and plasma is expressed.

Time for Procedure

One hour.

Summary of Procedure

This procedure describes the steps to reduce the volume of an HPC product. This procedure may be used to process marrow or HPCs from apheresis (HPC-A) to prepare for further processing, cryo-preservation, or infusion.

Equipment

1. Biological safety cabinet (BSC).
2. Centrifuge.
3. Scale.
4. Plasma expressor.
5. Sterile connection device.
6. Tubing sealer.

Supplies and Reagents

1. Sterile syringes: 60 mL, 20 mL, 10 mL, 3 mL, and 1 mL.
2. Sampling-site couplers.
3. Transfer packs: 600 mL, 300 mL, and 150 mL.
4. Plasma transfer set with spike and needle adapter.
5. Assay sample tubes.

Procedure

A. General

All open manipulations of HPC products must be performed using aseptic technique in the BSC.

B. Initial Evaluation

1. Weigh the product and record the weight on the worksheet. Calculate the volume.

2. Place the product in the BSC and remove appropriate samples for product testing and characterization.
3. Before manipulating the product, calculate and record the total nucleated cells (TNCs)/kg and total CD34+ cells/kg of recipient weight.
4. Sufficiently label the bags used during processing to ensure accurate product identification (unique unit number, name of product, patient name, identifiers, and modifiers such as "red cell," "plasma," etc).

C. Processing

1. Using the sterile connection device, attach an appropriately sized and labeled transfer pack to the product bag.
   a. For products >300 mL, use a 600-mL bag.
   b. For products <300 mL, use a 300-mL bag.
2. Drain the product into the transfer pack and heat-seal the tubing.
3. Determine the desired final volume according to protocol and calculations.
4. Centrifuge the product at room temperature at a speed of 1300 to 1800 rpm for 10 minutes.
5. Remove the product from the centrifuge and attach an appropriate transfer pack using the sterile connection device. Estimate the amount of plasma to remove to achieve the desired final product volume.
6. Carefully place the product in the plasma expressor with an attached empty transfer pack on a scale next to the expressor. Do not disrupt the red cell/plasma line.
7. Tare the empty transfer bag.
8. Slowly remove the predetermined volume of plasma.

Note: If the hematocrit of a product is particularly high, it may be difficult to reduce the product to a desired volume. Do not risk losing cells.

9. Clamp and remove the product from the plasma expressor. Heat-seal the tubing between the two transfer packs and disconnect.

10. Weigh the product to determine its volume.

11. Perform quality control testing according to the standard operating procedure (SOP).

Calculations

1. To determine the volume of a product:
   a. Tare the bag and weigh the product.
   b. A 1:1 ratio of mL to grams may be used, such that 53 g = 53 mL of product.

2. Calculate TNCs:
   a. TNCs in product = NC count (usually reported as WBC $\times 10^6$/mL) $\times$ product volume (mL).
   b. TNCs divided by recipient weight (kg) = NCs/kg.

3. If CD34 analysis is performed, calculate total CD34+ cells:
   a. CD34+ cells/mL = absolute CD34+ cells/μL $\times$ 103 μL/mL.
   b. Volume of product (mL) $\times$ CD34 cells/mL = total CD34+ cells.
   c. Total CD34+ cells divided by weight = CD34+/kg.

Anticipated Results

Recovery of TNCs in the final product should be >90% of the starting TNCs in the collected product.

Notes

If the product will be infused after processing, cell concentration may be adjusted by adding sterile infusible saline in place of a portion of plasma removed. For example, if 450 mL of plasma was removed, a transplant center might replace 225 mL of the harvested plasma with 225 mL of sterile saline to facilitate infusion and decrease cell concentration.

Quality control assays such as sterility, CD34 or other flow cytometry markers, ABO typing, etc may be performed on initial, intermediate, and final products as outlined in facility SOPs.

References/Resources

1. Padley D, ed. Standards for cellular therapy product services. 3rd ed. Bethesda, MD: AABB, 2008.

2. Code of federal regulations. Title 21, CFR Part 1271. Human cells, tissues, and cellular and tissue-based products. Washington, DC: US Government Printing Office, 2008 (updated annually).

3. FACT-JACIE international standards for cellular therapy product collection, processing, and administration. 4th ed. Omaha, NE: Foundation for the Accreditation of Cellular Therapy and the Joint Accreditation Committee of ISCT and EBMT, 2008.

Method 26-2. HES Sedimentation for Manual Red Cell Removal

Description

In this procedure, 6% hydroxyethyl starch (HES) is added to the hematopoietic progenitor cell (HPC) product to facilitate manual red cell removal after sedimentation and centrifugation.

Time for Procedure

From 1 to 3 hours.

Summary of Procedure

The hematopoietic progenitor cells from apheresis (HPC-A), marrow, or umbilical cord blood (UCB) product are mixed with HES solution and centrifuged, and the red cells are removed. The product is then available for further processing or infusion.

Equipment

1. Biological safety cabinet (BSC).
2. Tubing sealer.
3. Centrifuge.

Supplies

1. 6% HES.
2. Blood transfer packs: 150 mL, 300 mL, 600 mL.
3. Syringes.
4. Needles or needleless system.
5. Sampling site couplers.

Procedure

A. *Addition of HES*
    (HES should be stored at 2 to 8 C before the anticipated procedure.)
    1. Determine the HPC product volume. Transfer the HPCs into the appropriate size transfer bag. Do not disconnect the original bag.
    2. Add 20% HES by volume through the sampling site coupler into the original product bag.
    3. Rinse the bag thoroughly with HES and add HES rinse to the transferred product.

4. Thoroughly mix the HPC product and HES. Seal and discard the original bag.

B. *Sedimentation*
    1. Place HPC product/HES bag port down in a refrigerated centrifuge at 1 to 6 C for 45 minutes to 2 hours for red cell sedimentation by gravity. (Centrifuge is *off.*)
    2. After completion of RBC sedimentation time, centrifuge product gently for 7 minutes at approximately $50 \times g$ at 1 to 6 C to prepare for red cell removal.

C. *Removal of Red Cells*
    1. Determine the total volume of red cells in the product. Use the total red cell volume and red cell limits to guide red cell removal.
    2. Optionally, allow the bag to hang in the BSC after centrifugation for further separation for 15 to 20 minutes.
    3. Carefully insert a sampling site coupler and slowly remove red cell volume with a syringe.

Calculations

1. Volume of HES added (20%) = Total volume/5
   Example: 106 mL/5 = 21.2 mL
2. Total red cell volume in product:
   Total red cell volume = product volume × hematocrit
   Example: (106 mL × 33%) = 35 mL

Anticipated Results

Recovery of nucleated cells should be >70%.

References/Resources

1. FACT-JACIE international standards for cellular therapy product collection, processing, and administration. 4th ed. Omaha, NE: Foundation for the Accreditation of Cellular Therapy and the Joint Accreditation Committee of ISCT and EBMT, 2008.

2. Code of federal regulations. Title 21, CFR Part 1271. Human cells, tissues, and cellular and tissue-based products. Washington, DC: US Government Printing Office, 2008 (updated annually).

3. Rubinstein P. Processing and cryopreservation of placental/umbilical cord blood for unrelated bone marrow reconstitution. Proc Natl Acad Sci U S A 1995;92:10119-22.

4. Alonso JM. A simple and reliable procedure for cord blood banking, processing, and freezing: St Louis and Ohio Cord Blood Bank experiences. Cytotherapy 2001; 3:429-33.

Method 26-3. Volume Reduction of Peripheral Blood Progenitor Cells for Cryopreservation

Description

This procedure describes the processing of peripheral blood progenitor cells (PBPCs) to reduce volume by manual centrifugation, using blood collection bags.

Time for Procedure

Approximately 1 hour.

Summary of Procedure

The PBPCs are collected by apheresis. The product is centrifuged and plasma is removed for volume reduction before cryopreservation. Samples for quality control testing are removed from the initial product upon receipt and upon completion of centrifugation. The product cell concentration is adjusted to between 20×10^6 and 800×10^6 nucleated cells (NCs) per mL for cryopreservation.

Equipment

1. Biological safety cabinet (BSC).
2. Refrigerator at 2 to 8 C.
3. Refrigerated centrifuge.
4. Plasma expressor.
5. Sterile connection device.
6. Scale.
7. Tubing sealer.

Supplies and Reagents

1. Sterile container.
2. Injection site couplers.
3. Syringes.
4. 18-gauge needles or needleless adapters.
5. Transfer packs.

Procedure

1. Tare the scales for the collection bag. Weigh the collection product and convert grams to milliliters using a 1:1 ratio.

2. Record this on the cell processing worksheet for total nucleated cell (TNC) calculations.
3. Mix the product bag well, including around the edges of the bag.
4. Inside the BSC, aseptically remove the minimum amount of product to perform a preprocessing NC count and other quality control assays.
5. Obtain the NC count on the preprocessing specimen. Using this number and the desired cell concentration, calculate the cell volume to be frozen.
6. Divide the TNC by the desired NC count per mL to calculate the final volume and number of bags needed to freeze the cells for optimal viability.
7. Sterile-connect a properly labeled transfer bag to the product and transfer the product from the collection bag to the transfer bag.
8. Seal tubing and remove original container.
9. Centrifuge the product.
10. Using a sterile connection device, attach a labeled transfer pack to the product.
11. Using the plasma expressor, remove the plasma, making sure to retain the buffy coat layer inside the product bag. Stop expressing approximately one-half inch below the top of the bag.
12. Seal and cut the tubing. Weigh the product again on the scale and calculate the volume as described above.
13. Mix the product bag until the cells appear to be mixed uniformly.
14. Inside the BSC, aseptically remove the minimum amount of product to perform postprocessing quality control assays, including NC count.
15. Obtain the postprocessing TNC and calculate cell recovery.
16. Proceed to the controlled-rate freeze.

Anticipated Results

1. TNC recovery ≥90%.
2. Final NC concentration of 20 to 800×10^6/mL after processing, before addition of cryoprotectant solution.

Notes

1. Lot numbers and expiration dates of all critical supplies and reagents used in the processing procedure should be recorded.
2. Any material containing the patient's stem cells at any time during the processing procedure must have the following attached, at a minimum: the patient's name and identifier and the product's unit number and complete name.
3. The use of all equipment must be appropriately documented.

References/Resources

1. Gorin NC. Cryopreservation and storage of stem cells. In: Areman EM, Deeg HJ, Sacher RA, eds. Bone marrow and stem cell processing: A manual of current techniques. Philadelphia: FA Davis, 1992:130.
2. FACT-JACIE international standards for cellular therapy product collection, processing, and administration. 4th ed. Omaha, NE: Foundation for the Accreditation of Cellular Therapy and the Joint Accreditation Committee of ISCT and EBMT, 2008.
3. Padley D, ed. Standards for cellular therapy product services. 3rd ed. Bethesda, MD: 2008.

Method 26-4. Separating Bone Marrow Buffy Coat Using the COBE 2991

Description

Before processing or infusion, it may be desirable to remove the excess media, plasma, and red cells present in harvested marrow. The COBE 2991 Cell Processor (CaridianBCT, Lakewood, CO) may be used to prepare a buffy coat in a semiautomated procedure.

Time for Procedure

One hour.

Summary of Procedure

Marrow containing at least 125 mL of red cells is harvested into Plasma-Lyte A (Baxter Healthcare, Deerfield, IL) and preservative-free heparin (10 units heparin/mL marrow) containing at least 125 mL of red cells. See calculations section for determining red cell content.

Equipment

1. COBE 2991 Cell Processor.
2. Tubing sealer.
3. Scale.
4. Biological safety cabinet (BSC).
5. Centrifuge.

Supplies and Reagents

1. COBE 2991 processing set.
2. 2000 mL transfer packs.
3. Sampling site couplers.

Procedure

1. Perform daily instrument quality control according to the manufacturer's instructions. Load the COBE 2991 single processing set onto the machine according to manufacturer's instructions.
2. Confirm the following machine settings:
   a. Centrifuge speed: 3000 rpm.
   b. Supernatant out rate: not used.
   c. Minutes agitation time: not used.

d. Supernatant out volume: 600 mL.
   e. Spin time #1: not used.
   f. Spin time #2: not used.
   g. Auto/manual switch: MANUAL.
3. Install the processing set:
   a. Refer to the COBE 2991 Cell Processor operator's handbook.
   b. Using hemostats, clamp all colored lines and close off the main inlet line.
      Note: Valves and red cell sensor are not used for this procedure.
   c. Red line: Attach the marrow product bag.
   d. Blue line: Attach a 2000-mL transfer bag to this line for waste. (The waste bag provided with the processing kit cannot be used for this procedure because it cannot be accessed due to lack of ports.)
   e. Green line: Attach a 300-mL transfer pack for buffy coat collection.
   f. Yellow line: Use for collection of a lipid layer, if needed
   g. Purple line: not used.
   h. Seal the needle adapter line of the transfer pack unit containing the marrow collection. Disconnect excess tubing.
   i. In the BSC, pool the collected marrow into a 2000-mL transfer pack. Aseptically insert a sampling site coupler into a port in the transfer pack and remove samples for quality-control assays.
   j. Weigh the marrow and calculate the volume using a 1:1 ratio to convert grams to milliliters.
4. Connect the marrow to the red line. (Be sure that the inlet line is *not* in the red cell sensor.) Unclamp the red line and allow the marrow to fill the centrifuge bag. Expel the air out of the centrifuge bag into the marrow bag by pressing the START/SPIN button. Repeat this procedure until the centrifuge bag is filled. (It will hold approximately 600 mL of the marrow.) Then reclamp the red line.

5. Press the START/SPIN button and centrifuge the marrow at 3000 rpm for 10 minutes.

6. Unclamp the blue line and press the SUPER OUT button to remove the supernatant plasma. When the buffy coat reaches the inlet line, immediately press the HOLD button and reclamp the blue line. This procedure is done by watching the buffy coat in the centrifuge bag.

7. Unclamp the green line and press the CONTINUE button.

8. If the original volume of the marrow was greater than 600 ml—ie, not all marrow fit into the centrifuge bag—then *collect only approximately 20 mL of buffy coat.* Measure the volume by placing the buffy coat bag onto a tared scale. Press the HOLD button and reclamp the green line, then press the STOP button. Add more marrow by unclamping the red line until the bowl fills.

9. Repeat Steps 4 through 8 until all of the marrow has been processed.

10. If all of the original marrow fit into the bowl initially, then collect the entire visible buffy coat at once. The volume collected should be between 60 and 100 mL. When the buffy coat layer has been collected, press the HOLD button, reclamp the green line, then press the STOP button.

11. Unclamp the red and green lines and allow the marrow in the tubing to flow into the buffy coat collection bag. Reclamp both lines.

12. Carefully seal the green line above the hemostat, and seal the main inlet line on the COBE 2991 processing set. Make double seals before cutting the tubing.

13. Mix the product and remove samples for quality control testing.

Calculations

1. Calculate the percentage of the total nucleated cells (TNCs) recovered. To determine TNC recovery:

Initial nucleated cell count $\times$ initial volume = initial TNC content

Final product nucleated cell count $\times$ final volume = final TNC content

TNC final product / TNC initial $\times 100 = \%$ nucleated cell recovery

2. To determine red cell content in harvested marrow:

Marrow volume $\times$ HCT = red cell volume

Anticipated Results

TNC recovery of at least 70%. If recovery is <70%, it may be necessary to pool plasma/marrow and repeat the process.

Notes

1. The COBE 2991 requires a red cell volume ≥125 mL in the harvested marrow.

2. Because the final product of this procedure contains a significant number of red cells, this method is not recommended for red cell depletion in ABO-incompatible marrow transplants.

3. During centrifugation, lipids may be seen accumulating above the buffy coat. The number of nucleated cells in the lipid layer is usually quite low. However, if desired, the lipid layer may be collected in a bag attached to the yellow line, and a count may be performed at the end of the run to check for cell loss.

References/Resources

1. COBE 2991 Cell Processor operator's handbook. Deerfield, IL: Baxter Healthcare, 1991.

2. FACT-JACIE international standards for cellular therapy product collection, processing, and administration. 4th ed. Omaha, NE: Foundation for the Accreditation of Cellular Therapy and the Joint Accreditation Committee of ISCT and EBMT, 2008.

3. Code of federal regulations. Title 21, CFR Part 1271. Human cells, tissues, and cellular and tissue-based products. Washington, DC: US Government Printing Office, 2008 (updated annually).

4. Padley D, ed. Standards for cellular therapy product services. 3rd ed. Bethesda, MD: AABB, 2008.

Method 26-5. Processing Marrow on Fenwal CS3000 Plus for Mononuclear Cell Enrichment

Description

This method uses a closed system to separate plasma, red cells, and mononuclear cells from harvested marrow. The tubing kit is installed on the CS3000 Plus Cell Separator (Fenwal, Lake Zurich, IL) and primed with normal saline containing human serum albumin (HSA). Cells are pumped into a chamber at 25 mL/min until the sensors detect the change in the density of the plasma, which indicates the presence of MNCs. At that time, the machine will divert the cells to a separate collection chamber. At the completion of the procedure, the plasma, the red cells, and the MNCs will be in separate bags.

Time for Procedure

One hour.

Equipment

1. CS3000 Plus Cell Separator.
2. A-35 collection container holder.
3. GRANULO separation container holder.
4. Open system kit (Baxter).
5. Tubing sealer.

Supplies

1. Sodium chloride, 0.9% USP.
2. HSA (25%).
3. 16-g needles.
4. Sampling site coupler.
5. 1000-mL transfer bags with spikes.
6. Plasma transfer sets.
7. Acid (or anticoagulant)-citrate-dextrose formula A (ACD-A).

Procedure

1. Before beginning the set up, determine if the volume of red cells is greater than 300 mL to ensure marrow can be processed automatically.

2. Set up CS-3000+:
   a. The instrument should be set on Program SPECIAL 1. Verify this setting by checking the instrument menu display line.
   b. Follow the manufacturer's instructions to load the processing kit, separation chambers, and collection bags.
3. Set up the bags:
   a. Saline:
      i. Add a 50-mL bottle of 25% HSA to a 1-L bag of 0.9% saline.
      ii. Aseptically place the vent line needle into the rubber stopper on the front of the saline bag. Tape the needle in place. Squeeze the drip chamber unit until half full.
      iii. Insert the saline line into the center top port of the saline bag.
   b. Plasma bag:
      i. Attach 1 1000-mL transfer bag to the plasma collection line.
      ii. If necessary, attach a second bag, with a hemostat on the connecting tubing, to the plasma bag to allow transfer of excess plasma.
   c. Autoprime:
      Press MODE, then START/RESUME, and proceed with autoprime according to the manufacturer's instructions.
   d. Install and prime packed red cells prepared from marrow (PRBCs) and tubing:
      i. Label 1 1000-mL transfer bag "PRBC." Enter one port of the bag with the spike of a plasma transfer set and close the roller clamp.
      ii. Place the hemostat on the PRBC bag integral tubing (the one with numbers on it), between the bag and spike.
      iii. Aseptically insert the needle of the plasma transfer set into the PRBC line injection site located furthest to the

left from the air trap below the blue monitor box. Tape the needle in place.

iv. Open the roller clamp on the plasma transfer set and allow an amount of albumin solution to enter the PRBC bag that is approximately equal to the red cell volume (hematocrit × volume) in the starting marrow. A minimum of 200 mL is recommended.

v. Close the roller clamp.

vi. Hang the PRBC bag on the second IV hook from the right. Leave this bag hanging so that air does not enter the transfer set tubing.

vii. Open the hemostat on the integral tubing to allow the line to fill with solution. Close the hemostat once the line is full.

e. Connecting marrow and final set:

i. Mix the marrow with ACD-A 10% by volume.

ii. Hang the marrow bag with the coupler already inserted.

iii. Using aseptic technique, over a waste container, open the roller clamp on the inlet line and prime the line with saline until free of air. Close the roller clamp and insert the needle into the coupler site in the marrow bag. Tape the needle in place.

iv. Place a hemostat on the ACD-A line near the Y junction of the inlet line (the one that is not connected to the inlet clamp).

v. Before starting the procedure, allow the lipids in the marrow to float to the top by hanging the marrow bag for a few (<15) minutes.

vi. Spike one port of the marrow bag with the coupler from the PRBC bag, leaving the hemostat closed.

f. Using the following check list, check that all steps were properly performed:

i. Installation agrees with diagram.

ii. Interface detector is set at 120.

iii. There are no air bubbles >1 inch in diameter.

iv. There is a hemostat on the PRBC bag.

v. Roller clamps are closed on the return and ACD-A lines.

vi. Roller clamps are open to saline/HSA prime and vent lines and plasma collection line.

vii. Roller clamp to PRBC bag is open.

viii. Inlet line roller clamp is open.

4. Perform automated marrow processing:

a. Press MODE.

b. Press START/RESUME. (Code 84, ENTER SINGLE ACCESS CYCLE VOLUME, will appear, and a chime will sound.)

c. Press START/RESUME to clear this code.

d. Check to see that the marrow is entering the line. Check to see that fluid is entering the plasma collection bag (tilt and check).

e. Ensure whole blood flow rate (WBFR) is 25 mL/min.

f. After plasma appears in the plasma pump lines (approximately 150-200 mL blood processed), set the interface detector baseline as indicated below:

i. Press the DISPLAY/EDIT key.

ii. Use the UP/DOWN ARROW keys to display interface detector baseline in the message center.

iii. Press the ENTER key to set the value (eg, approximately 30 for marrow).

iv. Press the DISPLAY/EDIT key to exit.

5. No further attention is necessary until the marrow bag is almost empty. To calculate the time needed before emptying the PRBC bag into the starting marrow bag, use the following formula:

Total marrow volume / WBFR = minutes to transfer PRBCs
(Example: 1000 mL / 25 = 40 minutes.)

6. When the starting marrow bag is almost empty, transfer the PRBCs to the starting marrow bag.

a. Mix the contents in the PRBC bag, and lower the marrow bag to get ready to mix with PRBCs.

b. When the lipid layer is at the exit ports of the marrow bag, but not in the inlet line, remove the hemostat from the line between the PRBCs and the marrow bags. This step begins the transfer of the PRBCs to the starting marrow bag for the second cycle of processing.

c. When the PRBC bag is empty, replace the hemostat. Continue processing until the starting marrow bag is empty for the second time.

7. Autoreinfuse—initiate the reinfuse cycle.
   a. When the marrow bag is empty for the second time and fat/air is entering the inlet line, press HALT/IRRIGATE, then immediately press MODE and START/RESUME. This initiates the reinfuse cycle.
   b. The reinfuse cycle consists of a 5-minute soft spin followed by the final MNC harvest and the rinsing of the PRBCs from the separation chamber.
   c. Processing ends when CODE 25 (procedure complete) is displayed.

8. Removing the mononuclear product:
   a. When processing marrow on the CS3000 Plus Cell Separator, the final product volume is 200 mL. If a smaller volume is desired, approximately 90 mL of supernatant can be removed from the top of the product before disconnecting it from the machine.
      i. When the procedure is complete (code 25), close all roller clamps (5).
      ii. Press START/RESUME. This action will open the plasma collect clamp.
      iii. Open the centrifuge doors, lower the plasma collect bag (removing the tubing from the open clamp) below the centrifuge, and place the bag on a scale.
      iv. Tare the scale to the weight of the plasma collection bag.
      v. Open the roller clamp on the plasma collection line to begin plasma flow.
      vi. Once the scale indicates that the desired volume of plasma has been removed, close the roller clamp on the plasma collection line.
   b. The A-35 collection container can be sealed off and removed. Ensure that three hermetic seals are placed on each line, cutting the tubing to leave two seals on the end toward the product.

Anticipated Results

This procedure should yield 60% to 70% of the starting MNCs, with a product purity of approximately 80% MNCs. Red cell volume in the final product should be 2% to 5% of the starting red cell volume.

Calculations

1. Calculate TNCs as follows: WBCs/μL $\times$ conversion factor (1000 μL/mL) $\times$ product volume (mL) = **TNCs.**
   Example: WBCs = $35.7 \times 10^3/\mu$L; volume = 1437 mL
   $(35.7 \times 10^3/\mu L) \times (1000 \ \mu L/mL) \times 1438$ mL $= 51.3 \times 10^9$ TNCs
   where WBCs = white cells; TNCs = total nucleated cells. NC count is usually reported as WBC $\times 10^6$/mL.

2. TNCs $\times$ % MNCs = **total MNCs.**
   Example: TNC = 51.3×10^9; %MNC = 32%
   $(51.3 \times 10^9) \times 32\% = 16.4 \times 10^9$
   where MNCs = mononucleated cells.

3. Product volume $\times$ product Hct = red cell volume.
   Example: volume = 1438 mL; Hct = 32.7%
   $1438 \times 0.327 = 470$ mL of red cells

4. Final product TNC and MNC divided by initial TNC and MNC $\times$ 100 = **% recovery.**

References/Resources

1. Code of federal regulations. Title 21, CFR Part 1271. Human cells, tissues, and cellular and tissue-based products. Washington, DC: US Government Printing Office, 2008 (updated annually).
2. Areman EM, Cullis H, Bazar L, et al. Automated isolation of bone marrow mononuclear cells with the Fenwal CS3000 blood cell separator (abstract). Exp Hematol 1990;18:678.
3. Areman E, Cullis H. Automated mononuclear cell purification of marrow with the Fenwal CS3000 and CS3000 Plus, Version C. In: Areman EM, Deeg HJ, Sacher RA, eds. Bone marrow and stem cell processing: A manual of current techniques. Philadelphia: FA Davis, 1992:130.

Method 26-6. Processing Marrow Using the COBE Spectra for Mononuclear Cell Enrichment

Description

This procedure is used to isolate mononuclear cells (MNCs) from harvested marrow for cryopreservation or red cell depletion. This procedure describes the use of the COBE Spectra (CaridianBCT, Lakewood, CO) in processing marrow for immediate transplant or in preparation for further processing, including cryopreservation.

Time for Procedure

From 1 to 2 hours.

Summary of Procedure

Marrow is filtered through a blood administration set that is loaded onto a Spectra apheresis device fitted with a marrow processing set. Marrow passes from one bag, through the machine where cell separation occurs during centrifugation, and into the second bag. During this process, MNCs are collected into a collection bag. The marrow is continuously processed back and forth until the cell target is reached. Acid (or anticoagulant)-citrate-dextrose formula A (ACD-A) is added to the product to facilitate separation.

Equipment

1. COBE Spectra.
2. Biological safety cabinet (BSC).
3. Scale.
4. Plasma expressor.
5. Sterile connecting device.
6. Tubing sealer.

Supplies

1. Disposable white cell blood tubing set (CaridianBCT).
2. Bone marrow processing set (BMP) (CaridianBCT).
3. One 600-mL transfer bag for plasma collection (only for marrow with >215 mL red cells).

4. 0.9% sodium chloride for injection (1000 mL).
5. Plasma transfer set with two spikes.
6. Plasma transfer set with spike and needle adapter (for marrow with >215 mL red cells).
7. Plastic hemostats.
8. Transfer pack: 2 L.
9. ACD-A.

Procedure

1. Pool marrow into a 2-L transfer pack; mix and weigh. Calculate total volume of marrow. Calculate volume of red cells in the starting product.
2. Add ACD-A to a concentration of 10% of total marrow volume using a plasma transfer set. Subtract any ACD-A that was added during the collection process so that the final concentration is 10% ACD-A.
3. Remove the quality control samples and filter the marrow with the blood administration set (170-210 μ) to remove any clumps or particulates.
4. Set up and prime the Spectra according to COBE Spectra manual instructions.
5. Enter the total volume and the hematocrit using the keypad when the Spectra screen prompts.
   a. Total bag volume allowed range is 100 to 6000 mL, with a validated range of >300 mL.
   b. If the marrow starting volume is <100 mL, it must be processed by an alternate method.
6. The permissible hematocrit range is 10% to 80%, with a validated range of 15% to 45%. If marrow values fall outside these parameters, refer to the calculations section for instructions.
7. The red cell volume of the marrow must be at least 125 mL. If the red cell volume is less than that amount, then either additional red cells

must be added or the product must be processed by an alternate method.

8. The Spectra system uses data entered by the operator and microprocessor algorithms to calculate and show various parameters during the collection process.

9. Approve the marrow processing values:

   a. Press "yes" to exit data entry displays and continue to Step 10. Run parameters are listed in Table 26-6-1.

   b. For marrow with >215 mL red cells, attach a plasma transfer bag to the white cell set at the plasma line luer connection when prompted to do so. Press ENTER.

10. Transfer the marrow:

    a. Place a clamp at point 0 as marked on the bone marrow volume processed (BMP) set. (Refer to the Spectra manual.)

    b. Clamp all white pinch clamps on the administration lines of the BMP set. These include four spike lines and two luer connection lines.

    c. Use the spikes on the administration lines to enter the marrow product bag.

       Note: The air chamber below the spikes is not intended to filter the marrow. It allows the marrow product to flow into bag A. If the chamber clogs, additional filtering may be required.

    d. Open the clamp to the line (either spike or luer line) attached to the BMP set. The marrow is transferred to bag A.

    e. Connect the BMP set to the white cell set by connecting the red line to the white cell access line (also red).

    f. Connect the blue line to the white cell return line (also blue).

    g. Once the marrow has been transferred, seal off the administration line of the BMP set. This line may be removed at this time.

    h. Hang the bags and remove the hemostat from clamp point. Allow the BM access and return lines to prime.

    i. Close both the access and return saline lines.

    j. Open the white clamps on the access and return lines.

11. Start Run Mode:

    a. Press the CONTINUE key to start the system in RUN. All pumps will start, and the centrifuge speed will increase based on the parameters preset by the data and Spectra algorithms.

       Note: Anticoagulant (AC) infusion rate is not applicable to BMP. The AC pump is at 0 mL/minute throughout the procedure because the marrow has been previously anticoagulated.

Table 26-6-1. Spectra Procedure Run Parameters

Marrow Volume to Process Based on Red Cell Volume*	
Volume >215 mL red cells	3 × marrow volume
Volume = 170-215 mL red cells	4 × marrow volume
Volume = 125-170 mL red cells	5 × marrow volume
BMP ratio	1:99.9
BMP collection rate	1.5 mL/minute
BMP inlet flow (marrow volume = 1L)	90 mL/minute
BMP inlet flow (marrow volume <1L)	70 mL/minute

*Counted from the time the collection valve opens.
BMP = bone marrow volume processed.

b. The Spectra will now proceed with the automated Quick Start procedure to establish the correct red cell/plasma interface.

12. A message will display on the keypad when Quick Start is complete. Monitor the collection line for proper interface positioning.
    a. Use the COBE Spectra white cell Colorgram (CaridianBCT) to help determine when the red cell/plasma interface position is correct. (Refer to the Spectra manual.)
    b. For BMP, collect at 3% to 5% hematocrit until the target volume has been processed. Using the Colorgram, increase or decrease the plasma pump flow rate in small increments to obtain the correct color/cell layer.
13. As the marrow is processed, gently shake the bag from side to side to prevent settling of the cellular components.
14. Although the goal of this procedure is to collect a minimum number of red cells with the maximum number of marrow MNCs, there is some intermixing of red cells and MNCs at the interface. To collect the greatest possible number of marrow MNCs with this procedure, it is necessary to collect some of the red cell layer as well. The white cell collection tube in the centrifuge will contain streaks of red cells.
15. When the interface has been established, open the collection valve. During processing, the marrow is first drawn from bag A and returned to bag B. When the hemostat is moved, marrow is drawn from bag B and returned to bag A. This transfer between bags continues until the target volume has been processed.
16. A sample can be collected for cell count and differential to estimate recovery during processing.
17. Processing is continued until the target cell dose is reached.
18. When processing is complete, start rinse-back by pressing the CHANGE MODE key.
19. When rinse-back is complete, seal off the collection bag and remove the disposables. (Refer to the COBE procedure manual for detailed instructions.)

Calculations

1. Determine the volume of marrow using a 1:1 ratio of grams to milliliters.

2. To determine the volume of ACD-A to add to marrow: mL marrow/10 = mL ACD-A to add
Example: 945 mL marrow/10 = 94.5 mL ACD-A to add
Note: Total volume is now 1040 mL.

3. Remove sample and perform cell count to determine total nucleated cells (TNCs):
(WBCs $\times 10^6$ per mL) $\times$ (mL marrow + mL ACD-A) = TNCs
Example: $(15.0 \times 10^6/mL) \times 1040$ mL = 1.56×10^{10}

4. To determine total MNCs:
Obtain differential results (as a percentage). Add monocytes, lymphocytes, and immature MNCs to obtain the percentage of MNCs. Multiply the percentage of MNCs by TNCs for the total MNCs.
Example: % MNC = 34%; TNC = 1.56×10^{10}
$(1.56 \times 10^{10}) \times 0.34 = 5.3 \times 10^9$ total MNC

5. To determine the percentage of TNC and MNC recovery:
Perform calculations as above. Divide the final product TNC and MNC results by the initial product numbers. Multiply these values by 100 to obtain the percentage of recovery.

Anticipated Results

Recovery of at least 70% of the MNCs and approximately 25% to 30% of TNCs.

Note

If a minimum cell yield has not been reached in approximately 10 passes (bag A to B, B to A, A to B, etc), consult the laboratory director.

References/Resources

1. COBE Spectra apheresis system operator's manual. Version 6.0-6.9 software programs. Lakewood, CO: CaridianBCT, 1997.
2. FACT-JACIE international standards for cellular therapy product collection, processing, and administration. 4th ed. Omaha, NE: Foundation for the Accreditation of Cellular Therapy and the Joint Accreditation Committee of ISCT and EBMT, 2008.
3. Code of federal regulations. Title 21, CFR Part 1271. Human cells, tissues, and cellular and tissue-based products. Washington, DC: US Government Printing Office, 2008 (updated annually).
4. Padley D, ed. Standards for cellular therapy product services. 3rd ed. Bethesda, MD: AABB, 2008.

Method 26-7. Separating Marrow by the Density Gradient Method Using COBE 2991

Description

After a buffy coat preparation by centrifugation, marrow cells are layered onto a density gradient solution to isolate the mononuclear cell (MNC) layer.

Time for Procedure

Approximately 90 minutes.

Summary of Procedure

The procedure for processing the marrow can be divided into three steps: 1) preparation of the buffy coat, 2) MNC purification, and 3) washing of the MNC product. The COBE (CaridianBCT, Lakewood, CO) triple processing set consists of three processing bags, two spikes on the red line, five spikes on the green line, and capability for additional waste capacity on the purple line. A pump tubing segment is included on the longer yellow line for insertion into a peristaltic pump.

Equipment

1. Biological safety cabinet.
2. Scale.
3. Plastic hemostats.
4. Tubing sealer.
5. COBE 2991 Cell Processor.
6. Timer.
7. Peristaltic pump.

Supplies and Reagents

1. COBE 2991 triple processing set (#912647-901; CaridianBCT).
2. COBE 2991 double coupler adapter (#912647-912).
3. Optional COBE 2991 female luer coupler (#912647-904).
4. Transfer pack: 300 mL with coupler.
5. Transfer pack: 600 mL.
6. 1000 mL 0.9% sodium chloride (NaCl) for injection.
7. 200 mL of sterile density separation medium.
8. 1800 mL of wash solution [Plasma-Lyte A (Baxter Healthcare, Deerfield, IL) with albumin or other suitable solution].

Procedure

A. *Loading the COBE 2991 Triple Processing Set*
  1. Check hydraulic system prime on 2991 Cell Processor according to operator's handbook.
  2. Remove the triple set from packaging and orient it according to the color-coded pinch valves on the front panel. Load it onto COBE 2991 processor per the manufacturer's instructions.
     Note: Do not load tubing into the red cell detector. If the tubing is loaded, detection of red cells may result in premature shutdown of the SUPER OUT function.
  3. Place the other two processing bags to the left and rear of the centrifuge cover. Place a plastic hemostat on the line leading to these bags near the junction with the first bag, which has been loaded into the centrifuge.
  4. Using TUBE LOAD and the VALVE SELECTOR knob, load the tubing as follows:
     a. Place the red line into valve 1.
     b. Place the purple line into the SOV valves.
     c. Place the green line into valve 2.
     d. Place the yellow line into its holder. (Do not load it into the valve.)
     e. Attach a 2991 double coupler adaptor (#912647-912) to spike on the yellow line.

f. Close the clamps on the 2991 double coupler adaptor.

5. Press STOP/RESET to close the valves.

6. Close all in-line slide clamps on the red and green lines.

7. Place a hemostat on the yellow line approximately 0.5 inches from the center manifold.

8. Aseptically make the following transfers:
   a. Add 200 mL of density gradient separation medium to a 300-mL transfer pack.
   b. Transfer 250 mL of saline into an empty 300-mL transfer pack.
   c. Transfer 1800 mL wash solution to a 2000-mL transfer bag.

9. Attach the marrow product, wash solution, and density gradient separation solution to the appropriate lines and hang them from hanger bars on the instrument.
   a. Attach the transfer pack with the density gradient solution to the blue line.
   b. Attach the empty 300-mL transfer pack to the spike port on the purple line (plasma collection).
   c. Attach wash solution to the spike on the green line.
   d. Attach the empty 600-mL transfer pack to one spike of the double coupler adaptor attached to the yellow line (final buffy coat collection). Do not load the yellow tubing into peristaltic pump.
   e. Attach transfer pack with 250 mL of saline in the 300-mL transfer pack to

the other spike of the double coupler adaptor attached to the yellow line.
   f. Attach marrow product to the spike(s) on the red line.
   Note: If more than two bags of marrow are to be processed, use the 2991 double coupler adaptor (#912647-912) for the appropriate number of spikes.

B. *Cell Concentration Procedure*
   Note: Avoid letting the round processing bag remain stationary for more than 3 minutes in the centrifuge after the product has been introduced into the processing bag. This will minimize the risk of the disposable seal faces sticking together—a condition that may result in failure of the rotating disposable seal. COBE recommends not beginning processing until the entire marrow product is in the laboratory, allowing continuous processing to take place.

1. In the MANUAL mode, set the machine settings to the appropriate values (see Table 26-7-1).

2. Open up the slide clamps(s) on the red lines that are attached to the marrow.

3. Press BLOOD IN and allow the marrow product to flow into the processing bag.

4. When fluid has stopped flowing into the bag, press AIR OUT. When all of the air reaches the marrow bag, press BLOOD IN to allow the processing bag to completely fill with the product. Press STOP/RESET.

Table 26-7-1. Manual Mode Settings for Cell Concentration

Centrifuge Speed	Super-Out Rate	Minimum Agitate	Super-Out Volume	Valve Selector
3000	450	N/A	600	V1
Diode pins			N/A	
Red cell override			N/A	
Pump restore rate			450 mL/minute	

N/A = not applicable.

5. Press START/SPIN. Centrifuge the product for 10 minutes.

6. After 5 minutes of centrifugation, to prevent marrow cells from going into the waste bag, manually depress (with hemostat) the red line pinch valve until the cells that are in the tubing between the center manifold and the processing bag flow back into the red line (approximately 5 seconds).

7. To collect autologous plasma, perform the following steps in order:
   a. Place a hemostat on the clear line attached to the waste bag.
   b. Ensure there is an open line to the plasma collection bag.
   c. Press SUPER OUT.
   d. Collect an appropriate amount of plasma into the plasma collect bag.
   e. Press HOLD.
   f. Place a hemostat on the clear line leading to the plasma collection bag.
   g. Remove the hemostat from the clear line above the waste bag.
   h. Do not clamp and unclamp the lines while in the SUPER OUT mode. Instead, press HOLD first. Make the necessary change and then press CONTINUE. Failure to use the HOLD mode before clamping or unclamping lines may increase the risk of seal failure.
   i. Press CONTINUE to divert plasma into the waste bag until the buffy coat is 0.5 inches (1.3 cm) from the center plate in the centrifuge.
   j. Press AGITATE/WASH IN. When the last of the marrow product has reached the manifold, press STOP/RESET.

8. In order to rinse the marrow bag, perform the following steps in order (to maintain seal integrity, the following steps must be completed within 3 minutes):
   a. Place marrow bag on the centrifuge.
   b. Open the slide clamp on the wash solution on the green line.
   c. Place a hemostat on the clear tubing above the rotating seal.
   d. Press PRE-DILUTE.
   e. Allow saline to flow into the empty marrow bag (for rinse).
   f. Press STOP/RESET.
   g. Remove the hemostat from the clear tubing above the rotating seal.

   Alternate procedure:
   a. Clamp the tubing below the cell detector.
   b. Open the saline line manually by pressing on the V2 valve. The saline will start draining into the marrow bag. Drain approximately 50 cc of saline.
   c. Hang the marrow bag.
   d. Press START/SPIN, then SUPER OUT, then immediately press AGITATE/WASH IN. When the last of the rinse has reached the manifold, change the valve selector to V2.
   e. Allow the rinse solution to completely fill the processing bag.
   f. Press START/SPIN. Centrifuge for 10 minutes.
   g. Press SUPER OUT. When the buffy coat is 0.5 inches from the center plate in the centrifuge, press HOLD.

9. To collect the buffy coat, perform the following steps in order:
   a. Set the SUPER OUT rate to 100 mL/minute.
   b. Remove the hemostat from the yellow line.
   c. Place a hemostat on the purple line.
   d. Open the slide clamp to the 600-mL transfer pack on the yellow line.
   e. Press CONTINUE.
   f. Collect 100 mL (by weight or time) of buffy coat into the transfer pack.
   g. Press HOLD.
   h. Remove a hemostat from the purple line and put it back on the yellow line.
   i. Press STOP/RESET.

10. To flush cells from the yellow line into the transfer pack, perform the following steps in order:
   a. Place a hemostat on the clear tubing above the rotating seal.
   b. Press TUBE LOAD.
   Note: Make sure the valve selector is on V2.

Table 26-7-2. Manual Mode Settings for Density Gradient Separation

Centrifuge Speed	Super-Out Rate	Minimum Agitate	Super-Out Volume	Valve Selector
2000	100	N/A	600	N/A
	Diode pins		N/A	
	Red cell override		N/A	
	Pump restore rate		450 mL/minute	

d. Remove the hemostat from the yellow line.

e. As soon as the line is clear, press STOP/RESET.

f. Remove the hemostat from the clear tubing above the rotating seal.

g. Load the pump tubing segment on the yellow line into a peristaltic pump of the appropriate specifications and with an adjustable flow rate of 20 to 100 mL/minute.

h. To dilute the buffy coat, open the slide clamp on the saline bag attached to the yellow line and allow approximately 200 mL to flow into the buffy coat bag. Replace the slide clamp on the saline.

i. After dilution, the weight of the buffy coat bag should not be >350 g. If it is, it may be difficult to pump all of the cells into the gradient in the next step.

j. Clamp, seal off, and remove the used processing bag from the centrifuge.

C. *Density Gradient Separation Procedure*

1. In the MANUAL mode, set the machine settings to the appropriate values (see Table 26-7-2).

2. Load either of the two remaining processing bags into the centrifuge. Do not load into the red cell detector.

3. Set the appropriate layering speed (20 mL/minute) on the peristaltic pump.

4. Move the plastic hemostat from the clear line leading to the processing bags. Clamp off the remaining processing bag not in the centrifuge.

5. To load the density gradient separation medium into the centrifuge bag, perform the following steps in order:
   a. Remove the hemostat from the blue line.
   b. Allow the density gradient separation medium to enter the processing bag.
   c. Place a hemostat on the blue line.

Table 26-7-3. Automatic Mode Settings for Washing the MNC Product

Centrifuge Speed	Super-Out Rate	Minimum Agitate	Super-Out Volume	Valve Selector
2000	450	70	450	V2
	Diode pins		See Table 26-7-4	
	Red cell override		Not applicable	
	Pump restore rate		450 mL/minute	

d. Press START/SPIN, let the centrifuge come to speed, and then press SUPER OUT.

e. When the density separation medium enters the purple line, press STOP/RESET.

6. To load the 300 mL of buffy coat (BC) onto the separation medium, perform the following steps in order:

a. Press START/SPIN and allow the centrifuge to come up to speed.

b. Switch the pump to FORWARD and allow the cell product to pump into the processing bag.

c. Stop the pump when the last of the fluid reaches the "Y" connector of the adaptor coupler attached to the yellow line. Open the slide clamp on the saline attached to the yellow line, and allow 50 mL to flow into the buffy coat transfer pack. Close the slide clamp on the saline line.

d. Rinse the bag well, then switch pump to FORWARD.

e. Stop the pump when the last of the fluid reaches 3 inches (7.7 cm) above the rotating seal of the processing bag.

f. Continue centrifugation for 15 minutes.

7. To collect the MNC interface, perform the following steps in order:

a. Press SUPER OUT and allow the supernatant to flow into the waste bag until the interface with the desired cell fraction is 0.5 inches (1.3 cm) from the center plate in the centrifuge.

b. Press HOLD.

c. Remove the plastic hemostat from the third processing bag (outside of the centrifuge). Place a plastic hemostat below the manifold but above the junction leading to the two processing bags.

d. Press CONTINUE, allowing the desired cell fraction to flow into the remaining processing bag.

e. When the desired cell fraction is completely in the new processing bag, press HOLD.

f. Clamp the line to the processing bag that now contains the desired cell fraction.

g. Press STOP/RESET to stop the procedure.

h. Heat-seal the line leading to the processing bag that is in the centrifuge.

   Note: Do not seal the bag that contains the desired cell fraction.

D. *Washing the MNC Product*

   Note: Make sure the container with 1800 mL of wash solution is on the green line.

1. In the AUTOMATIC mode, set the machine settings to the appropriate values (see Table 26-7-3).

2. Set diode pins to the appropriate setting for spin times and valve selectors (see Table 26-7-4).

3. Load the third processing bag into the centrifuge.

   Note: Do not load clear line into red cell detector. If the line is loaded, detection of red cells may result in premature shutdown of the SUPER OUT function.

4. Remove the hemostat from the line leading to this bag.

5. Open the slide clamps on the appropriate wash solution containers on the green line.

6. To fill the centrifuge bag with the wash solution, perform the following steps in order:

a. Press TUBE LOAD.

b. Press STOP/RESET when the wash solution stops flowing.

7. To remove air from the bag, perform the following steps in order:

a. Press START/SPIN.

b. Press SUPER OUT.

c. When fluid reaches the purple line, press STOP/RESET.

8. To completely fill the bag, press TUBE LOAD. When the wash solution stops flowing, press STOP/RESET.

9. Press START/SPIN to begin the washing process.

10. When the machine alarm sounds (because of the double pin in the timer), change

Table 26-7-4. Diode Pin Settings for Spin Times and Valve Selectors*

	Timer			Valve				
Cycle	1†	2	PC	1	2	3	RC	RCO
1	●	○	○	○	●	○	○	○
2	●	○	○	○	●	○	○	○
3	●	○	○	○	●	○	○	○
4‡	●	●	●	○	○	○	○	○

*designates placement of diode pin.
†Timer 1: 2 minutes.
‡Timer is double-pegged for cycle 4.
PC = packed cells pin setting; RC = resuspended cells pin setting; RCO = red cell override pin setting.

SUPER OUT volume to 550 mL and remove the diode pin from Timer 2. Press CONTINUE.
11. When the machine alarm sounds the second time, press STOP/RESET.
12. Heat-seal the processing bag and remove it from the centrifuge.

Anticipated Results

1. Red cell volume in the final product is <5.0 mL.
2. MNC recovery is greater than 80%.

Reference/Resource

1. COBE 2991 Cell Processor essentials guide. (June 2008) Lakewood, CO: CaridianBCT, 2008. [Available at http://www.caridianbct.com/cps/rde/xbcr/SID-3916ADC2-9CC247B8/caridianbct/709016001-2991_Essentials_Guide_EN.pdf (accessed April 14, 2009).]

In: Areman EM, Loper K, eds
Cellular Therapy: Principles, Methods, and Regulations
Bethesda, MD: AABB, 2009

◆◆◆　27　◆◆◆

Umbilical Cord Blood Processing

Philip H. Coelho, BSME, and Kathy Loper, MHS, MT(ASCP)

STEM CELLS DERIVED FROM UMBILICAL cord blood (UCB) have proven to be a rich source of hematopoietic progenitor cells (HPCs) for hematopoietic reconstitution. Presently, the minimum acceptable range for the nucleated cell (NC) dose of UCB cells for transplantation is 2.0 to 3.0×10^7 NC/kg, which is a log less than that from other sources.[1] Although UCB stem cells appear to be more potent than a comparable number of marrow cells or HPCs from apheresis (HPC-A), more widespread use of single UCB units for transplantation remains limited by the available NC dose.[2] Because the likelihood and speed of engraftment correlate with the NC dose, single-unit transplantation has been performed primarily in the pediatric transplant population. More recently, cell expansion protocols and double-unit UCB transplants have been used more frequently in both pediatric and adult patients.[3-6]

As described in a previous chapter, UCB is collected either by in-utero or ex-utero techniques from consenting donors who were previously determined eligible by assessment of their medical history, physical examination, and risk factors.

Testing for infectious diseases is performed on maternal samples, and additional testing is performed on samples from the UCB unit, depending on the practices of the UCB bank. Safety and characterization testing are performed, with samples taken from UCB products after processing and before cryopreservation. Some testing may also be performed on samples taken from the unit before processing is performed. Processing of UCB units is performed either by manual or automated methods.

Manual Processing of Cord Blood

The manual method usually consists of red cell depletion with hydroxyethyl starch (HES) and plasma depletion by centrifugation. These methods are time consuming and, if performed in an open system, can result in contamination during processing. The use of a sterile connection device can greatly reduce contamination in the process, and, generally, minimal cell loss results when experienced personnel perform the procedure.

Philip H. Coelho, BSME, President, PHC Medical, Inc, Sacramento, California, and Kathy Loper, MHS, MT(ASCP), Director, Cellular Therapies, AABB, Bethesda, Maryland

The authors have disclosed no conflicts of interest.

Another platform, the PrepaCyte-CB Cord Blood Processing System (BioE, Inc, St Paul, MN), uses a single-step process to isolate MNCs. Prepa-Cyte-CB uses a proprietary non-density gradient reagent to separate UCB into red cell, TNC, and plasma layers. The technology combines gravity sedimentation with centrifugation. The system consists of three bags interconnected via tubing with attached sterile ports and clamps. One of the bags contains a proprietary reagent. A second bag is used for centrifugation, and a third container is used for cryopreservation. Modifications and other bag configurations are also available. Recoveries of 87% of TNCs, 88% of MNCs and CD34+ cells, and 98.5% red cell removal have been reported.[2] (See Method 27-3.)

Automated Processing of Cord Blood

Several manufacturers have developed automated platforms for UCB processing using microprocessor-controlled cell separators. The automated methods require less technologist time and occur in a closed system, which reduces the potential for product contamination and facilitates efficient laboratory operations. Automated methods also ensure a consistent product volume for more efficient liquid nitrogen storage and inventory management.

UCB banking began in 1992 at the New York Blood Center (NYBC), the first public cord blood bank. At that time, the entire CB unit that was collected, including red cells and plasma, was cryopreserved. The large volume of these units—

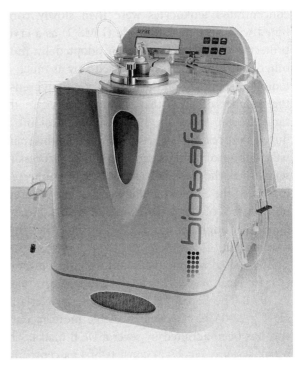

Figure 27-1. Sepax instrument (Biosafe, Eysins, Switzerland).

consisting primarily of red cells, plasma, and cryoprotectant—posed difficulties for banking because resources for long-term storage in liquid nitrogen (then as now) were both limited and costly. In October 1995, in the *Proceedings of the National Academy of Sciences*, the NYBC reported that almost all the hematopoietic colony-forming cells (CFCs) present in UCB units could be recovered in a uniform volume of 20 mL by using rouleaux formation induced by HES and centrifugation to reduce the bulk of erythrocytes and plasma.[7] The

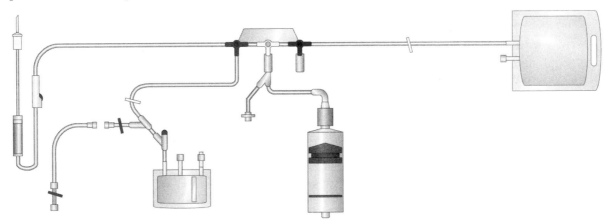

Figure 27-2. Sepax processing kit (Biosafe).

concentrated leukocytes were then slowly combined with dimethyl sulfoxide (DMSO) as a cryoprotectant. This method, soon adopted by most other cord blood banks, increased—by as much as tenfold, depending on the inventory system used—the number of units that could be stored in the same freezer space. In 1997, Pall Medical introduced a processing bag set that simplified this manual method of volume reduction. This processing set, with all the transfer bags and tubing connected, improved the ease of handling and quality of aseptic transfers of the UCB from the collection container, through processing, and into the final freezing bag.

Automated volume reduction with the Optipress (Baxter Healthcare, Deerfield, IL) was introduced in 1999. The Sepax (Biosafe, Eysins, Switzerland; see Fig 27-1) has become available more recently and has been adopted by several UCB banks. The Sepax system (Fig 27-2) consists of 1) a centrifuge system, composed of a pneumatic circuit, valve system, microcomputer, and LCD display and 2) a single-use kit, including a harness kit and separation chamber that serves as both centrifuge container and transfer piston. After attaching the collection container to the processing kit using a sterile connecting device, the process is initiated. The piston,

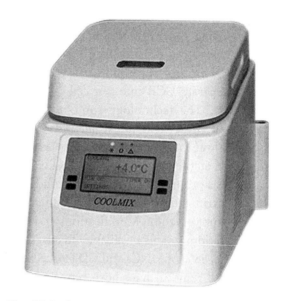

Fig. 27-3. Coolmix (Biosafe).

initially located in the upper part of the chamber, is forced down by negative pressure in the lower section of the chamber, thus pulling the UCB into the chamber. The chamber is then rotated at high speed along its axis, providing centrifugal force that separates the CB into its various components. Following a stand-by period to allow sufficient sedimentation of the cord blood components, a

1. Processing bag hanger
2. LED display panel
3. Processing bag cavity
4. Front cover
5. Level sensor
6. Valve actuator
7. Freezing bag carrier door
8. Main housing
9. Tubing/RBC bag cavity
10. Freezing bag carrier

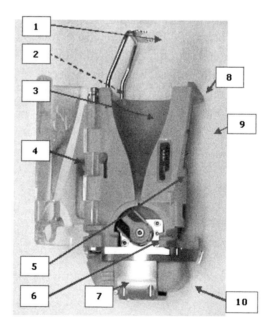

Figure 27-4. AutoXpress device (ThermoGenesis Corp, Rancho Cordova, CA).

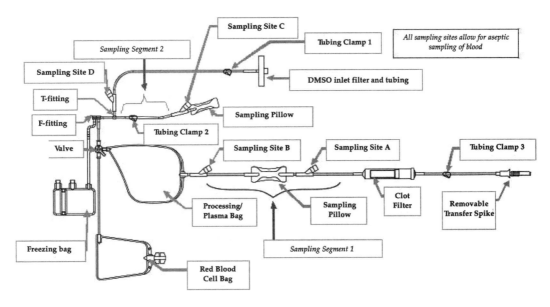

Figure 27-5. AXP processing bag set (ThermoGenesis).

positive pressure is applied to the piston that drives the separated fluids (plasma, red cells, and buffy coat) into the harness and into the appropriate collection bags. The fluid path is controlled by the automated rotary valves, which are part of the single-use kit but are driven and controlled by the main machine unit. Addition of HES to the starting material facilitates the automated concentration and separation of the fractions. A cryoprotectant solution can be added to the final UCB product using the optional Coolmix (Biosafe) device (Fig 27-3), which controls temperature and continually mixes the product in the cryopreservation bag. Air bubbles are extracted, quality control segments are created, and the process concludes with an over-wrap bag for the freezing process. Reported recoveries are 80% for TNCs and 86% for CD34+ cells.[8]

The AutoXpress system (ThermoGenesis Corp, Rancho Cordova, CA; see Fig 27-4) is another instrument used for automated processing. It is a compact, battery-powered device and disposable set that performs the volume reduction in a stan-

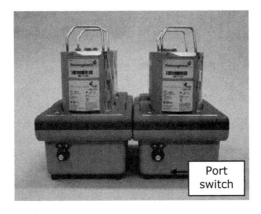

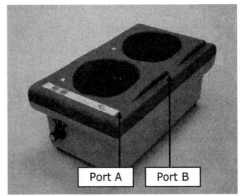

Figure 27-6. AutoXpress and docking station (ThermoGenesis). The main docking station has the following features: 1) capacity for holding two devices, 2) port for data transfer to and from a personal computer, 3) battery charging capabilities, and 4) ability to be electrically linked to a maximum of two satellite docking stations.

dard blood bank centrifuge cup. The AXP platform (Figs 27-5 and 27-6) consists of the microprocessor-controlled AXP device, docking stations, and disposable blood bag sets for closed processing. Light-sensitive sensors control the operation of a three-way valve at the intersection of the tubing that links the three bags of the bag set. The valve, which is operated individually for each UCB unit under sensor control, allows for separation of the buffy coat from the erythrocyte bulk and the excess plasma into discrete bags (components of the bag set). The bag set also includes the valve and small sampling segments for withdrawing pre- and post-processing samples in a closed system. The valve and other bag-set components fit into functional areas of the device that house, store, and functionally protect the bags and specimen sections. Up to six units of UCB can be processed at one time with a standard blood bank centrifuge. During centrifugation, blood is stratified into red cell, buffy coat, and plasma layers. The AXP device separates these components sequentially into the erythrocyte bag and the freezing bag, while keeping the excess plasma in the processing bag.

One recent report described UCB recoveries of 85% of total nucleated cells (TNCs), 98% of mononuclear cells (MNCs), and 95% of CD34+ cells.[9] The UCB MNC product is concentrated into a uniform volume in the freezing bag for cryopreservation and is compatible with a variety of storage freezers, including the BioArchive System (ThermoGenesis). This cryopreservation system provides automated controlled-rate freezing, robotic transfer to addresses in liquid nitrogen, and retrieval from those addresses into insulated sleeves for removal. It is described in detail in Method 28-2.

Current State of the Field and Future Directions

The authors estimated collections of UCB worldwide at approximately 400,000 units for 2007, with approximately 80% of these being processed by manual methods. UCB banks around the world are beginning to convert from manual to automated processing methods. Conversion to automated processing methods is expected to increase as UCB banks strive to meet regulatory requirements of safety, purity, and potency. The intent of automated

UCB processing is to standardize methods to ensure consistent and optimal MNC and CD34+ cell recoveries within a sterile single-use processing bag set, while reducing product handling and personnel time.

Ackowledgments

Method 27-1 was submitted by Anna Chiou, MS, Product Manager, Biosafe, Eysins, Switzerland. Method 27-2 was submitted by Philip H. Coelho, BSME, President, PHC Medical, Inc, Sacramento, California, and John Chapman, PhD, Vice President of Scientific Affairs, ThermoGenesis Corp, Rancho Cordova, California. Method 27-3 was submitted by Shari Tyler Root, MT(ASCP), PrepaCyte Product Manager, QC/QA, and David Miller, MT(ASCP), Technical Applications Specialist, BioE, Inc, St Paul, Minnesota.

References/Resources

1. Gluckman E, Rocha V. Donor selection for unrelated cord blood transplants. Curr Opin Immunol 2006;18: 565-70.
2. Long GD, Laughlin M, Madan B, et al. Unrelated umbilical cord blood transplantation in adult patients. Biol Blood Marrow Transplant 2003;9:772-80.
3. Navneet M, Brunstein C, Wagner J, et al. Double umbilical cord blood transplantation. Curr Opin Allergy Clin Immunol 2006;18:571-5.
4. Barker J, Wagner J. Umbilical cord blood transplantation: Current practice and future innovations. Crit Rev Oncol Hematol 2003;48:35-43.
5. Barker J, Davies S, DeFor T, et al. Survival after transplantation of unrelated donor umbilical cord blood is comparable to that of human leukocyte antigen-matched unrelated donor bone marrow: Results of a matched-pair analysis. Blood 2001;97:2957-61.
6. Barker J, Weisdorf D, DeFor T, et al. Transplantation of 2 partially HLA-matched umblical cord blood units to enhance engraftment in adults with hematologic malignancy. Blood 2005;105:1343-7.
7. Rubinstein P, Dobrila L, Rosenfield RE, et al. Processing and cryopreservation of placental/umbilical cord blood for unrelated bone marrow reconstitution. Proc Natl Acad Sci U S A 1995;92:10119-22.
8. Lapierre V, Pellegrini N, Bardey I, et al. Cord blood volume reduction using an automated system (Sepax) vs. a semiautomated system (Optipress II) and a manual method (hydroxyethyl starch sedimentation) for routine cord blood banking: A comparative study. Cytotherapy 2007;9:165-9.

9. Dobrila L, Shanlong J, Chapman J, et al. ThermoGenesis AXP AutoXpress platform and bioarchive system for automated cord blood banking (abstract). Presented at the EBMT/ASBMT Tandem meeting, Honolulu, HI, February 16-20, 2006. [Poster available at http://www.thermogenesis.com/CMSFiles/Pdf/Clinical/bmtposter.pdf (accessed March 11, 2009).]

Method 27-1. Automated Processing of Umbilical Cord Blood with Biosafe Sepax System and Related Accessories

Description

This procedure describes the processing of umbilical cord blood (UCB) with the Sepax automated system (Biosafe, Eysins, Switzerland) using its "UCB-HES" protocol with the sedimentation agent hydroxyethyl starch (HES) solution. It also includes automated addition of a cryopreservation solution with the Coolmix device (Biosafe).

Time for Procedure

From 40 to 60 minutes.

Summary of Procedure

Processing of UCB with Sepax and the "UCB-HES" protocol allows concentration of the stem cells in a fully automated and closed system performing the following steps:

1. Receipt and quality control of UCB.
2. Addition of HES.
3. Automated cell processing.
4. Automated cryopreservation preparation.

Equipment

1. Sepax device S-100 and accessories (Fig 27-1).
2. Coolmix device AS-210.
3. Syringe pump.
4. Sterile connection device.
5. Automated cell counter instrument for white cell (total nucleated cell, or TNC) content and percentage of hematocrit (HCT).
6. Tubing sealer: 3.0 × 4.0 mm diameter.
7. Standard 5-, 20-, and 60-mL syringes.

Supplies and Reagents

1. Sepax processing kit (Fig 27-2).
2. HES solution: 450/0.7/6% (molecular weight/molar substitution/HES percentage).
3. Dimethyl sulfoxide (DMSO).
4. Dextran 40.

Procedure

A. UCB Processing

1. Perform initial quality control testing, including volume determination.
2. Add 20% HES solution.
3. Connect the input bag to the Sepax kit.
4. Install the kit on the Sepax.
5. Begin automated processing with the Sepax. The process consists of the following steps:
   a. Kit test.
   b. Priming and sedimentation process.
   c. Extraction(s) of plasma, buffy coat, and red cells (in that order).

B. End of Processing

1. Perform a product assessment.
2. Remove the kit from the Sepax.

C. Cryopreservation Using Sepax Cryobags

1. A cryoprotectant solution is automatically added to the UCB product using the Coolmix device.
2. The Coolmix device continuously mixes the cells while monitoring the temperature and cooling the cryobag to approximately 5 C.
3. Remove air from the cryobag.
4. Seal the cord blood segments and bag.
5. Place the cryobag in an overwrap bag to prevent cross-contamination.
6. Remove air from between the two bags.
7. Place cryobag into a labeled metal storage canister.
8. Proceed with cryopreservation process.

Anticipated Results

1. Volume ranges of 20 to 50 mL.
2. TNC recovery >80%.
3. Hematocrit <40%.

References/Resources

1.　Sepax system. Eysins, Switzerland: Biosafe, 2009. [Available at http://www.biosafe.ch/article_pictures/article_1_104.pdf (accessed February 26, 2009).]

2.　Sepax system operator's manual (Biosafe, Eysins, Switzerland).

3.　Coolmix operator's manual (Biosafe, Eysins, Switzerland).

Method 27-2. Automated Volume Reduction of Umbilical Cord Blood Using the AutoXpress System

Description

The AutoXpress System (or AXP, ThermoGenesis Corp, Rancho Cordova, CA) is a compact, battery-powered device that performs umbilical cord blood (UCB) volume reduction by centrifugation in a standard blood bank centrifuge cup. The intent of this automated volume reduction is to recover the most possible mononuclear and CD34+ cells from each unit of collected UCB, to perform this process within the sterile single-use processing bag set, and to reduce labor, time, and variations in unit-to-unit cell recoveries.

Time for Procedure

Each volume reduction process takes approximately 45 minutes.

Summary of Procedure

1. Transfer UCB into the AXP processing set.
2. Add hydroxyethyl starch (HES).
3. Place the set inside the AXP device.
4. Centrifuge and collect the components.
5. Add dimethyl sulfoxide (DMSO) and prepare for cryopreservation.

Equipment

1. AXP device (Fig 27-4).
2. AXP processing bag sets (Fig 27-5).
3. AXP docking station (Fig 27-6).
4. Centrifuge.
5. Sterile connection device.
6. Tubing sealer.
7. Syringe pump.
8. Scale.

Supplies and Reagents

1. Syringe.
2. Canister.
3. HES.
4. DMSO.
5. Dextran.

Procedure

A. *UCB Requirement*
1. Volume is between 50 and 150 mL, not including anticoagulant.
2. HES is added at a volume of 20% (if used).
3. UCBs are processed at room temperature within 48 hours from the time they are collected.

B. *UCB Processing*
1. Inspect and prepare a disposable AXP set for processing (see Fig 27-4).
2. Label the freezing bag.
3. Connect and transfer the UCB to the AXP bag set.
4. Mix the plasma/processing bag and collect a sample for testing.
5. Load the AXP device.
    a. Add the HES to the plasma/processing bag using a sample site port.
6. Remove the AXP device from the docking station.
7. Open the freezing bag and load it by folding the minor compartment over the major compartment. Insert the freezing bag into the freezing bag carrier.
8. Align the tubing and ports with the channel on the freezing bag carrier door and close the door. Ensure that the tubing and ports are not kinked or twisted.
9. Turn the device so that the clear door is facing up. Orient the plasma/processing bag into the plasma/processing bag cavity.
10. While holding the F-fitting, place the bottom end into the round depression on

the device base plate. Gently insert the fitting into place.

11. Close the clear door.

12. Insert the DMSO tubing and filter into the storage cavity.

13. Close clamp 2 and insert it into the clamp cavity. Insert the tubing into the channel on device and hang sampling site D on the hook.

14. Insert the tubing from the Red Blood Cell (RBC) bag into the channel. Hang the RBC bag and ensure that the butterfly clamp is seated in the groove above the bag cavity. Tuck the RBC bag edges under the flanges in the cavity.

15. Tuck sampling site B between the plasma/processing bag and the cavity wall. Hang the plasma/processing bag.

16. Verify the tubing is properly seated and that there are no kinks.

17. Balance the devices.

18. Centrifuge to stratify the sample at 1400 RCF for 20 minutes.

19. To harvest cells, centrifuge for 10 minutes at 80 RCF.

C. *Sample Harvest*

1. Remove the disposable bag set.

2. Sample the harvested buffy coat.

Anticipated Results

1. Postprocessing UCB volume (mL; target volume = 20 mL): 19.7 ±0.3 mL.

2. Postprocessing UCB hematocrit (%): 29.8 ±2.6.

3. Total nucleated cells (TNCs) (% recovery): 84.8 ±9.2.

4. Mononuclear cells (MNCs) (% recovery): 97.9 ±4.9.

5. Viable CD34+ cells (% recovery): 98.2 ±8.0.

Reference/Resource

1. Dobrila L, Shanlong J, Chapman J, et al. ThermoGenesis AXP AutoXpress platform and bioarchive system for automated cord blood banking (abstract). Presented at the EBMT/ASBMT Tandem meeting, Honolulu, HI, February 16-20, 2006. [Poster available at http://www.thermogenesis.com/CMSFiles/Pdf/Clinical/bmtposter.pdf (accessed March 11, 2009).]

Method 27-3. Processing Cord Blood with the Prepacyte System

Description

The PrepaCyte-CB Cord Blood Processing System (BioE, Inc, St Paul, MN) is a sterile processing system that separates total nucleated cells (TNCs), including hematopoietic progenitor cells (HPCs), from human umbilical cord blood (UCB). The PrepaCyte-CB processing system depletes a majority of the red blood cells (>98%), while maintaining high TNC recovery.

Time for Procedure

Approximately 1 hour.

Summary of Procedure

PrepaCyte-CB is a non-density-based, one-step reagent designed specifically to aggregate and sediment erythrocytic components, recovering the nucleated cells and stem cells in the supernatant. PrepaCyte-CB is based on BioE's patented PrepaCyte technology platform. See Fig 27-3-1.

Equipment

1. Plasma expressor.
2. Centrifuge.

Supplies and Reagents

1. The PrepaCyte-CB processing system.
2. 5% human serum albumin (HSA).

Procedure

1. Assess the cord blood unit [collected in citrate-phosphate-dextrose (CPD) or citrate-phosphate-dextrose-adenine (CPDA)] to ensure that it meets acceptability requirements according to facility procedures.

2. Use the spike from bag 1 on the bag set to enter a port on the cord blood unit and drain the blood into bag 1, which is prefilled with PrepaCyte-CB reagent. A sterile connection device may also be used to connect the bag set to the cord blood unit.

3. Mix bag 1 by hand or on a rocker for 3 minutes.

4. Allow the bag to hang upright from a standard blood bank plasma expressor for 30 (±5) minutes.

5. During the 30 minutes of settling time, the red cells slowly fall out of solution and sediment to the bottom of bag 1. After 30 minutes, there is good definition between the supernatant (top layer containing white cells and stem cells) and the sediment (bottom layer containing red cells).

6. After the 30 minutes of settling, the supernatant is expressed from bag 1 through the tubing to bag 2. This process is accomplished by closing the expressor door and stopping the liquid flow just as the red cells are about to enter bag 2.

7. The bag set is centrifuged at $400 \times g$ for 10 minutes. After removal from the centrifuge, the white cells are pelleted in the bottom of bag 2. The bag is then placed back on the expressor.

8. The centrifuge waste (top layer now in bag 2) is expressed back into bag 1. The pelleted cells remain at the bottom edge of bag 2.

9. The pelleted cells are resuspended by agitating and mixing bag 2. A reagent (BioE recommends 5% HSA) is added to bring it to the desired volume.

10. Cells are transferred to bag 3 for cryopreservation.

11. A cryopreservative is added to the cells, and the unit is frozen according to facility procedures.

PrepaCyte-CB Bag Set Configurations

Bag 1: Cell separation bag containing 150 mL
PrepaCyte-CB reagent.
Bag 2: Empty supernatant centrifugation bag.
Bag 3: Cryopreservation bag.

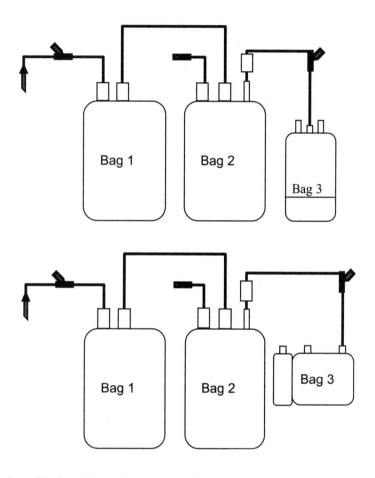

Figure 27-3-1. PrepaCyte-CB Cord Blood Processing System (BioE, Inc, St Paul, MN): bag set configurations.

Anticipated Results

PrepaCyteCB averages from the clinical study are as follows:

% TNC Recovery:	85.0%
% RBC Depletion:	98.6%
Hematocrit:	<3%
Volume:	5 to 15 mL, concentrate;
	24 to 26 mL, final volume

Reference/Resource

1. Wagner JE. Umbilical cord blood stem cell transplantation. Am J Pediatr Hematol Oncol 1993;15:169-74.

In: Areman EM, Loper K, eds
Cellular Therapy: Principles, Methods, and Regulations
Bethesda, MD: AABB, 2009

♦♦♦   **28**   ♦♦♦

Cryopreservation of Cellular Therapy Products

Allison Hubel, PhD

HUMAN CELLS, IN GREAT VARIETY, ARE being used therapeutically for a wide range of disorders, and the ability to preserve cellular therapy (CT) products is essential for their clinical utility. Specifically, preservation permits shipping of the cells from the site of collection to a processing facility, and then to the site of clinical use. A good example of the need for cryopreservation is the collection and storage of umbilical cord blood (UCB). UCB may be collected any time of the day or night and shipped in the liquid state to a central processing/banking facility, where it is processed and frozen. When needed for clinical use, the frozen UCB unit may be shipped in the frozen state to a third location where the unit is thawed and administered to the recipient.

An increasing number of cellular therapies require extensive manipulation of the cells, such as selection of subpopulations, ex-vivo culture, or even genetic modification. Safety and quality control (QC) testing of extensively manipulated cells may be more time consuming than for minimally manipulated products. Preservation permits the completion of all the necessary safety and QC testing before the product is administered to a patient. Cellular therapies are typically given to patients who are quite ill, and if cells are administered fresh, both the cells and the recipient must be ready at the same time. The ability to preserve cells facilitates the coordination of the therapy with patient care regimens. Additionally, the ability to preserve cells is important because the number of patients and the variety of disorders treated with cells only continue to increase. Expanding further the number of patients who can be treated requires developing a "manufacturing paradigm" for cellular therapies to maximize the number of products that a given facility can produce. The ability to preserve cells is an important element in that manufacturing paradigm because it permits full use of a given facility's capacity to produce a CT product, which can in turn be preserved until it is needed as therapy.

The objective of this chapter is to summarize the current understanding and practice of cryopreservation for cellular therapies. These strategies will help in developing cryopreservation protocols as

Allison Hubel, PhD, Associate Professor, Mechanical Engineering, University of Minnesota, Minneapolis, Minnesota

The author has disclosed no conflict of interest.

well as improving the outcomes of existing protocols.

Elements of a Cryopreservation Protocol

There are six elements of a cryopreservation protocol (as shown schematically in Fig 28-1). Five of these elements—introduction of a cryopreservative solution, cooling protocol, storage, warming, and post-thaw assessment—represent the core of the preservation protocol. The remaining element, prefreeze processing, influences post-thaw outcome and may or may not be specified as a part of the overall protocol.

Prefreeze Processing

It is noteworthy that what happens to a CT product between the time it is obtained from a donor and the time it is frozen can influence the product's response to the stresses of freezing and thawing. Prefreeze processing of cells may involve short-term liquid storage, selection of subpopulations, ex-vivo culture, or genetic modification. Any of these processes can influence the state of the cells before cryopreservation and, therefore, their ability to survive the stresses of freezing and thawing. For example, CB is usually collected in a hospital and shipped in the liquid state to a central processing facility, where its red cell and/or plasma content are reduced before cryopreservation. Studies have demonstrated that the liquid storage conditions (duration of storage, temperature, cell concentration, and storage solution) influence the ability of the cells to survive the stresses of freezing and thawing.[1-3]

Ex-vivo culture may also influence the freezing response of the cells by altering their biophysical properties (see Hubel[4] for review). Hubel and colleagues demonstrated that, for both hematopoietic progenitor cells (HPCs)[5] and mature lymphocytes,[6] ex-vivo culture altered the water transport characteristics for the cells. When compared to freshly isolated cells, even cells cultured for relatively short periods of time (72 hours) demonstrated significant shifts in water permeability. These studies suggest that optimum freezing protocols for cells that have been extensively cultured ex vivo may vary from those for freshly isolated cells.

These studies illustrate that the handling of the cells before freezing can influence their response to the stresses of freezing and thawing. Liquid storage protocols should be evaluated to ensure that the storage conditions (time, temperature, and duration) do not result in increased losses when compared to results of protocols that freeze cells immediately after isolation. Similarly, other pre-freezing processing (eg, culture or genetic modification) should be evaluated for its influence on post-thaw recovery. Monitoring cells for early signs of apoptosis or shifts in metabolism to stress pathways may also help in determining whether a pre-freezing processing protocol might harm the cells.

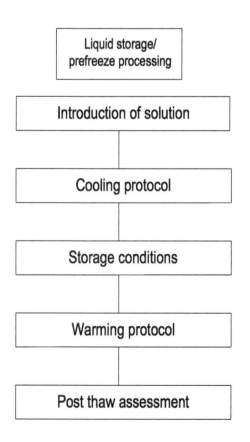

Figure 28-1. Elements of a cryopreservation protocol.

Formulation and Introduction of a Cryopreservation Solution

Cryopreservation solutions typically contain three different types of components: culture media (or a balanced salt solution), cryoprotective agents

(CPAs), and proteins. Polge and colleagues observed in 1949 that the addition of glycerol to a solution extended the survival of sperm.[7] This study led to the observation that certain additives improve cells' ability to survive the stresses of freezing and thawing. The most commonly used cryoprotective agents are glycerol (the additive found in the Polge study) and dimethyl sulfoxide (DMSO). Cryoprotective agents act through a variety of mechanisms. The addition of organic molecules reduces the concentration of salt at a given subzero temperature[8] (colligative effect). Certain cryoprotective agents have been shown to influence growth and structure of the ice phase (see Mazur[9] for review). Other protective agents, such as trehalose, have been shown to stabilize the cell membrane.[10-12] Recently, molecular dynamic simulations suggest that DMSO may also alter the fluidity and permeability of the cell membrane.[13] These studies suggest that CPAs influence both the biological cell and the structure of water in a manner that acts to protect the cells.

Cryopreservation solutions are specialized solutions that are not physiological. For example, a 10% DMSO solution is approximately 1.4 Osm (vs 270-300 mOsm for isotonic solutions). When transferred from an isotonic solution to a CPA solution containing DMSO, cells exhibit a rapid efflux of water as they attempt to reduce the difference in chemical potential between intracellular and extracellular solutions [Fig 28-2(A)]. Slowly,

the DMSO from the surrounding solution permeates the cell membrane. Both the rate of volume change and the absolute volume changes experienced by the cell can produce cell lysis (see Fahy et al[14] for review). Cells also experience volumetric excursions upon dilution or removal from a cryopreservation solution. Transfer of a cell equilibrated with a CPA solution into an isotonic solution will produce a rapid influx of water to decrease the chemical potential of the intracellular solution, followed by a slow efflux of DMSO [Fig 28-2(B)]. Because cells are much more sensitive to lysis upon expansion (than they are upon dehydration), post-thaw DMSO removal protocols can be critical for preventing cell losses.

Cell losses can result not only from introduction to or removal from CPA solutions but also from exposure to the solution over time. The time of exposure for cells becomes less of an issue if cells are maintained at a low temperature during or after exposure to the solution. Early cryopreservation studies documented the sensitivity of HPCs to DMSO (see Rowley[15] for review.) The conventional wisdom in cell-processing facilities is that, for both prefreeze and post-thaw periods, exposure time of the cells to DMSO must be minimized. As a result, many processing protocols specify that, after DMSO is added, the freezing process must start within 15 minutes. HPC products from marrow (HPC-M) and from apheresis (HPC-A) are often thawed at the bedside and infused directly into the

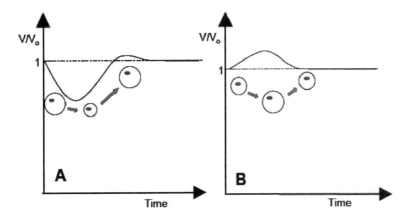

Figure 28-2. Normalized volume (volume at a given time/initial volume) as a function of time for cells being introduced and removed from a cryopreservation solution. (See text for full explanation.) V/V_0 = normalized spheroid volume fraction.

patient without post-thaw manipulation so that cell losses caused by time exposure are minimal.[16] Despite its limited cell dose, UCB remains the one source of HPCs that is often washed upon thawing. In this case, the cells are washed primarily to reduce infusion-related reactions in pediatric patients who have low body weight and who currently represent the majority of recipients.[17,18]

Current strategies for removal of DMSO from CT products are time consuming, labor intensive, and result in significant cell losses. Typically, cells are centrifuged to form a cell pellet at the bottom of a bag; the supernatant is expressed and replaced with fresh wash solution (eg, dextran/albumin solution for UCB). The centrifugation process is normally repeated in order to achieve approximately 95% DMSO reduction, and the entire washing process takes 1.5 to 2 hours in the clinical facility. Cell losses can occur as a result of mechanical stresses on the cells during both centrifugation and expression of the supernatant. Further, the centrifugation process requires significant intervention by an experienced and skilled operator to minimize cell losses. Finally, changes in the concentration of a cryopreservation solution that result from introducing the wash solution can also result in cell losses from osmotic stress as described previously. Antonenas and colleagues quantified losses of 27% to 30% of nucleated cells (NCs) resulting from post-thaw washing of UCB.[19] A more recent study by Perotti and colleagues[20] observed a similar loss in NC counts for UCB units washed with an automated cell washer.

Cooling Rate

The strong influence of cooling rate on post-thaw survival has been documented for a variety of cell types.[9] For most cells used therapeutically, the cooling rate is controlled by the use of a controlled-rate freezer (CRF). A typical CRF protocol is shown schematically in Fig 28-3 and is composed of three basic segments.

The first segment—an equilibration phase—permits the samples to reach equilibrium with the chamber before initiation of the freezing protocol. Insufficient time for equilibration will result in the samples not tracking with the chamber temperature for the initial portion of the freezing protocol. The end result is that samples placed in the cham-

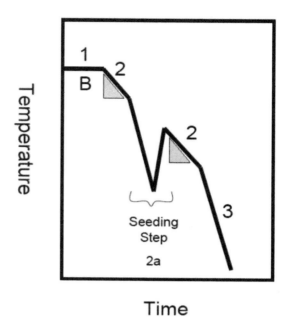

Figure 28-3. Temperature vs time for a typical controlled-rate freezing protocol.

ber and subjected to the same freezing protocols will have different temperature histories and, therefore, potentially different post-thaw recoveries.

The second segment typically consists of a constant cooling rate portion. When a protocol specifies a cooling rate (eg, 1 C/minute), the cooling rate in the second segment should correspond to this value. At some point during the second segment, ice will form in the extracellular solution. The temperature at which ice formation in the extracellular solution is observed is important. As a result of nucleation of ice in the extracellular solution, water is removed from the solution in the form of ice, and there is a corresponding increase in extracellular concentration.[8] The formation of ice in the extracellular solution also results in an increase in the solution's temperature because of the release of the latent heat of fusion. Studies by Toner and colleagues demonstrated elegantly that the temperature at which ice forms profoundly influences post-thaw viability.[21] Specifically, decreasing the temperature at which ice formed in the extracellular solution increased the fraction of cells with intracellular ice formation (and, therefore, the fraction of cells that were dead) for a given cooling rate. Controlled-rate freezing protocols may control the temperature at which ice forms in the extracellular solution by inserting a "hold" step to permit manual seeding of the sample, by using a chilled instrument, or by inserting a rapid cooling step followed by rapid warming.[18] Most CT protocols use an "automatic seeding" step (segment 2a in Fig 28-3) in the freezing protocol. In this step, the chamber is rapidly cooled, and then warmed again, to attempt to induce controlled nucleation of ice in the solution. This seeding step does not ensure that every sample in the controlled-rate freezer forms ice in the extracellular solution at the same temperature, but it increases the likelihood that it will. The ability to monitor and control the freezing process would be enhanced by the development of improved technology for temperature measurement and controlled ice nucleation during controlled-rate freezing.

The third segment of the freezing protocol involves cooling the sample to the final temperature, which is selected to prevent significant warming of the sample when it is transferred from the controlled-rate freezer to storage. Each element of the cooling protocol is important and can influence the post-thaw survival that is observed.

Storage

Samples that have been frozen are usually stored in liquid nitrogen (LN$_2$), in either liquid or vapor phase. Storage of products in LN$_2$ requires storage Dewars and access to a constant supply of LN$_2$. Although there is some interest in storage in mechanical freezers (–80 or –150 C), the risks of mechanical device failure must be considered. Storage conditions will influence product stability and shelf life. For example, the composition of the cryopreservation solution—a complex, multi-component mixture—is a factor. Unlike pure water, this type of solution does not freeze at a single temperature but over a range of temperatures.[8] The seeding of the extracellular solution removes water in the form of ice. There is a fraction of solution that is highly concentrated and does not freeze completely until the system reaches the eutectic temperature. For a 10% DMSO solution, the eutectic temperature is approximately –70 C.[22] Other cryopreservation solutions that are commonly used for cell preservation have eutectic temperatures as low as –120 C.[23] Storage of a product at or near the eutec-

tic temperature implies that the extracellular solution is not fully solidified, the cells will be surrounded by high concentration solutions, and ice crystals will continue to grow and coalesce.[24] These changes, in turn, can influence post-thaw recovery.

Stability of a frozen and stored CT product is also influenced by cellular activity at low temperatures. Much of the cells' activity, such as water transport, is minimal for temperatures below –40 C. However, enzymatic activity of cells persists to very low temperatures, and this activity can influence post-thaw recovery. Tappel studied the activity of common intracellular enzymes at low temperatures and observed that there is a threshold temperature below which the enzymatic activity is suppressed.[25] The actual threshold temperature depends on the enzymes present, but storage below –150 C is typically recommended. More recently, Fowke and colleagues[26] observed that post-thaw apoptosis levels increased when MNCs from peripheral blood were stored at higher temperatures (–70 C). These studies suggest that the storage of cells at temperatures above that of LN$_2$ may reduce the shelf life of the product.

Warming

When the cells that have been frozen and stored are to be used, they must be warmed to room temperature. The same dangerous chemical and mechanical environment that is observed during freezing is present during warming. For example, very small ice crystals present in the cells during cooling may have time to grow during warming and damage the cells. The growth of ice in the cells during warming is called recrystallization damage. As with cooling, the cells are exposed to very high extracellular concentrations during warming, and those concentrations can be damaging.[9] Thus, warming protocols are as critical as cooling protocols. The optimum warming protocol depends on the cooling protocol used.[27] For a conventional controlled cooling rate—freezing over the range of cooling rates used for most cell types (1 to 10 C/minute)—optimally, warming protocols should be as rapid as possible (>200 C/minute). Rapid warming rates are most commonly achieved by agitating the sample in a warm waterbath until a significant fraction of the visible ice crystals have melted. More rapid warming rates can also be achieved by increasing the temperature of the warm waterbath used for thawing, but using higher bath temperatures must be evaluated carefully to prevent cell damage resulting from exposure to supraphysiological temperatures.

Post-Thaw Assessment

Developing a cryopreservation protocol requires developing effective methods of assaying viability post-thaw. It is not possible to determine the influence of different factors (composition of cryopreservation solution, cooling protocol) on viability if an effective method of determining viability has not been developed. It is important to remember that determining the viability of a frozen and thawed cell presents some specific challenges that differ from determining the viability of a cell that has not been subjected to freezing and thawing. First of all, cells that have been frozen and thawed and are still intact have undergone extensive dehydration that may leave the cell membranes transiently leaky.[28] Similarly, cells that have been frozen and thawed have experienced suppression of metabolic activity, and there can be a delay between thawing and the resumption of normal metabolic activity.[29] Finally, in several cell types, the stresses of freezing and thawing have been shown to result in post-thaw apoptosis.[30] For example, frozen and thawed hematopoietic cells have been shown to exhibit post-thaw apoptosis.[31-33] The result of these influences implies that the viability of cells that have been frozen and thawed may vary with time after thawing.

Typically, more than one measure is used to establish the post-thaw viability of cells. Viability assays can be divided into different categories: physical/membrane integrity, metabolic activity, mechanical activity (attachment, contraction), mitotic activity (proliferation assay), and engraftment potential (see Pegg[28] for review). Each type of assay provides a different type of information on the post-thaw function of the cell and, for most primary cell types, using only one type of assay to establish post-thaw function may not be sufficient. For example, numerous studies have measured high levels of membrane integrity for frozen and thawed hepatocytes,[34-36] and yet, unless these cells attach to a surface and exhibit metabolic functions, the cells are not useful. Therefore, post-thaw mea-

sures of hepatocyte function will frequently involve assays measuring a variety of functions, including synthetic and detoxification functions of the cells. In general, the measurement of membrane integrity for a given cell type is typically not sufficient for determining post-thaw recovery.

Interpretation is another common source of error for viability assays. Most assays are performed on intact cells. For example, HPC products are commonly cultured in methylcellulose and, after a specified time in culture, the frequency of colonies is counted. Similarly, as a surrogate functional assay, the fraction of cells that express the CD34+ surface marker is also determined via flow cytometry. Functional recovery of the cells may then be determined by comparing the frequency of colonies or CD34+ cells after thawing with those obtained before freezing. The end result of this method is that it is common in the literature to see recoveries or post-thaw viabilities approaching 100% (see Glass and Hubel[37] for review). It is unlikely that the process of freezing and thawing has resulted in the proliferation of stem cells. It is more likely that the method of interpreting the data has led to the introduction of a measurement bias. A certain fraction of the cells that have been frozen and thawed has been destroyed and is no longer intact. Failing to account for the cells that have been destroyed during freezing and thawing may result in a bias in the post-thaw recoveries that are reported. Accurate and meaningful measures of post-thaw assessment are critical to the development of effective preservation protocols. The use of single measures to assay post-thaw recovery and improper interpretation of the data obtained from those measures can lead to the incorrect interpretation of results.

Summary

The growth in cellular therapies presents a tremendous opportunity to improve human health. The ability to preserve cells used therapeutically is critical to the clinical implementation and expansion of cellular therapies. A cryopreservation protocol can be identified and rationally developed with the following elements: formulation and introduction of cryopreservation solutions, controlled-rate freezing, storage, warming, and post-thaw assessment. Each element of the protocol is important and can have a strong influence on post-thaw recovery. Advances in preservation science as well as technology are needed to improve post-thaw recoveries for all cellular therapies.

Acknowledgments

Method 28-1 was submitted by Leigh Ann Stamps, MT(AMT), Cell Processing Technologist, Sarah Cannon Blood and Marrow Transplant Program at Centennial Medical Center, Nashville, Tennessee. Method 28-2 was submitted by Philip H. Coelho, BSME, President, PHC Medical, Inc, Sacramento, California, and John Chapman, PhD, Vice President of Scientific Affairs, ThermoGenesis Corp, Rancho Cordova, California.

References/Resources

1. Hubel A, Carlquist D, Clay M, McCullough J. Short term liquid storage of umbilical cord blood. Transfusion 2003; 43:626-32.
2. Hubel A, Carlquist D, Clay M, McCullough J. Cryopreservation of cord blood after liquid storage. Cytotherapy 2003;5:370-6.
3. Hubel A, Carlquist D, Clay M, McCullough J. Liquid storage, shipment, and cryopreservation of cord blood. Transfusion 2004;44:518-25.
4. Hubel A. Cellular preservation—Gene therapy, cellular metabolic engineering. In: Baust JG, ed. Advances in biopreservation. Boca Raton, FL: CRC Press, 2006:143-56.
5. Hubel A, Norman J, Darr TB. Cryobiophysical characteristics of genetically modified hematopoietic progenitor cells. Cryobiology 1999,38:140-53.
6. Hubel A, Darr TB, Norman JA. Freezing characteristics of genetically modified lymphocytes for the treatment of MPS II. Cell Transplant 1999; 8:521-30.
7. Polge C, Smith A, Parkes A. Revival of spermatozoa after vitrification and dehydration at low temperatures (letter). Nature 1949;164:666. [Available at http://www.nature.com/nature/journal/v164/n4172/abs/164666a0.html (accessed April 14, 2009).]
8. Cocks FH, Brower W. Phase diagram relationship in cryobiology. Cryobiology 1974;11:340-58.
9. Mazur P. Principles of cryobiology. In: Fuller BJ, Lane N, Benson E, eds. Life in the frozen state. Boca Raton, FL: CRC Press, 2004:3-66.
10. Crowe JH, Crowe LM, Chapman D. Infrared spectroscopic studies on interactions of water and carbohydrates with a biological membrane. Arch Biochem Biophys 1984;232:400-7.

11. Oliver AE, Hincha DK, Crowe LM, Crowe JH. Interactions of arbutin with dry and hydrated bilayers. Biochim Biophys Acta 1998;1370:87-97.
12. Garcia de Castro A, Tunnacliffe A. Intracellular trehalose improves osmotolerance but not desiccation tolerance in mammalian cells. FEBS Lett 2000;487:199-202.
13. Gurtovenko AA, Anwar J. Modulating the structure and properties of cell membranes: The molecular mechanism of action of dimethyl sulfoxide. J Phys Chem B 2007;111: 10453-60.
14. Fahy GM, Lilley TH, Linsdell H, et al. Cryoprotectant toxicity and cryoprotectant toxicity reduction: In search of molecular mechanisms. Cryobiology 1990;27:247-68.
15. Rowley SD. Hematopoietic stem cell processing and cryopreservation. J Clin Apher 1992;7:132-4.
16. Lasky LC. The role of the laboratory in marrow manipulation. Arch Pathol Lab Med 1991;115:293-8.
17. Rubinstein P, Dobrila L, Rosenfield RE, et al. Processing and cryopreservation of placental/umbilical cord blood for unrelated bone marrow reconstitution. Proc Natl Acad Sci U S A 1995;92:10119-22.
18. Fraser JK, Cairo MS, Wagner EL, et al. Cord blood transplantation study (COBLT): Cord blood bank standard operating procedures. J Hematother 1998;7:521-61.
19. Antonenas V, Bradstock K, Shaw P. Effect of washing procedures on unrelated cord blood units for transplantation in children and adults. Cytotherapy 2002;4:16.
20. Perotti CG, Fante CD, Viarengo G, et al. A new automated cell washer device for thawed cord blood units. Transfusion 2004;44:900-6.
21. Toner M, Cravalho E, Karel M. Thermodynamics and kinetics of intracellular ice formation during freezing of biological cells. J Appl Physics 1990;67:1582-93.
22. Pegg DE. Equations for obtaining melting points and eutectic points for the ternary systems dimethyl sulfoxide/sodium chloride/water. Cryo Letters 1988;7:387-94.
23. Fahy GM. Equations for calculating phase diagram information for the ternary systems NaCl-dimethyl sulfoxide-water and NaCl-glycerol-water. Biophys J 1980;32: 837-50.
24. Shepard ML, Goldston CS, Cocks FH. The H_2O-NaCl-glycerol phase diagram and its application in cryobiology. Cryobiology 1976;13:9-23.
25. Tappel A. Effects of low temperature and freezing on enzymes and enzyme systems. In: Meryman HT, ed. Cryobiology. New York: Academic Press, 1966:163-77.
26. Fowke KR, Behnke J, Hanson C, et al. Apoptosis: A method for evaluating the cryopreservation of whole blood and peripheral blood mononuclear cells. J Immunol Methods 2000;244:139-44.
27. Karlsson JO. A theoretical model of intracellular devitrification. Cryobiology 2001;42:154-69.
28. Pegg DE. Viability assays for preserved cells, tissues, and organs. Cryobiology 1989;26:212-31.
29. Borel Rinkes IH, Toner M, Sheeha SJ, et al. Long-term functional recovery of hepatocytes after cryopreservation in a three-dimensional culture configuration. Cell Transplant 1992;1:281-92.

30. Baust JM, Van B, Baust JG. Cell viability improves following inhibition of cryopreservation-induced apoptosis. In Vitro Cell Dev Biol Anim 2000;36:262-70.

31. Xiao M, Dooley DC. Assessment of cell viability and apoptosis in human umbilical cord blood following storage. J Hematother Stem Cell Res 2003;12:115-22.

32. de Boer F, Drager AM, Pinedo HM, et al. Early apoptosis largely accounts for functional impairment of CD34+ cells in frozen-thawed stem cell grafts. J Hematother Stem Cell Res 2002;11:951-63.

33. de Boer F, Drager AM, Pinedo HM, et al. Extensive early apoptosis in frozen-thawed CD34-positive stem cells decreases threshold doses for haematological recovery after autologous peripheral blood progenitor cell transplantation. Bone Marrow Transplant 2002;29:249-55.

34. Chesne C, Guillouzo A. Cryopreservation of isolated rat hepatocytes: A critical evaluation of freezing and thawing conditions. Cryobiology 1988;25:323-30.

35. Powis G, Santone KS, Melder DC, et al. Cryopreservation of rat and dog hepatocytes for studies of xenobiotic metabolism and activation. Drug Metab Dispos 1987;15: 826-32.

36. Gomez-Lechon MJ, Lopez P, Castell JV. Biochemical functionality and recovery of hepatocytes after deep freezing storage. In Vitro 1984;20:826-32.

37. Glass K, Hubel A. Cryopreservation of hematopoietic stem cells: Emerging science, technology and issues. Transfus Med Hemother 2007;34:268-75.

Method 28-1. Cryopreserving Cellular Therapy Products in Freezing Bags

Description

This procedure involves freezing cellular therapy products such as hematopoietic progenitor cells (HPCs) in a dimethyl sulfoxide (DMSO) cryoprotectant at a controlled rate using commercial freezing bags (eg, Cryocyte, Baxter, Deerfield, IL). The HPCs are frozen at a controlled rate until the product reaches –80 C. At that time, the product is transferred to a liquid nitrogen (LN$_2$) storage freezer and maintained at –175 C. Using slow, controlled-rate freezing helps to maintain the viability and functionality of the HPCs to provide the patient with viable stem cells for transplantation.

Summary of Procedure

Intracellular and extracellular ice crystal formation occurring during freezing can cause cell damage. By controlling the rate at which the cells freeze and with the addition of a DMSO-containing freezing medium, the process should yield a cryopreserved, viable product easily stored until needed for patient administration.

Equipment

1. Programmable controlled-rate freezer (CRF) with probe.
2. Freezing press.

3. Cryogloves.
4. LN$_2$ source.

Supplies and Reagents

Labeled freezing cassettes.

Procedure

After the HPCs have been processed and the DMSO freezing medium has been added, perform the following steps:

1. Place the bags flat on the freezing presses. Make sure the product is covered by the top plate and that the ports are free of the plate line.
2. Place the flat end of the temperature probe between a bag and the top plate or between two bags. Ensure that the probe is flat against the bag and centered over the central portion of bag (liquid, not label pocket).
3. Turn the rings on the plate corners to secure the bags.
4. If cryovials have been prepared, place them in the CRF with the product.
5. Perform controlled-rate freezing. Table 28-1-1 gives an example of a freezing program for the Cryomed CRF (model 7452).
6. Monitor the freezing and heat-release processes.

Table 28-1-1. Freezing Process for Cryomed CRF

Step	Rate	Desired Temperature	Location
1	WAIT	0 C	Chamber
2	1.0 C/minute	–4 C	Sample
3	25.0 C/minute	–55 C	Chamber
4	15.0 C/minute	–24 C	Chamber
5	1.0 C/minute	–45 C	Chamber
6	2.0 C/minute	–80 C	Chamber
7	END		

7. Identify locations in the storage freezer for cryobags and cryovials.
8. When the CRF process is complete, remove the frozen products from the freezing press and immediately transfer them and any cryovials to the appropriate freezer locations.
9. Review the freeze graph and file with the processing record.

Anticipated Results

A viable HPC product frozen to –80 C.

Notes

1. Be sure that the CRF is working properly before adding the DMSO freezing media to the cells.

2. If the controlled-rate freezing procedure is interrupted because of instrument malfunction, determine the status of the product and continue freezing according to a validated alternative procedure. Different procedures may be necessary depending on the point where the process was stopped.

References/Resources

1. Areman EM, Deeg HJ, Sacher RA, eds. Bone marrow and stem cell processing: A manual of current techniques. Philadelphia: FA Davis, 1992.
2. FACT-JACIE international standards for cellular therapy product collection, processing, and administration. 4th ed. Omaha, NE: Foundation for the Accreditation of Cellular Therapy and the Joint Accreditation Committee of ISCT and EBMT, 2008.
3. Padley D, ed. Standards for cellular therapy product services. 3rd ed. Bethesda, MD: AABB, 2008.

Method 28-2. Automated Controlled-Rate Freezing, Storage, and Retrieval of Volume-Reduced Cord Blood Units Using the BioArchive System

Description

Manual transfer of hematopoietic cord blood progenitor cell (HPC-C) units from a –80 C or free-standing, controlled-rate freezer (CRF) to a conventional storage Dewar and, subsequently, from storage to a shipping container exposes cryopreserved HPC-C to a wide range of temperatures. Moving one unit from one storage container to another can necessitate temporary removal of an entire rack of cord blood products, including units that are not intended for transfer. The multiple exposures of cryopreserved products to ambient air and to a range of cryogenic temperatures are referred to as transient warming events (TWEs). Because the BioArchive (ThermoGenesis, Rancho Cordova, CA; Fig 28-2-1) is an automated system with integrated modules for freezing, storing, and retrieving HPC-C products, it can reduce the frequency of TWE for individual HPC-C units.

Using this system, HPC-C reduced to a volume of 25 mL are placed in specially designed freezing bags, then frozen and stored in canisters at individ-

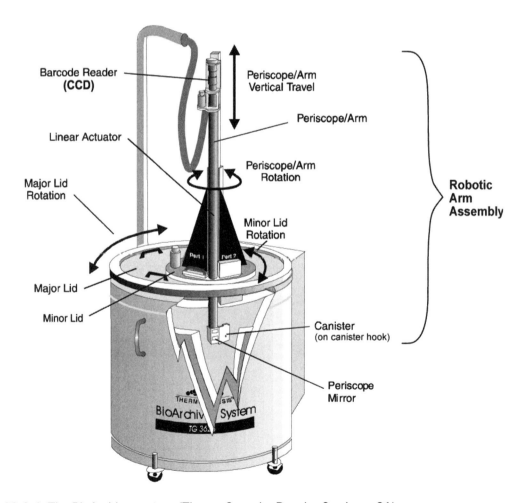

Figure 28-2-1. The BioArchive system (ThermoGenesis, Rancho Cordova, CA).

ual "addresses" in the BioArchive Dewar. The system performs the initial controlled-rate freezing in the gas phase above liquid nitrogen, records the freezing curves, and robotically transfers the unit to its assigned storage address under liquid nitrogen within the same Dewar. When units are retrieved for shipment, the BioArchive robotically removes the individual unit and transfers it from liquid nitrogen into insulated sleeves in the gas phase. The insulated unit is then transferred to a liquid nitrogen-cooled dry shipper for transport.

Time for Procedure

The controlled-rate freezing process for a 25-mL HPC-C unit typically takes 25 to 28 minutes. The user is provided with a chart showing a graph of the freezing curve and relevant details of the process.

Summary of Procedure

1. Activate BioArchive computer.
2. Insert canister into the CRF.
3. Activate controlled-rate freeze.
4. Store HPC-C at long-term storage address under LN_2 (automated storage).

Equipment

1. BioArchive System consisting of the following components:
   a. Liquid nitrogen (LN_2) Dewar and control module with storage rack.
   b. Two integral CRF modules that can be operated individually or simultaneously (Fig 28-2-2):
      i. CRF is inserted into a port in the BioArchive system.
      ii. CRF control module remains above the top surface of the minor lid.
      iii. CRF doors containing the canister are suspended in the LN_2 vapor inside the Dewar.
      iv. When fan mounted at the rear of the CRF doors is activated, nitrogen vapor is forced through the interior of the chamber and controlled cooling of the canister occurs. The rate of cooling of the canister is determined by the speed of the fan.
      v. The temperature on the surface of the freezing bag is monitored by a sensor.

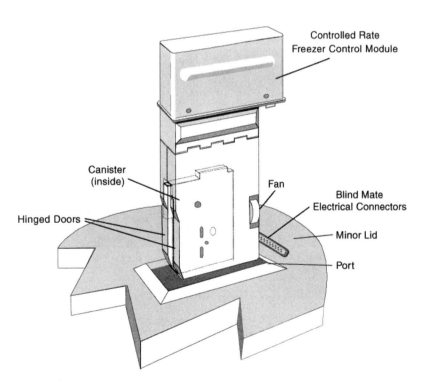

Figure 28-2-2. Controlled-rate freezer (ThermoGenesis).

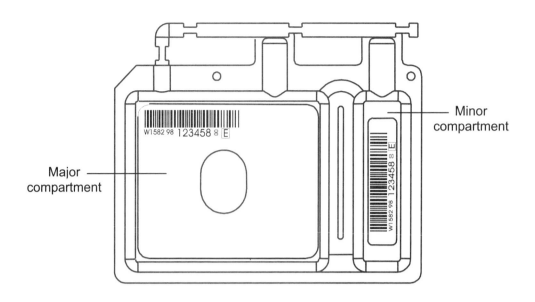

Figure 28-2-3. Freezing bag labeling (ThermoGenesis).

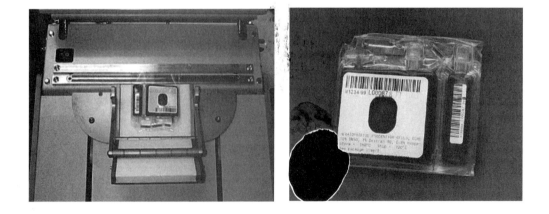

Figure 28-2-4. Overwrapping the freezing bag (ThermoGenesis).

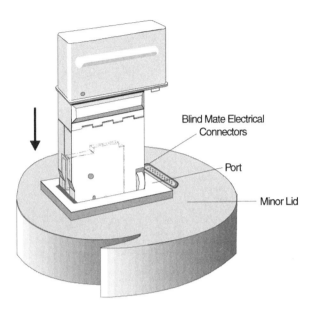

Figure 28-2-5. Controlled-rate freezer is inserted in a port in the BioArchive (ThermoGenesis).

c. Sample retrieval module:
    i. Used for retrieving frozen specimens, it is similar in appearance to the CRF except that the two doors and the fan are not present.
    ii. Contains a frame to hold a foam canister sleeve that slows the warming of the canister when it is removed.
d. Robotic arm assembly consisting of a bar code reader, periscope, and canister hook (see Fig 28-2-1):
    i. An electromechanical system that transports a specimen (contained in a protective canister) from the CRF module to a specific storage address in the Dewar.
    ii. The robotic arm also retrieves the frozen specimen from its storage address when it is needed.
e. Microprocessor and sample management software (SMS) control systems:
    i. Controls the robotic motions, monitors the storage temperature, and maintains records of freeze profiles and system inventory:

• Controls the motion of the robotic arm system and the opening and closing of the doors on the CRF.
• Assigns the specific addresses at which each canister containing a specimen is to be stored.
• Maintains the location of each specific specimen in the database.
• Stores the specimen identification, time and date the specimen was frozen, and temperature-vs-time data that are obtained during freezing.
2. Impulse sealer.

Procedure

1. Label the canister.
2. Label the freezing bag, both major and minor compartments (Fig 28-2-3).
3. Overwrap the freezing bag (Fig 28-2-4): place the labeled freezing bag in an overwrap bag and seal using the impulse sealer.
4. Place the bag into the canister and close the canister.
5. Place the canister in the CRF.
6. Store the product in the BioArchive.
    a. After the canister containing the overwrapped freezing bag is placed in the CRF, the freezing process can be initiated.
    b. To initiate the freeze:
        i. Select the port to be used. If both are available, either one can be used.
        ii. Remove the port plug from that port.
        iii. Gently insert the CRF in a port with the exposed side of the canister facing the periscope shaft (Fig 28-2-5).
    c. Fully seat the CRF gently in the port. Within a few seconds, the LED on the CRF will turn red and the system will move to read the bar code label on the canister. When complete, the identification of the sample will appear in the sample identification part of the display, and the port status will indicate "idle."
    d. Click on BIOARCHIVE, STORE.
    e. The store dialog box will appear. If you are using bar code verification, the system will automatically select the port by comparing

Table 28-2-1. Anticipated Results

No. Unit	Res Vol. (mL)	Final Vol. (mL)	Initial TNCs 10⁶	% TNC Recov. Post-proc.	Total Initial Ly+Mo 10⁶	% Ly+Mo Recov. Post-proc.	Total CD 34+ Initial 10³	CD 34+ Viab. Initial %	Total CD34+ Post-Proc. 10³	CD 34+ % Viab. Post-proc.	CD34+ % Recov. Post-proc.	Total CFUs Pre-proc. (Initial)	Total CFUs Post-proc. (Final)	% CFU Recov. Post-proc.	% CFU Recovery Post-thaw (from Final)	CD34+ % Viab. Post-thaw
Avg.	93	20	1150	85	453	98	3364.5	99.74	3256.9	99.75	98.2	2,625,043	2,471,223	94.6	96	94.3
SD	12.5	0.03		9.2		4.9		0.3		0.2	8.0			7.0	4.8	2.1

Avg = average; SD = standard deviation; Res Vol. = residual volume; TNCs = Total nucleated cells; Recov. Postproc. = recovered postprocessing; Viab. = viability; CFU = colony-forming unit; Preproc. = preprocessing.

the sample identification entered with the canister bar code.

Anticipated Results

See Table 28-2-1.

References/Resources

1. Kobylka, Ivanyi P, Breur-Vriesendorp BS. Preservation of immunological and colony-forming capacities of long-term (15 years) cryopreserved cord blood cells. Transplantation 1998;65:1275-8.
2. Donnenberg AD, Koch EK, Griffin DL, et al. Viability of cryopreserved BM progenitor cells stored for more than a decade. Cytotherapy 2002;4:157-63.
3. Broxmeyer HE, Cooper S. High-efficiency recovery of immature haematopoietic progenitor cells with extensive proliferative capacity from human cord blood cryopreserved for 10 years. Clin Exp Immunol 1997;107 (Suppl 1):45-53.
4. Broxmeyer HE, Srour EF, Hangoc G. High-efficiency recovery of functional hematopoietic progenitor and stem cells from human cord blood cryopreserved for 15 years. Proc Natl Acad Sci U S A 2003;100:645-50.
5. Mugishima H, Harada K, Chin M, et al. Effects of long-term cryopreservation on hematopoietic progenitor cells in umbilical cord blood. Bone Marrow Transplant 1999;23:395-6.
6. Dobrila L, et al. Transient warming events and cell viability of placental/umbilical cord blood (PCB). Presented at ISHAGE meeting, Quebec City, PQ, Canada, June 14-17, 2001.

In: Areman EM, Loper K, eds
Cellular Therapy: Principles, Methods, and Regulations
Bethesda, MD: AABB, 2009

◆◆◆   **29**   ◆◆◆

Cryopreservation Containers for Cellular Therapy Products

Herbert M. Cullis, MT, and Mary Dadone, PhD

BECAUSE THIS DISCUSSION IS LIMITED TO storage containers designed for clinical use, it does not address methods of storage and transport such as sperm delivery straws, screw-top containers, or vials that have removable caps and that can expose contents to the environment when opened. A freezing container for cellular therapy (CT) products must accommodate aseptic filling, reliable sterile containment, and aseptic product removal.

Freezing Bags: General Considerations

Selection of freezing bag sizes can be challenging, especially since bag manufacturers specify two volumes for their containers: 1) total capacity and 2) freezing capacity. The freezing capacity is based on the volume that can be accommodated between metal plates, used with some controlled-rate freezers (CRFs), that are between 4 and 10 mm apart. Ideally, the bags will have ports for filling that can be sealed off and removed before freezing. Ports for withdrawing the product should be hermetically sealed until entry after thawing. A means of containing label information that prevents loss or damage should be provided.

CT products may be cryopreserved before or after culture. Some freezing bags can be used directly for culture, thereby reducing risks of product loss or contamination that might occur in transferring the product to another bag. Sterile connecting devices should be considered for all transfers to maintain a sterile fluid path. Because some manufacturing conditions may require a specific shape or port configuration for optimal results, some manufacturers offer to provide customized containers upon request. Freezing bags should provide for retention of samples in the form of segments or aliquots that are available for pre-thaw testing without compromising the integrity of the primary bag contents.

Container Materials

Since the 1960s, red cells have been frozen in bags made of polyvinylchloride (PVC) plastic. However,

---

Herbert M. Cullis, MT, President, American Fluoroseal Corp, Gaithersburg, Maryland, and Mary Dadone, PhD, Consultant, Annapolis, Maryland

The authors have disclosed no conflicts of interest.

other materials may be required for bags used for freezing CT products such as hematopoietic progenitor cells (HPCs) and leukocytes for immunotherapy, because such products require different cryoprotectants, freezing conditions, and postprocessing manipulation.

Cryopreservation containers are made from several types of plastic that are broadly classified as either plasticized or plasticizer-free. Most bags are made from polyolefins and are frequently mixtures of these plastics. This group includes polyethylene (PE), polypropylene (PP), PVC, and ethyl vinyl acetate (EVA). Most of these materials, including those mentioned, are rigid unless plasticizer oils such as di(2-ethylhexyl)phthalate (DEHP) or citric adipate (CA) are added. However, these plasticizer oils do not provide flexibility below the crystalline temperature of the plastics (in the range of –42 C for nonfluorocarbon plastics), which will crack at temperatures below –42 C if flexed. Fluorocarbon plastics such as fluoroethylene propylene (FEP) and polyvinyl vinylidene fluoride (PVDF) are naturally flexible and remain flexible at liquid nitrogen (LN_2) temperatures without the addition of plasticizers.

Dimethyl sulfoxide (DMSO), a commonly used cryoprotectant for cells, is also a solvent for most common plastics, including PVC. DMSO has been routinely used at refrigerator temperatures to control its tendency to dissolve plastic and to counteract the large exothermal reaction that occurs when it is added to freezing solutions. DMSO has no effect on FEP plastics at any temperature. All bag materials must be certified to be safe and effective for the purpose of containing cryopreserved cells for human use. Although it is not possible for the plastic to guarantee the effectiveness of the CT product, it is possible for the plastic to influence or reduce the effectiveness of the product by adsorbing, absorbing, or leaching materials into the cryopreserved material. Although it is essential for bag materials to meet USP Class VI biological compatibility or an equivalent, some manufacturers can also provide more extensive testing information. It remains the responsibility of the user to demonstrate that the safety and effectiveness of the CT product are not impaired by the container material.

Freezer Cassette Size

Freezer cassettes are usually supplied by the manufacturer of the freezer or the manufacturer of the storage frame or "rack" inside the freezer. Because the cassettes and frames can be expensive, facilities usually establish a standard freezer cassette size and may already possess a large inventory of these materials. Cassette size is a consideration when selecting freezing containers and should be considered early on in the container selection process. Storage freezer manufacturers may offer several different sizes and configurations. Cassette thickness may be 4 mm or 10 mm. If the institution has an existing inventory system designed for a specific bag size, it may be limited in its new freezing bag selection options. Some freezing cassettes have additional features such as "windows" to view the label without opening the cassette. Validation of the cryopreservation process should include using the specific cassette that is planned for the clinical freezing procedure.

Freezer Temperature

The temperature of a "mechanical" (dual-stage Freon) storage freezer may be –70 or –80 C, whereas temperatures of the new "cascade" low-temperature mechanical freezers may be as low as –125 C. "Vapor-phase" LN_2 freezers may be between –125 and –175 C, and the temperature in LN_2 is –196 C. Bag storage conditions will influence bag selection, the need for an overwrap, and the chances of bag failure. At temperatures below –18 C, the water component of cryopreservation cell media freezes into pure water crystals, excluding gases such as carbon dioxide and oxygen into bubbles in the center of the freezing bag. At this point, the bag may still be flexible, but the contents are rigid. (See detailed discussion earlier in this chapter.) At freezing temperatures above –40 C, most bags will survive freezing, thawing, and moderate handling. However, at temperatures below –42 C, PVC, EVA, PP, polyolefin, and other nonfluorocarbon plastic bags become rigid and will fracture if flexed or mechanically shocked. At temperatures below –78 C, carbon dioxide solidifies into dry ice. As thawing temperatures rise above –78 C, solid dry ice changes into a carbon dioxide gas phase, increasing in volume 960 times. This expansion places extreme stress on non-fluorocarbon bags, which cannot flex to absorb this increase in volume.

The chance of contamination by cryopreserved organisms entering a port or a fracture in a freezing container would appear to be less for products stored in mechanical or nitrogen vapor freezers than in LN_2 freezers, where the liquid may act as a vehicle for microbial transfer. Even with vapor-phase nitrogen storage, there is a risk that failure of the LN_2 fill valve could allow the vapor-phase space to be flooded with LN_2. The submersion of screw-capped plastic vials may permit contact between contaminated LN_2 and the sample contained in the vial. Condensation of the atmosphere within a tube or vial can create a vacuum, drawing in LN_2. One study described a series of patients who became infected with the hepatitis B virus, apparently transmitted to products stored in a contaminated LN_2 storage tank.[1] The hepatitis B DNA detected in these patients matched that in the LN_2. Numerous studies have reported fungal and bacterial contamination of LN_2 freezers and of cryopreserved products.[2,3] LN_2 also presents the greatest risk of contamination by cryopreserved microbes because the potentially contaminated liquid contacts all parts of the bag and can seep under the port covers. The use of plastic overwrap bags as an additional barrier between the product and the LN_2 environment has been implemented in a number of cryopreservation facilities.

Container Filling

When available, the use of closed systems in CT product manufacturing is preferred over systems that are open to the environment. The use of a sterile connection device can extend the closed system from the introduction of the collected product through processing and cryopreservation stages. Although most freezing bags are available with filling ports such as luer fittings, connection by sterile docking might still be the optimal means of maintaining an aseptic environment. If it is necessary to cryopreserve multiple aliquots of frozen cells, a manifold device for filling bags could be considered.

A sterility assurance level (SAL) of 10^{-3} has been demonstrated with the sterile connection devices manufactured by Terumo, Fenwal, and Haemonetics.[4,5] The freezing bag should be equipped with PVC tubing that is 4 mm (0.158 inches, outside diameter) by 3 mm (0.118 inches, inside diameter) to fit the sterile connection device. Most other plastics cannot be sterile-docked because either the materials do not melt at the temperature of the sterile connection device or the materials do not become sticky when melted. Most intravenous tubing and most blood bank tubing is 4 mm PVC, whereas the tubing in dialysis equipment is usually a larger size and is not appropriate for use with the sterile connection device.

Container Volume

Freezing containers should be selected to contain a volume that can be frozen at a thickness that can be accommodated by freezing cassettes and CRFs. The most commonly used bags for freezing CT products are generally limited to a volume of 70 mL per bag, but larger and smaller volume containers are also available. It is advisable to work with manufacturers if special volumes are needed.

Container Overwraps

If cells are stored in LN_2, bags should be hermetically sealed to prevent contact with the liquid environment. LN_2 is not sterile, and, as previously mentioned, a report from 1995[1] described viral transmission to cryopreserved products and their recipients through an LN_2 storage tank. One safety measure that can be used to protect the frozen product from nitrogen penetration is to place the bag in an overwrap before or after freezing. Overwrap materials include the plastics mentioned above from which freezing bags are commonly made, as well as Kapton (apolyamide, DuPont, Wilmington, DE). Kapton is orange colored, can be written on, and remains strong and flexible in LN_2. Kapton does not seal to itself but can be obtained in a laminate in which Kapton is bonded to FEP, which can be heat-sealed. This FEP/Kapton combination provides protection against the external force of nitrogen penetration.

Product Removal

Removal of CT products from their cryopreservation containers requires use of aseptic techniques to recover the thawed cells because PVC tubing suitable for sterile docking is not considered to be reliable after freezing. It also may be advisable to sanitize or disinfect the exterior of the freezing bag before transferring the product.

References/Resources

1. Tedder RS, Zuckerman MA, Goldstone AH, et al. Hepatitis B transmission from a contaminated cryopreservation tank. Lancet 1995;346:137-40.

2. Fountain D, Ralston M, Higgins N, et al. Liquid nitrogen freezers: A potential source of microbial contamination of hematopoietic stem cell components. Transfusion 1997;37:585-91.

3. Klein M, Kadidlo D, McCullough J, et al. Microbial contamination of hematopoietic stem cell products: Incidence and clinical sequelae. Biol Blood Marrow Transplant 2006;12:1142-9.

4. AuBuchon JP, Pickard C, Herschel L. Sterility of plastic tubing welds in components stored at room temperature. Transfusion 1995;35:303-7.

5. European Committee for Standardization (CEN). European Standard EN 556-1:2001. Sterilization of medical devices—Requirements for medical devices to be designated "STERILE." Part I: Requirements for terminally sterilized medical devices. Brussels, Belgium: CEN, 2001.

In: Areman EM, Loper K, eds
Cellular Therapy: Principles, Methods, and Regulations
Bethesda, MD: AABB, 2009

♦ ♦ ♦   30   ♦ ♦ ♦

Transportation and Shipping of Cellular Therapy Products

Donna Regan, MT(ASCP)

SAFE TRANSPORTATION OF CELLULAR therapy (CT) products is an essential component of successful patient treatment. Hematopoietic progenitor cell (HPC) products are frequently collected from unrelated donors who are not in the same location as the recipient and are often processed and/or cryopreserved at a facility in another city, state, or country. The cells need to be shipped to the infusion site in a manner that ensures the safety of personnel and property who come in contact with the product and its packing material, while protecting the integrity of the cellular components. In addition, the shipping container must conform to both the shipper's and receiver's local regulations regarding the mode of transport.

Product Procurement

Multiple factors are critical to patient outcome. Identification of a suitable HPC product for transplant is accomplished by searching worldwide data-

bases of volunteer donors. Sources of unrelated donor cells include anticoagulated marrow and peripheral blood stem cells or umbilical cord blood (UCB). Freshly collected products may be processed before infusion. The specific processing procedures are determined by the treatment protocol and can be as simple as plasma depletion and cryopreservation or as extensive as CD34+ selection, T cell depletion, or genetic manipulation (ie, viral transduction or gene therapy). Increasingly stringent and evolving standards have greatly escalated the cost of operating a compliant, dedicated processing facility. Health-care restrictions and insurance reimbursement policies have also encouraged the centralization of these services, which necessitates the shipping of HPC products to transplant centers.

Unrelated donors are selected based on a comprehensive assessment of their medical and social history to qualify them as safe donors, and they are thoroughly tested for infectious diseases using the latest techniques. Therefore, the majority of collected products are considered nonhazardous.

Donna Regan, MT(ASCP), Executive Director, St Louis Cord Blood Bank and Cellular Therapy Laboratory at SSM Cardinal Glennon Children's Medical Center, St Louis, Missouri

The author has disclosed no conflicts of interest.

Fresh Products

Shipment of fresh products directly to a transplant center is typical for a patient who has already received high-dose immunosuppressive therapy in preparation for transplant. In these cases, products are hand-carried by a properly trained courier, and a plan is in place for alternative transport in case of an emergency. Fresh products generally travel at cool temperatures, facilitated by frozen or refrigerated gel packs, via a dedicated representative of the registry or transplant center. Products that leave the collection facility or are shipped on public roads are carried in an outer shipping container. This container can be a simple, thermally insulated cooler adequate to withstand leakage of contents, shocks, pressure changes, and other conditions incident to ordinary handling in transportation. Because couriers are in direct control of the containers at all times, incidents that occur during their transport can be immediately addressed. If a problem should arise, adequate time and resources are often available to restore the proper conditions for transport.

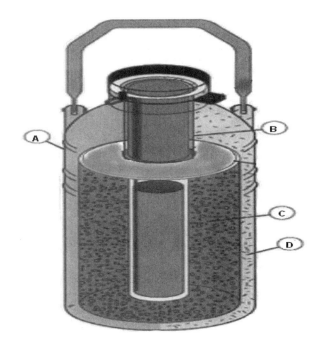

Figure 30-1. Cross section of a dry shipper.[1] A = outer aluminum wall; B = foam lid; C = hydrophobic absorbent material; D = vacuum space (insulation).

Cryopreserved Products

HPCs may be frozen in a cryoprotectant solution at temperatures that place the cells in metabolic stasis. The frozen product may be stored immersed in liquid nitrogen (LN_2), in the vapor phase of LN_2, or in mechanical freezers. A temperature maintained below −150 C is generally recommended for long-term storage. Products can be frozen in specially designed cryobags or vials capable of withstanding these low temperatures for prolonged periods.

Equipment and Cautions

Dry Shippers

LN_2 dry shippers are designed and constructed to ship HPC products safely at very cold temperatures. Dry shippers are constructed of an internal cylinder that hangs from the neck of the vessel, surrounded by an absorbent layer, a vacuum-jacketed insulation layer, and an outer container that houses the vessel (Fig 30-1). The absorbent layer is designed to absorb LN_2 within the walls of the shipper, removing the risks associated with LN_2 contact. Therefore, as long as they are completely drained of

excess LN_2, dry shippers are not considered hazardous and are not regulated. Dry shippers contain sufficient absorbed LN_2 to maintain the storage chamber temperature below −150 C for an extended period of time, usually 5 to 15 days. This period is well within the requirement that they maintain temperature for at least 48 hours beyond the expected time of arrival at the receiving facility.

LN_2 vapor is heavier than air. When the shipper is stored upright in the cargo space of an aircraft or transport vehicle, the escape of LN_2 vapor from the vessel into the surrounding environment occurs at a rate that does not pose a risk to personnel handling the shipper, animals in small cargo, or passengers. The outer shell allows for safe handling of the inner vessel, protects the shipper from physical injury, and is designed to ensure that the shipper will be maintained in an upright position (see Figs 30-2 and 30-3). The outer shell should be sealed or locked in a way that opening or tampering of the shipper is evident. This can be accomplished with a padlock (either on the inner vessel or on the outer shell) or with tie tags or tape.

Vessels must be charged according to the manufacturer's instructions[2] for most effective function.

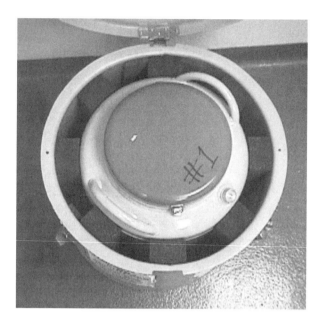

Figure 30-2. View of a dry shipper's opened outer shell, showing the foam packing that helps to stabilize the transport vessel and protect it from impact.

Typical charging instructions specify that the operator perform the following steps:

1. Fill the dry shipper cavity just above the upper cavity holes. The LN_2 will be absorbed into the sides of the container where the absorbent material is located.
2. Wait at least 3 hours and refill the dry shipper cavity just above the upper cavity holes. Caution should be taken not to overfill the vessels because dangerous spillage can occur when the lid is placed back into the necktube.
3. Allow the dry shipper to hold the LN_2 until the following day.
4. Pour off the remaining LN_2. The dry shipper is now ready for use.

Vessels and shippers are designed to operate with little or no internal pressure build-up. The use of tight-fitting stoppers or plugs in the necktube that do not allow venting of the gas causes pressure build-up that can damage or rupture the inner vessel.

Data Loggers

Data loggers are electronic recording instruments that monitor environmental conditions over time. For cryogenic transport, these devices allow continuous measurement and tracking of temperature

throughout the duration of shipment. Combined with shipping records, data loggers can designate location, indicating when the vessel was opened for retrieval of the product or whether it was tampered with during shipment. Software allows the downloading of information from the device, providing a temperature-tracing graph for a shipping facility's records.

Limitations and Recommendations

Dry Shippers

Though LN_2 dry shippers are sturdy and able to handle the normal bumps of transit, certain circumstances can compromise their function. For example, shippers that have been dropped and their vacuum compromised will lose their temperature control very quickly since the vacuum provides the insulation. All cryogenic vessels must be transported in an upright position. If allowed to tip, shippers on their sides cannot properly regulate the rate at which LN_2 vapor escapes from the vessel. In

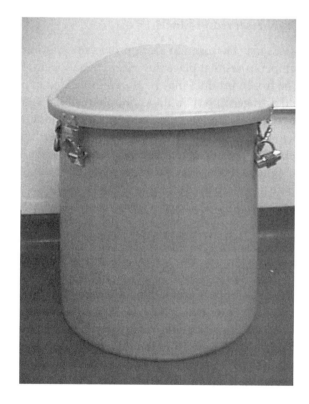

Figure 30-3. A typical dry shipper's outer shell, which helps maintain the package in an upright position.

this position, LN_2 dry shippers lose their charge in a matter of hours. Manufacturer's instructions should always be followed. Shippers improperly or not fully charged will not hold temperatures for the time originally validated by the facility. Transportation of products in dry shippers is generally very safe; however, handling LN_2 and cryobiologic shippers can be extremely hazardous if proper precautions are not taken. Personal protective equipment is necessary for handling products stored at very low temperatures. Cryogloves are used to protect the hands from the cold as well as exposure of the products to body temperature while transferring products from storage into the shippers. Impervious lab coats and face shields should be worn to protect the eyes, face, and body from LN_2 splashes and spills.

Liquid Nitrogen

Two basic properties of LN_2 must always be understood and respected:

1. LN_2 is extremely cold. At atmospheric pressure, LN_2 boils at −196 C (−320 F).
2. LN_2 is an asphyxiant. It vaporizes into large amounts of gas (1 L of liquid produces 25 cubic feet of gas), displacing oxygen in the surrounding air.

In consideration of these characteristics, LN_2 should never be allowed to touch bare skin because serious frostbite injury can result; human tissues freeze almost instantaneously upon contact. When working with LN_2 or items cooled by LN_2, handlers must always wear insulated gloves that are loose fitting for quick removal should they become saturated or liquid splash into them. Objects cooled by LN_2 will stick to bare skin and may tear the skin when removed. Always use forceps or tongs to remove objects from storage vessels. Medical help should be sought immediately in the event of exposure to LN_2 or cold nitrogen gas or in the event that a worker becomes dizzy or loses consciousness. Because it is tasteless, odorless, and colorless, the gas can easily reduce the air's oxygen content below the level needed for safe breathing before it has been detected. Thus, LN_2 must be stored and used only in a well-ventilated area. Enclosed trucks and vans should be used with caution as transport vehicles because of the potential for nitrogen gas build-

up, which can result in suffocation. The cloud of vapor observed when working with LN_2 is condensed water vapor and cold nitrogen gas. When exposed to cold nitrogen gas, delicate tissues such as those of the eyes can be damaged even when the contact is too brief to affect the skin of the hands and face. Always wear a face shield when working with or around LN_2 or cold nitrogen gas. Even high gas concentrations can burn exposed skin and cause frostbite.

Blood-Borne Pathogens

Although HPC donors are thoroughly screened and tested, all infectious disease test results may not be available before product shipment. HPC products should be handled as though they were capable of transmitting disease, including the use of secondary containers such as sealable bags and wearing gloves when directly handling the product.

General Guidelines

Most CT product shipments are medically urgent in nature, and all personnel involved with this activity must understand the importance of timely delivery. With air transport, the number of connecting flights should be minimized to reduce transit time and excessive handling of the package. Products should not be exposed to x-ray or irradiation devices designed to detect metal objects. Some studies have shown that exposure to standard airport security x-ray machine radiation does not decrease cell viability or the content of colony-forming unit (CFU) or long-term culture-initiating cell (LT-CIC) activity.[3] However, the effect of airport radiation exposure on long-term engraftment potential has yet to be determined. Accordingly, although the effect of radiation exposure at these levels is thought to be negligible, the calibration of these x-ray devices and the delivery of radiation may not be consistent. Therefore, exposure to these devices is discouraged.

Airports require x-ray or physical examination of packages and their contents. It is permissible for the contents of the container to be inspected by hand. However, inspection of dry shippers poses a potential safety hazard for airline employees who may lack proper training and equipment such as cryogloves for examination of products. Inspection also poses a risk of physical trauma to frozen cellular products if improperly handled.

Requirements regarding the temperature at which HPCs should be shipped vary by the cell source and applicable regulations or standards. To provide an additional margin of safety, frozen units are generally transported in dry shippers capable of maintaining a temperature substantially below that required. An advantage of shipping frozen products is that they can be stored at the infusion facility before conditioning the patient for transplant. Alternatively, if an immediate need exists—for example, for a second product for an already ablated patient whose primary graft has failed—the product can be immediately thawed, processed, and infused. Because there are so many opportunities for unexpected changes to arise in any transplant agenda, it is important to procure the product as soon as possible after confirming the transplant date.

Responsibilities of Personnel Involved with Transport

The responsibilities of all personnel involved with the transportation of CT products do not end until the package has safely reached its destination. All personnel should be available for contact throughout the duration of the trip.

Consigner

A consigner is the company, hospital, or laboratory that is responsible for dispatching the shipment. The shipping facility may not necessarily be the consigner but, rather, may be an employee or company hired by the consigner. The shipping facility should be familiar with shipping requirements, recognize the hazards presented by the transport of the products, understand procedures for safe handling of the materials associated with the shipments, and plan for emergency procedures in case of an accident. Additionally, the shipper should have training specific to the products being transported.

Only the consigner has first-hand knowledge of what the package contains. Therefore, the shipping facility is responsible for properly classifying the package as nonhazardous material and identifying its contents in detail. The shipping facility should pack the product in a manner that protects it from physical trauma, maintains the temperature throughout transport, and ensures the safety of all individuals who come in contact with the package. The package must be clearly labeled with the name and address of the destination, as well as a contact name and number, in case communication regarding transport is necessary. Additionally, the package should be marked as "medically urgent" and be accompanied by instructions describing its proper handling. After being notified of a product request, the shipping facility should communicate first with the courier to arrange shipment and then with the receiving institution to transmit the transport agenda in preparation for the product's arrival. In the case of international shipments, the shipping facility must also prepare customs documents as required by the local government for importation into a foreign country. Details of shipping activity should be well documented and retained at the shipper's facility for easy reference.

When the shipping facility prepares to retrieve the product from storage, the identity of the product should be verified against the requesting facility's documents to ensure shipment of the correct component. This task is routinely carried out by two members of the shipping facility staff. A final review of the product documents should be performed for last-minute qualification of the unit before its export.

The shipping facility is responsible for validating the integrity of the transport vessel and its ability to maintain proper temperature. Appropriate qualification of the vessel should be performed before each use to ensure that it is operating as expected. The dry shipper is prepared according to manufacturer's instructions.

Operator (Courier)

The operator is an individual, company, or airline that agrees to transport a package from its point of origin to its destination. Couriers are professionals who ensure that airline regulations and security and customs requirements are resolved before the actual shipment. Upon presentation of the package, the courier inspects it and its accompanying documents. The courier's responsibility begins when the acceptance checklist has been completed. The courier has the right to open or inspect any package if he or she believes the package has been classified incorrectly and should be considered dangerous, or if he or she suspects the package may be improperly prepared for shipment. The courier can request a signed statement from the shipper that the package contents are not dangerous and can consult with an outside authority for clarification if necessary. During transport, the courier is responsible for properly storing and loading the package, protecting it from physical trauma, and ensuring the safety of all who come in contact with it. The courier delivers the package and its associated documents to its destination.

Consignee (Receiving Facility)

The consignee is the receiving institution, most likely a processing facility or transplant center. When shipping frozen products, it is essential that the receiving laboratory have proper facilities for storage. It is also imperative to inspect the container upon its arrival and to transfer the product to a suitable storage location as soon as possible. The consignee documents the condition of the package and its contents and relays that information to the shipping facility.

Procedure

Shipping arrangements are made before the day of transport, usually through a courier, which may be a same day/overnight delivery service. Timing of collections and delivery should be mutually agreed upon by consigner and consignee, in accordance with the patient transplant conditioning regimen and the anticipated time of infusion.

The shipping agenda should be communicated in detail to the receiving facility so that preparations can be made to accept and inspect the shipping container immediately on arrival. Communication is vital, both in terms of arranging shipment with the courier and advising the transplant center of what to expect and at what time. Occasionally, this itinerary is communicated to the registry that is coordinating transfer of the product. Delivery of the unit is scheduled with the receiving facility at a time when qualified personnel are available to transfer the product to appropriate storage. Arrangements should also be made for prompt return of the dry shipper for quality control and maintenance of the shipper inventory.

Noncryopreserved Products

A CT product that is not cryopreserved is placed in a secondary plastic bag that is sealed to prevent leakage. The product is then surrounded by absorbent material that is capable of containing the entire contents of the product in the event that the primary and secondary containers become compromised during transit.

Cryopreserved Products

Delivery of cryopreserved products is usually arranged before inititation of patient conditioning for transplant. The shipping facility should notify the receiver of the type (cryobags or vials) and dimensions of the container to be shipped to permit proper handling and storage by the receiving institution. Frozen products are placed in a LN_2 dry shipper as described above and surrounded by styrofoam or similar packing material to absorb any impact in transit. Dry shipper characteristics that can be monitored are weight, temperature, and appearance. All should be checked before leaving the shipping facility and again when received at the facility that is to store and administer the product. If continuous monitoring is desired to track the temperature of the vessel during shipment, an electronic data logger can be used.

Upon receipt, the facility verifies the presence of cryogenic material in the shipper by recording the weight and temperature of the internal vessel. Receiving personnel must inspect the product labeling and container integrity. This review should be done while the product is in the vapor phase of LN_2 to avoid rapid warming and a potential rupture of the product container.

International Export

International exports pose unique issues. Different languages can be a barrier to effective communication. Additional infectious disease tests may be required by the health ministry or other agency for acceptance into a particular country.

Importation papers are prepared by the consignee/receiver and provided to the shipping facility to accompany the product in transport. Supplementary customs papers may be prepared by the shipping facility and should also accompany the product. All documents must be made available to the appropriate personnel during shipment.

Potential Problems

Flight delays or cancellations can occur as a result of weather or a variety of other conditions. For instance, delivery of products in transit during the September 11th, 2001 emergency were rerouted when all flights were cancelled for several days. Ground transit became especially important during this time, as did flexibility in travel agenda and preparation of the patient for transplantation. Communication of delays and cancellations is critical for alleviating anxiety in both shippers and receivers.

Shipping Validation/Qualification

Whether shipping unfrozen or cryopreserved products, it is important that the shipping process and procedures be validated. The purpose of the validation is to demonstrate that the method and all of its related procedures result in acceptable product recovery. Additionally, a proper validation can be useful for providing a reference for those shipping excursions outside the norm. For example, typical shipments of a UCB unit may take <24 hours from collection to receipt at the processing laboratory, or from the cryopreservation facility to the transplant center. However, a delay might be encountered that results in a 42-hour transport. Validation data extending beyond the range of the typical time frame can provide assurance that the proper temperature was maintained, which leads to expected product viability and cell recovery.

When preparing a validation plan for a thermal insulated container or an LN_2 dry shipper, the following items should be considered:

1. Shipping temperature range. As much as is feasible, extremes at both ends should be tested. Does the outer container maintain an appropriate temperature for the required number of hours or days at both 90 F and 0 F, representing extreme weather conditions? This question will be important if the shipping occurs year-round and from several parts of the country or internationally. Minimum/maximum thermometers and data loggers may be especially helpful.
2. Length of shipment. Holding studies can be performed to emulate shipping conditions. If a stability study was performed with a fresh product to determine expiration date, for example, the baseline information may already exist. It is best to test the system for longer time periods than anticipated in case excursions from the shipment protocol are encountered.
3. Weight. LN_2 contributes additional weight to a dry shipper and may be a good indicator of the rate of LN_2 loss from a dry shipper over time.
4. Sturdiness. Both the exterior and interior shipping container should be inspected and documented so that physical changes can be detected.

Clinical cell sources for validation studies may not be readily available. In some situations, bags of water or media can be used to simulate temperature conditions. Certain CT products not acceptable for clinical use because of donor eligibility issues or nonconforming product characteristics may be adequate for use in holding studies for determining stability over time and under various conditions. Colleagues in other cell processing facilities may be willing to receive, open, and return a package, or one could even ship a product to one's own facility to monitor courier performance.

Just as initial validation is important in ensuring that CT products arrive in good condition, maintaining container integrity, which can be affected by a number of factors during transport, is crucial. Dry shippers that may have sustained damage undetectable by physical examination should be requalified before reuse to ensure that the integrity of the shipper was maintained throughout the transport and is in good condition for the next trip. If performance does not meet expectation, a full revalidation is appropriate.

Quality Control: Dry Shippers

Good laboratory practice mandates that dry shippers be validated before being placed in service and qualified upon return to ensure that the shipper's integrity was not compromised in transit. Monitoring the length of time the nitrogen charge is maintained for each shipper and comparing it to the initial validation will help detect the degradation of shipper quality.

Weight

Before a dry shipper is placed into service, it should be weighed before and after being properly charged. Noting that 1 L of LN_2 weighs 1.78 pounds, the laboratory can determine the amount of LN_2 absorbed by the shipper. This value helps to establish a baseline rate of LN_2 evaporation for a particular dry shipper. Once established, this measurement can serve to gauge shipper integrity upon return and to indicate deterioration as the vessel ages.

Temperature

Colorimetric thermal indicators were once regarded as the optimal devices for ensuring proper temperature throughout shipment. Once activated, these indicators change color from green to red when their temperature limit has been exceeded, and indicators with different temperature limits are available. For instance, if a –120-C indicator is placed into the bottom of a shipping container and the temperature within rises above that tolerance limit, an activated indicator will turn from green to red. When the indicator turns red, it remains red. Location of the indicator within the shipper is important, and its placement should take into account the storage conditions of the frozen product. If set at the top of the vessel, the indicator may turn red as the shipper lid is removed and warm air from the room rushes across the top of the shipper. In this instance, the indicator does not reflect the true interior temperature of the vessel and could cause unnecessary alarm. Personnel unpacking the shipping container should immediately, upon opening the container, note the color of the indicator. They should not wait to check it until after it has been unpacked and placed at room temperature. Because these indicators are not designed to reflect the temperatures required for cryogenic shipping, the use of colorimetric thermal indicators has recently been discontinued for shipping frozen CT products.

Data loggers are electronic monitors that permit continuous measurement of temperature throughout the duration of shipment. When set to intervals of seconds to minutes, they can track temperature and location, indicating when the vessel was opened for retrieval of the product or whether the container was tampered with during shipment. The device allows the shipping facility to download the recorded data once the shipping container is returned to the site. The use of data loggers does not preclude the need for the receiving facility to assess the container temperature upon receipt. When the data logger is equipped with a temperature display, the receiving facility can record the temperature before unpacking the vessel. Alternatively, the facility can use a calibrated thermometer probe to measure the internal vessel temperature. Because not all receiving facilities possess equipment that can accurately measure such extreme temperatures, data logging devices with visual displays may be preferred. Whether or not a data logger enables visual temperature reading, most shipping facilities forward a temperature tracing to the receiving facility after the dry shipper has been returned and the data downloaded.

Appearance

A visual check of the shipper's condition must be performed regularly, and any evidence of damage should prompt immediate evaluation of the container (see Fig 30-4). Also, the bottom should be examined for an increase in concavity indicating loss of vacuum, possibly from the impact of being dropped (see Fig 30-5). A shipper whose vacuum has been compromised will bubble excessively or "boil" for an extended period of time after being filled with LN_2, even when the temperature of the vessel stabilizes. Excessive condensation may appear on the outside of the vessel if the vacuum has been compromised or if the insulation has been lost.

Problem Documentation and Corrective Action

All incidents and accidents that occur during transit must be documented, and a corrective action plan must be implemented to prevent their recurrence.

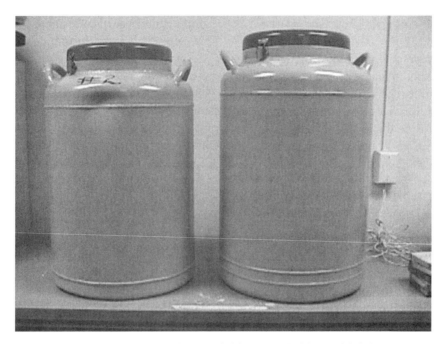

Figure 30-4. Damage evident to the side of a shipper (left); normal shipper (right).

Paperwork and Labeling

Therapeutic indications and contraindications for the use of CT products can be found in the *Circular of Information for Cellular Therapy Products* and should be made available to the patient by the transplant center.

Product labeling and/or supplemental paperwork accompanying the product should provide a detailed description, including all materials used in the collection, processing, and/or cryopreservation of the product. These documents should include the most recent infectious disease testing results, the cellular characteristics of the products, and reg-

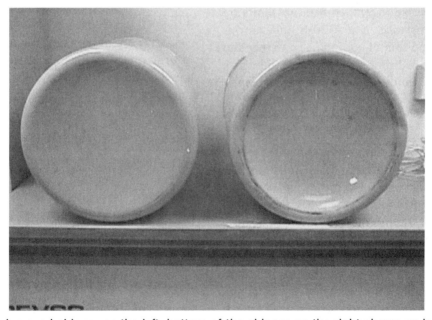

Figure 30-5. Undamaged shipper on the left; bottom of the shipper on the right shows an increase in concavity. Damage to the vacuum jacket could have resulted from an impact, such as from the package's being dropped from an extreme height.

ulatory language regarding identification of and warning to the recipient. These materials should be available to anyone with authority to inspect the product for the purpose of protecting the carriers and the general public. The outer container should be clearly labeled to identify the product and any special shipping instructions to those handling the container during transit.

Shipping records and labels permit tracking of the product from the shipping facility to the consignee and should contain the information in Table 30-1. These records designate the date and time that the product is shipped and received. They also identify the source facility, the receiving facility, and the personnel responsible for shipping and receiving the product. Contact names and phone numbers for both the shipping and receiving facilities must be clearly identified on the shipping label so that issues involved with transport can be properly communicated and addressed. The records should document the identity of the courier and any delays or problems occurring during transportation of the product. Often a courier will request that a recipient identifier be documented on the shipping container to verify the identity of the shipment, but this should be done in a manner that maintains confidentiality. It should be clearly evident on the outside of the package that this is a "medically urgent" situation in which the package contains human cells for transplant. Labeling on the outside of the package should indicate that the package cannot be dropped, tipped, opened, or x-rayed. It is important to protect the individuals

requesting to inspect the shipper by informing them of the hazards associated with the cold temperatures inside the container. Unless the contents of the package have not been tested or are repeatedly reactive for an infectious disease marker, the package is not considered biohazardous. If the contents have not been tested or are reactive for any infectious disease markers—if, for example, the contents are serologically positive for hepatitis B virus—the package must be clearly marked as biohazardous.

For the safety of both the product and the personnel handling shipment, a minimum storage temperature appears on the outside of the shipper so that all who are associated with the transport are aware the shipper contains a product that is stored at very cold temperatures.

Regulation

CT products can be shipped by a single mode or a combination of modes of transportation. Air shipments are regulated by the International Air Transport Association (IATA), International Civil Aviation Organization (ICAO), and Food and Drug Administration (FDA); ground shipments are regulated by the Department of Transportation (DOT): the Research and Special Programs Administration (RSPA) and the Federal Highway Association. Air shipment regulations are more restrictive than ground transport regulations. Therefore, by complying with IATA regulations, shipment safety and

Table 30-1. Content of Shipping Records and Labels

Shipping Facility	Consignee
Date/time product shipped	Date/time product received
Source facility	Receiving facility
Personnel responsible for shipping: names and phone numbers	Personnel responsible for receiving: names and phone numbers
Courier identity	Recipient identifier
Minimum storage temperature of product	"Medically Urgent" label

Special Instructions

Do Not Drop—Risk: vacuum could be compromised
Do Not Tip—Risk: rapid nitrogen evaporation
Do Not Open—Risk: injury to untrained personnel
Do Not X-ray—Risk: radiation damage to product

compliance in both modes (air and ground) can be ensured.

ICAO governs all civil aviation matters. Its *Technical Instructions for the Safe Transport of Dangerous Goods by Air*[4] is based on recommendations of the United Nations Committee of Experts and incorporated into Canadian and US law. IATA is the agency that developed the first regulations for the transport of dangerous goods by air, published in 1956. This publication provides procedures for shippers and operators by which shipments with hazardous properties can be safely transported by air on commercial air carriers. These regulations apply to anyone who handles, offers for transport, or transports dangerous goods—or causes dangerous goods to be transported. IATA defines dangerous goods as "articles or substances which are capable of posing a significant risk to health, safety, or . . . property when transported by air."[5]

Within the United States, the DOT, through the RSPA, is the federal agency that regulates the handling of dangerous goods. The divisions of the DOT that enforce DOT and RSPA hazardous materials regulations include the US Coast Guard, the Federal Aviation Administration, the Federal Highway Administration, and the Federal Railroad Administration.[6] Professional organizations, such as the AABB and the Foundation for the Accreditation of Cellular Therapy, provide standards for proper shipping temperatures and minimum documentation for the control of shipping and receipt of CT products. Programs involved with the transportation of fresh or frozen products should refer to the specific guidelines of the organization under which they are accredited.

Export activities may be coordinated by a registry such as the National Marrow Donor Program or the Caitlin Raymond International Registry, which have their own guidelines that the shipping facility must follow.

Conclusion

Safe transportation of CT products to their designated recipients is an essential component of the therapeutic process. The safety of all personnel involved in shipping and handling is as important as the safety of the product itself. It is expected that standards and security issues will continually evolve. Shipping facilities must be vigilant and adhere to the appropriate standards and regulations to prevent complications, and even disaster, in transport. Flexibility and communication are vital to the transport process.

References/Resources

1. Cryopreservation equipment: Storage and transport systems for biological materials. Ballground, GA: Chart Industries, 2009. ["Literature" at www.chartbiomed.com (accessed April 14, 2009).]

2. Vapor shipper series technical manual. Part number VSS.TM0600. (January 2004) Romeo, MI: Custom Bio-Genic Systems, 2004.

3. Petzer AL, Speth HG, Hoflehner E, et al. Breaking the rules? X-ray examination of hematopoietic stem cell grafts at inernational airports. Bood 2002;99:4632-3.

4. International Civil Aviation Organization. Technical instructions for the safe transport of dangerous goods by air. Doc 9284. 2005-2006 ed. Montreal, PQ, Canada: ICAO, 2005.

5. Comprehensive guide to shipping infectious substances. Edmonton, AB: SafTPak, 2001.

6. Code of federal regulations. Title 49, CFR Part 171. Research and Special Programs Administration, Department of Transportation: General information, regulations, and definitions. Washington, DC: US Government Printing Office, 2008 (revised annually).

Method 30-1. Shipping Cord Blood Units

Description

Cryopreserved products are shipped in liquid nitrogen (LN_2) dry shippers at a temperature below −150 C to preserve cellular integrity. When properly charged, dry shippers will maintain appropriate transport temperature for at least 5 days. Export must be well documented to ensure that the correct product is selected and it arrives at the transplant center in good condition.

Time for Procedure

Approximately 24 hours.

Summary of Procedure

Upon request for shipment, a validated dry shipper is charged and subsequently packed with a selected product for transplant. The shipment's itinerary is arranged through a courier and communicated to the receiving facility. Shipping conditions are documented before leaving the shipping facility and upon receipt in the receiving facility, and the shipping container's temperature is continuously monitored during transit.

Equipment

1. Dry shipper.
2. Data logger.
3. Scale.

Supplies and Reagents

1. LN_2.
2. Cryogloves.

Procedure

1. Upon receipt of the Request for Shipment form, preparations will be made for product transport.
2. Charge the dry shipper with LN_2 according to the manufacturer's directions, overnight before the ship date.
3. Verify the availability of a validated data logger. Make sure that any previous data are stored and cleared and that the device is activated to record data for the current shipment.
4. Initiate fulfillment of the shipping documents.
5. Complete the airbill for the courier service that will transport the product.
6. Call the courier to arrange the shipment. Document the job number and itinerary.
7. Prepare the notification of shipment and receipt instructions. Fax these to both the receiving facility and the transplant center.
8. Organize a package including the following items to accompany the product:
   a. Notification of shipment.
   b. National Marrow Donor Program (NMDP) product insert (for NMDP shipments).
   c. Receipt instructions.
   d. Unit receipt form.
   e. Comprehensive matched cord blood report.
   f. Copy of patient and product confirmatory testing results.
   g. Thawing procedure.
   h. Follow-up forms.
   i. *Circular of Information for the Use of Cellular Therapy Products.*
9. Prepare the shipping label and apply it to the outer shipping container. The label includes the following:
   a. Product description.
   b. Name and address of the receiving institution.
   c. Name and phone number of the contact person responsible for the handling and receipt of the component.
   d. Name, address, and phone number of the emergency contact at the bank.
   e. Name of courier and shipping date.
   f. Food and Drug Adminstration product code 57M01.

10. Apply the additional labels to the outer shipping container:
    a. Dry shipper label (nonregulated, nonhazardous indications).
    b. Cold warning label.
    c. Medical urgency label.
    d. X-ray warning label.
    e. Large red arrow, pointing upward, with warning to keep shipper upright.
11. Verify product identifier with the request for the shipment. Inspect the container integrity and document it.
12. Remove the product from the freezer and place it in the charged dry shipper, inserting additional styrofoam racks tightly around the cassette to reduce jarring and prevent damage during transit.
13. Obtain all ancillary samples and place them into the vessel (if applicable).
14. Insert the probe of the activated data logger into the area of the dry shipper that the product will occupy in transport. Allow the temperature to stabilize and record it.
15. Weigh the shipper and document the weight.
16. Request that the receiving facility examine and document the condition of the shipper, product, and temperature monitor immediately upon arrival and that the receiving facility communicate this information to the shipping facility to acknowledge acceptable receipt of the product.

Notes

1. Once a product has been exported from the program, it becomes the property of the requesting transplant center and cannot be returned to inventory.

2. Dry shippers are considered nonhazardous and, therefore, are unregulated by the Department of Transportation. The secondary container will indicate this information for all personnel involved with transit.
3. Review the product receipt information to ensure safe arrival to the transplant center. Follow up on any comments or unexpected problems with the shipment.

Quality Assurance

1. The director reviews the product record, including information on the product's processing, test results, and medical history before the product's release.
2. Information from the data logger will be downloaded upon return.
    a. The data logger graph will be printed and placed in the product folder.
    b. Printed tracing is forwarded to the transplant center.

References/Resources

1. NetCord-FACT international standards for cord blood collection, processing, testing, banking, selection and release. 3rd ed. Omaha, NE: FACT, 2006. [Available at http://www.factwebsite.org/uploadedFiles/Standards/CB%20Stds_3rd%20Ed_FINAL%201%2029%2007.pdf (accessed April 4, 2009).] .
2. Padley D, ed. Standards for cellular therapy product services. Bethesda, MD: AABB, 2008.
3. AABB, America's Blood Centers, American Association of Tissue Banks, et al. Circular of information for the use of cellular therapy products. Bethesda, MD: AABB, 2007. [Available at http://www.aabb.org/Content/About_Blood/Circulars_of_Information/aabb_coi.htm (accessed March 18, 2009).]

In: Areman EM, Loper K, eds
Cellular Therapy: Principles, Methods, and Regulations
Bethesda, MD: AABB, 2009

♦♦♦ **31** ♦♦♦

Thawing and Infusing Cellular Therapy Products

Meghan Delaney, DO, and Richard L. Haspel, MD, PhD

ALTHOUGH THAWING OF CRYOPRESERVED cellular therapy (CT) products may appear to be a straightforward process, attention to detail is important to ensure sterility and optimal cell viability. The CT product container is usually placed in a clean plastic bag and submerged in a bath at 37 C filled with sterile water or 0.9% (normal) saline. The product container may be massaged to facilitate thawing, and it should be removed from the bath just as ice crystals disappear. At this time, samples may be obtained for quality control testing to assess cell viability, cell recovery, and other characteristics that might have been affected by freezing and thawing. Dry warming devices have also been used to thaw stem cell products.[1]

Considerations

Bags

Several issues can arise when thawing a CT product. One study of 377 thawed apheresis products reported a bag rupture rate of 1.06%.[2] Although not all causes of ruptured bags have been identified, these events may occur when the frozen product is accidentally punctured during transfer, or when placement into the storage cassette causes stress on the tubing and bag edges.[2,3] Therefore, extreme care should be exercised when placing the bag in the cassette for freezing/storage and when handling a frozen bag.

To mitigate the extreme temperature change from storage at −196 C to thawing at 37 C, some facilities transfer products (that are stored in the liquid phase of nitrogen) from the liquid phase to the vapor phase for a period before removal for thawing. If interim vapor storage is performed, care should be taken to maintain inventory control and proper documentation.

Before the thawing process begins, the stored bag should be carefully inspected for cracks or chips that might cause problems during thawing. If damage is noted, it should be reported to the laboratory director and the transplanting physician so that other products can be selected, if available, or so that appropriate antibiotic therapy can be pre-

Meghan Delaney, DO, Assistant Medical Director, Puget Sound Blood Center, Seattle, Washington, and Richard L. Haspel, MD, PhD, Medical Director, Stem Cell Processing Laboratory, Beth Israel Deaconess Medical Center, Boston, Massachusetts

The authors have disclosed no conflicts of interest.

scribed for administration when the product is infused. Even if no damage to the frozen container is observed, it is advisable to use an overwrap bag during thaw to facilitate salvage of the product and reduce contamination in case of an unanticipated problem. If salvage of a ruptured bag is necessary, small leaks or tears can be sealed off with hemostat clips, and the product can be transferred to a labeled syringe. If the tear is larger and allows leakage into the overwrap bag entirely, the product may be transferred via sterile syringe inside a biological safety cabinet (BSC) into a new container.[3,4] A stocked salvage kit should be readily available for use in these situations. Postsalvage sterility testing should be performed to assess contamination and aid with the choice of antibiotic therapy.

In one study, although the rate of positive cultures from 24 bag breakages was 42%,[3] none of the product recipients had positive blood cultures or serious sequelae following infusion. This occurrence may have been because all patients were either already receiving or were immediately placed on broad-spectrum antibiotic coverage before infusion. It is clear that the integrity of freezing bags is critical to the quality of hematopoietic progenitor cell (HPC) products, and as such, freezing containers are discussed in greater detail in Chapter 29 of this section.

Thawing Environment

Thawing occurs either at the bedside, in an adjacent area, or in the stem cell laboratory. Thawing products at the bedside decreases the time from thaw to infusion. However, it may place the product in a less-controlled environment, creating the opportunity for contamination or other issues. Although, at some institutions, laboratory staff with experience handling HPC products participate in the bedside thawing process, such additional laboratory staff may not always be readily available to assist, especially in an ancillary location. Bedside thawing also creates logistical difficulties for post-thaw sampling because there may not be suitable working areas. Another negative aspect of thawing at the bedside is that any problems that may arise with the product must be discussed within audible range of patients and families.

Thawing in a controlled laboratory environment provides appropriate equipment and supplies for post-thaw sampling and/or bag rescue, as well as dedicated space and personnel for product preparation. Regardless of which environment is used for thawing CT products, the entire process requires excellent organization of all parties involved, as well as consistent communication between the laboratory and patient care team.

DMSO

Because of purported dimethyl sulfoxide (DMSO) cytotoxicity, thawed CT products are infused as soon as possible. Many laboratories assign an expiration time for thawed HPC products ranging from 1 to 4 hours.[5] Products released after the expiration time has been reached should be infused only as exceptions, under institutional policies for exceptional products and deviations. DMSO, a polar, osmotically active solvent used extensively as a cryoprotectant, can be toxic to HPC products in the liquid phase over time. Data are inconclusive regarding the impact of short-term, post-thaw exposure of HPC products to DMSO. Rowley et al found no loss in the progenitor cell activity of marrow, as measured by progenitor colonies [colony-forming unit—granulocyte-macrophage (CFU-GM) and burst-forming unit—erythrocyte (BFU-E)] after incubation at 4 C for 1 hour in 10% DMSO.[6] Branch et al also did not find significant decrease in the progenitor cell activity (CFU-GM and CFU total) of marrow products incubated for up to 2 hours in 8% DMSO. However, a modest loss of mononuclear cells after the first 30 minutes of incubation (26%) was noted.[7] In a more recent study of HPCs from apheresis (HPC-A), Rodriguez et al observed a significant decrease in CFU-GM, but not in CFU total or CD34+ cells, after a 1-hour incubation at 4 C in 10% DMSO.[5] Overall, while HPCs appear relatively stable in DMSO, it seems prudent to infuse products as soon as possible after thaw. In emergency cases when there is a substantial time between thaw and infusion, products can be washed to remove DMSO, thereby minimizing any potential cellular toxicity. However, because of the potential for cell loss, the washing practice is usually used only when extreme toxicity is a concern. (See "Prevention of Adverse Events from CT Product Infusion" later in this chapter.)

As new therapies and storage containers are developed, some modifications of the thawing process may be needed. Vials with frozen CT products should not be immersed in waterbaths because their lids may not be watertight. Other containers, such as the straws used in sperm banking, may have unique requirements of their own. As novel containers and freezing techniques become available, consideration of the same previously mentioned parameters, such as maintaining sterility, should be considered. (See Method 31-1.)

Process for Infusion of Thawed Cellular Therapy Products

Most centers prepare recipients for CT product infusion with some combination of hydration, antihistamines, antipyretics, and anti-inflammatory agents. Medications such as diphenhydramine, acetaminophen, and hydrocortisone are administered to prevent allergic, DMSO-related, and febrile nonhemolytic transfusion reactions. Administering fluids before infusion may decrease the risk of kidney damage from red cell stroma and hemoglobin in the product. Hard candies such as mints are often provided to help reduce DMSO-induced nausea. Practices vary widely, and there are no published studies comparing different preinfusion regimens and their ability to prevent adverse events.[8]

Infusion of CT products is usually handled by the clinical staff caring directly for the patient. The procedure for infusion is similar to that used for most blood components.[9] Patient and product identity must be verified before initiating the process. Normal saline is usually the only fluid administered concomitantly with the CT product and can also be used to flush the IV line at the end of the procedure to ensure that all cells are infused. A standard blood filter is sometimes used, but CT products should never be leukocyte reduced or irradiated. As described in the *Circular of Information for the Use of Cellular Therapy Products*,[9] HPC infusion should "begin slowly and with sufficient observation to detect symptoms . . . . Thereafter, the rate of infusion may be as rapid as tolerated."

The patient's physician must be notified of any unexpected and/or severe reactions to a CT product; then, these reactions should be reported immediately to the CT facility. Because reactions are not uncommon with infusion of CT products, clear guidelines should be available for clinical and laboratory staff that define and describe the reactions that require communication to the laboratory for investigation. As an example, mild adverse events such as nausea and pruritis are often tolerated by the recipient without significant medical intervention and may not need to be reported to the laboratory for investigation. Because of the dangers associated with immunosuppressed transplant patients and bacteremia, all fevers, chills, and hypotensive episodes following CT product infusion should be investigated and reported to the laboratory. In many centers, blood cultures are collected and prophylactic antibiotics administered when these signs/symptoms are noted. Overall, the medical team overseeing the CT product infusion should be vigilant in detecting infusion reactions and treating them appropriately. For example, fluid overload should be treated with diuretics, whereas anaphylaxis should be treated with epinephrine.[9]

Problems during Infusion

Product Issues

In the CT facility, there are several ways to manage the problem of visible clumps or clots in a CT product during processing. Clumps and clots may be caused by inadequate anticoagulation, platelets, or DNA released by ruptured granulocytes. Standard blood filters (170-260-micron pore size) have been shown to have no adverse effect on the CD34+ cell dose[9,10] and are frequently used to prevent clumps in the product from reaching the patient. DNAse has also been used in the past to treat the product before infusion to dissolve DNA fragments that may mediate cell aggregation.[11] Although there is a pharmaceutical DNAse, it is not currently approved for this indication and may not be readily available to the laboratory.

If platelet clumping is noted during collection of HPC-A, the anticoagulant can be increased to greater than the usual 1:9 ratio in the collection bag. Additional anticoagulant can also be added to the product upon receipt or during thawing in the laboratory. Some centers report up to 10% addition of acid (or anticoagulant)-citrate-dextrose formula

A (ACD-A) to avoid additional platelet clumping. Some centers also report using heparin, either in the cryopreservation media or as needed during thawing.

Adverse Events

As is the case with blood components, CT product infusion may be associated with allergic, febrile, hemolytic, and septic reactions, as well as fluid overload.[9] There are also adverse events unique to CT products, such as reactions to DMSO. Fortunately, severe infusion-related reactions are uncommon. The largest study investigating severe adverse events following HPC infusion reported only five severe reactions in 1410 infusions (0.4%).[12] In this study, the severe reactions were either neurologic, leukostatic, or anaphylactic in nature, and all of the affected patients recovered. Case reports have also documented severe reactions related to infusion, including cardiac and neurologic events.[13-17]

The reported rates of mild adverse events vary greatly among published studies. For example, one study reported nausea in 50% of patients, whereas others found rates of 7% to 14%.[12,18,19] This variability likely reflects differences in product processing, patient monitoring, premedication, and adverse event classification. Moreover, study design differences (eg, retrospective chart review vs concurrent clinician reporting of significant adverse events) may yield varying rates of detection. Overall, it appears that most adverse events are mild, with limited to no associated morbidity.

DMSO-Related Adverse Events

Though infusions containing DMSO are usually well tolerated, DMSO is often cited as a cause of CT-product infusion-related adverse events.[9] The exact dose for toxicity in humans is not known, but the LD_{50} (lethal dose in 50% of tested animals) for IV DMSO is 2.5g/kg (dogs) and >11g/kg (monkeys).[8] Interestingly, DMSO has been used safely to treat a variety of ailments, including skin conditions and interstitial cystitis.[20,21] In one study of stroke patients, doses of 0.56 g/kg of DMSO twice a day, combined with a glycolytic intermediate, were infused without any adverse effects.[22] It is routinely recommended that adult and pediatric transplant recipients receive <1g/kg DMSO per 24-hour period.[12,23] An HPC unit containing 100 mL total volume at the concentration of 10% DMSO will contain 10 g DMSO, well below the threshold DMSO dose for adult patients.

Adverse reactions to DMSO infusion are highly variable and are thought to be secondary to histamine release and mast cell degranulation. Animal studies have also demonstrated DMSO-induced negative chronotropic effects on cardiac tissue.[17] In the clinical setting, the most common reactions attributed to DMSO are mild and include nausea and shivering. Patients also frequently report a "garlic" or "sweet cream corn" taste.[8,9] Several case reports have described severe reactions thought to be caused by DMSO, including cardiovascular, neurologic, and pulmonary events.[13-17] Pain at the IV insertion site, ascribed to the viscous quality of DMSO (molality = 1.42 mol/L), has also been reported. Consequently, it is recommended that HPC products containing DMSO be given intravenously through the largest bore available, preferably through a central venous catheter.[8] Because of the presumed cytotoxicity of DMSO, cells are often infused as quickly as they can be tolerated. However, DMSO-related symptoms can often be moderated with a reduction of the infusion rate.

There is considerable discrepancy in reported rates of DMSO-related adverse events. Stroncek et al compared autologous cryopreserved HPCs from marrow (HPC-M) to fresh allogeneic HPC-M infusion and found patients experienced emesis (but not nausea) in a DMSO dose-dependent manner. Nausea, vomiting, fever, and chills were also significantly more frequent in the administration of cryopreserved HPC-M compared to fresh HPC-M (76.1%), but the rate of reactions associated with fresh products was also quite high (26.8%).[74] Regarding apheresis products, Donmez et al performed an analysis of 219 transplants and found autologous cryopreserved products had significantly more side effects than fresh allogeneic HPC-A (25.3% vs 0%). DMSO content, total nucleated cell (TNC) content, and median product volume were all found to correlate with this finding.[25] Both of these studies partially attribute adverse events to DMSO; however, more specifically, they compare differences in reaction rates of cryopreserved vs fresh products. It is possible that other variables, including TNC, hematocrit, total product volume, and amount of cellular debris may contribute to the observed differences in reaction rates.

In contrast to the relatively high rates of adverse events attributed to DMSO listed above, a study by Alessandrino et al looking at 126 patients receiving autologous marrow or apheresis infusions did not find adverse events related to the dose of DMSO.[18] Moreover, a survey of DMSO use by European stem cell processing laboratories reported that only 1 in 70 transplant recipients experienced a DMSO-related adverse event.[23] Finally, as noted above, high doses of DMSO have been infused in nontransplant settings without serious side effects.[22] In summary, while DMSO may be associated with adverse events during CT product infusions, it appears that most reactions are mild and tolerable at the standard doses given to adults. Potential methods to reduce DMSO toxicity are discussed later in the section "Washing of Thawed CT Products."

Hemolysis-Related Adverse Events

ABO-incompatible transplants are frequently performed with good results.[26,27] The classification for ABO mismatches is based on donor/recipient ABO typing. In HPC transplants with major ABO incompatibility, the recipient has anti-A and/or anti-B isoagglutinins that are directed at the donor's red cell antigens. In minor ABO incompatibility, the donor's plasma has anti-A and/or anti-B isoagglutinins that are directed at recipient red cell antigens. There can also be bidirectional mismatches (eg, an A donor and a B recipient), with both major and minor ABO incompatibility.

No severe immediate hemolytic transfusion reactions have been reported as a result of blood group incompatibility of a CT product. In the largest published study of ABO-incompatible transplants, 158 recipients of ABO-incompatible HPC-M and HPC-A did not exhibit laboratory or clinical findings consistent with immediate hemolysis.[28] The low rate of hemolytic reactions may be the result of preinfusion processing of ABO-incompatible products, including red cell and plasma reduction (see "Prevention of Adverse Events from CT Product Infusion"), or possibly caused by the immunosuppressed condition of recipients.

Free hemoglobin in the CT product can cause adverse reactions. In two cases with ABO-identical grafts at the author's institution, infusion of free hemoglobin is thought to have contributed to clinical manifestations of a hemolytic reaction, including hemoglobinuria, back pain, chest pain, nausea, and vomiting. In one case, an ABO-identical cryopreserved HPC-A product that contained 55 mL of hemolyzed red cells was infused without washing the product after thawing. In the second case, an ABO-identical fresh unit of HPC-M with prolonged time from harvest to infusion contained 478 mL of hemolyzed red cells. The hemolysis was not recognized and the product was released for infusion. Following onset of symptoms, the product infusion was halted. The remaining product was promptly returned to the processing laboratory, washed, and subsequently infused without further symptoms.

Adverse Events Related to Bacterial Contamination

Contamination of CT products can occur during collection (via skin flora or a bacteremic donor), processing, thawing, or sampling. Positive bacterial cultures from HPC products are relatively common, with the largest and most recent studies (encompassing >9000 products) reporting a contamination rate of 1.2% to 1.6%.[4,19] Higher rates of contaminated products are found with monoclonal antibody-selected products and products with extensive open-system processing steps or bag breakage.[3,24,29] These results support the intuitive notion that increased product manipulation leads to increased risk for microbial contamination. Not all organisms detected before freezing are detected after thawing. It appears that products from a bacteremic donor or those with positive pre- and postprocessing samples have a higher likelihood of having post-thaw recovery of the organism.[19]

In contrast to red cell or plasma products, CT products with positive bacterial cultures are often infused. In several large studies that transfused culture-positive HPCs, very few patients had clinically significant bacteremia that matched the product isolate.[3,4,19,24,29] Overall, it seems that recipient survival does not differ between culture-positive and culture-negative stem cell infusions if appropriate antibiotics are given early.[19] In the recent literature, one fatal infection from stem cell infusion has been documented. In this case, the contamination with *Pseudomonas cepacia* likely occurred during laboratory processing.[4] This patient experienced symptoms of a septic transfusion reaction, including fever, tachypnea, chest pain, and a decline in urine output. Subsequently, the patient required blood pressure support and later developed disseminated intravascular coagulation and renal failure before death on posttransplant day 7. Outbreaks originating from stem cell laboratories are also possible. In 2001, there was an outbreak of an actinomycete derived from a stem cell laboratory and traced to a multiple-use cryopreservation media bottle.[30]

Cardiovascular, Embolic, and Pulmonary Events

Although serious cardiovascular events such as heart block and cardiac arrest have occurred following infusion of CT products, the most often encountered cardiac effects are mild and include clinically insignificant bradyarrhythmias and minimal alterations in blood pressure.[16-18,31-34] Etiologic theories include volume-mediated vagal stimulation or toxicity related to DMSO or cellular debris.[17,18,33,34] Milone et al, in a large prospective study involving 157 HPC-A and 22 HPC-M transplants, found that patients with higher total infused product volumes and longer infusion times had significantly more cardiovascular side effects.[34] Alessandrino et al found in their study of 126 patients that bradycardia was significantly more common during HPC-M infusion than HPC-A infusion. The authors hypothesized the higher red cell content in the marrow may have played a role.[18] Several studies have found that the type of chemotherapy or the patient's ejection fraction may affect the number of cardiovascular adverse events.[16,31,32] Overall, however, it seems there is no clear way to predict severe cardiac events following HPC infusion.[31]

Although rare, embolic events have also been reported with HPC infusion. Fat contamination from a marrow harvest can cause pulmonary fat embolism.[35] Additionally, thromboembolic events from thawed HPC particulate matter are thought to have caused three cerebrovascular accidents in patients with patent foramen ovales (PFOs). The PFOs allowed the particles to pass to the left side of the heart and gain access to the systemic circulation.[10] In regard to pulmonary events, as with any blood product, dyspnea caused by circulatory overload can occur with CT product infusion.[9] A single case of transfusion-related acute lung injury (TRALI) from a CT product infusion has also been reported. In 2003, a patient experienced hypoxia,

necessitating oxygen and steroids during infusion of an allogeneic marrow product. Laboratory testing found that the patient's serum contained anti-neutrophil antibodies that may have reacted with neutrophils in the graft. Specific anti-HLA antibodies were not found.[36]

Prevention of Adverse Events from CT Product Infusion

Washing of Thawed CT Products

To prevent adverse events related to cellular debris, free hemoglobin, and additives such as DMSO, some laboratories wash cryopreserved products before infusion. There are many methods to wash CT products. In general, washing consists of adding a sterile liquid such as saline, albumin, or dextran to the product, and then centrifuging and expressing off the supernatant. This step is followed by resuspension in albumin, plasma, or dextran, or a combination of these materials. Washing can be done by an automated machine or manually.[5,11,37-42] A widely accepted manual washing method for thawed umbilical cord blood (UCB) has been adopted from the New York Blood Center protocol, which uses 2.5% albumin and 5% dextran with centrifugation at 10 C.[38,41] Automated devices like the COBE 2991 (CaridianBCT, Lakewood, CO) and the CytoMate (Baxter, Deerfield, IL) use closed or semiclosed systems that offer speed and decreased risk for contamination.[37,40] Whereas the COBE uses centrifugation to separate the plasma layer by density, the CytoMate employs a spinning membrane for filtration against a counterflow of buffer solution.[40]

Washing can be detrimental to CT product integrity, and most studies of manual or automated washing demonstrate some degree of cell loss ranging from approximately 10% to 30%.[37,40,42] Washing also increases the time, up to several hours, from thawing to infusion; introduces opportunities for contamination; creates extra costs; and increases the workload of the CT facility.

Studies examining the benefits of washing are not definitive, and there have been no randomized studies comparing washed vs nonwashed products. In one report of a group of 95 patients, automated washing reduced adverse reaction rates from 81%

to 54%.[40] As more data were accumulated, however, this difference was no longer apparent.[43] In a large survey of transplant centers, 22 centers that either used a final DMSO concentration of <10% or washed their products had lower transfusion reaction rates compared to 78 centers that used 10% DMSO (0.3% vs 1.5% adverse reaction rates, respectively).[23] A survey, however, cannot distinguish between other methodologic differences in the various laboratories.

In determining whether to wash a CT product, the risks of adverse events from DMSO or cellular debris and DMSO cytotoxicity need to be weighed against the added cost, processing time, and potential cell loss. On the basis of the available data, it appears that most HPC products do not need to be washed if the DMSO dose remains below the threshold of <1 g/kg over a 24-hour period and can be infused soon after thawing. In cases of multiple product infusion leading to a DMSO dose greater than the threshold, the products can be infused over several hours or 2 days.[44] Given the potential cytotoxicity issues, an example of a product that might be washed is a cryopreserved donor lymphocyte infusion (DLI), which may have to undergo lengthy testing (eg, flow cytometry to calculate CD3+ cell dose) before infusion.[5-7]

Because UCB products were initially used only in pediatric transplants, UCB units were washed to prevent DMSO from reaching toxic levels in these smaller patients. Recent data demonstrate that washing UCB may cause significant cell loss.[45] Because low CD34+ dose is a major barrier to the use of UCB in large patients, several groups have demonstrated that a wash step may be omitted for UCB without serious adverse events or an effect on engraftment.[46,47]

Red Cell and Plasma Reduction

As described earlier in this chapter, red cell and plasma reduction procedures are often performed to prevent hemolysis caused by ABO or other blood group incompatibility.[28,48] There are no published, evidence-based thresholds for red cell or plasma reduction. In one large study, processing procedures were guided by recipient and donor isoagglutinin titers (IgM and/or IgG) and type of ABO mismatch. Recipients of major ABO-incompatible HPC-M with titers >1:16 received products that were red cell reduced. HPC-M products with minor incompatibility and titers >1:128 were plasma reduced. HPC-A products were not red cell or plasma reduced. Although the authors did not present any evidence to support their choice of this strategy, no immediate hemolytic events were reported.[28]

With limited data, stem cell laboratories are forced to use self-determined thresholds for red cell and plasma reduction, and there is wide variation among institutions. In an informal survey of six stem cell laboratories, the threshold of incompatible red cells permitted before undertaking a red cell reduction procedure for HPC-A ranged from 15 to 40 mL.[49] In determining a threshold, the risk of hemolytic reactions must be balanced against the deleterious effects of extensive processing, such as an increased risk of microbial contamination, the potential for cell loss, time commitment, and expense.[3,24,29] Further studies to determine the threshold at which to manipulate a product are clearly necessary.

Aside from cases of minor incompatibility, plasma reduction can also be done to reduce the volume of an HPC product. Typically, volume reduction is performed in pediatric cases where the desired infusion volume is <10 mL/kg. Methods for volume reduction are similar to those for red cell reduction described above and in Chapter 26.

Contamination (Nonsterile Products)

To detect potential microbial contamination, all products should be tested upon receipt in the laboratory and following processing and thawing steps (when possible).[30] In products with known bacterial contamination or those with a high probability of contamination (eg, bag rupture), the laboratory director and transplant physician should be contacted to weigh the risks and benefits of infusion. Important considerations include the type of organism, ability to repeat the collection from the donor, and whether there is a critical need for the product.[19] Fortunately, it appears the risks are typically small, given the relatively high rate of reported incidents of contamination but infrequent reporting of serious adverse events. This situation may be the result of the initiation of appropriate antibiotic treatment after an event such as a container break or once contaminating organisms are identified.[3,4,16,22,27]

Acknowledgments

Methods 31-2 and 31-4 were submitted by Deborah Lamontagne, MT(ASCP), Tech Leader, Stem Cell Laboratory, Department of Pathology, Division of Laboratory Medicine, Beth Israel Deaconess Medical Center, Boston, Massachusetts. Method 31-3 was submitted by Janice Davis-Sproul, MAS, MT(ASCP)SBB, Manager, Cell Therapy and Development Laboratories, Sidney Kimmel Comprehensive Cancer Center at Johns Hopkins, Baltimore, Maryland. Method 31-5 was submitted by Donna Regan, MT(ASCP), Executive Director, St Louis Cord Blood Bank and Cellular Therapy Laboratory at SSM Cardinal Glennon Children's Medical Center, St Louis, Missouri. Method 31-6 was submitted by Denise Cummings, RN, Coordinator, Bone Marrow Transplant Center, Beth Israel Deaconess Medical Center, Boston, Massachusetts.

References/Resources

1. Rollig C, Babatz J, Wagner I, et al. Thawing of cryopreserved mobilized peripheral blood—comparison between waterbath and dry warming device. Cytotherapy 2002;4:551-5.
2. Mele L, Dallavalle FM, Verri MG, et al. Safety control of peripheral blood progenitor cell processing—eight-year survey of microbiological contamination and bag ruptures in a single institution. Transfus Apher Sci 2005; 33:269-74.
3. Khuu HM, Cowley H, vid Ocampo V, et al. Catastrophic failures of freezing bags for cellular therapy products: Description, cause, and consequences. Cytotherapy 2002;4:539-49.
4. Klein MA, Kadidlo D, McCullough J, et al. Microbial contamination of hematopoietic stem cell products: Incidence and clinical sequelae. Biol Blood Marrow Transplant 2006;12:1142-9.
5. Rodriguez L, Velasco B, Garcia J, et al. Evaluation of an automated cell processing device to reduce the dimethyl sulfoxide from hematopoietic grafts after thawing. Transfusion 2005;45:1391-7.
6. Rowley SD, Anderson GL. Effect of DMSO exposure without cryopreservation on hematopoietic progenitor cells. Bone Marrow Transplant 1993;11:389-93.
7. Branch DR, Calderwood S, Cecutti MA, et al. Hematopoietic progenitor cells are resistant to dimethyl sulfoxide toxicity. Transfusion 1994;34:887-90.

8. Sauer-Heilborn A, Kadidlo D, McCullough J. Patient care during infusion of hematopoietic progenitor cells. Transfusion 2004;44:907-16.
9. AABB, America's Blood Centers, American Association of Tissue Banks, et al. Circular of information for the use of cellular therapy products. Bethesda, MD: AABB, 2007. [Available at http://www.aabb.org/Content/About_Blood/Circulars_of_Information/aabb_coi.htm (accessed March 18, 2009).]
10. Berg A. Impact of filtering thawed hematopoietic progenitor cells (HPC) with routine blood filter on CD34+ cell number (abstract). Transfusion 2006;46(Suppl):61A.
11. Del ML, Venturini M, Viscoli C, et al. Intensified chemotherapy supported by DMSO-free peripheral blood progenitor cells in breast cancer patients. Ann Oncol 2001; 12:505-8.
12. Graves V, Danielson C, Abonour R, et al. How to ensure safe and well-tolerated stem cell infusions (abstract). Transfusion 1998;38(Suppl):30S.
13. Benekli M, Anderson B, Wentling D, et al. Severe respiratory depression after dimethylsulphoxide-containing autologous stem cell infusion in a patient with AL amyloidosis. Bone Marrow Transplant 2000;25:1299-301.
14. Dhodapkar M, Goldberg SL, Tefferi A, et al. Reversible encephalopathy after cryopreserved peripheral blood stem cell infusion. Am J Hematol 1994;45:187-8.
15. Hoyt R, Szer J, Grigg A. Neurological events associated with the infusion of cryopreserved bone marrow and/or peripheral blood progenitor cells. Bone Marrow Transplant 2000;25:1285-7.
16. Styler MJ, Topolsky DL, Crilley PA, et al. Transient high grade heart block following autologous bone marrow infusion. Bone Marrow Transplant 1992;10:435-8.
17. Zenhausern R, Tobler A, Leoncini L, et al. Fatal cardiac arrhythmia after infusion of dimethyl sulfoxide-cryopreserved hematopoietic stem cells in a patient with severe primary cardiac amyloidosis and end-stage renal failure. Ann Hematol 2000;79:523-6.
18. Alessandrino P, Bernasconi P, Caldera D, et al. Adverse events occurring during bone marrow or peripheral blood progenitor cell infusion: Analysis of 126 cases. Bone Marrow Transplant 1999;23:533-7.
19. Padley DJ, Dietz AB, Gastineau DA. Sterility testing of hematopoietic progenitor cell products: A single-institution series of culture-positive rates and successful infusion of culture-positive products. Transfusion 2007;47: 636-43.
20. Bookman AA, Williams KS, Shainhouse JZ. Effect of a topical diclofenac solution for relieving symptoms of primary osteoarthritis of the knee: A randomized controlled trial. CMAJ 2004;171:333-8.
21. Peeker R, Haghsheno MA, Holmang S, et al. Intravesical bacillus Calmette-Guerin and dimethyl sulfoxide for treatment of classic and nonulcer interstitial cystitis: A prospective, randomized double-blind study. J Urol 2000;164:1912-5.
22. Karaca M, Kilic E, Yazici B, et al. Ischemic stroke in elderly patients treated with a free radical scavenger-glyco-

lytic intermediate solution: A preliminary pilot trial. Neurol Res 2002;24:73-80.

23. Windrum P, Morris TC, Drake MB, et al. Variation in dimethyl sulfoxide use in stem cell transplantation: A survey of EBMT centres. Bone Marrow Transplant 2005; 36:601-3.

24. Stroncek DF, Fautsch SK, Lasky LC, et al. Adverse reactions in patients transfused with cryopreserved marrow. Transfusion 1991;31:521-6.

25. Donmez A, Tombuloglu M, Gungor A, et al. Clinical side effects during peripheral blood progenitor cell infusion. Transfus Apher Sci 2007;36:95-101.

26. Kim JG, Sohn SK, Kim DH, et al. Impact of ABO incompatibility on outcome after allogeneic peripheral blood stem cell transplantation. Bone Marrow Transplant 2005; 35:489-95.

27. Maciej ZJ, Mielcarek M, Takatu A, et al. Engraftment of early erythroid progenitors is not delayed after non-myeloablative major ABO-incompatible haematopoietic stem cell transplantation. Br J Haematol 2002;119:740-50.

28. Rowley SD, Liang PS, Ulz L. Transplantation of ABO-incompatible bone marrow and peripheral blood stem cell components. Bone Marrow Transplant 2000;26:749-57.

29. Webb IJ, Coral FS, Andersen JW, et al. Sources and sequelae of bacterial contamination of hematopoietic stem cell components: Implications for the safety of hematotherapy and graft engineering. Transfusion 1996; 36:782-8.

30. Hirji Z, Saragosa R, Dedier H, et al. Contamination of bone marrow products with an actinomycete resembling *Microbacterium* species and reinfusion into autologous stem cell and bone marrow transplant recipients. Clin Infect Dis 2003;36:e115-e121.

31. Hertenstein B, Stefanic M, Schmeiser T, et al. Cardiac toxicity of bone marrow transplantation: Predictive value of cardiologic evaluation before transplant. J Clin Oncol 1994;12:998-1004.

32. Keung YK, Lau S, Elkayam U, et al. Cardiac arrhythmia after infusion of cryopreserved stem cells. Bone Marrow Transplant 1994;14:363-7.

33. Lopez-Jimenez J, Cervero C, Munoz A, et al. Cardiovascular toxicities related to the infusion of cryopreserved grafts: Results of a controlled study. Bone Marrow Transplant 1994;13:789-93.

34. Milone G, Mercurio S, Strano A, et al. Adverse events after infusions of cryopreserved hematopoietic stem cells depend on non-mononuclear cells in the infused suspension and patient age. Cytotherapy 2007;9:348-55.

35. Lipton JH, Russell JA, Burgess KR, et al. Fat embolization and pulmonary infiltrates after bone marrow transplantation. Med Pediatr Oncol 1987;15:24-7.

36. Urahama N, Tanosaki R, Masahiro K, et al. TRALI after the infusion of marrow cells in a patient with acute lymphoblastic leukemia. Transfusion 2003;43:1553-7.

37. Beaujean F, Hartmann O, Kuentz M, et al. A simple, efficient washing procedure for cryopreserved human hematopoietic stem cells prior to reinfusion. Bone Marrow Transplant 1991;8:291-4.

38. Berz D, McCormack EM, Winer ES, et al. Cryopreservation of hematopoietic stem cells. Am J Hematol 2007;82: 463-72.

39. Kurtzberg J, Laughlin M, Graham ML, et al. Placental blood as a source of hematopoietic stem cells for transplantation into unrelated recipients. N Engl J Med 1996; 335:157-66.

40. Lemarie C, Calmels B, Malenfant C, et al. Clinical experience with the delivery of thawed and washed autologous blood cells, with an automated closed fluid management device: CytoMate. Transfusion 2005;45: 737-42.

41. Rubinstein P, Dobrila L, Rosenfield RE, et al. Processing and cryopreservation of placental/umbilical cord blood for unrelated bone marrow reconstitution. Proc Natl Acad Sci U S A 1995;92:10119-22.

42. Syme R, Bewick M, Stewart D, et al. The role of depletion of dimethyl sulfoxide before autografting: On hematologic recovery, side effects, and toxicity. Biol Blood Marrow Transplant 2004;10:135-41.

43. Calmels B, Lemarie C, Esterni B, et al. Occurrence and severity of adverse events after autologous hematopoietic progenitor cell infusion are related to the amount of granulocytes in the apheresis product. Transfusion 2007; 47:1268-75.

44. Martino M, Morabito F, Messina G, et al. Fractionated infusions of cryopreserved stem cells may prevent DMSO-induced major cardiac complications in graft recipients. Haematologica 1996;81:59-61.

45. Laroche V, McKenna DH, Moroff G, et al. Cell loss and recovery in umbilical cord blood processing: A comparison of postthaw and postwash samples. Transfusion 2005;45:1909-16.

46. Hahn T, Bunworasate U, George MC, et al. Use of non-volume-reduced (unmanipulated after thawing) umbilical cord blood stem cells for allogeneic transplantation results in safe engraftment. Bone Marrow Transplant 2003;32:145-50.

47. Nagamura-Inoue T, Shioya M, Sugo M, et al. Wash-out of DMSO does not improve the speed of engraftment of cord blood transplantation: Follow-up of 46 adult patients with units shipped from a single cord blood bank. Transfusion 2003;43:1285-95.

48. Tsang KS, Li CK, Wong AP, et al. Processing of major ABO-incompatible bone marrow for transplantation by using dextran sedimentation. Transfusion 1999;39:1212-9.

49. Delaney M, Shaz BH, Lamontagne D, et al. The threshold for red cell volume in major ABO incompatible donor-recipient pairs: Experience from one tertiary care center (abstract). Transfusion 2006;46(Suppl):4A.

Method 31-1. Thawing of Hematopoietic Progenitor Cells: Laboratory and Bedside

Description

This method describes the process used in the cellular therapy facility for thawing cryopreserved hematopoietic progenitor cells from marrow (HPC-M), HPCs from apheresis (HPC-A), or HPCs from cord blood (HPC-C). The procedure does not contain details such as protocols for clerical checks or labeling of products.

Time for Procedure

Approximately 30 minutes.

Summary of Procedure

1. Cryopreserved products are thawed at 37 C in a waterbath.
2. Samples are obtained for testing before product release.

Equipment

1. Waterbath at 37 C.
2. Biological safety cabinet (BSC).

Reagents and Disposables

1. Clean plastic bags.
2. Sterile water or 0.9% saline.
3. Sampling site couplers.
4. 18-gauge needles.
5. 3-cc syringes.
6. Blood culture bottles.
7. 60-cc syringes.
8. Plastic tubes: 6 mL.
9. 300-mL transfer packs and labels (used only if leakage occurs).

Procedure

A. *Laboratory Thaw*
   1. Clean the BSC before the procedure.
   2. Clean and fill the waterbath with sterile saline (or water). Confirm the temperature setting of 37 C.

3. Prepare disposables for quality control of the post-thaw product.
4. Perform the following thaw steps:
   a. Before thawing, confirm the infusion with the patient's physician or designee.
   b. Thaw only one bag at a time: remove the product from the canister and verify the product/recipient identification.
   c. Place the frozen product in a clean bag. Place it in a 37-C waterbath, keeping the top seal of the outer clean bag out of the water.
   d. Observe the product bag for any sign of leakage. If no leakage is detected, then proceed.
      - If leakage is detected, clamp off the affected area, place the bag in the BSC, and transfer thawed contents to an appropriate transfer bag using a syringe or sample site port.
      Note: Once the product is thawed, it is important to work quickly. Dimethyl sulfoxide (DMSO) at a concentration of 10% may be toxic to the cells.
      - Label the transfer pack so that the information is identical to that on the freezing bag.
      - Notify a supervisor and a laboratory medical director. The laboratory medical director will determine if the product is acceptable for infusion. File an occurrence report.
      - If the product is acceptable for infusion, the laboratory medical director will discuss potential contamination with the transplanting physician.

- If the product is unacceptable for use, the laboratory medical director will discuss other options with the transplanting physician and communicate follow-up instructions to the laboratory staff.

e. Once the product is thawed to a slushy consistency, remove it from the waterbath. Transfer the product to the BSC and, following aseptic technique, sample the product for quality.

f. Complete product label:
    - Expiration date/time.
    - Storage temperature.

B. Bedside Thaw

1. Clean and fill the waterbath. Confirm the temperature setting of 37 C.
2. Prepare the disposables for quality control of the post-thaw product.
3. Before thawing, confirm the infusion with the patient's physician or designee.
4. Before transport, remove the product from the canister and verify the following:
    a. Patient's name, medical record number (MRN), and National Marrow Donor Program (NMDP) number or donor registry number, if applicable.
    b. Donor's name and MRN (or NMDP or donor registry number, if applicable).
    c. Component number and product type [autologous or allogeneic; HPC-A, HPC-M, HPC-C, or therapeutic cells, T cells (TC-T)].
5. Transport the product to the bedside in an appropriate container.
6. Place the frozen product in a clean plastic bag.
    a. Place the bag in a waterbath at 37 C, keeping the top seal of the outer clean bag out of the water.
    b. Observe the product bag for any sign of leakage. If no leakage is detected, proceed.
    c. If leakage is detected, clamp off the affected area, transfer the thawed contents to an appropriately sized syringe using a needle or sample site port. Care must be used to prevent contamination when possible.

        Note: Once the product is thawed, it is important to work quickly. DMSO at a concentration of 10% may be toxic to the cells.

        - Notify the laboratory medical director or designee who will determine whether the product is acceptable for infusion. File an occurrence report.
        - If the product is acceptable for infusion, the laboratory medical director will discuss potential contamination with the patient's physician.
        - If the product is unacceptable for use, the laboratory medical director will discuss other options with the patient's physician and communicate follow-up instructions to the laboratory staff.
    d. Once the product is thawed to a slushy consistency, remove it from the waterbath and sample it for quality control tests.

References/Resources

1. FACT-JACIE international standards for cellular therapy product collection, processing, and administration. 4th ed. Omaha, NE: Foundation for the Accreditation of Cellular Therapy and the Joint Accreditation Committee of ISCT and EBMT, 2008.
2. Code of federal regulations. Title 21, CFR Part 1271. Human cells, tissues, and cellular and tissue-based products. Washington, DC: US Government Printing Office, 2008 (updated annually).
3. Padley D, ed. Standards for cellular therapy product services. Bethesda, MD: AABB, 2008.
4. Code of federal regulations. Title 21, CFR Parts 200-299. Washington, DC: US Government Printing Office, 2008 (updated annually).
5. Code of federal regulations. Title 21, CFR Parts 600-799. Washington, DC: US Government Printing Office, 2008 (updated annually).
6. Snyder E, Haley NR, Triulzi D, eds. Cellular therapy: A physician's handbook. 1st ed. Bethesda, MD: AABB, 2004.

Method 31-2. Filtration of Cellular Therapy Apheresis Products

Description

Platelet clumps that do not disperse during processing can be filtered with a standard 170- to 210-micron blood filter. This method describes the filtering process.

Time for Procedure

Approximately 5 to 10 minutes to set up and filter 100 mL of concentrated cells.

Summary of Procedure

1. Hematopoietic progenitor cell (HPC) products are concentrated during processing by centrifugation and observed for platelet clumping.
2. Platelet clumps that do not disperse are filtered out using a standard blood filter.
3. Infusion or a cryopreservation process using filtered concentrated cells is continued.
4. The procedure can also be performed with thawed HPC products.

Equipment

1. Biological safety cabinet (BSC).
2. Sterile connecting device.
3. Heat-sealer.

Supplies and Reagents

1. 170- to 210-micron standard blood filter.
2. Transfer pack.

Procedure

1. Properly label an appropriately sized transfer pack, but do not seal off the tubing.
2. Close roller clamp on the blood filter. Use sterile connecting device to connect the filter tubing to the tubing of the transfer pack.
3. Inside the BSC, following aseptic technique, insert a blood administration filter into the transfer pack containing the HPCs.
4. Open the roller clamp and squeeze the filter to create a siphon (or follow the manufacturer's instructions). Allow the concentrated product to flow through the filter into the new transfer pack.
5. When complete, close the roller clamp, heat-seal the tubing, discard the filter, and empty the transfer pack.
6. Continue with the processing or infusion.

Reference/Resource

1. Snyder E, Haley NR, Triulzi D, eds. Cellular therapy: A physician's handbook. 1st ed. Bethesda, MD: AABB, 2004.

Method 31-3. Washing Cellular Therapy Products Using the COBE 2991

Description

This procedure describes the use of the COBE Spectra 2991 (CaridianBCT, Lakewood, CO) to wash cellular therapy products. Various techniques have been developed for use in cell processing that require the removal or depletion of reagents. During processing, the removal or reduction of processing reagents can be accomplished by washing on the COBE 2991.

Time for Procedure

Approximately 25 minutes.

Equipment

1. COBE 2991 Cell Processor.
2. Tubing sealer.

Supplies

1. COBE 2991 Processing Set: COBE #912647-819.
2. Hemostats.
3. Wash solution (usually procedure dependent).

Procedure

A. *COBE 2991 Setup*
   1. Check the hydraulic system prime on the 2991 Cell Processor according to the operator's handbook. (See the sections "Priming Hydraulic System" and "Checking the Prime" in the handbook).
   2. Take the tubing set out of the bag, and orient it according to the color-coded pinch valves on the front panel.
   3. Place the clear tube in front of the red cell detector assembly. (Do not insert the tube all the way into the detector.)
   4. Load the processing bag into the 2991 as the operator's handbook instructs. Place lines into the corresponding pinch valves.
   5. Place hemostats on the blue and yellow lines and on the line leading to the processing bag. Make the following fluid connections:
      a. Red line: cellular product.
      b. Green line: wash solution.
      c. For older COBE devices that are controlled by pins (not electronic), set the panel as in Tables 31-3-1 and 31-3-2.

   Note: See instructions in the operator's handbook for creating a program to perform the same actions as described by the pins shown in Table 31-3-1.

Table 31-3-1. Pin Settings for COBE Devices Controlled by Pins*

Pin Settings						Super Out Volume
Timer		PC†	Valve			
1	2	1	1	2	3	
●	○	○	○	●	○	450
●	○	○	○	●	○	450
●	○	●	○	○	○	600

*● designates placement of diode pin.
†Packed cells pin setting.

Table 31-3-2. Dial Settings for COBE Devices Controlled by Pins*

Centrifuge Speed[†]	Super Out Rate	Minimum Agitate	Super Out Volume
3000	450	90	450
	Spin timer 1		2 minutes
	Spin timer 2		Not applicable
	Auto/manual		AUTO
	Pump restore rate		450 mL/minute
	Red cell override		Not applicable

*For newer COBE devices in which the automatic program is preprogrammed, press the appropriate program number and check that cycle LED is "1."
[†]Some wash procedures will use a centrifuge speed of 2000 rpm.

Note: If the total volume of the product is >650 mL, it must be concentrated before washing.

B. *Washing with COBE 2991*
1. Press TUBE LOAD and prime the green line with wash solution (for 5 seconds).
2. Press STOP/RESET and turn the valve selector to V2. Place the product on the top of the centrifuge.
3. If the total volume is <500 mL, press PREDILUTE and allow 100 mL of wash solution to enter the bag of cells.
4. Press STOP/RESET. Mix the cells.
5. Hang the product on the left hanger. Remove the clamp on the line leading to the processing bag. Press BLOOD IN and allow the processing bag to fill.
6. Press AIR OUT and allow air to be pushed into the product bag.
7. Press BLOOD IN, and as the cells reach the central line, press STOP/RESET. Press TUBE LOAD and allow wash solution to finish filling the bag.
8. Press START/SPIN and the machine will wash the product.
9. When the timer light or LED is on the third cycle, increase the SUPER OUT VOLUME dial to 600 mL, unless otherwise defined in the product-specific standard operating procedure.
10. The machine will beep when the procedure is complete.
11. Place a clamp on the line close to the processing bag. Seal the line.
12. Remove the cells from the machine.
13. Mix the cells and complete the appropriate processing procedure.

Anticipated Results

The nucleated cell recovery should be 70% to 100%. Consult with the laboratory director if it is less than 70%. Products other than marrow may yield different results, depending on the starting material.

References/Resources

1. McMannis JD. Use of the COBE 2991 Cell Processor for bone marrow processing. In: Gee AP, ed. Bone marrow processing and purging: A practical guide. Boca Raton, FL: CRC Press, 1991:73-85.
2. Rowley S. Bone marrow stem cells. In: Anderson N, ed. Scientific basis of transfusion medicine: Implications for clinical practice. Philadelphia: WB Saunders, 2000:357-75.
3. COBE 2991 Cell Processor essentials guide. (June 2008) Lakewood, CO: CaridianBCT, 2008. [Available at http://www.caridianbct.com/cps/rde/xbcr/SID-3916ADC2-9CC247B8/caridianbct/709016001-2991_Essentials_Guide_EN.pdf (accessed April 14, 2009).]
4. COBE 2991 Cell Processor protocols guide. (June 2008) Lakewood, CO: CaridianBCT, 2008. [Available at http://www.caridianbct.com/cps/rde/xbcr/SID-3916ADC2-6CE55F09/caridianbct/709017001-2991_Protocols_Guide_EN.pdf (accessed April 14, 2009).]

Method 31-4. Washing Cryopreserved Hematopoietic Progenitor Cells to Remove Dimethyl Sulfoxide

Description

Some hematopoietic progenitor cells (HPCs) are frozen in dimethyl sulfoxide (DMSO). For therapeutic cells (non-HPCs)—such as therapeutic cells, T cells (TC-T, also known as donor lymphocyte infusions or DLI)—the product may need to be retested to calculate the T-cell dosage. Because retesting may require several hours, it may be advisable to wash the product free of DMSO after thawing to prevent excessive cytotoxicity. Thawed cells are washed and resuspended in a solution of dextran 40 and 5% human serum albumin (HSA). A similar procedure could be applied to other cellular therapy (CT) products. This procedure does not contain protocols for clerical checks or labeling of products.

Time for Procedure

Approximately 2 hours.

Summary of Procedure

1. The product is thawed in a waterbath containing sterile saline or sterile water at 37 C. Saline may be preferable because it is isotonic and may cause less cell lysis if there is damage to the container during thawing.
2. A sample is removed for viability testing.
3. The product is washed and resuspended in dextran/HSA.
4. Samples are removed for additional testing (eg, flow cytometry to calculate the T-cell dose).

Equipment

1. Blood storage refrigerator at 4 C.
2. Biological safety cabinet (BSC).
3. Waterbath at 37 C.
4. Balance.
5. Sterile connection device.
6. Heat sealer.
7. Centrifuge.
8. Plasma expressor.
9. Adjustable pipettes.
10. Microscope.
11. Hemacytometer.
12. Cell counter.

Reagents and Disposables

1. 18-gauge needles.
2. Syringes (3 mL).
3. Sterile zipper-top bags.
4. Blood culture bottles.
5. Sampling site couplers.
6. Transfer packs (600 mL).
7. Dextran 40.
8. Sterile saline (or water).
9. HSA 5%.
10. Alcohol wipes.
11. Red-top tubes (3 mL).
12. Plastic tubes (6 mL).
13. Pipette tips (sterile filtered).
14. Trypan blue (0.4%).

Procedure

A. Setup

1. Gather reagents and disposables for each product:
   a. 4 plastic tubes (6 mL).
   b. 2 red-top tubes (3 mL).
   c. 1 set blood culture bottles.
2. Ready the equipment:
   a. Confirm that the waterbath is clean and filled with sterile saline. Bring to 37 C.
   b. Clean the BSC before use.

B. Thaw

1. Chill the dextran 40 and 5% HSA to 4 C before use.
2. Thaw the product in the 37-C waterbath according to the institutional standard operating procedure for thawing.

3. Once the product is thawed, draw off a sample for viability testing.

4. Immediately after thawing, slowly add (at 5 mL/minute) *cold* dextran 40 equal to half the volume of the thawed product.

5. Follow the dextran 40 by a similar volume of *cold* 5% HSA at 5 mL/minute.

6. Transfer the cells to a 300-mL transfer pack using the sterile connection device. Leave 6 to 8 inches of tubing between the bags when sterile-connecting.

7. Sterile-connect another properly labeled 300-mL transfer pack to the bag containing the cells. Leave at least 18 inches of tubing between the bags. *Do not open the sterile-connected seal.* Fold the tubing several times and secure it with a rubber band.

   Note: Be careful not to fold the tubing on the sterile connection device seal because this action may damage the seal.

8. Place the product and the empty transfer pack in a sterile bag and seal it. Centrifuge the product at 400 ×g for 10 minutes at 10 C.

9. Carefully remove product from the centrifuge and place it on the plasma expressor with the label facing away from the operator. Express off as much plasma as possible. Seal and disconnect the tubing.

10. Insert a sampling site coupler into the bag containing the cells. Using a syringe, add *cold* dextran 40, equal to the volume in Step 4.

11. Using a syringe, add *cold* 5% HSA, equal to the volume in step 5.

12. Mix the product well and obtain samples for postwash cell counts as follows:
    a. 0.7 mL for flow cytometry.
    b. Draw off from this dilution:
       • 100 µL for CBC and automated differential.
       • 100 µL for viability.

13. Perform the trypan blue viability test and calculate the percent viability.

Note: Notify supervisor of any viability that is <50% for a cryopreserved product.

14. Perform the CBC and automated differential. Using the percent viability, calculate the total (viable) nucleated cells (TNCs).

15. Bring the specimen to the flow cytometry laboratory for CD3, CD19, and CD45 analysis and manual differential. When the results are complete, calculate the total T cells and determine the volume for the cell dose.

16. Transfer the appropriate volume for the dose to a labeled transfer pack. Bring the total volume to a minimum of 25 mL with 5% HSA.

17. Draw off two 1-mL samples (using separate syringes) for blood cultures (anaerobic and aerobic) and inoculate the blood culture bottles.

18. Label the product. The expiration date is 24 hours from the date and time of the thaw.

19. Store the product at 4 C in a blood storage refrigerator until the product is issued.

References/Resources

1. Code of federal regulations. Title 21, CFR Parts 200 to 299 and 600 to 799. Washington, DC: US Government Printing Office, 2008 (revised annually).

2. Food and Drug Administration. Draft document concerning the regulation of peripheral blood hematopoietic stem cell products intended for transplantation or further manufacture into injectable products. (February 1996) Rockville, MD: CBER Office of Communication, Training, and Manufacturers Assistance, 1996.

3. Padley D, ed. Standards for cellular therapy product services. 3rd ed. Bethesda, MD: AABB, 2008.

4. FACT-JACIE international standards for cellular therapy product collection, processing, and administration. 4th ed. Omaha, NE: Foundation for the Accreditation of Cellular Therapy and the Joint Accreditation Committee of ISCT and EBMT, 2008.

5. Areman EM, Deeg HJ, Sacher RA, eds. Bone marrow and stem cell processing: A manual of current techniques. Philadelphia: FA Davis, 1992.

Method 31-5. Reconstitutive Thawing: Preparing Frozen Cord Blood Products for Infusion

Description

Cord blood products must be prepared for infusion in a manner that achieves a high cell recovery, maintains cellular integrity and viability, and avoids contamination of the product.

Time for Procedure

Approximately 1 hour.

Summary of Procedure

Frozen cord blood products are reconstituted with equal or greater amounts of a diluent composed of albumin and Gentran (Baxter, Deerfield, IL), which allows stabilization of cellular components before infusion for laboratory testing and transport. Because centrifugation and expression of supernatant are not required, product safety is increased through fewer manipulations, cell loss is potentially decreased, and preparation time is reduced.

Equipment

1. Biological safety cabinet (BSC).
2. Waterbath at 37 C.
3. Scale.
4. Automated cell counter.

Reagents and Supplies

1. Clean or sterile sealable bag.
2. Syringes: 1 mL, 3 mL, 5 mL, 30 mL.
3. 16-gauge needles.
4. Albumin (human): USP, 25% solution.
5. 10% Gentran 40 (dextran 40) and 5% dextrose or saline.
6. Alcohol wipes.
7. Sampling site couplers.
8. Transfer packs: 150 mL, 300 mL.
9. Hemostat.
10. Cryogloves.
11. Gloves.

Specimen

Cryopreserved cord blood product.

Procedure

1. Verify the product identity, labeling, and container integrity.
2. Prepare reconstitution solution by combining 250 mL Gentran 40 and 50 mL 25% albumin in a 300-mL transfer bag.
3. Using an appropriately sized syringe and 16-gauge needle, withdraw an amount of reconstitution solution equal to the volume of the cord blood unit (including cryoprotective cocktail), plus an additional 5 mL of reconstitution solution for final rinse.
4. Thaw the progenitor cell product:
   a. Move the progenitor cell product from liquid-phase storage to vapor-phase storage. Leave the product in the gas phase for 5 to 10 minutes before proceeding.
   b. Remove the canister from the vapor phase and open it.
   c. Remove any segment attached to the product bag before thawing and store at <−80 C.
   d. Remove the bag from the canister using cryoprotective gloves. Be careful not to bend the bag because the plastic is very brittle at this temperature and will break if bent. Examine the bag for breaks or cracks.
   e. Carefully place the product inside a sealable bag, partially seal the bag, and submerge it in the 37-C waterbath, keeping the port dry and above water.
   f. To accelerate thawing, gently knead contents of bag.

   Note: Inspect for leaks! The most common location where container integrity may be compromised is where the segment was removed

from the unit. Clamping with hemostats as the product thaws can prevent leakage from this site. If product leaks out into the sealed bag, find the site of the break in the freezing bag and position the unit in a way that prevents further escape of product. While maintaining that position, open the sealed bag, and insert the spike of a plasma transfer bag into the freezing bag's port. Let the entire contents drain into the transfer bag and seal the tubing.

5. When the bag's contents become slushy, remove the bag from the 37-C waterbath.

6. Insert a sampling site coupler into the cryobag.

7. Slowly introduce half of the reconstitution solution to the thawed product while mixing the fluids in the bag. Rinse well to remove cells from the bag's ports.

8. Insert the spike of a properly labeled 150-mL transfer bag into the cryobag's second port and drain the contents from the cryobag into the transfer bag.

9. Clamp the tubing between the bags with a hemostat.

10. Add the remaining reconstitution solution to the cryobag through the sampling site coupler. Mix well to rinse the cells from the bag.

11. Drain the reconstitution solution into the transfer bag. Mix well. Note the volume for calculating cell numbers.

12. Allow a small amount of the product to drain back into the cryobag. Through the sampling site coupler, using three 1-mL syringes and 16-gauge needles, remove the following:

    a. Sample of 0.5 mL of product for quality control testing. Deliver it into labeled aliquot tube.

    b. Two 0.5-mL aliquots and inoculate aerobic and anaerobic blood culture bottles.

13. Drain the remaining product into the transfer bag. Clamp the tubing with a hemostat.

14. Add the 5 mL of reconstitution solution into the cryobag for a final rinse. Mix well and drain the contents into the transfer bag. Remember to consider this amount when documenting the infusion volume.

15. Seal the tubing between the cryobag and the transfer bag. Cut the tubing at the seals and separate the bags.

    Note: Upon completion of the following steps, which will take approximately 30 minutes, the product will be ready for infusion. It is standard practice in some centers to page the patient's physician and notify the transplant unit before performing Steps 16 and 17 so that the patient may receive pre-infusion medications.

16. Perform and document a nucleated cell count.

17. Prepare the product for transport or shipping, as appropriate.

Quality Control

From the aliquot of thawed product, the following are performed:

1. Nucleated cell count used to calculate the total nucleated cell (TNC) count and nucleated cell recovery.

2. CD34 analysis by flow cytometry.

3. Colony-forming unit (CFU) assay.

4. Trypan blue and 7-amino-actinomycin D (7-AAD) viability.

5. ABO/Rh type.

6. Aerobic/anaerobic and fungal cultures, which are obtained directly from product.

Calculations

1. TNCs = (WBCs + NRBCs) × (reconstituted product volume – 1.5 mL)

2. Cell recovery =

$$\frac{\text{TNC count of final product} \left[\text{WBCs} + \text{NRBCs} (\times 10^6/\text{mL})\right] \times 100}{\text{TNC count of original product} (\times 10^6/\text{mL})}$$

(TNC = total nucleated cell; WBC = white cell; NRBC = nucleated red cell.)

Anticipated Results

The following are expected results derived from multi-institutional reports of post-thaw activity:

1. Nucleated cell recovery >78%.

2. CD34 recovery >67%.

3. CFU recovery (not quantitative).

4. Trypan blue and 7AAD viability >60%.

5. Aerobic/anaerobic and fungal cultures: no bacterial or fungal growth.
6. ABO/Rh type: consistent with the product record.

Notes

1. This procedure applies to red cell and plasma-reduced products only.
2. Gentran and albumin should be prepared and used at room temperature.
3. Expiration date of thawed cord blood units is 4 hours from time of thaw.
4. If more than 4 hours elapse between thawing and infusion, an aliquot of the product should be removed immediately before infusion to determine the cellular characteristics of the infused product.
5. Any deviation from the standard operating procedure must be approved by the medical director or transplant center's attending physician. The authorization must be documented, retained in the patient and product files, and copied and sent to the transplanting physician. Also, a deviation report should be initiated.
6. Initially, cord blood transplantations were performed primarily in the pediatric setting. The conventional wash procedure was developed because units were not red cell- or plasma-reduced, were of larger volumes, and required greater amounts of dimethyl sulfoxide. With the expanding applications, this may not be

necessary (D Wall, personal communication). With newer processing and storage techniques, it has been demonstrated that simple reconstitution of units accomplishes the following (D Regan, unpublished observations):
a. Stabilizes the product coming out of thawing.
b Eliminates the safety risks involved with centrifugation.
c. Provides material for characterization studies without adversely affecting the transplant dose.
d. Increases confidence that cells are not lost in the expression step.
e. Increases recovery of hematopoietic progenitor cells after thawing.
f. Improves clinical outcomes from transplant centers with limited experience in manipulating frozen cord blood products.

References/Resources

1. Areman EM, Deeg HJ, Sacher RA. Bone marrow and stem cell processing: A manual of current techniques. Philadelphia: FA Davis Company, 1992.
2. Rubinstein P, Dobrila L, Rosenfield RE, et al. Processing and cryopreservation of placental/umbilical cord blood for unrelated bone marrow reconstitution. Proc Nat Acad Sci U S A 1995;92:10119-22.
3. Hahn T, Bunworasate U, George MC, et al. Use of non volume-reduced (unmanipulated after thawing) umbilical cord blood stem cells for allogeneic transplantation results in safe engraftment. Bone Marrow Transplant 2003;32:145-50.

Method 31-6. Infusion of Hematopoietic Progenitor Cells in Adult Patients

Description

Hematopoietic progenitor cells (HPCs) are harvested and processed, but may or may not be cryopreserved, before infusion. For autologous transplants and cord blood transplants, the HPC product will have been cryopreserved and then thawed before infusion. For allogeneic transplants, the HPC product is usually infused "fresh" on the same day of the collection, although cryopreservation of allogeneic HPC-A products is not rare. This procedure describes infusion of the HPC product either "fresh" or following thawing.

Time for Procedure

Approximately 30 minutes for infusion.

Summary of Procedure

1. The patient is premedicated and hydrated.
2. Positive identification of the recipient and the product is performed.
3. The HPC product is infused, usually through a central venous catheter, but occasionally through a peripheral line by qualified medical personnel. The procedure is usually performed with a physician immediately available in case the recipient should experience an adverse reaction to the infusion.

Equipment and Supplies

1. Normal saline.
2. Nonfiltered Y-site tubing.
3. Electrocardiogram (EKG) machine.
4. Pulse oximeter.
5. Oxygen setup.
6. Adverse reaction kit: epinephrine, Benadryl (Pfizer, New York, NY), hydrocortisone.
7. Atropine.
8. 60-cc syringe with 19-gauge needle.
9. Three 12-cc syringes filled with normal saline (NS).
10. 19-gauge needles.
11. Nonsterile gloves.
12. Hard candy.

Procedure

A. *Transplantation Planning*
   1. For cryopreserved HPCs, avoid infusing >1 g of DMSO per kilogram of recipient weight per day. Each bag of 100 cc of cryopreserved cells in 10% DMSO contains 10 g of DMSO. Therefore, a 55-kg patient can receive 5 bags.
   2. When the DMSO load exceeds 1 g/kg recipient weight, the infusion may be divided and infused with several hours between infusions (or the remaining infusion on following day).

B. *Premedication and Preparation*
   1. Prehydrate patients according to physician's orders over 2 to 3 hours before infusion. Continue hydration between infusions and, once the infusions are completed, administer an additional liter of intravenous (IV) fluid.
   2. Preinfusion medications may include acetaminophen, diphenhydramine, and antiemetics.
   3. The laboratory should confirm infusion times with nursing staff to ensure that the recipient is prepared (ie, premedications administered, vital signs monitored, and IV set up). It takes approximately 5 to 10 minutes for HPCs to be thawed.
   4. The HPCs are usually transported to the infusion location by the cellular therapy (CT) facility staff.
   5. The designated infusionist must be ready to infuse the HPCs when the CT staff member arrives with the HPC products.

C. *Identification of the HPC Unit and Patient*

Note: The recipient and the HPC container must be positively identified by two persons immediately before the infusion.

1. The infusionist and, in most cases, the nurse caring for the patient, in the presence of the recipient, should verify the following:

   a. Recipient name, identification number, and HPC product ordered.

   b. Recipient name, identification number, and ordered HPC product number match the HPC container information, if applicable, as well as the laboratory slip attached to the bag.

2. For allogeneic transplant patients, donor information, when available, should be verified in the same manner and at the same time.

3. The laboratory slip attached to the HPCs must be signed by the person administering the HPCs and the second person verifying the identification.

D. *Infusion of the HPC Product*

Note: HPCs must be infused using sterile, pyrogen-free tubing. Leukocyte-reduction filters or microaggregate filters must not be used.

1. Before beginning the infusion, the recipient must be connected to EKG monitoring and a pulse oximeter.

2. To begin the infusion, connect the HPCs to one side of the Y-tubing. The other side must have a 250-cc or 500-cc bag of NS attached.

3. Monitor the patient's vital signs and record them immediately before the infusion, 5 minutes after initiation of the infusion, every 10 to 15 minutes during the infusion, and at the completion of the infusion.

4. Administer the HPCs via a central line through the largest lumen. Do not administer HPCs through a needle or cap because it may slow infusion and/or cause lysis of cells.

5. Recipients may be offered hard candy during the infusion to minimize the unpleasant taste and nausea from the HPCs preserved in DMSO.

6. All identification attached to the HPC bag should remain attached at least until the infusion has been completed.

7. HPCs should be infused at a rate determined by the type of HPC infused:

   a. Usual infusion rates for HPC-A: 10 to 30 minutes.

   b. Red-cell- or plasma-depleted HPCs: 5 to 30 minutes.

   c. Nondepleted HPCs: varies according to volume.

8. HPCs may be diluted with a small amount of NS using the Y-tubing setup.

9. When more than one HPC bag is infused, the subsequent bag(s) should be thawed while the current bag of HPCs is being infused. If an adverse event or delay occurs while infusing HPCs, notify the CT facility as soon as possible to halt the thawing of subsequent HPC bags.

E. *Completion*

1. When each HPC infusion is complete, the HPC bag should be rinsed with a small amount of NS, using the Y-tubing setup, and administered to the recipient to ensure the administration of most of the HPCs. NS infusion should be continued until the IV tubing is clear of HPCs.

2. Each HPC bag, along with the IV tubing setup, should be discarded in a biohazard waste receptacle or returned to the CT facility in the case of an adverse reaction.

F. *Documentation*

1. Ensure the laboratory slip attached to the HPCs shows the date, start and end times of each infusion, and the signatures of both the person administering the HPCs and the witness.

2. Record the volumes of NS and HPCs infused on the recipient's flow sheet.

3. The member of the transplant team supervising the HPC infusion should document the infusion and patient response, including adverse reactions, in a progress note.

4. For serious adverse events, return the HPC container to the CT facility for additional testing, along with the appropriate documentation. Notify the medical director of the CT facility.

References/Resources

1. AABB, America's Blood Centers, American Association of Tissue Banks, et al. Circular of information for the use of cellular therapy products. Bethesda, MD: AABB, 2007. [Available at http://www.aabb.org/Content/About_Blood/Circulars_of_Information/aabb_coi.htm (accessed March 18, 2009).]

2. Brecher ME, Lasky LC, Sacher RA, et al, eds. Hematopoietic progenitor cells: Processing, standards, and practice. Bethesda, MD: AABB, 1995.

3. Davis JM, Rowley SD, Braine HG, et al. Clinical toxicity of cryopreserved bone marrow graft infusion. Blood 1990;75:781-6.

4. Sacher RA, AuBuchon JP, eds. Marrow transplantation: Practical and technical aspects of stem cell reconstitution. Bethesda, MD: AABB, 1992.

5. Sauer-Heilborn A, Kadidlo D, McCullough J. Patient care during infusion of hematopoietic progenitor cells. Transfusion 2004;44:907-16.

Production: Complex or Extensive Processing

THIS SECTION DISCUSSES CELLULAR THERapy (CT) production methods that are more complex than those termed "basic" in the previous section. These processes require more training, more laboratory resources, and a greater time commitment than those described earlier. Because many of these methods entail extensive manipulation of the CT product, they pose a greater risk of contamination or product damage than the more basic methods do. Nevertheless, the novel therapies described in this section, as well as others in various stages of development, may hold the key to the successful treatment and cure of a wide variety of serious, even life-threatening, conditions.

The methods presented here are a few examples of the constantly expanding repertoire of CT products painstakingly translated from small-scale research laboratory procedures to large-scale methods appropriate for clinical use. As explained more fully in Section VI, all methods are presented as examples, and details of aseptic processing steps have been omitted for the sake of brevity and consistency.

The cell-processing facility's main goal is to provide patients and clinical programs with safe, potent, and pure cellular products. It is important to validate and practice any procedure a laboratory performs. Because, not uncommonly, some of these techniques are performed only rarely, mock products are often the only way to train staff and maintain competency. Any procedure should be performed in a reliable and reproducible manner and result in a pure, potent cell product of the highest quality for administration. In summary, in the process of evaluating various production methods, it is important to consider factors such as hematopoietic cell recovery, purity of the final product, procedure time and labor, availability of clinical reagents and equipment, and relevant regulations. Ultimately, the product's success will be determined by its clinical efficacy for patients.

Section Editors: Melissa Croskell, MT(ASCP), Manager of Regulatory Compliance, Department of Pathology and Laboratory Services, and BMT Program Quality Manager, The Children's Hospital–Aurora, Aurora, Colorado; Kathy Loper, MHS, MT(ASCP), Director, Cellular Therapies, AABB, Bethesda, Maryland; and David H. McKenna, Jr, MD, Scientific and Medical Director, Molecular and Cellular Therapeutics, University of Minnesota, St Paul, Minnesota

M. Croskell and K. Loper have disclosed no conflicts of interest. D. McKenna has disclosed a financial relationship with BioE, Inc.

In: Areman EM, Loper K, eds
Cellular Therapy: Principles, Methods, and Regulations
Bethesda, MD: AABB, 2009

◆ ◆ ◆ **32** ◆ ◆ ◆

Graft Modification: Cell Enrichment or Depletion

Safa Karandish, MT(ASCP)

GRAFT-VS-HOST DISEASE (GVHD) HAS been a major complication of allogeneic hematopoietic progenitor cell (HPC) transplantation. The incidence and severity of GVHD may depend on the degree of HLA matching between donor and recipient; whether the donor is unrelated or is a related, matched donor; and the source of HPCs used for transplantation. It has been shown that reducing the number of T lymphocytes in the graft lowers the risk of GVHD. However, patients transplanted with T-cell-depleted grafts have experienced higher incidences of graft failure, rejection, or relapse, as well as delayed immune reconstitution and greater risk of infection. To reduce the risk of GVHD and graft failure, several clinical studies have explored such interventions as infusion of a limited number of T cells and transplantation of "mega doses" of HPCs.

In the autologous transplant setting, the risks of both graft failure and disease relapse have been a major concern. Graft failure has been attributed to such factors as poor product quality, inadequate progenitor cell dose, and suboptimal cellular function, especially in the case of tumor-depleted products, whereas residual tumor cells in the graft may contribute to disease relapse.[5-7] It is unclear to what extent a contaminated graft contributes to relapse and to what extent residual tumor in the host is responsible. Studies on these issues suggest some answers, but their conclusions often disagree.[8,9] The need for and effectiveness of ex-vivo tumor purging to lower the risk of relapse are still debated among scientists and clinical investigators. Other challenges include accurately determining tumor cell contamination in the graft, as well as demonstrating the relationship between residual tumor cells and clinical outcome.

Immunotherapy may be defined as treatment to stimulate or restore the immune system's ability to function properly or fight disease. Cellular therapies have the potential to serve as biologic immune modulators. Dendritic cells, mesenchymal stromal cells, and graft manipulation for transplant are all potential platforms for immunotherapy and are discussed later in this section.

Safa Karandish, MT(ASCP), Field Application Scientist, Pall Life Sciences, Houston, Texas

The author has disclosed no conflicts of interest.

Cell Isolation Methods

Various approaches to reduce the number of T cells or tumor cells in the graft, using immunologic, nonimmunologic, or combination techniques, have been evaluated. A few examples of these techniques are cell depletion or purging using monoclonal antibodies, tumor cell depletion with chemotherapeutic agents, T-cell depletion using counterflow centrifugal elutriation (CCE), and sheep red blood cell (SRBC) rosetting with soybean agglutinin. More recently, techniques combining immunomagnetic beads and monoclonal antibodies specific for various T-cell or tumor cell populations have also been used to remove target cells from the product. All of these strategies aim for "negative selection"—the removal or destruction of the unwanted cells in the graft.

Monoclonal antibody techniques generally involve the addition of antibody to cells. Cells are then removed either by physical methods (such as immunomagnetic selection, described below) or by the addition of complement to destroy target cells. Human serum as a complement source has replaced rabbit complement over the years because of regulatory concerns regarding animal products. Antibodies to CAMPATH-1 (CD52) have been used for T-cell depletion because it binds to lymphocytes and monocytes (but not progenitor cells). These procedures are cumbersome and lengthy, often requiring 4 to 8 hours of processing time after the initial product preparation, such as a buffy coat preparation. Although variable, the outcomes of a number of investigational trials employing these processes, performed primarily in the HLA-mismatched setting, demonstrated reduced risk of GVHD without an increased risk of graft failure.[10] Many of the early cell purging techniques have been replaced with more automated methods such as antibody-specific immunomagnetic selection.

Tumor purging has been tried in the autologous setting as a means to prevent relapse. Several studies, including some incorporating gene marking, have demonstrated the presence of tumor cells in autologous marrow and HPCs from apheresis (HPC-A) products.[5-7,11] This negative selection approach has most often used a variety of pharmacologic agents or tumor-specific antibodies to remove the undesirable cell population. Because trials using chemotherapeutic agents have resulted in delayed engraftment, these procedures are rarely performed in common clinical practice. Monoclonal antibody procedures require tumor-specific antibodies, which may not always be available. Furthermore, because of the heterogeneity of most tumors, all of the tumor cells may not be removed or destroyed by the procedure.[11] Finally, current thinking that residual disease in the patient contributes to relapse as much as or more than reinfused tumor cells has reduced enthusiasm for these methods as effective means of preventing cancer recurrence.[8,9]

Cell Enrichment

Also referred to as cell selection or positive selection, cell enrichment may be performed to decrease the concentration of dimethyl sulfoxide (DMSO) or other additives in a product, to remove unwanted cells from a product by selecting and retaining all but the undesirable cell population, or as a preparative step for further manipulation. For HPC transplantation, one strategy is to enrich for the HPC population in the graft as an indirect means of removing the unwanted cells. HPCs express CD34 antigen on their cell surface. Presence of this identifying marker has allowed the development of CD34-positive cell selection methods using anti-CD34 monoclonal antibodies bound to immunomagnetic beads. In the autologous transplant setting, this methodology may not be suitable for all disorders because the CD34 antigen is expressed on certain tumor or leukemic cells. However, for patients with CD34-negative tumors, such as lymphoma and multiple myeloma, CD34-positive cell enrichment has been used as an invitro graft purging technique.[12]

Device manufacturers have developed automated clinical-scale devices for cell selection based on immunomagnetic bead technology. Currently, in the United States, one device is FDA-approved for processing autologous HPC-A products to obtain a CD34+ cell-enriched population intended for hematopoietic reconstitution after myeloablative therapy in patients with CD34-negative tumors (Isolex 300i Magnetic Cell Selection System, Baxter, Deerfield, IL—see Fig 32-1).

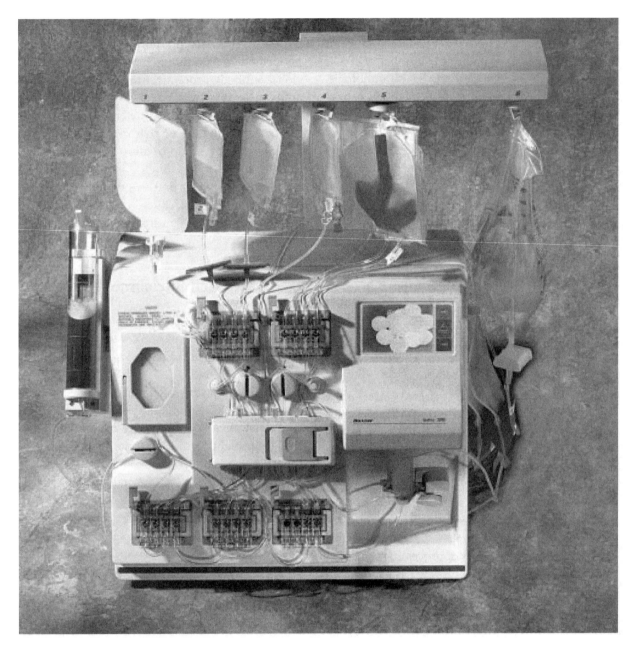

Figure 32-1. Isolex 300i Magnetic Cell Selection System (Courtesy of Baxter, Deerfield, IL).

The Baxter Isolex 300i system is CE-marked (Conformité Européenne) and approved for use in Europe. In this system, CD34-positive cells are first sensitized with a murine anti-human CD34 monoclonal antibody. The sensitized cells are then captured with immunomagnetic beads that have been conjugated to sheep anti-murine immunoglobulin. The captured cells are placed in a magnetic field to retain the CD34-positive cells/antibody/bead complexes while removing the nontarget (CD34-negative) cells. The CD34-positive cells are nonen-zymatically released from the antibody/bead complexes using an octapeptide-releasing agent. CD34-positive and CD34-depleted fractions are collected in separate containers. Up to 8×10^{10} total nucleated cells (TNCs) can be loaded onto the device. Total cell yields of 50% to 60% with 80% to 90% purity have been reported.[11,13-15] Generally, facilities target a minimum CD34 dose preselection of 5×10^6 CD34-positive cells/kg, with delayed platelet engraftment reported in patients receiving $<2 \times 10^6$/kg CD34-positive cells.[16] Product age, red cell content, and platelet concentration may affect yield and purity. Earlier investigative studies were performed with marrow, but more recent applications primarily focus on CD34-positive cells in mobilized peripheral blood for CD34-positive selection.[17] Combined positive and negative selection of allogeneic products resulting in 3 to 4 $\log^{10}$ T-cell depletion has been reported in some research trials.[18]

Another automated device available from a different manufacturer (CliniMACS Cell Selection System, Miltenyi Biotec, Bergisch Gladbach, Germany—see Fig 32-2) is also CE-marked for international distribution and can be used within the United States under FDA-approved clinical protocols and for research purposes. For HPC applications, up to 6×10^{10} total cells can be processed. The CD34-positive cells are labeled with CD34 monoclonal antibody that has been directly coupled to small super-paramagnetic particles. The labeled cells are then passed over a strong magnet, which generates a magnetic field for retaining the target cells and allowing the unwanted cells to be removed from the graft. Once the magnet is removed, the retained cells are released and collected. Purities >90% and yields of 55% to 60% have been reported.[15,19] Other monoclonal antibodies are also available for selection of other cell types such as monocytes, dendritic cells, natural killer cells, and T-cell subsets. Not all reagents are currently approved for human use, and several trials are under way comparing CD34-positive and CD 133-positive (another progenitor cell marker) selected products in engraftment and expansion studies.[20]

Both of these devices also result in a product that has a significantly smaller volume than the starting material and that would require the use of less DMSO for cryopreserved products. While yield, purity, and viability results are similar with both instruments, at least one study reported a difference in functionality for cell culture applications.[15] Results with starting products containing higher CD34+ cell numbers are generally better than those from products with lower starting values.[21]

References/Resources

1. Ho VT, Soiffer RJ. The history and future of T-cell depletion as graft-versus-host disease prophylaxis for alloge-

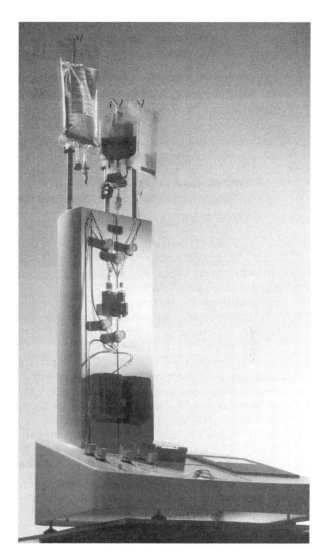

Figure 32-2. CliniMACS Cell Selection System (Courtesy of Miltenyi Biotec, Bergisch Gladbach, Germany).

neic hematopoietic stem cell transplantation. Blood 2001;98:3192-204.

2. Berger TG, Strasser E, Smith R, et al. Efficient elutriation of monocytes within a closed system (Elutra) for clinical-scale generation of dendritic cells. J Immunol Methods 2005;298:61-72.

3. Beckman Instruments, Inc. The JE-5.0 Elutriation System: Instructional manual. Palo Alto, CA: Spinco Division of Beckman, 1989.

4. Kim S, Kim HO, Baek EJ, et al. Monocyte enrichment from leukapheresis products by using the Elutra cell separator. Transfusion 2007;47:2290-6.

5. Lundell BI, Vredenburgh JJ, Tyer C, et al. Ex vivo expansion of bone marrow from breast cancer patients: Reduction in tumor cell content through passive purging. Bone Marrow Transplant 1998;22:153-9.

6. Simpson SJ, Vachula M, Kennedy MJ, et al. Detection of tumor cells in the bone marrow, peripheral blood, and apheresis products of breast cancer patients using flow cytometry. Exp Hematol 1995;23:1062-8.

7. Burgess J, Mills B, Griffith M, et al. Breast cancer contamination of PBSC harvests: Tumor depletion by positive selection of CD34(+) cells. Cytotherapy 2001;3:285-94.

8. Matthay KK, Atkinson JB, Stram DO, et al. Patterns of relapse after autologous purged bone marrow transplantation for neuroblastoma: A children's cancer group pilot study. J Clin Oncol 1993;11:2226-33.

9. Cristofanilli M, Budd G, Ellis M, et al. Circulating tumor cells, disease progression, and survival in metastatic breast cancer. N Engl J Med 2004;351:781-91.

10. Hale G, Zhang M, Burnes D, et al. Improving the outcome of bone marrow transplantation by using CD52 antibodies to prevent graft versus host disease and graft rejection. Blood 1998;92:4581-90.

11. Paulus U, Dreger P, Viehmann K, et al. Purging peripheral blood progenitor cell grafts from lymphoma cells: Quantitative comparison of immunomagnetic CD34+ selection systems. Stem Cells 1997;15:297-304.

12. Dyson P, Horvath N, Joshua D, et al. CD34+ selection of autologous peripheral blood stem cells for transplantation following sequential cycles of high dose therapy and mobilization in multiple myeloma. Bone Marrow Transplant 2000;25:1175-84.

13. Gryn J, Shadduck R, Lister J, et al. Factors affecting purification of CD34+ peripheral blood stem cells using the Baxter Isolex 300i. J Hematotherapy Stem Cell Res 2002;11:719-30.

14. Hildebrandt M, Serke S, Myer O, et al. Immunomagnetic selection of CD34+ cells: Factors influencing component purity and yield. Transfusion 2000;40:507-12.

15. Watts MJ, Somervaille T, Ings SJ, et al. Variable product purity and functional capacity after CD34 selection: A direct comparison of the CliniMACS (v2·1) and Isolex 300i (v2·5) clinical scale devices. Br J Haematol 2002;118:117-23.

16. Bensinger W, Applebaum F, Rowley S, et al. Factors that influence collection and engraftment of autologous peripheral-blood stem cells. J Clin Oncol 1995;13:2547-55.

17. Kasow K, Sims-Poston L, Eldridge P, et al. CD34+ hematopoietic progenitor cell selection of bone marrow grafts for autologous transplantation in pediatric patients. Biol Blood Marrow Transplant 2007;13:608-14.

18. Martin-Henao G, Picon M, Amill B, et al. Combined positive and negative cell selection from allogeneic peripheral blood progenitor cells (PBPC) by use of immunomagnetic methods. Bone Marrow Transplant 2001;27:683-7.

19. Arpaci F, Cetin T, Ozet A, et al. The excessive numbers of total nucleated cells does not affect the performance of CliniMACS. J Clin Apher 2004;19:197-201.

20. Lang P, Bader P, Schumm M, et al. Transplantation of a combination of CD133+ and CD34+ selected progenitor cells from alternative donors. Br J Haematol 2004;124:72-9.

21. Perotti C, Del Fante C, Viarengo GL, et al. Impact of leukapheresis cell composition on immunomagnetic cell selection with the Baxter Isolex 300i device: A statistical analysis. Stem Cells Dev 2004;13:350-6.

Method 32-1. Selecting CD34+ Cells Using the Isolex 300i Magnetic Cell Selection System

Description

The Isolex 300i Magnetic Cell Selection System (Baxter, Deerfield, IL) is a fully automated device used for processing cellular therapy products to obtain a population that is CD34+ enriched.

Time for Procedure

From 3.5 to 4 hours, including advance cell and reagent preparation.

Summary of Procedure

1. Sensitization step: Cells are mixed with anti-human CD34 murine IgG monoclonal antibody, which binds to CD34+ cells.
2. Rosetting step: Following wash steps to remove the unbound antibody, cell suspension is mixed with immunomagnetic beads coated with sheep anti-mouse IgG antibody that recognizes the murine CD34 antibody bound to the cells. This step results in formation of bead/cell rosette complexes.
3. Releasing step: The rosettes are separated from the rest of the cell suspension by applying the magnetic field to the chamber containing the cells. Following several wash steps to remove the unbound cells, the PR34+ stem cell releasing agent (octapeptide) is added to separate the CD34+ cells from the murine antibody and the Dynabeads.
4. Collection step: The magnetic field is applied to the chamber again to retain the bead/antibody complexes and collect the released CD34+ cells.
5. The selected cells are then concentrated and washed.

Equipment

1. Isolex 300i Magnetic Cell Separator, software version 2.5 (Baxter #4R9771).

2. Dynal MPC-1 magnetic particle concentrator [Invitrogen (#120-01D), Carlsbad, CA].
3. Automated cell counter or microscope and hemacytometer for nucleated cell count.
4. Tubing sealer.
5. Electronic balance.
6. Biological safety cabinet (BSC).

Supplies and Reagents

1. Isolex stem cell reagent kit (Baxter #4R9734):
   - 1 vial anti-CD34 monoclonal antibody (2.5 mL).
   - 1 vial sheep anti-mouse (SAM) IgG-coated Dynabeads (10 mL).
   - 1 vial PR34+ stem cell releasing agent (20 mL).
2. Dulbecco's phosphate-buffered saline (DPBS; Ca++ and Mg++ free): 3-L bag (Baxter #EDR9865 or equivalent).
3. Immune globulin intravenous (IVIG, human): Gammagard (0.5g/vial; Baxter #060384 or equivalent).
4. Human serum albumin (HSA): 25% solution.
5. Sodium citrate anticoagulant: 4% solution, 250-mL bag [Fenwal (#4B7867Q), Lake Zurich, IL].
6. Isolex 300i magnetic cell separator disposable set (Baxter #R4R9850): includes Lifecell bag with in-line filter.

Procedure

A. *Working Buffer and Reagent Preparation*
   1. Aseptically prepare the following in the BSC:
      a. Working buffer: 3-L DPBS supplemented with 1% HSA and 0.41% sodium citrate (weight/volume).
      b. 5% IVIG solution: Prepare solution following the manufacturer's instruc-

tions. After the lyophilized IVIG is dissolved completely, transfer the solution into a 10-mL syringe and store it at room temperature until use.

c. Dynabeads:
- Transfer the contents of 1 vial of Dynabeads (10 mL) to a 50-mL centrifuge tube.
- Add 10 mL of working buffer to the beads. After gentle mixing, place the tube on the Dynal MPC-1 magnet for 2 minutes.
- While holding the tube against the magnet, remove the supernatant using a pipette.
- Remove the tube from the magnet and resuspend the beads in 10 mL working buffer.
- Draw the beads into a syringe.

2. Draw the contents of the PR34+ release agent vial (20 mL) and the CD34 antibody vial (2.5 mL) into the syringes.

B. Preparation of Cells

1. Aseptically obtain preprocessing quality control (QC) samples (for cell count, viability, flow cytometry analysis, and sterility as required).

2. Perform cell counts and calculate total nucleated cells (TNCs) in the product. The maximum cell number for each selection procedure is 8×10^{10} nucleated cells. The product may be split for two procedures.

3. Aseptically add the 10 mL dissolved IVIG to the cell suspension and incubate it for 15 minutes at room temperature. Transfer the cells into the Lifecell bag with the in-line filter (provided with the disposable tubing set).

C. Instrument and Disposable Tubing Set Setup

1. Refer to the operator's manual for detailed instructions on the instrument and disposable tubing setup.

2. After installing the disposable set, the instrument automatically tests the integrity of the set and the proper installation. Connect the buffer bag to the set when

prompted, and begin the automatic prime step.

3. Follow the instructions on the screen for adding reagents and connecting the cell product bag.

D. Automated Selection Procedure: Major Automated Steps

1. Buffer addition: Buffer is added to the reagent and cell source bags.

2. Platelet wash: Cells are concentrated and washed with buffer in the recirculation wash bag and spinner.

3. Antibody transfer: CD34 antibody is added to the bag containing the washed cells.

4. Antibody incubation: Cells are recirculated through the spinner during the 15-minute antibody incubation period.

5. Antibody wash: Cells are washed with buffer to remove unbound antibody.

6. Transfer of cells: Cells are transferred to the chamber and the volume is brought up to the minimum of 100 mL.

7. Rosetting: Cells are mixed with Dynabeads and incubated for 30 minutes. After completion of the incubation time, cell/bead rosettes are captured by the magnet, and nontarget cells are drained out of the chamber and collected in the negative fraction bag.

8. Chamber cell wash I to III: Cell/bead rosettes are washed with the buffer. Wash solution is collected in the negative fraction bag.

9. Release agent transfer and cell release, incubation, and rinse: The release agent is transferred from the weight scale to the chamber. The chamber is filled with buffer up to approximately 100 mL. Cell/bead rosettes are incubated with the release agent for 30 minutes. After completion of incubation time, released cells are transferred from the chamber into the second wash bag. The chamber is then rinsed once with buffer, and wash solution is added to the cells in the second wash bag.

10. Release agent wash: Released cells (CD34+ cells) are concentrated and washed with buffer.

11. Cell transfer to end-product bag: Washed/concentrated CD34+ cells are transferred to the final bag, and the volume is brought to approximately 100 mL.

E. *Procedure Completion*
   1. Heat-seal and remove the positive fraction bag. Determine the final volume and aseptically remove QC samples (for cell count, viability, flow cytometry analysis, and sterility). Selected cells are ready for either fresh infusion or further manipulation such as cryopreservation. If volume reduction is necessary, cells should be transferred into centrifuge tube(s) for manual concentration using a centrifuge.
   2. Heat-seal and remove the negative fraction bag. Determine the final volume and asep-

tically remove QC samples (cell count and flow cytometry analysis).
   3. Remove the disposable set by following the instructions in the operator's manual.

Anticipated Results

1. CD34+ cell recovery >50%.
2. Purity >85%.
   Note: Unsuccessful mobilization and a low number of CD34+ cells in the preselection product may negatively affect the results.

References/Resources

1. Isolex 300i magnetic cell selection system operator's manual. Version 2.5. Deerfield, IL: Baxter Healthcare, 2004.
2. Isolex 300i magnetic cell separator package insert. Deerfield, IL: Baxter Healthcare, 2004.

Method 32-2. Selecting CD34+ Cells Using the CliniMACS System

Description

The CliniMACS system (Miltenyi Biotec, Bergisch Gladbach, Germany) is used for processing of cellular therapy products to obtain a cell population that is CD34+ enriched.

Time for Procedure

From 3.5 to 4 hours, including preliminary cell and reagent preparation.

Summary of Procedure

The CD34+ cells are labeled by incubation with the CliniMACS CD34 reagent (iron dextran super-paramagnetic particles conjugated with CD34 monoclonal antibody). After unbound reagent is removed by washing the labeled cell suspension, the cells are ready for the automated selection process. The CliniMACS system passes the antibody-labeled cell suspension through a column in which strong magnetic field gradients are generated. The selection column retains the magnetically labeled CD34+ cells, while unwanted cells flow through and are collected in the negative fraction bag. After completion of several washing steps, the selected CD34+ cells are released from the column by removing the column from the magnetic field and eluting the cells into the cell collection bag.

Equipment

1. CliniMACS instrument (Miltenyi #151-01).
2. COBE 2991 Cell Processor (CaridianBCT, Lakewood, CO).
3. Automated cell counter or microscope and hemacytometer for nucleated cell count.
4. Tubing sealer.
5. Electronic balance.
6. Biological safety cabinet (BSC).
7. Sterile connection device.
8. Centrifuge.
9. Orbital rotator.

10. Plasma extractor.

Supplies and Reagents

1. CliniMACS CD34 reagent: 1 vial (7.5 mL; Miltenyi #171-01).
2. CliniMACS phosphate-buffered saline (PBS)/EDTA: 1000-mL bag (Miltenyi #700-25).
3. Human serum albumin (HSA): 25% solution.
4. CliniMACS tubing set (Miltenyi #161-01).
5. Blood transfusion filter: 40 μ [Pall (#SQ40S or equivalent), East Hills, NY].
6. 300-mL and 600-mL transfer packs.
7. Transfer sets with spike–to-needle adapter [Fenwal (#4C2240 or equivalent), Lake Zurich, IL].
8. COBE 2991 single processing set (CaridianBCT #912-647-819).
9. COBE 2991 single coupler (CaridianBCT #912-647-904).
   Note: The above product codes are for clinical investigational materials available in the United States.

Procedure

A. Buffer and Apheresis Product Preparation
1. Aseptically prepare three 1-L CliniMACS PBS/EDTA buffer bags supplemented with 0.5% HSA (final concentration) in the BSC.
2. Determine the volume of the cell product and aseptically remove QC samples (for cell count, viability, flow cytometry analysis, and sterility).
3. Perform cell counts and calculate the total nucleated cells (TNCs) in the product. The maximum cell number for each selection procedure is 6×10^{10} nucleated cells and 0.6×10^9 CD34+ cells with one reagent vial.
   Note: For cell products containing a higher cell number (up to 12×10^{10} nucleated cells and 1.2×10^9 CD34+ cells), two reagent vials may be

used. Labeled cells can be either split in half after labeling, for processing with two standard tubing sets, or kept together for processing with one large-scale tubing set (CliniMACs tubing set #LS 162-01).

B. *Platelet Depletion*

1. Transfer the cells to a 600-mL transfer pack using the sterile connection device.
2. Close the roller clamp on a plasma transfer set, and insert the spike into one of the ports in one of the buffer bags. Using the sterile connection device, connect the tubing on the transfer set to the 600-mL transfer pack containing the cells.
3. Add buffer to fill the 600-mL bag (approximately 600 mL). A 1:3 dilution of cells with buffer is recommended for the platelet-depletion step. Determine the final volume using the electronic balance.
4. Using the sterile connection device, connect an empty 600-mL transfer pack to the diluted cell bag. Do not open the weld.
5. Centrifuge the bag at $200 \times g$ for 15 minutes at room temperature and low or no brake.
6. Determine the volume of supernatant to be removed after centrifugation.
   a. The target volume of cell suspension remaining in the bag is 95 mL if using one reagent vial, or 190 mL if using two vials.
   b. The volume of diluted cells (Step 3 above) minus 95 or 190 mL (Step 6a above) is the volume of supernatant to remove.
7. After completion of centrifugation, place the cell bag on the plasma extractor and the empty transfer pack on the balance.
8. Open the tubing weld, and transfer the amount of supernatant calculated above into the empty transfer pack. Seal the tubing and disconnect the supernatant bag.
9. Determine the volume of platelet-depleted cells and obtain QC samples for cell count and other needed tests.

C. *Magnetic Labeling of the Cells*

1. Depending on the starting cell number, aseptically add the contents of one or two

CliniMACS CD34+ reagent vial(s) (7.5 mL per vial). Mix the cells with the reagent.
2. Place the bag on an orbital rotator at approximately 25 rotations per minute, or manually mix the cell suspension every 5 minutes. Incubate the cells with the reagent for 30 minutes at room temperature.

D. *Post-Antibody-Incubation Wash (COBE 2991 Method)*

Note: Cells may be washed twice using a manual centrifugation method if the COBE 2991 is not available. (centrifuge settings used for the platelet-depletion step may be used.)

1. Following the manufacturer's instructions, install the COBE 2991 tubing set, but do not load the inlet line in the red cell detector.
2. Set the following instrument settings:
   a. Centrifuge speed: 1500 rpm.
   b. SUPER OUT rate: 250 mL/minute.
   c. Minimum agitate time: not applicable.
   d. SUPER OUT volume (SOV): 550.
   e. Valve selector: V2.
   f. Collect/SOV light: SOV (green).
   g. Auto/manual light: manual (yellow).
   h. Attach a bag of CliniMACS buffer (1000 mL) to the spike on the green line, and after completion of the antibody incubation time, attach the cell bag to the red line.
3. Press BLOOD IN to transfer cells to the donut bag. Press STOP/RESET.
4. Place a hemostat on the line going into the donut bag, lower the cell bag, press PREDILUTE, and add approximately 300 mL of buffer to the cell bag. Press STOP/RESET. Rinse the bag and rehang it on the solution pole.
5. Remove the hemostat from the line going to the donut, and press BLOOD IN to transfer the rinse volume to the donut bag. Press AIROUT, and when the fluid reaches the cell bag, press BLOOD IN. Place a hemostat on the red line as soon as the fluid reaches the tubing manifold. Press STOP/RESET.
6. Press PREDILUTE to fill the donut bag with buffer. Press STOP/RESET.

7. Remove the hemostat from the red line, set the timer for 8 minutes, and press START/SPIN. Centrifuge the product for 8 minutes.

8. Press SUPER OUT, and express supernatant for approximately 2 minutes. Then press AGITATE/WASH IN to fill the donut bag with buffer.

9. Set the timer for 8 minutes and press START/SPIN. Centrifuge the product for 8 minutes.

10. Press SUPER OUT and express the supernatant for approximately 2 minutes. Press STOP/RESET.

11. Heat-seal the inlet line, remove the donut bag, resuspend the cells, and attach the sampling site coupler to the donut bag.

12. Aseptically transfer the cells from the donut bag into an empty 300-mL transfer bag. Rinse the donut bag with approximately 20 mL of CliniMACS buffer. Add the rinse solution to the transfer pack. Repeat two to three times or until the donut bag is sufficiently rinsed.

13. Adjust the final cell volume to 150 to 300 mL by adding buffer, and obtain QC samples for the cell count and other needed tests.

> **Note:** If the cells were labeled with two reagent vials, adjust the volume to 300 mL. Either use a large-scale tubing set to perform one run, or split the product in half for two runs using the standard tubing set.

E. CliniMACS CD34+ Cell Selection

1. Heat-seal and remove the tubing on an empty 300-mL transfer pack. Insert the spike end of a COBE 2991 single coupler into one of the ports on the 300-mL transfer pack. Do not close the clamp.

2. Under the BSC, open the tubing set packaging and connect the bag to the male luer on the CliniMACS tubing set.

3. Turn the instrument on, select the program, and install the tubing set following the manufacturer's instructions and screen prompts.

4. When prompted, connect the CliniMACS buffer (1-L) bag to the processing set, and hang it on adjustable left bag hanger.

5. Connect the 40-μ filter to the bubble trap, and adjust the support to hold the filter in an upright position. Follow the screen prompts to begin priming the set.

6. After completion of prime, connect the cell bag to the filter and place the bag on the bag hanger.

7. Ensure that the liquid sensor tubing is properly inserted and press RUN to begin the automated procedure. The following are the automated steps:

    a. Loading cells: The filter is primed with buffer. The cells are loaded onto the selection column after passing through the precolumn. Labeled cells are retained in the selection column, and the unlabeled cells are collected in the negative fraction bag. When the cell bag is empty (as detected by the liquid sensor), the cell bag is rinsed twice. The magnet is exposed during this step.

    b. Column wash I: The selection column and fluid pathway are rinsed with buffer to remove unlabeled cells. Wash buffer is collected in the buffer waste bag. The magnet is exposed during this step.

    c. Release of cells I: Cells are released, circulated, and rinsed within an internal tubing cycle. The magnet is retracted during this step.

    d. Reloading of cells I: The cells are loaded onto the selection column. The magnet is exposed during this step.

    e. Column wash II, release of cells II, reloading of cells II, and column wash III: Repeat above steps.

    f. Final elution of the cells: Selected cells are eluted off the selection column and are collected in the positive fraction bag. The magnet is retracted during this step.

8. At the SELECTION COMPLETED screen, close the clamp on the positive fraction bag. The final volume is 45 mL.

F. Procedure Completion

1. Heat-seal and remove the positive fraction bag. Determine the final volume and aseptically remove QC samples (for cell count, viability, flow cytometry analysis, and sterility). Selected cells are ready for either fresh infusion or further manipulation such as cryopreservation. If volume reduction is necessary, cells should be transferred into centrifuge tube(s) for manual concentration using a centrifuge.

2. Heat-seal and remove the negative fraction bag. Determine the final volume and aseptically remove QC samples (for cell count and flow cytometry analysis).

3. Remove the disposable set following the instructions in the operator's manual.

Anticipated Results

Unsuccessful mobilization and a low number of CD34+ cells in the preselection product may negatively affect the results, but generally a CD34+ cell recovery of >50% and purity >85% can be expected.

Reference/Resource

1. CliniMACS system operator's manual. Bergisch Gladbach, Germany: Miltenyi Biotec.

In: Areman EM, Loper K, eds
Cellular Therapy: Principles, Methods, and Regulations
Bethesda, MD: AABB, 2009

◆◆◆   *33*   ◆◆◆

Cell Separation by Counterflow Centrifugal Elutriation

Julie Edwards, BS, MT(ASCP)

DEPLETION OF T CELLS FROM A HEMATO-poietic progenitor cell (HPC) graft can result in a decrease in the incidence and severity of graft-vs-host disease (GVHD). Counterflow centrifugal elutriation (CCE) is one technique that has been used for T-cell depletion of allogeneic marrow grafts. CCE can also be used to separate monocytes from peripheral blood for generating dendritic cells (DC).[2]

CCE is the process of separating cells by both size and density. Separation is obtained when two opposing forces, centrifugal force (a constant force) and media flow, work in conjunction to cause cells to separate.[3] Alternatively, a change in centrifuge speed while maintaining a constant flow rate may be used but is more difficult to control. The standard method uses a floor model centrifuge with a specialized rotor and a series of tubing, pumps, and collection bags controlled by clamps and hemostats. The elutriation chamber is in the shape of a *V* (Fig 33-1). The starting material is most often a mononuclear cell (MNC) preparation from bone marrow, although other cellular preparations have

also been used. While the centrifuge is spinning, the cells and media enter the narrowest part of the chamber. Medium is continuously pumped into the chamber and the flow rate remains constant. Centrifugal force and medium flow forces oppose one another, thus reaching an equilibrium. Cells separate into layers based on size and density.[3] The uppermost layer contains the smaller or lightest cells, and the denser and larger cells settle in the bottom section of the chamber. The system has proven to be consistent and reproducible.

Once the cells are completely loaded, equilibrium is reached, and the cells pack into the chamber forming layers as previously described. The media flow rate can be slowly increased, causing the uppermost layer of cells to be collected in a separate container. This process of collecting different fractions can be repeated at various flow rates by increasing the media flow. After the desired fractions are collected, the centrifuge is stopped, and the remaining large cells in the chamber can be evacuated to another collection container while maintaining a constant media flow. As many as 1 ×

Julie Edwards, BS, MT(ASCP), Hematopoietic Technical Specialist, Cell Therapy Laboratory, Sidney Kimmel Comprehensive Cancer Center, Johns Hopkins Hospital, Baltimore, Maryland

The author has disclosed no conflicts of interest.

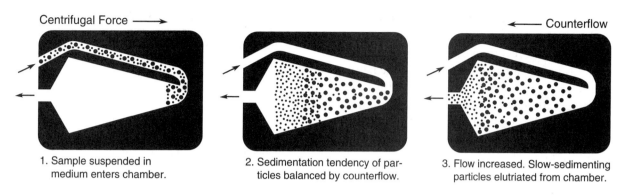

Centrifugal Force ———▶   ◀——— Counterflow

1. Sample suspended in medium enters chamber.

2. Sedimentation tendency of particles balanced by counterflow.

3. Flow increased. Slow-sedimenting particles elutriated from chamber.

Figure 33-1. Diagrammatic representation of the elutriation process. (Courtesy of Beckman Instruments, Inc.)

10^{11} total cells may be loaded into some chambers. The starting material must be a single-cell suspension free of clumps, which can cause turbulence during the separation. Successful procedures should result in a 2- to 4-$\log^{10}$ T-cell depletion. Although assembly of the instrument and associated materials is complicated, CCE is a rapid method for separating cells. The time for the procedure is approximately one-half to 1 hour, not including the time needed to set up the elutriator. Some products may require processing before elutriation to reduce the volume of the starting material and the red cell concentration. A variety of cell sizes (fractions) may be isolated and collected, such as monocytic cells, large lymphocytes, and smaller lymphocytes (including nucleated red cells).

The larger HPCs in marrow products contribute to early engraftment and are often infused immediately. The remaining fractions can be combined, and a CD34+ selection procedure can be performed to recover the remaining 30% to 50% of HPCs. This product can be used to augment the initial dose, decreasing the risk of engraftment failure. Although technically complex, this procedure has stood the test of time and continues to be performed by a handful of experienced CT facilities. An additional application for this procedure is the isolation of monocytes for subsequent processing (such as for dendritic cell applications). A significant drawback is the nondisposable chamber and other instrument parts. After cleaning, these materials, along with the plastic tubing, must be sterilized before use.

A functionally closed system has been developed by CaridianBCT (Lakewood, CO) for elutriation. The Elutra (Fig 33-2) uses a modified apheresis kit

as a disposable tubing set. Up to 3×10^{10} nucleated cells may be loaded into the semiautomated system. The instrument works best with leukapheresis products that contain few red cells.[2] The device uses

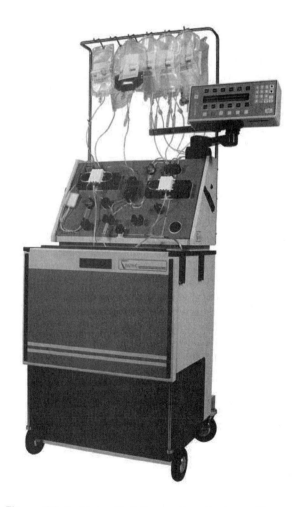

Figure 33-2. Elutra Cell Separation System. (Courtesy of CaridianBCT.)

a buffered saline (usually with albumin added), similar to the manual method, and the process is reported to take less than 60 minutes for complete separation of an apheresis product.[4] In the hands of experienced technologists, both elutriation methods result in good cell recovery and monocyte enrichment, although the automated system brings the benefits of automation and presterilized and assembled kits.

Acknowledgment

Method 33-2 was supplied by Linda Taylor, BS, Research and Development, CaridianBCT, Lakewood, Colorado.

References/Resources

1. Ho VT, Soiffer RJ. The history and future of T-cell depletion as graft-versus-host disease prophylaxis for allogeneic hematopoietic stem cell transplantation. Blood 2001;98;3192-204.
2. Berger TG, Strasser E, Smith R, et al. Efficient elutriation of monocytes within a closed system (Elutra) for clinical-scale generation of dendritic cells. J Immunol Methods 2005;298:61-72.
3. Beckman Instruments, Inc. The JE-5.0 elutriation system: Instructional manual. Palo Alto, CA: Spinco Division of Beckman, 1989.
4. Kim S, Kim HO, Baek EJ, et al. Monocyte enrichment from leukapheresis products by using the Elutra cell separator. Transfusion 2007;47:2290-6.
5. Lundell BI, Vredenburgh JJ, Tyer C, et al. Ex vivo expansion of bone marrow from breast cancer patients: Reduction in tumor cell content through passive purging. Bone Marrow Transplant 1998;22:153-9.
6. Simpson SJ, Vachula M, Kennedy MJ, et al. Detection of tumor cells in the bone marrow, peripheral blood, and apheresis products of breast cancer patients using flow cytometry. Exp Hematol 1995;23:1062-8.
7. Matthay KK, Atkinson JB, Stram DO, et al. Patterns of relapse after autologous purged bone marrow transplantation for neuroblastoma: A childrens cancer group pilot study. J Clin Oncol 1993;11:2226-33.
8. Cristofanilli M, Budd G, Ellis M, et al. Circulating tumor cells, disease progression, and survival in metastatic breast cancer. N Engl J Med 2004;351:781-91.
9. Burgess J, Mills B, Griffith M, et al. Breast cancer contamination of PBSC harvests: Tumor depletion by positive selection of CD34(+) cells. Cytotherapy 2001;3:285-94.
10. Hale G, Zhang M, Burnes D, et al. Improving the outcome of bone marrow transplantation by using CD52 antibodies to prevent graft versus host disease and graft rejection. Blood 1998;92:4581-90.
11. Paulus U, Dreger P, Viehmann K, et al. Purging peripheral blood progenitor cell grafts from lymphoma cells: Quantitative comparison of immunomagnetic CD34+ selection systems. Stem Cells 1997;15:297-304.
12. Dyson P, Horvath N, Joshua D, et al. CD34+ selection of autologous peripheral blood stem cells for transplantation following sequential cycles of high dose therapy and mobilization in multiple myeloma. Bone Marrow Transplant 2000;25:1175-84.
13. Kasow K, Sims-Poston L, Eldridge P, et al. CD34+ hematopoietic progenitor cell selection of bone marrow grafts for autologous transplantation in pediatric patients. Biol Blood Marrow Transplant 2007;13:608-14.
14. Gryn J, Shadduck R, Lister J, et al. Factors affecting purification of CD34+ peripheral blood stem cells using the Baxter Isolex 300i. J Hematother Stem Cell Res 2002;11:719-30.
15. Hildebrandt M, Serke S, Myer O, et al. Immunomagnetic selection of CD34+ cells: Factors influencing component purity and yield. Transfusion 2000;40:507-12.
16. Watts MJ, Somervaille T, Ings SJ, et al. Variable product purity and functional capacity after CD34 selection: A direct comparison of the CliniMACS (v2·1) and Isolex 300i (v2·5) clinical scale devices. Br J Haematol 2002;118:117-23.
17. Arpaci F, Cetin T, Ozet A, et al. The excessive numbers of total nucleated cells does not affect the performance of CliniMACS. J Clin Apher 2004;19:197-201.
18. Lang P, Bader P, Schumm M, et al. Transplantation of a combination of CD133+ and CD34+ selected progenitor cells from alternative donors. Br J Haematol 2004;124:72-9.
19. Martin-Henao G, Picon M, Amill B, et al. Combined positive and negative cell selection from allogeneic peripheral blood progenitor cells (PBPC) by use of immunomagnetic methods. Bone Marrow Transplant 2001;27:683-7.

Method 33-1. Counterflow Centrifugal Elutriation Using a Floor-Model Centrifuge

Description

A marrow mononuclear cell (MNC) preparation is loaded via tubing and bags into an elutriation chamber. Under constant media flow and with centrifugation, equilibrium is reached, and cell fractions are evacuated from the chamber by increasing media flow rates. Each fraction is collected into a separate bag.

Time for Procedure

From 30 to 45 minutes (excluding setup).

Equipment

1. Beckman centrifuge (J-6M) and rotor J 5.0 (Spinco Division of Beckman, Palo Alto, CA).
2. Elutriation chamber and balance.
3. Two sample reservoirs (30-mL and 70-mL capacity).
4. Pressure gauges.
5. Media pumps.
6. Mettler balance (or equivalent; Mettler-Toledo, Columbus, OH).
7. Computer with Mettler Balance Link software.
8. Masterflex tubing (14-inch and 16-inch; Cole-Parmer, Vernon Hills, IL).
9. Clamps.
10. Cell counter.
11. Collection containers.
12. pH meter.
    Note: All material and equipment coming into contact with cells intended for infusion must be sterile. Reusable equipment parts should be sterilized before the procedure.

Reagents

1. Media compatible with cells that are to be separated.
2. EDTA to prevent cell clumping.

3. 25% Human serum albumin (HSA): 20 mL needed per liter of media solution to prevent cell adherence to the chamber.

Procedure

A. *Preparation for Separation Procedure*
   1. Prepare the elutriation media and sample for appropriate pH.
   2. Before elutriation, an MNC concentrate may need to be prepared to reduce the volume of the starting material and red cell volume present in the product.
   3. Working in a biological safety cabinet (BSC), aseptically assemble the chamber and counterbalance it with transfer tubes according to the manufacturer's instructions. Sterilization indicators should be observed for proper color change.
   4. Place the chamber assembly into the rotor of the centrifuge.
   5. Attach the elutriator assembly to the media and sample lines that are connected to the pumps.
   6. Attach the retaining cable to the rotor to prevent the media lines from becoming tangled.
   7. Turn on the media pump and prime the system with elutriation medium. The media air trap should be filled half way, and the sample air trap should be filled one-third of the way with medium.
   8. Purge the system of all air in the lines and chamber by turning on the media pump at a low flow rate. Turn the rotor by hand to evacuate any remaining air, and pinch the outlet tubing until the pressure rises to 5 psi. Release the tubing to allow air to exit.
   9. Turn on the centrifuge to a low speed (1000 rpm). Repeat the finger clamping until the pressure is at 5 psi. Check for any

tubing or connection leaks. Increase the media pump setting to a higher flow rate, and repeat the finger clamping until 10 psi is reached.

10. Stop the centrifuge and observe for any leaks in the chamber or rotor tubing.

11. Place the empty calibration bag on the balance, and calibrate the pumps using the computer program.

B. Separation Procedure

1. Turn the media pump on, start the centrifuge, and adjust the media pump to the calibrated setting (ie, 30 mL/minute).

2. Check that there is no air in the system and that the pressure is <2 psi. Set the sample pump to the desired flow rate needed to load the cells. For instance, for loading the cells in the elutriator at 50 mL/minute, the sample flow rate would be set at 20 mL/minute and medium at 30 mL/minute. Simultaneously, turn the sample pump on and remove the clamp where the medium and sample lines join each other. Move the clamp from the first empty (load) bag to the calibration bag, and collect any cells that may not remain in the chamber during loading.

3. Check that the sample is entering the system. Cells should not be seen in the return line until the chamber has completely filled.

4. When 10 mL of sample remains in the bag, rinse with approximately 10 mL of medium to flush the remaining cells from the bag. Continue to add small amounts of medium until all cells are loaded. At the end of the

rinse, place the clamp back on the sample line and turn off the pump.

5. Remove the clamp from the next collection bag and place it on the load bag. Start a timer for the desired time of collection, and slowly increase the media flow rate to the next setting. Place the bag on the balance to determine whether the flow rate is within the desired range.

6. Continue performing Step 5 until all desired fractions are collected. Each fraction is collected by increasing the pump rate on the media line.

7. At the end of the collection, remove the clamp from the last bag and place it on the previous bag. Stop the centrifuge and start the timer for the desired collection time. This is the rotor-off fraction, and it will contain the larger cells.

References/Resources

1. Santos GW. Bone marrow transplantation in hematologic malignancies. Cancer 1990;65;786-91.

2. Ho VT, Soiffer RJ. The history and future of T-cell depletion as graft-versus-host disease prophylaxis for allogeneic hematopoietic stem cell transplantation. Blood 2001;98:3192-204.

3. Berger TG, Strasser E, Smith R, et al. Efficient elutriation of monocytes within a closed system (Elutra) for clinical-scale generation of dendritic cells. J Immunol Methods 2005;298:61-72.

4. Pandita TK. Enrichment of cells in different phases of the cell cycle by centrifugal elutriation. In: Lieberman HB, ed. Methods in molecular biology. Vol 241. Cell cycle checkpoint control protocols. Totowa, NJ: Humana Press Inc, 2003.

5. Beckman Instruments, Inc. The JE-5.0 elutriation system: Instructional manual. Palo Alto, CA: Spinco Division of Beckman, 1989.

Method 33-2. Monocyte Enrichment Using the Elutra Cell Separation System

Description

The Elutra Cell Separation System (CaridianBCT, Lakewood, CO) is a laboratory instrument that uses counterflow centrifugal elutriation (CCE) to separate cells based on size and density. Its intended application is monocyte enrichment.

Time for Procedure

The default monocyte enrichment procedure is completed in less than 1 hour.

Summary of Procedure

The Elutra procedure consists of an elutriation phase, which separates cells into multiple fractions based on size and density, and an optional red cell debulking phase (RBC debulking). In the elutriation phase, the starting cell (leukapheresis) product is pumped into a conical chamber, which is mounted on a centrifuge rotor. The flow of media and cells is in opposition to the centrifugal force of the rotor. Increasing the media flow through the chamber aligns the cells according to size and density and then selectively elutes them from the chamber into different fraction collection bags. After the removal of the small, less dense cells, the monocytes are recovered by turning the centrifuge rotor off.

An optional RBC debulking phase provides consistent monocyte enrichment from leukapheresis products that contain more than 7.5 mL of red cells. During the RBC debulking phase, the red cells are separated from the other cellular components by centrifugation and then pumped from the bottom of the separation chamber into a dedicated debulk bag.

The functionally closed disposable tubing set includes a preconnected separation chamber, tubing, and fraction collection bags. The separation chamber can process up to 3×10^{10} nucleated cells in a single elutriation procedure.

The Elutra cell separation system consists of a control panel, front panel, and centrifuge compartment. The Elutra allows the operator to perform a semiautomatic procedure, either using the default monocyte-enrichment profile or an operator-configured profile. The profile controls the pump flow rates, centrifuge speed, and volume processed during each step of the elutriation procedure.

Equipment

1. Elutra Cell Separation System.
2. Tubing sealer or sterile docking device.

Supplies and Reagents

1. Elutra Cell Separation disposable tubing set.
2. Hanks' balanced salt solution plus 1% human serum albumin: 4 L.

Procedure

1. Before the semiautomatic procedure, the Elutra system prompts the operator to load the disposable tubing set and then primes the set with media solution. Next, the operator is asked to select an elutriation profile and enter the starting cell product data. The Elutra system uses the starting cell product data to determine whether the white cell (WBC) content exceeds the capacity of the separation chamber and whether RBC debulking is recommended. The system provides the operator with an estimate of the procedure time and the media volume required.

2. At the start of the semiautomatic elutriation procedure, the system dilutes the starting cell product with media and loads the media and cells into the separation chamber. The flow of media and cells into the chamber is in a direc-

tion that opposes the centrifugal force. After loading is completed, the system adjusts the media flow rate and processes a set volume of fluid, as defined by the configured profile.

3. With the default monocyte-enrichment profile, the media flow rate is slowly increased to elute successively larger/denser cell populations. During this process, the eluted cell populations are diverted to different fraction collection bags.

4. Once the platelets, red cells, and lymphocytes are eluted, the monocytes are recovered from the separation chamber by turning the centrifuge rotor off. The enriched monocytes are diverted to the last fraction collection bag.

Anticipated Results

The goal of the monocyte-enrichment procedure is to generate an enriched monocyte product with an average purity of 80% and an average recovery of 60%. To achieve this goal, the starting cell (leukapheresis) product should meet the following specifications:

- WBC content: $\geq 5 \times 10^9$ to 30×10^9.
- Monocyte content: $\geq 1 \times 10^9$.
- Granulocyte content: <3%.
- RBC content: <7.5 mL. Otherwise, RBC debulking is recommended.

Notes

A caveat to US laboratories: CaridianBCT considers the Elutra cell separation system appropriate for laboratory use and, therefore, not subject to premarket clearance or approval by the US Food and Drug Administration (FDA). However, cells processed on this system—that are intended for direct transfusion or used in the production of a therapeutic product or vaccine for clinical use—may require advance approval by the FDA. Securing FDA approval is the sole responsibility of the user.

References/Resources

1. Elutra Cell Separation System operator's manual. P/N 777093-462. Lakewood, CO: CaridianBCT, 2005.
2. Chen Y, Hoecker P, Zeng J, Dettke M. Combination of COBE AutoPBSC and Gambro Elutra as a platform for monocyte enrichment in dendritic cell (DC) therapy: Clinical study. J Clin Apher 2008;23:157-62.
3. DiGiusto DL, Cooper LJ. Preparing clinical grade Ag-specific T cells for adoptive immunotherapy trials. Cytotherapy 2007;9:613-29.
4. Erdmann M, Dörrie J, Schaft N, et al. Effective clinical-scale production of dendritic cell vaccines by monocyte elutriation directly in medium, subsequent culture in bags and final antigen loading using peptides or RNA transfection. J Immunother 2007;30:663-74.
5. Lemarie C, Sugaye R, Kaur I, et al. Purification of monocytes from cryopreserved mobilized apheresis products by elutriation with the Elutra device. J Immunol Methods 2007;318:30-36.
6. Garlie N, et al. Enrichment of CD14+ cells for dendritic cell production using the Elutra cell separation system. J Immunother 2004;27:22.
7. Rouard H, Leon A, De Reys S, et al. A closed and single-use system for monocyte enrichment: Potential for dendritic cell generation for clinical applications. Transfusion 2003;43:481-7.
8. Voss CY, Albertini MR, Malter JS. Dendritic cell-based immunotherapy for cancer and relevant challenges for transfusion medicine. Transfus Med Rev 2004;18:189-202.
9. Noga SJ, et al. Development of a high capacity semi-automated monocyte isolation system for the generation of dendritic cells (DC). Blood 2001;98:658a.
10. Perseghin P, D'Amico G, Dander E, et al. Isolation of monocytes from leukapheretic products for large-scale GMP-grade generation of cytomegalovirus-specific T-cell lines by means of an automated elutriation device. Transfusion 2008;48:1644-9.

In: Areman EM, Loper K, eds
Cellular Therapy: Principles, Methods, and Regulations
Bethesda, MD: AABB, 2009

♦♦♦ 34 ♦♦♦

In-Vitro Cell Culture and Expansion

John D. McMannis, PhD

THE CURRENT SOURCES OF HEMATOPOI-etic progenitor cells (HPCs) for clinical use are marrow, mobilized peripheral blood, and umbilical cord blood (UCB). With all of these sources, product dose is critical, and complications arise when sufficient numbers of CD34+ cells and colony-forming cells (CFCs) are not present. Successful expansion techniques have the potential to improve engraftment kinetics, in turn reducing the need for transfusion support, the rate of infectious complications, and the length of hospital stays. The technology could also be adapted for such other potential clinical applications as tumor cell purging of autologous products, gene therapy protocols, and immunotherapies.

HPC Expansion Overview

Historically, the most common approaches to expansion culture in the field of cellular therapy (CT) have used mobilized HPCs from apheresis (HPC-A) that have been CD34+ selected. Expansion protocols for HPCs from cord blood (HPC-C), which appear to have a higher proliferative capacity than those from marrow (HPC-M) or blood, have outpaced those of mobilized HPC-A products in recent years. UCB has become the logical target for expansion because of the finite quantity of HPCs available from a single UCB unit. Although the cytokine and growth factor combinations reported in published studies differ, stem cell factor (SCF), flt-3 ligand, and thrombopoietin (TPO) play a key role in most expansion protocols. Culture conditions also vary and include use of a variety of cell culture media, supplementation with human serum and/or albumin, and culturing for durations of 4 to 14 days. Results of early expansion trials involving autologous breast cancer patients were not uniformly promising in regard to engraftment, transfusion independence, and length of hospital stay. However, with the recent increase in UCB expansions, it may be too early to draw definitive conclusions. Also, it has not yet been shown whether long-term repopulating cells that maintain capacity for multilineage differentiation and self-renewal can be reliably expanded.

Another issue of concern with ex-vivo expansion is the physical removal of the primitive HPCs from their hematopoietic microenvironment and their

John D. McMannis, PhD, Professor of Medicine and Director, Cell Therapy Laboratory, Department of Stem Cell Transplantation, The University of Texas M.D. Anderson Cancer Center, Houston, Texas

The author has disclosed no conflicts of interest.

subsequent culture in an artificial environment with exogenous growth factors added to prevent apoptosis and stimulate proliferation. This artificial setting may create the potential to drive differentiation at the expense of self-renewal because the cells may require the hematopoietic microenvironment niche to maintain their "stemness." More recent efforts have focused on simulating the in-vivo microenvironment in an attempt to improve results. Therefore, an alternative approach for ex-vivo expansion is the use of a feeder layer to provide a three-dimensional microenvironment for the HPCs.

Studies are currently under way to determine whether the co-culture of UCB cells with mesenchymal stromal cells (MSCs) enhances the yield of primitive HPCs (see Chapter 38) The MSC secretion of several different cytokines [SCF, flt-3, interleukin-6 (IL-6) and -11, leukemia inhibitory factor, and TPO] could contribute to and enhance UCB expansion produced by the recombinant growth factors routinely added exogenously to the cultures [eg, SCF, granulocyte colony-stimulating factor (G-CSF), and TPO]. Another benefit to this culture system is that the UCB-MSC co-culture does not require the isolation of CD34+ or CD133+ cells before expansion, minimizing the manipulation and loss of HPCs as a result of selection techniques. In this process, marrow-adherent cells are plated in tissue culture flasks for 21 to 30 days in order for the MSCs to reach a confluent monolayer. The UCB, in defined media containing SCF, G-CSF, flt-3 ligand, and TPO, is then added to the culture and allowed to expand for 14 days. Using an MSC co-culture expansion technique, McNiece et al[1] have demonstrated a 10- to 20-fold increase in total nucleated cells (TNCs), a 7- to 18-fold increase in committed progenitor cells (CFCs), a two- to five-fold increase in primitive progenitor cells (high-proliferative-potential CFCs, or HPP-CFCs), and a 16- to 37-fold increase in CD34+ cells.

All expansion cultures, whether involving HPC or other cell types, theoretically may alter the inherent cellular properties and are therefore considered high-risk "351" biological drug products by the US Food and Drug Administration. In the United States, an investigational new drug (IND) exemption must be obtained before initiation of clinical trials using these products. In addition, these cultures are dependent on the availability of growth factors and culture media that are appropriate for use in clinical trials. Production in compliance with current good manufacturing practice (cGMP) and complete characterization of these reagents should be in place before the initiation of Phase III trials, and these are strongly recommended to be in place as early as Phase I and Phase II trials. Because the growth factors may be manufactured by different pharmaceutical companies, the qualification process is often expensive and may involve challenging negotiations when engaging in simultaneous collaboration with multiple pharmaceutical companies.

Umbilical Cord Blood Expansion

Although HPC-C are more limited than HPC-M or HPC-A in total numbers of cells, there are benefits to using UCB as a source of HPCs rather than either marrow or peripheral blood. Fewer T cells and/or fewer developed T cells present in UCB compared to marrow[2] allows for the possibility that UCB grafts will produce less GVHD, the major cause of morbidity and mortality in the allogeneic transplant setting.[3] Furthermore, the placenta is a byproduct of the birthing process and—were it not used as a source of HPCs—would be discarded as biomedical waste. Because of the wide availability and ease of collecting UCB from placental veins before disposal of the placenta, the unrelated-donor HPC pool and, thus, the number of potential transplant recipients can be markedly increased with this allograft source. Because of the ethnic diversity of this source of HPCs, some UCB banks have been able to target collection of units with specific HLA types found more commonly in African-American, Hispanic, and other minority populations. Donors for patients with these tissue types are underrepresented in the National Marrow Donor Program Registry that recruits and types adult HPC-M and HPC-A volunteer donors.[4]

UCB recipients receive approximately 1 log fewer MNCs and substantially fewer myeloid progenitors measured as colony forming units—granulocyte-macrophage (CFUs-GM) than marrow recipients. Data from numerous published studies support the theory that there is a threshold relationship between the TNC dose of UCB infused and time to engraftment. Patients who received doses above the median for each study appeared to experience more rapid engraftment than patients who received TNC doses below the median. Gluckman et al demonstrated that engraftment and survival were superior in UCB recipients who received >3.7 × 10[7] TNCs/kg.[5] However, because of the amount of UCB available in most placentas, such a large cell dose is not generally available to patients weighing more than 45 kg. For adult patients, it appears that recipients of >1.0 × 10[7] TNCs/kg had more favorable engraftment than recipients of lower cell doses.[5,6] Kurtzberg et al reported a linear correlation between the number of UCB nucleated cells infused and the time to neutrophil engraftment (p <0.002) in the unrelated UCB transplant setting.[7] These data suggest that giving more UCB cells may result in faster neutrophil engraftment. Hence, recent efforts in ex-vivo expansion have focused on the expansion of HPC-C.

Methods

Several different strategies are undergoing evaluation for ex-vivo expansion of HPC-C. As with T cells, the types of cells obtained at the completion of culture are highly dependent on the growth factors that are added to the cultures. One strategy is to increase the number of committed progenitor cells that would have short-term benefits (ie, shorter time to engraftment) but might not increase the pool of pluripotent stem cells. For these studies, CD34+ cells are selected from either a fraction (20% or more) of the UCB allograft or an allograft in its entirety and cultured ex vivo in defined media with SCF, G-CSF, and megakaryocyte growth and differentiation factor (MGDF) for 10 to 14 days before transplantation.[8] It is hoped that these cells will provide short-term and rapid engraftment of neutrophils and platelets. In addition, the remainder of the unmanipulated UCB graft or a second UCB product is infused as a source of long-term engrafting pluripotent cells.[9]

Another expansion technology involves the use of a copper chelating agent, which has been shown by Peled et al to enhance the expansion of a more primitive CD34+ UCB population when combined with early-acting growth factors.[10] In these expansion cultures, the CD133+ cells are isolated from the smaller UCB fraction of a multipart freezing bag using the CliniMACS device (Miltenyi Biotec, Bergisch Gladbach, Germany) 21 days before infusion and are cultured for 3 weeks in media containing IL-6, TPO, flt-3, SCF, and the copper chelator tetraethylenepentamine (TEPA). Again, the larger, unmanipulated fraction is given to the patient as a source of pluripotent stem cells.

Culture Vessels and Devices

In research and development laboratories, cultures are often performed in tissue culture flasks (T-flasks) or even culture well trays. These vessels come in a variety of sizes and materials; T-flasks come with several other options, such as vented and unvented caps, etc. As cell dose and product volume increase, scaling up for clinical application requires more (or larger) vessels. For this reason and because of the need to increase system integrity, many clinical-scale CT culture methods have been translated from flasks and trays to cell culture bags. These containers are available in a variety of sizes, materials, and configurations to meet specific culture requirements, such as gas exchange, adherence, and nonadherence. The use of sterile docking and aseptic processing techniques are especially critical for these products, which may be incubated for days or weeks with several manipulations (medium exchange, cell counting, etc) occurring at various intervals. Cell factories offering "stacked" flasks present another option for larger scale production. Finally, roller bottles may be used in commercial manufacturing of extremely large volumes such as those needed for vaccine production.

Several device manufacturers have attempted to automate the expansion and perfusion aspects of CT culture. Aastrom Biosciences (Ann Arbor, MI) developed a closed system bioreactor that provides continuous perfusion after cell inoculation. The device is not available commercially at the time of writing but is finding applications in the regenerative medicine arena. The Replicell System (Aastrom Biosciences) was used for cell expansion trials in breast cancer[11] and has been replaced with the Aastrom's Tissue Repair Cell technology. Some researchers have legacy systems and use them for large-scale dendritic cell expansion (see Chapter 39).

The WAVE bioreactor (GE Healthcare, Chalfont St Giles, United Kingdom) incorporates a sterile, disposable chamber (Cellbag) that is placed on a rocking platform. The rocking motion of this platform induces waves in the culture fluid, providing mixing and oxygen transfer. Culture densities of 20×10^6 cells/mL have been reported. The bioreactor requires no cleaning or sterilization and uses disposable bags. Applications have included T-cell expansion under cGMP conditions.[12] Caridian-BCT (Lakewood, CO) is developing a hollow fiber bioreactor.[13] As this field expands, innovation and automation will continue to increase the options and efficiency for cell culture and expansion technologies.

T-Cell Expansion and Immunotherapies

In 1985, Stephen Rosenberg and colleagues at the US National Institutes of Health reported on their clinical studies with lymphokine activated killer (LAK) cells. In summary, white cells were removed by apheresis from patients who had either metastatic renal cell cancer or melanoma.[14] The MNC fraction (primarily T-lymphocytes) was enriched, and the cells were incubated with high levels of IL-2 for 3 to 4 days.[15] The cells were harvested, washed, and then reinfused into the patient, marking the first reported use of adoptive immunotherapy in humans. Between 20% and 30% of the subjects responded to this treatment.

Since this initial report, Rosenberg's group has modified and improved the method of isolating T-lymphocytes. They argued that T-lymphocytes found within the tumor should have a higher frequency of tumor antigen specificity and possibly greater lytic activity. These cells have been called tumor-infiltrating lymphocytes (TILs).

The procedure being evaluated by Rosenberg and others is the following: The tumor is resected in the operating room and delivered to the cell-processing facility where it is cut up into small fragments of approximately 1 cm³. These fragments are then put into a culture with high doses of IL-2. Growth is monitored, and between day 28 and day 40, the cells are removed and evaluated for tumor specificity. TILs derived from resected tumors that were expanded in vitro were shown to be capable of specifically recognizing tumor-associated antigens, particularly MART-1, in more than two-thirds of melanoma patients.[16,17] When administered in vivo to patients with metastatic melanoma, 35% of the patients had an objective response. This response rate was nearly twice that observed with IL-2 alone and was also seen in patients who were refractory to IL-2 treatment. However, most responses were transient, and it was difficult to identify the persistence of the circulating TILs in vivo.[18]

Since these original reports of "adoptive immunotherapy," many investigators have evaluated the role of activated lytic cells in vivo. These studies include either activated natural killer (NK) cells or antigen-specific T cells reactive against cytomegalovirus, Epstein-Barr virus (EBV), or tumor-associated antigens.[19-22] NK cells have been produced by incubating MNCs, CD56-enriched cells, or T- and B-cell-depleted MNCs with IL-2 overnight. These cells have demonstrated cytolytic activity against the NK-sensitive cell line, K562, and some reactivity to the NK-resistant cell line, Daudi. Antigen-specific T cells have been generated by the long-term culture of MNCs with either dendritic cells or EBV-transduced cell lines that express either the antigen of interest or tumor-associated antigens. These cultures require frequent restimulation of the T cells and the addition of exogenous IL-2. Antigen-specific cells are obtained after approximately 6 to 8 weeks of culture.

References/Resources

1. McNiece I, Harrington J, Turney J, et al. Ex vivo expansion of cord blood mononuclear cells on mesenchymal stem cells. Cytotherapy 2004;6:311-17.
2. Broxmeyer HE, Kurtzberg J, Gluckman E, et al. Umbilical cord blood hematopoietic stem and repopulating cells in human clinical transplantation. Blood Cells 1991; 17:313-29.
3. Barker JN, Wagner JE. Umbilical cord blood transplantation: Current state of the art. Curr Opin Oncol 2002; 14:160-4.
4. Kollman C, Abella E, Baitty RL, et al. Assessment of optimal size and composition of the US National Registry of Hematopoietic Stem Cell Donors. Transplantation 2004; 15:89-95.
5. Gluckman E, Rocha V, Boyer-Chammard A. Outcome of cord-blood transplantation from related and unrelated donors. Eurocord Transplant Group and the European Blood and Marrow Transplantation Group. N Engl J Med 1997;337:373-81.

6. Laughlin MJ, Barker J, Bambach B, et al. Hematopoietic engraftment and survival in adult recipients of umbilical-cord blood from unrelated donors. N Engl J Med 2001;344:1815-22.

7. Kurtzberg J, Laughlin M, Graham ML, et al. Placental blood as a source of hematopoietic stem cells for transplantation into unrelated recipients. N Engl J Med 1996; 335:157-66.

8. Shpall EJ, Quinones RB, Giller R, et al. Transplantation of expanded cord blood. Biol Blood Marrow Transplant 2002;8:368-76.

9. de Lima M, St John L, Wieder E, et al. Double-chimerism after transplantation of two human leukocyte antigen mismatched unrelated cord blood units. Br J Haematol 2002;119:773-6.

10. Peled T, Landau E, Mandel J, et al. Linear polyamine copper chelator tetraethylenepentamine augments long-term ex vivo expansion of cord blood-derived CD34+ cells and increases their engraftment potential in NOD/SCID mice. Exp Hematol 2004;32:547-55.

11. Chabannon C, Novakovitch G, Blache JL, et al. The role of autologous hematopoietic progenitor and cell reinfusion for intensive chemotherapy in women with poor-prognosis breast cancer. Clinical studies with ex-vivo expanded cells produced with the Aastrom Replicell technology. Hematol Cell Ther 1999;41:78-81.

12. Hami LS, Green C, Leshinsky N, et al. GMP production and testing of Xcellerated T cells for the treatment of patients with CLL. Cytotherapy 2004;6:554-62.

13. Antwiler D, Deppisch R, Neubauer, et al. Successful culture of both adherent multipotent bone marrow stromal cells (MSC) and cells in suspension, using a novel, closed, cell expansion system (CES). Cytotherapy 2008; 10(Suppl 1):221.

14. Rosenberg, SA, Lotze MT, Muul LM, et al. Observations on the systemic administration of autologous lymphokine-activated killer cells and recombinant interleukin-2 to patients with metastatic cancer. N Engl J Med 1985; 313:1485-92.

15. Boldt D, Mills BJ, Gemlo BT, et al. Laboratory correlates of adoptive immunotherapy with recombinant interleukin-2 and lymphokine-activated killer cells in humans. Cancer Res 1988;48:4409-16.

16. Kawakami Y, Eliyahu S, Sakaguchi K, et al. Identification of the immunodominant peptides of the MART-1 human melanoma antigen recognized by the majority of HLA-A2-restricted tumor infiltrating lymphocytes. J Exp Med 1994;180:347-52.

17. Kawakami Y, Eliyahu S, Jennings C, et al. Recognition of multiple epitopes in the human melanoma antigen gp100 by tumor-infiltrating T lymphocytes associated with in vivo tumor regression. J Immunol 1995;154: 3961-8.

18. Dudley ME, Wunderlich JR, Robbins PF, et al. Cancer regression and autoimmunity in patients after clonal repopulation with antitumor lymphocytes. Science 2002; 298:850-4.

19. Miller JS, Soignier Y, Panoskaltsis-Mortari A, et al. Successful adoptive transfer and in vivo expansion of human haploidentical NK cells in patients with cancer. Blood 2005;105:3051-7.

20. Bollard CM, Aguilar L, Straathof KC, et al. Cytotoxic T lymphocyte therapy for EBV-positive Hodgkin's disease. J Exp Med 2004;200:1623-33.

21. Leen A, Myers GD, Sili U, et al. Monoculture-derived T lymphocytes specific for multiple viruses expand and produce clinically relevant effects in immunocompromised patients. Nat Med 2006;12:1160-6.

22. Molldrem J, Dermime S, Parker K, et al. Targeted T-cell therapy for human leukemia: Cytotoxic T lymphocytes specific for a peptide derived from proteinase 3 preferentially lyse human myeloid leukemia cells. Blood 1996; 88:2450-7.

Method 34-1. Ex-Vivo Expansion of Selected Hematopoietic Progenitor Cells from Cord Blood

Description

Published reports suggest that the speed of neutrophil engraftment is related to the dose of HPCs from cord blood (HPC-C) infused. Because HPC-C units generally have low cell numbers, ex-vivo expansion of the cells should generate a higher number of HPCs available for transplantation. Ex-vivo expansion data have demonstrated a higher cell yield when a selected rather than unselected HPC product is cultured. Selected HPC-C products increase in total cell and progenitor cell content when cultured for 14 days in supplemented minimum essential medium (MEM)-Alpha containing 100 ng/mL of stem cell factor (SCF), granulocyte colony-stimulating factor (G-CSF), and thrombopoietin (TPO).

Time for Procedure

1. Setup: 4 to 6 hours on day 1.
2. Culture: 14 days with a 3- to 4-hour manipulation on day 7.
3. Harvest and reinfusion: 4 to 6 hours.

Summary of Procedure

This procedure is for the expansion of HPC-C in static culture:

1. The HPC-C unit is obtained from a public cord blood bank.
2. CD133+ enrichment is performed.
3. Cells are placed in a culture with appropriate growth factors.
4. Additional growth factors may be added during the culture period.
5. Cell density may be adjusted during the culture period.
6. After the culture period, the cells are harvested using the COBE 2991 Cell Processor (Caridian-BCT, Lakewood, CO).

7. Quality control (QC) assays are performed before release of the product for reinfusion.

Equipment

1. Biological safety cabinet (BSC).
2. Centrifuge.
3. Electronic balance.
4. Tubing sealer.
5. Waterbath.
6. Sterile connection device (TSCD, Terumo, Somerset, NJ, or equivalent).
7. Microscope.
8. Plasma expressor.
9. Intravenous (IV) solution pole.
10. CO_2 incubator.
11. COBE 2991 Cell Processor.

Supplies and Reagents

1. COBE 2991 single-set processing set (Caridian-BCT #912-647819).
2. Teflon-coated culture bag: large [volume = 290-985 mL; AFC 2P-0290 (American Fluoroseal Corporation, Gaithersburg, MD)].
3. Teflon-coated culture bag: small (volume = 72-130 mL; AFC 2P-0072).
4. 150-mL transfer pack (Baxter/Fenwal, Lake Zurich, IL; #4R2001 or equivalent).
5. 300-mL transfer pack with coupler (Baxter/Fenwal #4R2014).
6. 600-mL transfer pack with eight leads (Baxter/Fenwal #4R-2027 or equivalent).
7. Plasma transfer set with spike and needle adapter (Baxter/Fenwal #4C22240 or equivalent).
8. Sterile zipper-top bags.
9. Plasma transfer set with two spikes (Baxter/Fenwal #4C2243 or equivalent).
10. Sample site coupler (Baxter/Fenwal #4C2405 or equivalent).

11. Syringes: 1 mL, 3 mL, 5 mL, 10 mL, 30 mL, 60 mL.
12. Pipettes: 2 mL, 5 mL, 10 mL.
13. Aspirating pipette (Becton Dickinson, Franklin Lakes, NJ; #357558 or equivalent).
14. 18-g needle.
15. Alcohol pads.
16. Three-Lead Filter (Baxter, Deerfield, IL; #4C7784).
17. 2-mL cryovials.
18. Sterile 15-mL (17 × 100 mm) conical tubes.
19. Spinal needle.
20. 175-mL and 250-mL centrifuge tubes.
21. MEM-Alpha (Hyclone, Logan, UT; #SH30265.01).
22. Irradiated fetal bovine serum (FBS; Hyclone #SH30070.02 or equivalent).
23. L-glutamine (Hyclone #SH30034 or equivalent).
24. Gentamicin sulfate (Irvine Scientific, Santa Ana, CA; #9354).
25. Filgrastim (G-CSF, 0.3 mg/mL; Amgen, Thousand Oaks, CA; #BB0468-00).
26. SCF: 1875 µg/vial (Amgen #BB0508-00).
27. TPO: 25 µg/vial (R&D Systems, Minneapolis, MN; #288-TP-025/CF).
28. 5% and 25% human serum albumin (HSA).
29. 10% dextran-40.
30. DNAse (Genentech, South San Francisco, CA; #10039/10040).
31. Magnesium chloride.
32. Sterile water for injection.

Procedure

I. Day 0—Culture Initiation

A. *Media Preparation*
  Note: Only unopened bottles or vials of reagents should be used for the preparation.
  1. Prepare 60 mL of supplemented MEM-Alpha in a transfer pack:
     a. 54 mL of MEM-Alpha.
     b. 0.6 mL of 200 mM L-glutamine (final concentration = 2mM/mL).
     c. 0.3 mL of 10 mg/mL gentamicin sulfate (final concentration = 0.05 mg/mL).
     d. 6 mL of irradiated FBS.

2. Leave the transfer pack in the BSC, and allow it to warm to room temperature.

B. *Cell Preparation*
  1. Thaw and wash the HPC-C unit as instructed in the facility's standard operating procedure (SOP; see Fig 34-1-1).
  2. Remove samples for QC assays (for cell count, sterility, flow cytometry, etc).
  3. Perform CD133+ enrichment using the CliniMACS instrument (Miltenyi Biotec, Bergisch Gladbach, Germany) and following the facility's SOP.
  4. Transfer the selected cells into a 175-mL conical tube.
  5. Centrifuge the tube at 450 × g for 10 minutes at ambient temperature, with low or no brake.
  6. After the spin, remove the supernatant, leaving 5 mL in the conical tube.

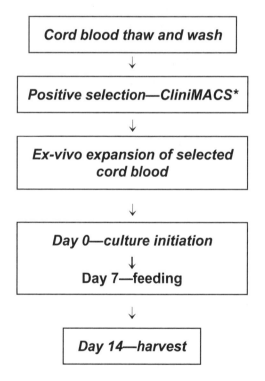

Figure 34-1-1. Schema for ex-vivo expansion of selected hematopoietic progenitor cells from cord blood.
*Miltenyi Biotec, Bergisch Gladbach, Germany.

7. Resuspend the cells well, and obtain a 0.2-mL QC sample for cell count, viability, and flow cytometry.

8. Add 20 mL of supplemented MEM-Alpha (prepared above) to the cells (final volume = 25 mL).

9. Label a 50-mL Teflon (DuPont, Wilmington, DE) culture bag with the required information.

10. Transfer the cells into the Teflon bag.

11. Add 25 mL of MEM-Alpha to the tube to rinse it. Add the rinse to the Teflon bag.

C. Cytokine Preparation and Addition

Note: Each vial of cytokine can be used for only one patient.

1. Resuspend and aliquot cytokines.
   a. The cord blood expansion requires three cytokines: SCF (0.281 mg/mL), G-CSF (0.300 mg/mL), and TPO (0.25 mg/mL).
   b. Because the amounts of the cytokines required for the culture are very small and require use of a micropipette, the three cytokines must be transferred from the original injection vials into sterile 2-mL vials.
   c. The SCF must first be resuspended in 6.67 mL of sterile water to yield a solution of 0.281 mg/mL.
   d. Lift off the top cover on the SCF vial, and wipe the injection port with alcohol.
   e. Resuspend the cytokine according to the manufacturer's instructions.
   f. Label two 2-mL sterile cryovials with the patient information and cytokine name, concentration, lot number, and expiration date.
   g. Aseptically transfer approximately 1.5 mL of reconstituted SCF to each of the labeled vials.
   h. Repeat the above steps for all cytokines.

2. The cytokines can then be added directly to the Teflon bag (if the quantity is feasible), or further dilutions can be performed. Ideally, 0.1 mL or more of each cytokine (at the appropriate concentration) should be added to the bag.

3. Mix the bag very well.

4. Place the culture bag in an alarm-monitored, humidified incubator at 37 C with 5% CO_2.

II. Day 7—Culture Expansion

Note: Culture media will be expanded from the initial 50 mL to 800 mL. The cultured cells will be transferred from a 50-mL Teflon culture bag into a 1000-mL Teflon culture bag.

A. Media and Bag Preparation

Note: If available, a sterile septum cap (Nalgene/Thermo Fisher Scientific, Rochester, NY; #342178-0384) may be used instead of a syringe for transferring media from the bottle.

1. Prepare 800 mL of supplemented culture medium in a culture flask:
   a. 20 mL of MEM-Alpha.
   b. 8.0 mL of 200 mM L-glutamine (final concentration = 2 mM/mL) and 4.0 mL of 10 mg/mL gentamicin sulfate (final concentration = 0.05 mg/mL).
   c. 80 mL of irradiated FBS.

2. Transfer 12 mL of the expansion medium into a 30-mL syringe for rinsing the day 0 culture bag and set it aside.

3. Label one 1000-mL Teflon culture bag with the HPC-C identification number, recipient name and identification number, and date.

4. Replace the blue vent cap on the culture bag with the clear cap provided.

5. Transfer 730 mL of the expansion medium into the culture bag using a balance and a transfer set with two spikes.

6. Seal and detach the transfer set tubing.

7. Leave the culture bag in the BSC and allow it to warm to room temperature.

B. Cultured Cell Transfer

1. Take out the culture bag setup on day 0 and check for signs of turbidity, media color change, or visible contamination.

2. Remove the 0.2-mL QC sample with a 1-mL syringe to verify cell count and viability.
   a. Perform a manual cell count and viability test.
   b. Calculate the total nucleated cell (TNC) fold expansion:
   Harvest TNCs (day 7) ÷ day 0 TNC = fold expansion
   Example:
   Day 0 TNCs = 5×10^6
   Harvest TNCs (day 7) = 200×10^6
   $(200 \times 10^6) \div (5 \times 10^6)$ = 40-fold expansion
   Note: If the culture has not shown significant growth (>two-fold expansion), notify the laboratory director or designee.
3. Draw the cell solution into a 60-mL syringe connected to the luer adaptor on the day 0 culture bag.
4. Inject the cell solution into the 1000-mL Teflon culture bag.
5. Rinse the original cell culture bag with the reserved 12 mL of media, and add the rinse to the 1000-mL culture bag.
6. Mix the 1000-mL culture bag.

C. *Cytokine Preparation and Addition*
   1. Calculations: Based on the current cytokine concentrations, the volume of each cytokine required for each culture bag on day 7 will be as follows:
      a. SCF: 800 mL × 0.1 μg/mL (100 ng/mL) ÷ 281 μg/mL = 0.285 mL (285 μL).
      b. G-CSF: 800 mL × 0.1 μg/mL (100 ng/mL) ÷ 300 μg/mL = 0.266 mL (266 μL).
      c. TPO: 800 mL × 0.1 μg/mL (100 ng/mL) ÷ 250 μg/mL = 0.320 mL (320 μL).
   2. Repeat the steps performed on day 0 to add the appropriate cytokines to the 1000-mL culture bag.
   3. Place the culture bag in an alarm-monitored, humidified incubator at 37 C with 5% CO_2.

Note: Unused reagents should be stored until after final product has been harvested.

III. **Day 14—Harvest**

A. *Reagent Preparation*
   1. Prepare two 1-L bags of CliniMACS buffer (phosphate-buffered saline/EDTA), each supplemented with 1% HSA.
   2. Remove the culture bag from the incubator. Verify that the bag information matches the information on the patient order form.
   3. Mix the bag well. Observe the bag for turbidity, media color change, or visible contamination.
   4. Remove a 0.2-mL sample for cell count and viability.

B. *Cord Blood Concentration and Wash on the COBE 2991*
   1. Aseptically attach the appropriate bags to the tubing set:
      a. Blue line: not used in this procedure.
      b. Green line: buffer bags (piggyback with a transfer set, hung on the right solution pole).
      c. Red line: cell product bag.
      d. Purple line: waste bag (already attached).
      e. Yellow line: not used in this procedure.
   2. Concentrate cells using the COBE 2991. Minimum spin time should be 5 minutes per cycle. Wash twice with saline.
   3. After removal of second wash supernatant, press STOP/RESET.

C. *Procedure Completion*
   1. Place a hemostat on the inlet line and open the centrifuge lid.
   2. Heat-seal the inlet line above the hemostat and remove the donut bag.
   3. Heat-seal and remove the buffer bag containing excess buffer.

4. Resuspend the cell pellet by gently massaging the bag. Be sure to target cells that may be trapped in the creases of the bag.

5. Determine the final volume and obtain the final samples:
   a. 0.2 mL for sample for manual cell count and viability.
   b. 0.2 mL for immunophenotyping (CD34+, CD34+/38–, CD133+, CD33+).
   c. 0.5 mL for sterility.
   d. 1.0 mL for mycoplasma assay.
   e. 1.0 mL for endotoxin assay.
   f. 0.2 mL for STAT Gram's stain.
   g. 0.2 mL for CFU [1500 nucleated cells per plate (refer to SOP)].

Anticipated Results

A. *Expected Values*
   1. TNC fold expansion, day 7: >twofold.
   2. TNC fold expansion, day 14: >fourfold.

B. *Critical Limits*
   1. Viability: <70%, day 7 or day 14.
   2. Endotoxin: >5 EU/kg.
   3. Mycoplasma: positive.
   4. Gram's stain: positive.
   5. Sterility: positive.

Notes

1. For products under investigational device exemption/investigational new drug (IDE/IND) status, refer to the certificate of analysis (COA) for final release criteria and approval. An approved COA from the quality assurance (QA) coordinator and reviewed batch records must be available before the product's release.

2. Worksheets should be reviewed by a supervisor and by QA after each day of processing.

Quality Control Assays

A. *Day 0—Postselection*
   1. TNC counts and viability.
   2. Immunophenotyping (CD34+, CD34+/38–, CD133+, CD3+, CD33+, viability).
   3. CFU.

B. *Day 0—Negative Fraction*
   1. TNC counts and viability.
   2. Immunophenotyping (CD34+, CD34+/38–, CD133+, CD3+, CD33+, viability).
   3. Sterility (after addition of DMSO).

C. *Day 7—Culture*
   TNC counts and viability.

D. *Day 14—Preharvest*
   TNC counts and viability.

E. *Day 14—Postharvest*
   1. TNC counts and viability.
   2. Immunophenotyping (CD34+, CD34+/38–, CD133+, CD33+, viability).
   3. CFU.
   4. Gram's stain.
   5. Sterility.
   6. Mycoplasma.
   7. Endotoxin.

Safety

1. Wear protective gloves and an impermeable lab coat when handling reagents, blood, and blood products.

2. Use a sterile technique and work under a BSC whenever possible.

3. When working in classified suites, follow appropriate gowning requirements.

4. Perform the appropriate environmental monitoring.

References/Resources

1. Robinson S, Niu T, de Lima M, et al. Ex vivo expansion of umbilical cord blood. Cytotherapy 2005;7:243-50.
2. Robinson SN, Ng J, Niu T, et al. Superior ex vivo cord blood expansion following co-culture with bone marrow-derived mesenchymal stem cells. Bone Marrow Transplant 2006;37:359-66.
3. de Lima M, McMannis J, Gee A, et al. Transplantation of ex vivo expanded cord blood cells using the copper chelator tetraethylenepentamine: A phase I/II clinical trial. Bone Marrow Transplant 2008;41:771-8.
4. CliniMACs operator's manual. Bergisch Gladbach, Germany: Miltenyi Biotec.
5. Rubinstein P, Dobrila L, Rosenfield RE, et al. Processing and cryopreservation of placental/umbilical cord blood for unrelated bone marrow reconstitution. Proc Natl Acad Sci U S A 1995;92:10119-22.

In: Areman EM, Loper K, eds
Cellular Therapy: Principles, Methods, and Regulations
Bethesda, MD: AABB, 2009

♦ ♦ ♦   35   ♦ ♦ ♦

T-Cell Expansion: Cytotoxic T Cells

Jerome Ritz, MD

MONOCLONAL ANTIBODIES (MoAbs) ARE now commonly used as therapeutic agents in various diseases, including many types of cancer, where MoAbs directly target tumor cells, as well as various autoimmune diseases, where antibodies directly target immune cells or inflammatory mediators. Although T cells represent an equally specific and potent arm of the immune system, adoptive T-cell therapies remain largely experimental and have not yet been proven to be effective treatments. Despite the many challenges to the development of effective T-cell therapies, adoptive T-cell therapies have great potential, and many different approaches are currently being evaluated in early-phase clinical trials for various indications.

Unlike antibodies that specifically bind to target antigens in soluble form or when expressed on the cell surface, T cells bind only to peptide epitopes when expressed on the cell surface by major histocompatibility complex (MHC) molecules. CD4+ T cells specifically recognize peptide epitopes presented by MHC Class II molecules (eg, HLA-DR), and CD8+ T cells recognize only peptide epitopes presented by MHC Class I molecules (HLA-A, -B, and -C). Almost all cells express MHC Class I mol-

ecules, and these molecules primarily present peptides derived from endogenous proteins. In contrast, MHC Class II molecules are primarily expressed by antigen-presenting cells (APCs), and these molecules are used by these specialized cells to present peptides derived from exogenous sources. In both cases, recognition by CD4+ and CD8+ T cells is mediated by clonally rearranged T-cell receptors (TCRs) expressed on the T-cell surface, complexed with CD3 proteins and either CD4 or CD8 proteins. During T-cell maturation in the thymus, only those T cells that recognize endogenous HLA molecules survive to be exported to the periphery. As a result, T-cell recognition is also restricted to target cells that express the same HLA alleles that are present in the patient.

Applications

Many applications of adoptive T-cell therapy are currently being evaluated in different patient populations, involving a variety of viral infectious diseases where endogenous T-cell responses to peptide epitopes derived from the infectious virus have not

Jerome Ritz, MD, Professor of Medicine, Harvard Medical School, and Director, Connell and O'Reilly Families Cell Manipulation Core, Dana-Farber Cancer Institute, Boston, Massachusetts

The author has disclosed no conflicts of interest.

been sufficient to control the infection and eliminate normal host cells that have been infected with the virus. In most of these instances, the patient's natural response to viral antigens has been compromised by administration of immune suppressive medications, or immune function has not reconstituted after allogeneic hematopoietic stem cell transplantation (HSCT). Examples involve patients with cytomegalovirus (CMV) or adenovirus infections or Epstein-Barr virus (EBV)-induced B-cell lymphoproliferative disease after either solid-organ transplantation or HSCT.[1,2]

Adoptive T-cell therapy is also being evaluated in patients with tumors that express viral antigens. In these instances, latent viral infections in the cancer cells result in the expression of peptide epitopes derived from the viral genome. Examples of such tumors include those from head and neck cancers and Hodgkin disease that express EBV antigens.[3,4] Although these latent infections result only in the expression of a limited set of viral genes, they are sufficient for recognition by normal T cells, and adoptive T-cell therapies directed against such epitopes have suggested that this may be an effective therapeutic approach.

In patients with hematologic malignancies undergoing allogeneic HSCT, donor T cells recognize minor histocompatibility antigens (mHAs) expressed on recipient cells. To the extent that residual leukemia cells express these antigens, the immune response directed against these epitopes facilitates the elimination of leukemia cells after transplantation. Targeting these mHAs with adoptive T-cell therapy is also being evaluated in clinical trials. In that application of T-cell therapy, normal cells in the recipient that express mHA can also be recognized, and targeting the normal cells can lead to substantial toxicity. For that reason, this approach has been used mainly to target the mHAs that are expressed primarily by hematopoietic cells and not other tissues in the recipient.[5-7]

Perhaps the most common use of adoptive T-cell therapy has been to target specific antigens expressed by tumor cells. Many clinical trials have evaluated the effect of cytotoxic T-lymphocyte (CTL) therapy directed against either melanoma or renal cell cancer antigens, with varying degrees of success. In these applications, investigators have infused either polyclonal T cells or expanded T-cell clones with specificity for single epitopes. CD4+

and CD8+ T cells have been evaluated, and dramatic tumor responses have been observed in some individuals.[8] However, it is also evident from most trials that the vast majority of infused cells do not persist for prolonged periods, and only limited numbers of infused cells are able to migrate to sites of tumor in vivo. Depletion of endogenous T cells to create a lymphopenic environment before infusion of exogenously expanded cells has been reported to improve expansion of infused cells in vivo and prolong the persistence of these cells.[9] However, tumors also maintain the ability to suppress T-cell responses directed at the tumor in vivo, and this remains an important mechanism for tumor resistance to CTL therapy.

One novel approach to improve the ability to generate larger numbers of more effective CTLs in vitro is to artificially create large numbers of otherwise normal CTLs that express surface receptors capable of recognizing broadly expressed tumor antigens. In this method, normal T cells are transduced with genetic vectors encoding chimeric antigen-specific receptors linked to transmembrane and intracellular domains of other molecules capable of initiating T-cell activation, proliferation, and target cell lysis. The chimeric antigen receptors (CARs) use the specific binding of immunoglobulin receptors directed against tumor-associated antigens such as CEA or CD19 to redirect the specificity of normal T cells toward tumor cell targets.[10-12] This approach obviates the need to target only small peptides that are endogenously processed by tumor cells and presented by their own HLA Class I molecules, and targeting a wide array of other molecules on the tumor cell surface becomes possible. Further, this approach precludes the need to select small numbers of epitope-specific CTLs and expand them in vitro for subsequent infusion. Instead, large numbers of antigen-specific T cells are created through genetic engineering approaches and more readily expanded to large numbers in vitro.

Methods for In-Vitro Isolation and Expansion

Donor Selection

Because no approaches for adoptive T-cell therapy have achieved Food and Drug Administration

(FDA) approval at this point, methods for isolation and expansion of these cells remain highly variable and experimental. In most of the instances described above, CTL therapy involves the use of autologous cells. Using autologous cells reduces the risk of immunologic rejection as well as other potential toxicities. However, when patients who have undergone allogeneic HSCT receive CTL therapy, CTLs can usually be obtained from the original HPC donor. Once patients have engrafted with allogeneic donor stem cells, further infusions of cells from the same donor are not recognized as foreign, and immune suppressive therapy is not required to prevent rejection of the infused cells.

Allogeneic cells have also been used to treat uncontrolled viral infections in patients with immune deficiency. In this application, complete HLA matching is not required, but the allogeneic donor and recipient must share at least some HLA alleles to ensure that the donor cells will be able to recognize at least some viral epitopes expressed by shared HLA alleles. The use of allogeneic cells that are not HLA-identical makes it possible to generate these cells from normal donors and to establish a large cryopreserved bank of such cells for immediate use when needed by individual patients with documented viral infections. Infusion of these cells in patients with active viral infections facilitates the elimination of recipient cells infected with the virus and control of the infection in vivo. However, because the allogeneic cells are not HLA-identical, infused cells will eventually be rejected by the recipient, and long-term engraftment is not anticipated.

Cell Selection and Expansion

The initial steps in the generation of CTLs involve the isolation of lymphocytes followed by methods to selectively stimulate and expand CTLs with the desired specificity. Many different approaches are currently being used, and the schema in Fig 35-1 illustrates only one method used in the Cell Manipulation Core Facility (CMCF) at the Dana-Farber Cancer Institute and Harvard Medical School. This method is adapted from an approach initially developed at the Center for Cell and Gene Therapy (CAGT) at the Baylor College of Medicine.[4] The goal of this method is to expand a polyclonal population of autologous CTLs that are specific for EBV epitopes. Tumor cells from patients with nasopha-

ryngeal carcinoma express these epitopes, and previous results from investigators at the CAGT have suggested that infusion of autologous CTLs manufactured with this method can induce tumor responses in vivo.

As outlined in this schema, mononuclear cells (MNCs) are first isolated from peripheral blood by ficoll hypaque density centrifugation. The majority of PMNCs are cryopreserved, and an aliquot is incubated with a supernatant containing high-titer EBV. The cells are incubated at 37 C to allow EBV-infected normal B cells to transform and begin autonomous proliferation. Typically, 8 to 9 weeks of incubation are required for B-cell transformation and expansion of sufficient numbers of polyclonal lymphoblastoid cell lines (LCLs) for cryopreservation and subsequent use as T-cell stimulators. In the second phase of manufacturing, thawed LCLs are irradiated and used as stimulators for thawed autologous lymphocytes. Multiple stimulations with irradiated LCLs are required to generate sufficient numbers of CTLs specific for EBV epitopes. Polyclonal EBV-specific CTLs are cryopreserved while aliquots of the manufactured cells undergo extensive testing to ensure safety and satisfy multiple release criteria. If all criteria are met, cryopreserved CTLs are thawed and prepared for intravenous infusion. The entire manufacturing procedure for each of these products typically takes approximately 3 months.

Also as outlined in the schema, multiple quality control analyses are performed during the lengthy and complicated process for manufacturing both LCLs and CTLs. These ensure the safety and sterility of the product as well as the adequacy of expansion and functional capacity for recognizing EBV-infected cells. The final product is expected to be heterogeneous, consisting of both CD8+ and CD4+ T cells specific for a variety of different EBV epitopes. It is also expected that only a fraction of the T cells generated will have any EBV reactivity because normal T cells with other specificities can also be stimulated and expanded with this method. The final product is therefore characterized by multiparameter flow cytometry using a panel of fluorescence-conjugated MoAbs specific for T-cell subsets and other lymphocytes, as well as for reactivity against known EBV epitopes.

In other clinical trials, various modifications have been developed to improve the lengthy manu-

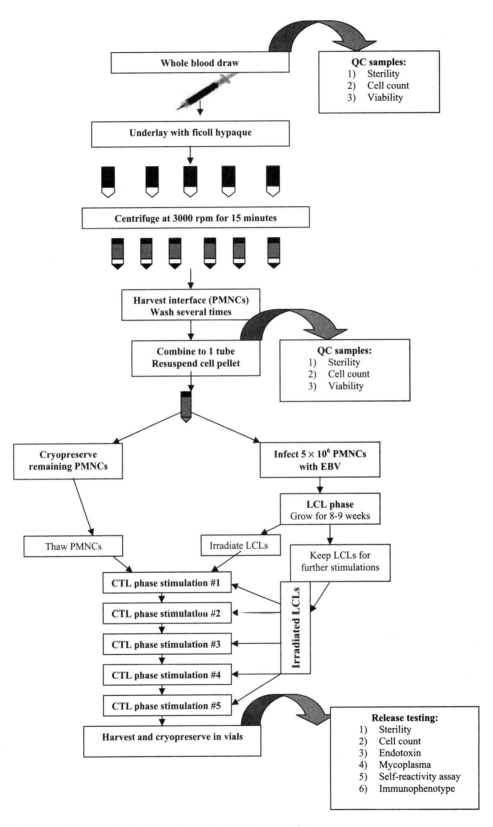

Figure 35-1. Schema for cytotoxic T-lymphocyte (CTL) generation.
QC = quality control; PMNCs = peripheral blood mononuclear cells; EBV = Epstein-Barr virus; LCL = lymphoblastoid cell line.

facturing process outlined in this schema. To do away with the need for manufacturing unique types of stimulator cells for each product, newer procedures have used genetically engineered APCs that can present specific T-cell epitopes and also stimulate T-cell growth.[13,14] These cells have the advantage of being manufactured in bulk and cryopreserved for subsequent use in multiple patients for various applications. Improvements are also being made in developing defined media and cytokines for more rapid expansion of CTLs, as well as in developing closed gas-permeable culture systems for more efficient use and exchange of culture media.

Conclusion

Although no extensively manipulated adoptive T-cell therapy has yet received FDA approval, numerous clinical trials and individual reports have suggested that infusions of specific T-cell populations can result in dramatic and long-lasting benefit in some patients. The most current studies have focused on the application of adoptive T-cell therapies for cancer, but other indications, especially for infectious diseases, also seem appropriate.

Although they can potentially benefit many patients, T-cell therapies remain in the very early stages of investigation. Different T-cell populations are unique in their specificity and functional attributes, and it is likely that very different methods will be needed to isolate and expand different functional cell types. Such complex manufacturing procedures will be difficult to standardize and bring to large-scale applications in large numbers of patients. Nevertheless, many investigators and cellular therapy manufacturing laboratories are actively engaged in this important new therapeutic area, and steady progress is being made on many fronts. This progress includes the development of efficient methods for isolation and expansion of different cell types with distinct functional capacities, as well as the definition of the most appropriate clinical indications for adoptive cell therapy.

References/Resources

1. Fujita Y, Rooney CM, Heslop HE. Adoptive cellular immunotherapy for viral diseases. Bone Marrow Transplant 2008;41:193-8.
2. Leen AM, Myers GD, Sili U, et al. Monoculture-derived T lymphocytes specific for multiple viruses expand and produce clinically relevant effects in immunocompromised individuals. Nat Med 2006;12:1160-6.
3. Bollard CM, Aguilar L, Straathof KC, et al. Cytotoxic T lymphocyte therapy for Epstein-Barr virus+ Hodgkin's disease. J Exp Med 2004;200:1623-33.
4. Straathof KC, Bollard CM, Popat U, et al. Treatment of nasopharyngeal carcinoma with Epstein-Barr virus-specific T lymphocytes. Blood 2005;105:1898-904.
5. Marijt E, Wafelman A, van der Hoorn M, et al. Phase I/II feasibility study evaluating the generation of leukemia-reactive cytotoxic T lymphocyte lines for treatment of patients with relapsed leukemia after allogeneic stem cell transplantation. Haematologica 2007;92:72-80.
6. Riddell SR, Bleakley M, Nishida T, et al. Adoptive transfer of allogeneic antigen-specific T cells. Biol Blood Marrow Transplant 2006;12:9-12.
7. Warren EH, Tykodi SS, Murata M, et al. T-cell therapy targeting minor histocompatibility Ags for the treatment of leukemia and renal-cell carcinoma. Cytotherapy 2002;4:441.
8. Hunder NN, Wallen H, Cao J, et al. Treatment of metastatic melanoma with autologous CD4+ T cells against NY-ESO-1. N Engl J Med 2008;358:2698-703.
9. Dudley ME, Wunderlich JR, Yang JC, et al. Adoptive cell transfer therapy following non-myeloablative but lymphodepleting chemotherapy for the treatment of patients with refractory metastatic melanoma. J Clin Oncol 2005;23:2346-57.
10. Beecham EJ, Ortiz-Pujols S, Junghans RP. Dynamics of tumor cell killing by human T lymphocytes armed with an anti-carcinoembryonic antigen chimeric immunoglobulin T-cell receptor. J Immunother 2000;23:332-43.
11. Cooper LJ, Topp MS, Serrano LM, et al. T-cell clones can be rendered specific for CD19: Toward the selective augmentation of the graft-versus-B-lineage leukemia effect. Blood 2003;101:1637-44.
12. Brentjens RJ, Latouche JB, Santos E, et al. Eradication of systemic B-cell tumors by genetically targeted human T lymphocytes co-stimulated by CD80 and interleukin-15. Nat Med 2003;9:279-86.
13. Butler MO, Lee JS, Ansen S, et al. Long-lived antitumor CD8+ lymphocytes for adoptive therapy generated using an artificial antigen-presenting cell. Clin Cancer Res 2007;13:1857-67.
14. Suhoski MM, Golovina TN, Aqui NA, et al. Engineering artificial antigen-presenting cells to express a diverse array of co-stimulatory molecules. Mol Ther 2007;15:981-8.

In: Areman EM, Loper K, eds
Cellular Therapy: Principles, Methods, and Regulations
Bethesda, MD: AABB, 2009

◆◆◆   **36**   ◆◆◆

Regulatory T Cells: Allograft Augmentation with Rapamycin-Generated Donor CD4+ Th2 Cells

*Daniel H. Fowler, MD; Vicki Fellowes, MT(ASCP); and
Hanh Khuu, MD*

ALLOGENEIC HEMATOPOIETIC STEM CELL transplantation (HSCT) represents a potentially curative therapy for patients with hematologic malignancy. Donor T cells play a crucial role in the immune-mediated antitumor response that is typically referred to as the graft-vs-leukemia (GVL) effect.[1] However, it has been difficult to clinically separate beneficial GVL effects from detrimental graft-vs-host disease (GVHD) because of the shared biology of these immune reactions.[2] In addition, donor T-cell promotion of alloengraftment has been difficult to clinically separate from GVHD.[3] To address this issue, researchers have evaluated the potential role of the donor Th1/Th2 cell cytokine balance to allow T-cell mediation of GVL effects or promotion of alloengraftment with reduced GVHD.

In initial studies, the authors [at the National Cancer Institute (NCI)][4] and other laboratories[5] found that augmentation of murine T-cell-replete allografts with donor Th2-type cells prevented GVHD reactions. In further studies, NCI characterized the role of such Th1/Th2 cell balance in the mediation of GVL and graft-vs-tumor (GVT) effects.[6,7] This latter study evaluated murine donor T cells that were generated ex vivo through magnetic bead-bound costimulatory antibodies and exposure to cytokines essential for Th2-type polarization, namely, interleukin-4 (IL-4) and IL-2.[8] Results showed that Th1-type cells generated potent allogeneic antitumor effects but induced severe GVHD. By comparison, donor Th2-type cells reduced GVHD but were less effective antitumor effectors. These data indicate that it is not

---

Daniel H. Fowler, MD, Head, Cytokine Biology Section, Experimental Transplantation and Immunology Branch, National Cancer Institute, National Institutes of Health; Vicki Fellowes, MT(ASCP), Medical Technologist, Experimental Transplantation and Immunology Branch, National Cancer Institute, National Institutes of Health; Hanh Khuu, MD, Assistant Medical Director, Cell Processing Section, Department of Transfusion Medicine, National Institutes of Health, Bethesda, Maryland

The authors have disclosed no conflicts of interest.

strictly possible to separate GVL/GVT effects from GVHD purely on the basis of Th1/Th2 biology. Given this information, for the therapy of patients with refractory hematologic malignancy, the authors have pursued a clinical strategy that aims to achieve a balance of Th1- and Th2-type populations after transplantation.[9] Because unmanipulated donor T cells differentiate primarily along a Th1-type pathway in vivo after transplantation,[4] the approach to induction of a Th1/Th2 balance involves the augmentation of T-cell-replete allografts with ex-vivo-generated donor Th2 cells.

In 1999, a pilot clinical trial at NCI and the National Institutes of Health (NIH) Clinical Center was initiated to translate this strategy of allograft augmentation with donor Th2 cells. Data regarding Th2 cell manufacturing, clinical results, and immune endpoints were recently published.[10] This chapter does not greatly detail the methods of Th2 cell manufacturing in this initial study but, rather, emphasizes current second-generation methods of manufacturing Th2 cells in rapamycin. Summarily, donor Th2 cells were manufactured by the following method:

1. Mononuclear cell collection by steady-state leukapheresis.
2. Elutriation to enrich for lymphocytes.
3. Enrichment for CD4+ T cells by negative selection using anti-CD8 and anti-B-cell antibodies and sheep anti-mouse bead removal.
4. Costimulation of the enriched donor CD4+ T cells using anti-CD3- and anti-CD28-coated tosyl-activated magnetic beads by the approach described by Levine and June[11] and subsequently evaluated in several adoptive T-cell immunotherapy trials.[12-15]
5. Expansion of costimulated cells in IL-4 and IL-2 for approximately 20 days through the use of a repeat costimulation step at approximately day 12 of the culture.

Donor Th2 cells were successfully manufactured in all 28 cases, with Th2 cell graft augmentation performed in a Phase I manner at doses of 5, 25, or 125×10^6 Th2 cells per kg of recipient body weight (n = 3, 19, and 6 subjects per dose level, respectively). The Th2 cells generated by this method were indeed shifted toward a Th2 cytokine phenotype relative to the culture input donor CD4+ cells; however, the Th2 shift was somewhat incomplete because residual IFN-γ secretion was detected and

the Th2 cytokine IL-10, which has been implicated as an anti-GVHD effector molecule,[16] was not produced in significant amounts by the donor Th2 cells. From a clinical perspective, the Th2 cell infusions were administered without specific toxicity, even in recipients of the highest dose of Th2 cells; however, a comparison of Th2 cell recipient results with the protocol control cohort demonstrated that the Th2 cell infusion did not reduce acute GVHD. Posttransplant immune monitoring demonstrated that Th2 cell recipients expressed a mixed pattern of Th1 and Th2 cytokine secretion.

In parallel with this first-generation Th2 cell clinical trial, an improved method of Th2 cell manufacturing was developed in a murine model that involved the ex-vivo use of high-dose rapamycin.[9] An ability to generate highly functional Th2 cells in rapamycin may seem unexpected because rapamycin has been associated with the induction of T-cell anergy[17] and the promotion of a regulatory T-cell phenotype.[18-20] However, in these experiments, rapamycin was relatively unbiased in terms of T-cell cytokine phenotype. The laboratory was able to generate potent effector cells, of either CD4+ Th1, CD8+ Tc1 phenotype or CD4+ Th2, CD8+ Tc2 phenotype, in supra-pharmacologic doses of rapamycin.[21] In addition, studies have shown that rapamycin-generated effector T cells do not express an abundance of the Foxp3 transcription factor associated with regulatory T cells (<5% CD4+Foxp3+ cells). Furthermore, rapamycin-generated Th1/Tc1 cells, which expressed a T-cell central memory state of differentiation that has been associated with an increased efficacy of adoptive T-cell therapy,[22] actually induced a greater degree of acute GVHD relative to control Th1/Tc1 cells.[21] In a murine model that used a fully MHC-mismatched, T-cell-replete allograft augmented with donor Th2 cells, data showed that rapamycin-generated Th2 cells were more potent than control Th2 cells, with respect to the reduction of GVHD, while preserving a component of the GVT effect. Significantly, Th2 cell prevention of GVHD was abrogated by use of IL-4-deficient donor Th2 cells. This result is consistent with a classical Th2-type mechanism that has not been attributed to regulatory T cells.

One additional finding from this work has implications for adoptive T-cell therapy efforts using donor Th2 cells—namely, there was an inverse correlation between the magnitude of Th2 cell cytokine production before infusion and the degree of cytokine polarization in vivo after transplantation (see Fig 36-1). As a result, in part, of this observation, subsequent clinical translation efforts using rapamycin-exposed Th2 cells prioritized a manufacturing method that incorporated a shorter time in culture (~12 days rather than ~20 days) and a single T-cell costimulation that permitted cytokine polarization, yet limited the magnitude of Th2 cell differentiation and cytokine secretion.

Current State of the Field

In light of results from the first-generation Th2-cell clinical trial and murine experiments, the authors

initiated a translational effort to evaluate the strategy of allograft augmentation with rapamycin-generated donor Th2 cells. A more detailed description of the method used in this second-generation Th2-cell clinical trial is provided in Method 36-1. Summarily, this method includes the following steps:

1. Mononuclear cell collection by steady-state leukapheresis.
2. CD4+ T-cell isolation by positive selection.
3. A single round of T-cell costimulation.
4. Approximately 12 days of T-cell expansion in media containing IL-4, IL-2, and high-dose rapamycin.

This new method has several practical advantages relative to the initial method, including the lack of requirements for elutriation, reduced use of

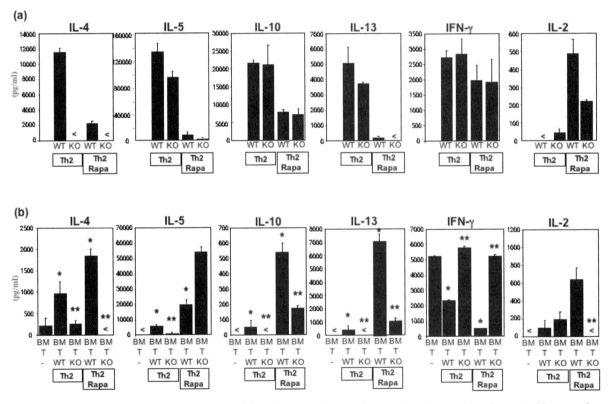

Figure 36-1. Inverse correlation between Th2 cell product cytokine production and in-vivo cytokine production. Murine Th2 cells were generated without ex-vivo rapamycin (Th2) or with ex-vivo rapamycin (Th2 Rapa). CD4+ cells were obtained from wild-type donors (WT) or interleukin-4 (IL-4) knock-out donors (KO). The top row (a) shows cytokine production from four different Th2 cell products before in-vivo administration, including the Th1 cytokines IL-2 and IFN-γ and the Th2 cytokines IL-4, -5, -10, and -13. The rapamycin-generated Th2 cell product had reduced magnitude of Th2 cell cytokine secretion relative to control Th2 cells. The bottom row (b) shows in-vivo cytokine production in murine recipients of semiallogeneic marrow and unmanipulated T-cells (T) either alone or with one of four generated Th2 cell products. Adoptive transfer of rapamycin-generated Th2 cells induced a more potent shift toward the Th2 cytokines after transplantation; this in-vivo effect was dependent on Th2 cell IL-4 secretion. (Reprinted from Foley et al.[9])

monoclonal antibody reagents with the positive selection method, and lower labor and reagent costs as a result of the reduced culture interval involving only a single round of costimulated expansion.

Reduced Th2 cell yield represents one potentially limiting factor for the manufacturing of Th2 cells in rapamycin. Figure 36-2 illustrates representative Th2 cell expansion curves with a side-by-side evaluation of cultures, both with and without rapamycin. Typically, the addition of rapamycin results in a 1- to 2-log reduction in Th2 cell yield over a 12- to 20-day culture interval. In the current clinical trial, rapamycin-exposed Th2 cells have been successfully generated in 33 of 34 donors to allow Th2 Rapa cellular therapy at a dose of 2.5×10^7 Th2 cells per kg recipient body weight. The median Th2 cell expansion over 12 days in culture has been 12.2-fold (n = 34; range = 2.2- to 21.9-fold).

One important advance in the current Th2-cell manufacturing method involving ex-vivo rapamycin relates to the use of CD4+ cell selection by the Miltenyi method (Miltenyi Biotec, Bergisch Gladbach, Germany). Prior methods used CD4+ cell

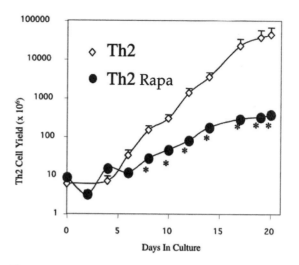

Figure 36-2. Rapamycin significantly reduces Th2 cell yield. Human CD4+ T-cells were isolated, costimulated, and expanded in media containing IL-4 and IL-2 either with rapamycin (1 μM; Th2 Rapa) or without rapamycin (Th2).

enrichment by elutriation and subsequent by negative selection using anti-CD8 and anti-B cell antibodies. Initial protocol implementation with ex-

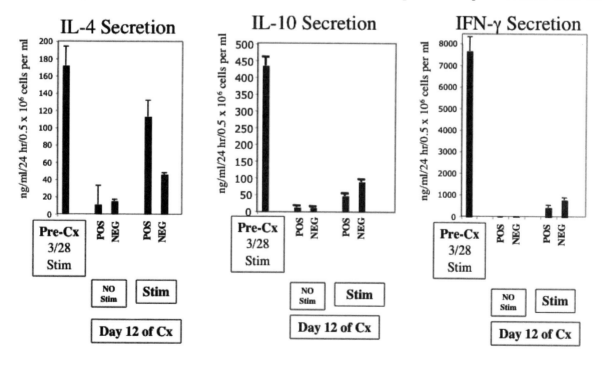

Figure 36-3. Cytokine phenotype of rapamycin-exposed Th2 cells generated from human CD4+ cells isolated by either positive selection (POS) or negative selection (NEG). Supernatants were obtained by costimulation of T cells at culture input (Pre-Cx) or after 12 days of culture in IL-4, IL-2, and rapamycin; control supernatants were obtained from T cells that did not receive costimulation (No Stim).

vivo rapamycin involved CD4+ enrichment by negative selection (n = 10 donors), whereas current protocol implementation involves CD4+ enrichment by positive selection (n = 24 donors). The positive selection method resulted in greater CD4+ purity at culture input relative to the negative selection method [mean and range for the percentage of CD4+ purity: 98% (64-99) vs 87% (74-95), respectively]; for both positively and negatively selected cell input populations, the percentage of CD4+ purity at the end of the Th2 cell culture was >99% in all 34 cases. To evaluate the two methods for potential influence on the Th2 cell cytokine phenotype, the authors performed a side-by-side comparison of positive vs negative selection and subsequent Th2 cell generation in rapamycin (results shown in Fig 36-3). CD4+ cells isolated by positive or negative selection yielded final Th2 cell products with similar cytokine profiles (preservation of Th2 cytokines and reduction in Th1 cytokines).

Future Directions

Clinical endpoints (toxicity, engraftment, GVHD, and GVT data) and immune endpoints (posttransplant cytokine profile) from the current Th2 cell protocol will help determine future translational efforts in this area. The current second-generation Th2-cell manufacturing method that uses high-dose rapamycin exposure is greatly simplified relative to the initial Th2 cell method. Also, it is hypothesized that the Th2 cell product will more effectively polarize patients to the Th2-type cytokine profile after transplantation. With respect to Th2 cell manufacturing, it is possible that further modification of the methodology would improve either the feasibility of manufacturing or the Th2 cell purity or function. For example, consideration should be given to evaluating the removal of CD4+ regulatory T cells from the input CD4+ cell population, because the authors have found, in a murine GVHD model, that such regulatory T cells have the potential to inhibit Th2 cell effector function.[23]

References/Resources

1. Weiden PL, Flournoy N, Thomas ED, et al. Antileukemic effect of graft-versus-host disease in human recipients of allogeneic-marrow grafts. N Engl J Med 1979;300:1068-73.

2. Fowler DH. Shared biology of GVHD and GVT effects: Potential methods of separation. Crit Rev Oncol Hematol 2006;57:225-44.

3. Martin PJ, Rowley SD, Anasetti C, et al. A phase I-II clinical trial to evaluate removal of CD4 cells and partial depletion of CD8 cells from donor marrow for HLA-mismatched unrelated recipients. Blood 1999;94:2192-9.

4. Fowler DH, Kurasawa K, Smith R, et al. Donor CD4-enriched cells of Th2 cytokine phenotype regulate graft-versus-host disease without impairing allogeneic engraftment in sublethally irradiated mice. Blood 1994; 84:3540-9.

5. Krenger W, Cooke KR, Crawford JM, et al. Transplantation of polarized type 2 donor T cells reduces mortality caused by experimental graft-versus-host disease. Transplantation 1996;62:1278-85.

6. Fowler DH, Breglio J, Nagel G, et al. Allospecific CD8+ Tc1 and Tc2 populations in graft-versus-leukemia effect and graft-versus-host disease. J Immunol 1996;157: 4811-21.

7. Jung U, Foley JE, Erdmann AA, et al. CD3/CD28-costimulated T1 and T2 subsets: Differential in vivo allosensitization generates distinct GVT and GVHD effects. Blood 2003;102:3439-46.

8. Le Gros G, Ben-Sasson SZ, Seder R, et al. Generation of interleukin 4 (IL-4)-producing cells in vivo and in vitro: IL-2 and IL-4 are required for in vitro generation of IL-4-producing cells. J Exp Med 1990;172:921-9.

9. Foley JE, Jung U, Miera A, et al. Ex vivo rapamycin generates donor Th2 cells that potently inhibit graft-versus-host disease and graft-versus-tumor effects via an IL-4-dependent mechanism. J Immunol 2005;175:5732-43.

10. Fowler DH, Odom J, Steinberg SM, et al. Phase I clinical trial of costimulated, IL-4 polarized donor CD4+ T cells as augmentation of allogeneic hematopoietic cell transplantation. Biol Blood Marrow Transplant 2006;12:1150-60.

11. Levine BL, Bernstein WB, Connors M, et al. Effects of CD28 costimulation on long-term proliferation of CD4+ T cells in the absence of exogenous feeder cells. J Immunol 1997;159:5921-30.

12. Levine BL, Bernstein WB, Aronson NE, et al. Adoptive transfer of costimulated CD4+ T cells induces expansion of peripheral T cells and decreased CCR5 expression in HIV infection. Nat Med 2002;8:47-53.

13. Laport GG, Levine BL, Stadtmauer EA, et al. Adoptive transfer of costimulated T cells induces lymphocytosis in patients with relapsed/refractory non-Hodgkin lymphoma following CD34+-selected hematopoietic cell transplantation. Blood 2003;102:2004-13.

14. Porter DL, Levine BL, Bunin N, et al. A phase 1 trial of donor lymphocyte infusions expanded and activated ex vivo via CD3/CD28 costimulation. Blood 2006;107:1325-31.

15. Levine BL, Humeau LM, Boyer J, et al. Gene transfer in humans using a conditionally replicating lentiviral vector. Proc Natl Acad Sci U S A 2006;103:17372-7.

16. Blazar BR, Taylor PA, Panoskaltsis-Mortari A, et al. Interleukin-10 dose-dependent regulation of CD4+ and CD8+ T cell-mediated graft-versus-host disease. Transplantation 1998;66:1220-9.

17. Powell JD, Lerner CG, Schwartz RH. Inhibition of cell cycle progression by rapamycin induces T cell clonal anergy even in the presence of costimulation. J Immunol 1999;162:2775-84.

18. Zheng XX, Sanchez-Fueyo A, Sho M, et al. Favorably tipping the balance between cytopathic and regulatory T cells to create transplantation tolerance. Immunity 2003;19:503-14.

19. Battaglia M, Stabilini A, Roncarolo MG. Rapamycin selectively expands CD4+CD25+FoxP3+ regulatory T cells. Blood 2005;105:4743-8.

20. Valmori D, Tosello V, Souleimanian NE, et al. Rapamycin-mediated enrichment of T cells with regulatory activity in stimulated CD4+ T cell cultures is not due to the selective expansion of naturally occurring regulatory T cells but to the induction of regulatory functions in conventional CD4+ T cells. J Immunol 2006;177:944-9.

21. Jung U, Foley JE, Erdmann AA, et al. Ex vivo rapamycin generates Th1/Tc1 or Th2/Tc2 effector T cells with enhanced in vivo function and differential sensitivity to post-transplant rapamycin therapy. Biol Blood Marrow Transplant 2006;12:905-18.

22. Klebanoff CA, Gattinoni L, Torabi-Parizi P, et al. Central memory self/tumor-reactive CD8+ T cells confer superior antitumor immunity compared with effector memory T cells. Proc Natl Acad Sci U S A 2005;102:9571-6.

23. Foley JE, Mariotti J, Amarnath S, et al. Th2.rapa cell treatment of established murine acute GVHD is abrogated by IL-2 therapy and T regulatory cells (abstract). Blood 2007;110:2169.

Method 36-1. General Overview of Current Th2 Cell Manufacturing: Rapamycin-Generated Donor Th2 Cells

Description

This procedure achieves ex-vivo T-cell expansion and cytokine polarization.

Time for Procedure

1. CD4+ cell isolation: approximately 6 hours.
2. Th2 cell expansion: 12 days.

Summary of Procedure

Donor CD4+ cells are isolated, costimulated, and expanded ex vivo in media containing Th2-polarizing cytokines and rapamycin.

Equipment

1. Apheresis instrument [CS-3000 (Fenwal, Lake Zurich, IL) or equivalent].
2. Selection device [CliniMACS (Miltenyi Biotec, Bergisch Gladbach, Germany)].
3. Humidified incubator (37 C, 4%-10% CO_2).
4. Coulter multisizer [for monitoring cell volume (Beckman Coulter, Fullerton, CA)].
5. Flow cytometer (for release assays).

Supplies and Reagents

1. Miltenyi CD4+ T-cell isolation kit.
2. Autologous (donor) plasma.
3. LifeCell sterile culture bags (LifeCell, Chennai, India). Anti-CD3- and anti-CD28-coated tosyl-activated magnetic beads (manufactured by Bruce Levine, PhD, University of Pennsylvania Abramson Family Cancer Research Institute).
4. Recombinant human interleukin-4 (IL-4) and IL-2.
5. Rapamune [(Wyeth, Madison, NJ) or rapamycin (FDA-approved source; oral suspension)].

Procedure

1. Collect the mononuclear cell (MNC) product from a donor using a standard steady-state apheresis method (typically, 5- to 10-L collection); a total nucleated cell (TNC) count of ~5 $\times 10^9$ cells will be sufficient.
2. Subject the TNC product to CD4+ cell selection using Miltenyi anti-CD4 microbeads and the CliniMACS device; the target number of CD4-enriched cells should be >3 $\times 10^8$ cells.
3. Initiate the Th2 cell culture in LifeCell bags using an initial cell concentration of 1.5 $\times 10^6$ cells/mL and a total CD4+ cell number of 3 $\times 10^8$ cells. The media of choice is X-VIVO 20 (Lonza Group, Basel, Switzerland) supplemented with 5% autologous, heat-inactivated plasma. Other additives include IL-4 (1000 IU per mL), IL-2 (20 IU per mL), and rapamycin (1 μM).
4. Propagate the Th2 cell culture by adding cytokines at day 2 of the culture (same concentrations), then by splitting cultures with cytokine- and rapamycin-replete media from days 4 through 9 to maintain a cell concentration of 0.5 $\times 10^6$ cells per mL.
5. At day 12 of the culture, harvest and concentrate cells using the Cytomate instrument (Baxter, Deerfield, IL), the COBE 2991 Cell Processor (CaridianBCT, Lakewood, CO), or the CS3000 cell separator (Fenwal, Lake Zurich, IL). The final volume of the Th2 cell product should be cryopreserved by a slow-rate method in approximately 250 mL of freezing medium media that contains 5% dimethyl sulfoxide and 5% pentastarch.
6. Test an aliquot of the final product for standard microbiological assays, for T-cell surface phenotype, and for T-cell cytokine phenotype.

Anticipated Results

The final Th2 cell product should be >99% pure with respect to the CD3+CD4+ flow cytometry panel. The cytokine phenotype of the final product is tested by repeat costimulation and testing of the 24-hour supernatant for cytokine content by enzyme-linked immunosorbent assay or Luminex methodology (Luminex, Riverside, CA). The Th2 cells should secrete greatly reduced IL-2 and IFN relative to the day 0 culture input cells and have detectable but relatively low-level secretion of the Th2 cytokines IL-4, -5, -10, and -13. Th2 cells will typically expand approximately 10-fold during the 12-day culture interval.

In: Areman EM, Loper K, eds
Cellular Therapy: Principles, Methods, and Regulations
Bethesda, MD: AABB, 2009

◆◆◆   **37**   ◆◆◆

Natural Killer Cells

David H. McKenna, Jr, MD, and Jeffrey S. Miller, MD

NATURAL KILLER (NK) CELLS ARE A DIS-tinct subset of lymphocytes within the innate immune system that mediate nonspecific lysis of target cells and produce a variety of cytokines. They play critical roles in the defense against viral infection and malignancy and in the regulation of hematopoiesis. NK cells comprise approximately 10% to 20% of peripheral blood lymphocytes. They have the morphology of large granular lymphocytes, and they are characterized immunophenotypically as negative for T-cell markers (eg, CD3, CD4) and positive for CD56, an isoform of a neural cell adhesion molecule.[1,2]

NK cells do not require expression of self-MHC (major histocompatibility complex) molecules by target cells for induction of cytolysis. In fact, downregulation of the expression of MHC Class I molecules—a phenomenon of malignantly transformed and virally infected cells—increases susceptibility to NK cell lysis.[3] For this reason, NK cells are a logical candidate for cancer immunotherapy. NK cells have shown promise in early-phase trials for the treatment of acute myeloid leukemia and myelodysplastic syndrome.[4] Further, a report by Ruggeri

et al[5] has suggested a clinical utility for NK cells in the setting of mismatched hematopoietic stem cell (HSC) transplantation. Trials using NK cells alone or in combination with HSCs are under way at several institutions.

The standard method for the manufacture of NK cell products involves immunomagnetic selection (CD3-depletion with or without CD56 enrichment) of a mononuclear cell (MNC) apheresis collection, possibly followed by a culture. Method 37-1 describes one such method: CD3-depletion of MNCs followed by an overnight incubation with interleukin-2 (IL-2). This method results in a mean purity, recovery, and viability of 38%, 79%, and 86%, respectively. Addition of a CD56-enrichment step results in equivalent viability (mean = 85%) and a greater purity (mean = 90%), as expected; however, the recovery is much lower (mean = 19%).[6] It remains to be determined whether an alternative cell source and/or different approach to cell selection and culture may be optimal.

Umbilical cord blood (UCB)-derived NK cells have been characterized with results suggesting therapeutic advantages over marrow and/or

David H. McKenna, Jr, MD, Scientific and Medical Director, Molecular and Cellular Therapeutics, University of Minnesota, St Paul, Minnesota, and Jeffrey S. Miller, MD, Professor of Medicine, Hematology, Oncology, and Transplantation, and Associate Director of Experimental Therapeutics, University of Minnesota Masonic Cancer Research Center, Minneapolis, Minnesota

D. McKenna has disclosed a financial relationship with BioE, Inc. J. Miller has disclosed no conflicts of interest.

peripheral-blood-derived NK cells.[7,8] Although most basic science studies on UCB-derived NK cells have involved fresh UCB, banked UCB units are the likely source of UCB for clinical applications and may also be used. Aside from the need for thawing and the addition of a few reagents, such as DNAse, the methods used with UCB-derived NK cells are very similar to those for apheresis MNC products.

One potential modification to current cell selection strategies would be the inclusion of a CD19-depletion step. Removal of B cells may prevent adverse B-cell-mediated phenomena such as Epstein-Barr virus infection and disease[4] and passenger lymphocyte syndrome-related hemolysis.[9] Culture length and conditions vary widely among studies, from immediate infusion after selection to several-day culture with multifold expansion of cells using more elaborate culture conditions.[10] Because there are few completed NK cell trials at this point, it is clear that further studies are necessary to elucidate the optimal methods of production.

Acknowledgments

The implementation of Method 37-1 was a collaborative effort between the University of Minnesota Cancer Center (JS Miller, Principal Investigator) and the clinical, technical, and quality teams of the Clinical Cell Therapy Laboratory and Molecular and Cellular Therapeutics of the University of Minnesota.

References/Resources

1. Chiorean EG, Miller JS. The biology of natural killer cells and implications for therapy of human disease. J Hematother Stem Cell Res 2001;10:451-63.

2. Miller JS. Biology of natural killer cells in cancer and infection. Cancer Invest 2002;20:405-19.

3. Ljunggren HG, Karre K. In search of the "missing self": MHC molecules and NK cell recognition. Immunol Today 1990;11:237-44.

4. Miller JS, Soignier Y, Panoskaltsis-Mortari A, et al. Successful adoptive transfer and in vivo expansion of human haploidentical NK cells in cancer patients. Blood 2005; 105:3051-7.

5. Ruggeri L, Capanni M, Urbani E, et al. Effectiveness of donor natural killer cell alloreactivity in mismatched hematopoietic transplants. Science 2002;295:2097-100.

6. McKenna D, Sumstad D, Bostrom N, et al. GMP-production of natural killer cells for immunotherapy: A six year single institution experience. Transfusion 2007;47:520-8.

7. Gardiner CM, O'Meara A, Reen DJ. Differential cytotoxicity of cord blood and bone marrow-derived natural killer cells. Blood 1998;91:207-13.

8. Dalle JH, Menezes J, Wagner E, et al. Characterization of cord blood natural killer cells: Implications for transplantation and neonatal infections. Pediatr Res 2005;57: 649-55.

9. Skeate RC, Miller JS, Eubanks J, et al. Acute hemolytic transfusion reaction due to anti-A in a type-A patient who received type-A red cells: Passenger lymphocyte syndrome post-NK cell infusion? (abstract) Cytotherapy 2005;7:132.

10. Lundqvist A, Abrams SI, Schrump DS, et al. Bortezomib and depsipeptide sensitize tumors to tumor necrosis factor-related apoptosis-inducing ligand: A novel method to potentiate natural killer cell tumor cytotoxicity. Cancer Res 2006;66:7317-25.

Method 37-1. Production of Peripheral-Blood-Derived, CD3-Depleted, IL-2-Activated Natural Killer Cells

Description

There are several strategies that can be followed to manufacture natural killer (NK) cell products, including positive and negative immunomagnetic selection-based methods. The following is a description of a procedure that involves CD3+ (T-cell)-depletion of a nonmobilized, peripheral blood, mononuclear cell apheresis collection followed by overnight culture and activation with interleukin-2 (IL-2).

Time for Procedure

1. Preculture processing: approximately 4 hours.
2. Postculture processing: approximately 3 hours.
3. Release testing: approximately 2 hours.

Summary of Procedure

A. *Day 1 (Preculture) Processing*
   1. Pre-CD3-depletion:
      a. Product receipt and inspection.
      b. Sampling for quality control (QC) testing.
      c. Total nucleated cell (TNC) adjustment for further processing.
   2. CD3+ depletion:
      a. Culture medium preparation.
      b. CD3+ cell labeling.
      c. CD3 depletion.
      d. Culture preparation and QC testing of CD3– and CD3+ fractions.
   3. Overnight culture in X-VIVO 15/IL-2 (Lonza Group, Basel, Switzerland).

B. *Day 2 (Postculture) Processing*
   1. Wash and resuspension.
   2. Volume reduction/wash (twice).
   3. Sampling for QC/lot release testing.
   4. Dose adjustment (if necessary).
   5. Final labeling and release.

Equipment

1. CliniMACS cell selection system (Miltenyi Biotec, Bergisch Gladbach, Germany).
2. COBE 2991 Cell Processor (CaridianBCT, Lakewood, CO).
3. Incubator: 5% CO_2, 37C.
4. Equipment related to QC/lot release testing.

Supplies and Reagents

A. *Day 1 (Preculture) Processing*
   1. CliniMACS phosphate-buffered saline/EDTA buffer.
   2. CliniMACS CD3 microbeads.
   3. CliniMACS tubing set [large scale (LS)].
   4. COBE 2991 processing set.
   5. Human serum albumin (HSA, 25%).
   6. Pall SQ40S filter (Pall Corp, East Hills, NY).
   7. Transfer bags: 150 mL, 300 mL, 600 mL, 1000 mL, 2000 mL.
   8. IL-2.
   9. FluoroEthylenePropylene (FEP) bags: 290 mL, 500 mL, 730 mL.
   10. Human AB serum: heat inactivated.
   11. X-VIVO 15 medium.

B. *Day 2 (Postculture) Processing*
   1. COBE 2991 processing set.
   2. HSA (5%).
   3. HSA (25%).
   4. Double coupler adapter.
   5. Transfer bags: 150 mL and 300 mL.
   6. Plasma-Lyte A.
   7. Dimethyl sulfoxide (DMSO).

Procedure

A. *Day 1 (Preculture) Processing*
   1. Pre-CD3 depletion:

a. Product receipt and inspection:
  - Documentation of arrival time and collection center.
  - Review of label information, including confirmation of product identity.
  - Gross inspection of product/bag.
  - Review of donor infectious disease testing and donor eligibility determination.
b. Sampling for QC testing:
  - Nucleated cell (NC) count.
  - Differential.
  - ABO/Rh confirmatory testing.
  - Flow cytometry [CD3, CD56, 7-amino-actinomycin D (7-AAD) viability].
c. Determination of volume and initial NC count:
  - TNC adjustment for further processing (if necessary).
  - The maximum number of NCs to be loaded on the CliniMACS is 2.5 $\times 10^{10}$.
2. CD3+ depletion:
  a. Culture the medium preparation:
    - Inspect bottles of X-VIVO 15 and heat-inactivated type AB human serum for part number, expiry date, container integrity, and appearance of reagent.
    - Add 110 mL of heat-inactivated type AB human serum to each 1000-mL bottle of X-VIVO 15.
    - Filter the prepared medium with a 0.22-micron filter unit, label accordingly, and place it into a 37-C incubator to warm.
  b. Supplement the CliniMACS buffer with 0.5% HSA:
    - Add 20 mL of 25% HSA to each buffer bag and label them accordingly.
  c. Wash the cells.
    - Inspect a COBE 2991 processing set for expiry date and integrity.
    - Load the processing set onto the COBE 2991 for the wash procedure and attach hemostats to all lines.

- Attach the bag of cells and one bag of CliniMACS buffer/0.5% HSA to the processing set.
- In manual mode, set the COBE 2991 settings as follows:
  - Centrifuge speed: 1200 rpm.
  - Super out rate: 450 mL/minute.
  - Minimum agitate time: 30 seconds.
  - Super out volume: 600 mL.
- Open the hemostat on the cell suspension line and transfer the cells to the COBE processing bag.
- Fill the COBE processing bag with CliniMACS buffer/0.5% HSA.
- Perform one wash (15 minutes at 1200 rpm), and expel as much supernatant as possible into the waste bag.
d. Label CD3+ cells:
  - Remove one vial of CliniMACS CD3 microbeads from the refrigerator; inspect the vial and 150-mL transfer bag for expiry date and integrity.
  - Label the bag appropriately and insert the dispensing pin into one port.
  - Add 52 mL CliniMACS buffer/0.5% HSA and the entire vial of CD3 microbeads to the transfer bag; inject approximately 90 mL of air from the biological safety cabinet (BSC) into the bag and mix well.
  - Attach the transfer bag to the blue line of the COBE processing set, remove the hemostat attached to blue line tubing, add the microbeads/buffer solution to the processing bag, clear the blue line of as many microbeads as possible using air from transfer bag, and place the hemostat on the blue line.
  - Lift the seal weight and open the sliding covers to remove the COBE processing bag from the instrument.
  - Resuspend cells in the bag by gently massaging it.
  - Return the bag to the centrifuge bowl, close the sliding covers, and replace the seal weight.

- In rapid succession, push START/ SPIN, SUPER OUT, and AGITATE/ WASH IN; incubate the product with constant agitation for approximately 30 minutes.
- Fill the COBE processing bag with CliniMACS buffer/0.5% HSA; remove air from the processing bag, and hemostat all lines.
- Press START/SPIN. Wash the product once at 1500 rpm for 15 minutes. At the end of the wash, press SUPER OUT; express as much supernatant as possible into the waste bag, and press STOP.
- Heat-seal all tubing lines except the line attached to the buffer bag.
- Remove the COBE processing bag and the attached buffer bag from the COBE 2991, and place them into the BSC. Detach and remove the remainder of the processing set and discard it.
- Transfer the cell suspension from the COBE processing bag into the transfer bag. Rinse the COBE processing bag with a small amount of CliniMACS buffer/0.5% HSA, and add the diluted cells to the transfer bag. Dilute the cell suspension with CliniMACS buffer/0.5% HSA to a final volume of approximately 100 mL.
- Remove the sample for NC count.

e. CliniMACS processing:
- Turn on the CliniMACS and choose DEPLETING PROGRAM 2.1.
- When prompted, indicate the LS tubing set, NC concentration, percentage of labeled cells (60%), and product volume.
- The CliniMACS program will calculate the volume of buffer needed for the depletion process and the volumes expected for collection in the negative fraction bag, buffer waste bag, and cell fraction bag. Adjust the bags accordingly (if >400 mL).

- Inspect the CliniMACS LS tubing set and the transfer bag for expiry date and integrity.
- Label the bags accordingly. The transfer bag will be the cell collection bag and should be labeled "CD3−." Label the bag on the tubing set designated "negative fraction" as "CD3+."
- Load the tubing set onto the CliniMACS instrument and attach the required amount of buffer solution.
- Perform prime and integrity testing by following the prompts.
- Connect the bag containing washed cells to the Pall filter and proceed with the cell separation.
- Once the separation is completed, heat-seal and detach both fractions (ie, CD3− and CD3+) and set them aside for further processing. Discard the remainder of the tubing set.

f. Volume reduction of the CD3− fraction:
- Weigh and calculate the volume and perform an NC count.
- Inspect the COBE processing set for expiry date and integrity.
- Load the set onto the COBE 2991. Place hemostats on all lines.
- In manual mode, input the COBE 2991 settings as follows:
  - Centrifuge speed: 1500 rpm.
  - Super out rate: 450 mL/minute.
  - Minimum agitate time: not applicable.
  - Super out volume: 600 mL.
- Open the hemostat on the cell suspension line and transfer the cells to the COBE processing bag.
- Process the product at 1500 rpm for 3 minutes per spin. At the end of SUPER OUT, expel as much supernatant as possible into the waste bag.
- Remove the COBE processing bag from the COBE 2991 and place it in the BSC. Discard the remainder of the processing set.
- Transfer the cell suspension into a transfer bag. Add warmed cell cul-

ture medium (X-VIVO 15) to the drained COBE processing bag, and add rinse to the transfer bag.

3. Culture preparation and QC testing of CD3– and CD3+ fractions:

    a. Determine the product volume and perform an NC count.

    b. Inspect the vial of IL-2 for expiry date, integrity, and gross appearance.

    c. Add warmed cell culture medium (X-VIVO 15) to obtain a target cell concentration of 2×10^6 nucleated cells/mL.

    d. Add IL-2 to obtain a concentration of 1000 U/mL of culture medium.

    e. Remove samples for QC testing of the CD3– fraction (eg, flow cytometry, cytotoxicity, sterility) and CD3+ fraction (eg, NC count, flow cytometry).

4. Culture overnight in X-VIVO 15/IL-2:

    a. Inspect appropriately sized culture bags (FEP) for expiry date and integrity.

    b. Transfer cells into culture bags and incubate at 37 C with 5% CO_2 for 8 to 16 hours.

B. *Day 2 (Postculture) Processing*

1. Wash and resuspension:

    a. Volume reduction/wash (twice):

    • Remove bags of cells from the incubator.

    • Inspect an appropriate number of bottles of 5% HSA for expiry date, integrity, and gross appearance.

    • Inspect the COBE processing set for expiry date and integrity.

    • Load the set onto the COBE 2991, placing hemostats on all lines.

    • In manual mode, input the COBE 2991 settings as follows:

    – Centrifuge speed: 1500 rpm.

    – Super out rate: 450 mL/minute.

    – Minimum agitate time: 30 seconds.

    – Super out volume: 600 mL.

    • Open the hemostat on the cell product line and transfer the cells to the COBE processing bag.

    • Process the product at 1500 rpm for 3 minutes per spin. At the end of the SUPER OUT, expel as much supernatant as possible into the waste bag.

    • Fill the processing bag with 5% HSA. Remove air from the processing bag. Wash the product twice at 1500 rpm for 3 minutes per spin, and expel as much supernatant as possible into the waste bag.

    • Heat-seal and remove the processing bag from the COBE 2991. Detach and discard the remainder of the processing set.

    • Transfer the cells into an appropriately sized transfer bag Rinse the processing bag with 5% HSA, and add the rinse to the transfer bag.

    b. Dilute the final product to a total volume of approximately 100 mL with 5% HSA.

2. Sampling for QC and lot release testing:

    a. NC count, flow cytometry (CD3, CD56, 7-AAD viability), sterility, Gram's stain, endotoxin, cytotoxicity.

    b. Adjust the cell dose, if necessary. Calculate the available dose and determine whether a portion of cells needs to be removed.

    c. Complete final labeling and release:

    • Label the product appropriately and include the following statement: "Caution: New Drug—Limited by Federal Law to Investigational Use" according to US federal regulations.[2]

    • Release NK cell product once lot release testing has been completed and passed.

References/Resources

1. McKenna D, Sumstad D, Bostrom N, et al. GMP-production of natural killer cells for immunotherapy: A six year single institution experience. Transfusion 2007;47:520-8.

2. Code of federal regulations. Title 21 CFR, Part 312.6. Washington, DC: US Government Printing Office, 2009 (revised annually).

In: Areman EM, Loper K, eds
Cellular Therapy: Principles, Methods, and Regulations
Bethesda, MD: AABB, 2009

♦♦♦ **38** ♦♦♦

Human Mesenchymal Stromal Cells

Karen Bieback, PhD, and Hermann Eichler, MD

MESENCHYMAL STEM OR STROMAL CELLS (MSCs) are cell-culture-expanded, adherent, fibroblastoid, multipotent stem-like cells. They are capable of extensive proliferation in ex-vivo culture and of differentiation into various tissues—probably even beyond the mesodermal germ layer.[1-3] Both attributes, in combination with the relative ease of isolation, ensure that the therapeutic capacities of MSCs will be intensely investigated for the treatment of a number of human diseases.[4] Indeed, MSCs have already demonstrated efficacy in a variety of cellular therapies, including treatment of children with osteogenesis imperfecta, bone regeneration, and hematopoietic support.[5-7]

MSCs have been isolated from different human tissues, including marrow, synovium, periosteum, muscle, liver, dermis, spleen, thymus, blood, umbilical cord/placental blood (UCB), cord matrix, amniotic fluid, placenta, fetal liver, and adipose tissue.[8] Despite the fact that every organ seems to contain MSCs, the precise identity of in-vivo MSC correlates in the adult remains elusive.[9-13] Among the different types of cells that assemble the marrow stroma, nonhematopoietic, multipotent stem cells have been identified using the colony-forming unit—fibroblastoid (CFU-F) assay.[14] This assay identifies adherent spindle-shaped cells forming colonies when marrow mononuclear cells are cultured in minimal medium containing fetal bovine serum (FBS). Cells within these colonies can be induced to differentiate into mesodermal and, possibly, endodermal and ectodermal lineages.[15,16]

At present, complications in defining these cells arise from the fact that no single marker has been identified to clearly define and prospectively isolate MSCs, as is possible with CD34 as an identifier of hematopoietic progenitor cells (HPCs). Although MSCs were initially thought to be a distinct population, some data indicate that either CD45low/CD133+ selected cells or clonally derived HPCs can give rise to MSCs.[17-20] Thus, many controversies remain regarding the phenotype and origin of the MSC in-vivo correlate.

In contrast, the immunophenotype of culture-expanded MSCs seems to be basically well characterized. A panel of different cell-surface markers is in use to specify culture-expanded MSCs using flow

Karen Bieback, PhD, Head of Research Laboratory, Institute for Transfusion Medicine and Immunology, Medical Faculty Mannheim, University of Heidelberg, Mannheim, Germany; and Hermann Eichler, MD, Director, Institute for Clinical Hematology and Transfusion Medicine, Saarland University Hospital, Homburg/Saar, Germany

The authors have disclosed no conflicts of interest.

cytometry.[21,22] Regarding MSCs derived from different tissue sources, there seem to be only small variations. Minimal criteria to define MSCs include the expression of CD73 as well as CD90 and the absence of hematopoietic markers on plastic-adherent fibroblastoid cells, with a differentiation capacity for at least three tissue lineages.[23]

Adding to the complexity surrounding MSCs is the fact that a variety of different cells have been named or described as MSCs—often based on different isolation protocols or different tissue sources. In addition, the nomenclature has been inconsistent, with "mesenchymal stem cells" and "mesenchymal stromal cells" used interchangeably.[23] MSC populations might be heterogeneous and/or affected by different isolation and expansion protocols. Furthermore, different tissues that might contain similar, but not identical, types of cells may result in variable phenotypes and functions of multipotent stem cell populations.[24] It is also possible that some tissues contain a higher percentage of immature cells, or that special culture conditions favor the outgrowth of more primitive subsets of progenitor cells, as has been suggested for multipotent adult progenitor cells (MAPCs) or unrestricted somatic stem cells (USSCs) from UCB.[25] Data indicate that these populations are in constant genetic (or epigenetic) transition, enabling them to easily shift phenotypes.[26]

Production of Human MSCs

Isolation of MSCs

Once primary tissues have been processed, isolation of MSCs derived from different tissues follows a similar protocol by 1) culturing adherent cells in the appropriate medium (normally solely a basal medium plus FBS, glutamine, and antibiotics), 2) subculturing fibroblastoid cells (to produce a CFU-F) upon appearance, and 3) characterizing them upon completion of the culture. Of course, initial processing to obtain primary cultures varies for the different tissues, but once MSCs are established as a CFU-F or a subconfluent monolayer, a secondary culture can be performed using a standardized process. The following discussion focuses exclusively on MSCs derived from bone marrow, adipose tissue, and UCB. Optimal in-vitro culture conditions

may be attained by selecting serum supplements and/or growth factors that may enhance MSC clinical utility.

Critical Steps in the General Processing of MSCs

In general, there are a few critical steps in the processing of MSCs:

1. **Depletion of Contaminating Cells.** This process may be performed by one of the following techniques:
   - Dilution.
   - Density gradient centrifugation.
   - Immune depletion techniques (such as rosette separation).
   - Enrichment of putative precursors by single markers using immunomagnetic techniques.
   - Adherence to plastic: In minimal medium containing no growth factors other than those provided by serum, only MSCs adhere to a plastic surface, so by removing all non-adherent cells, an initial enrichment can be performed.[27] Within hematopoietic tissues, there are only a few cells that tend to adhere to plastic: myeloid cells and B-cell precursors. These can be depleted by a short incubation with trypsin/EDTA, which is sufficient to detach MSCs but not the contaminating cells.[22]

2. **Selection of the Appropriate Batch of Serum.** Serum severely affects the expansion, and also the differentiation, of MSCs; thus, it is critical to select an appropriate batch of serum.[28,29] The proliferative support of sera has to be evaluated in vitro in early passages, and cells must be subjected to differentiation assays to evaluate the extent of differentiation at least qualitatively, or even quantitatively. The ultimate control for sera quality is the in-vivo ceramic tube assay to control osteo- and chondrogenesis.[30] Laboratories that cannot afford these tests may either very carefully conduct the in-vitro testing or may rely on commercially available MSC growth media kits that contain preselected FBS lots. In addition, some groups add exogenous growth factors—such as basic fibroblastoid growth factor (FGF), epidermal growth factor (EGF), and others—to accelerate expansion.[31]

MSCs from Marrow

Bone marrow is harvested from volunteer donors who give informed consent. A standard procedure is to aspirate marrow from the posterior iliac crest using a Jamshidi needle and to transfer it into a heparin-containing syringe, as described in Chapter 22.

Aseptic processing of the marrow aspirate is performed within a biological safety cabinet (BSC). Samples should be processed with caution to avoid contamination and checked for microbial contamination at appropriate processing steps.

Various protocols have been developed to process the marrow aspirate:

1. A very small volume of marrow aspirate is diluted in a culture medium. Various media have been proposed, including minimal essential medium (MEM)-alpha, Dulbecco's modified eagle medium (DMEM)—low glucose, and various other commercially available media.[32] The culture medium is supplemented with preselected FBS or human alternatives such as human serum or platelet-derived factors, penicillin/streptomycin, and L-glutamine. Cells are then directly transferred to a tissue culture (TC)-treated flask for an adherence period of 1 to 4 days. A CFU-F assay should be performed in parallel to evaluate the individual donor capacity to form colonies. Subsequently, the nonadherent cells are discarded, and the adherent cells are cultivated with a biweekly change of medium until fibroblastoid cells appear. Upon reaching a subconfluent monolayer, cells are trypsinized and replated to further expand MSCs. In parallel, cells from either passage 1 or 2 should be assayed by flow cytometry and in-vitro differentiation assays to characterize the cells as MSCs. This is probably the simplest strategy.

2. Mononuclear cells are separated by using either Ficoll (GE Healthcare, Chalfont St Giles, United Kingdom) or Percoll (GE Healthcare) density gradient centrifugation.[30,33] The marrow aspirate is diluted either with medium or phosphate-buffered saline (PBS)/EDTA and carefully layered onto the density gradient medium and centrifuged. The cells of the interface are collected, washed, and subsequently diluted in culture medium. After

transfer into TC-treated flasks, the cells are subjected to the same procedure as described in item 1 above.

3. Laboratories have tried to enrich MSCs by immunomagnetic depletion of lineage-positive cells or by selection, using different antibodies or methods, including anti-STRO-1, anti-CD49a, anti-CD271, anti-CD105, anti-CD133, anti-SSEA-4, anti-fibrin microbeads, anti-fibroblast, and aldehyde dehydrogenase activity.[17,20,34-42] After putting cells in TC-treated flasks, procedures as described in item 1 above can be performed. See Section VIII on characterization for additional detail on immunophenotyping of MSCs.

MSCs from Umbilical Cord Blood

UCB is harvested from the placenta of consenting mothers into blood bags containing citrate-phosphate-dextrose (CPD) anticoagulant. Within a BSC, the UCB is drained into a 50-mL polypropylene tube and diluted 1:1 with PBS/EDTA.[43,44] Again, different methods have been tested:

1. Mononuclear cells are separated using Ficoll density gradient centrifugation. The interface buffy coat cells are collected, washed, and subsequently suspended in culture medium and put into TC-treated flasks.[45,46] After 1 to 7 days of primary culture, all nonadherent cells are discarded, and flasks are incubated for up to 4 weeks, with a weekly change of medium. Flasks must be carefully screened at intervals to assess the development of fibroblastoid colonies. Once colonies develop, cultures should be split as soon as possible because contact inhibition within the densely packed colonies can occur, minimizing the yield of UCB MSCs within subsequent cultures.

2. In UCB, because of a very low concentration of MSCs, contaminating monocytes frequently overgrow the cultures, preventing development and expansion of MSCs. To alter the adherence kinetics of myeloid cells, the TC-treated flasks can be precoated with FBS. Adhering monocytes can be significantly reduced using this approach.[43]

3. Another technique depletes mature hematopoietic cells with a commercially available kit (RosetteSep, Stemcell Technologies, Vancou-

ver, BC, Canada).[47] UCB is mixed with a tetrameric antibody cocktail cross-linking unwanted cells with red cells. These immunorosettes are subsequently removed by pelleting during Ficoll density gradient centrifugation. The resulting cells are cultured as described in item 1 above. Similarly, Multi-Lineage Progenitor Cells (MLPC, BioE, St Paul, MN) have been isolated using a proprietary reagent. This reagent, PrepaCyte-MLPC, stimulates the aggregation of undesired cell types, which can then be removed by centrifugation.

4. Selection of MSCs has been performed by two additional methods: 1) immunomagnetic selection for CD133+ cells and 2) osmotic selection using the high resistance of MSCs to osmotic lysis.[17,48]

MSCs from Adipose Tissue

Initial studies were aimed at isolating adipocyte precursors. Epidermal fat pad tissue was minced and digested using collagenase. Cellular subfractions were separated by centrifugation to yield mature adipocytes within the supernatant and progenitor cells, plus HPCs in the pellet.[49]

In humans, lipoaspirates derived from tumescence liposuction frequently serve as starting material.[50] The lipoaspirate is washed intensely with sterile PBS (volume 1:1) to remove cellular debris and erythrocytes. Washed aspirates are digested by adding collagenase under gentle agitation. The digested aspirates are then centrifuged at increased centrifugal force to obtain the stromal vascular fraction within the pellet. Remaining erythrocytes may be removed using a lysing buffer. The stromal vascular cells are cultured in a complete medium overnight. All nonadherent cells are discarded by extensive washing, and the remaining adherent cells appear as fibroblastoid cells (Fig 38-1). These are cultivated for about 10 days until a 60%- to 70%-confluent monolayer has developed and the cells can be split to initiate the subsequent culture passage.

MSC Expansion

To purify large numbers of cells for experimental approaches or, ultimately, for clinical therapies, MSCs must be expanded ex vivo. During expansion culture, MSCs exert a highly variable self-renewal capacity. Mitotic divisions mainly depend on serum growth factors. In general, without further additions, 30 to 40 population doublings can be achieved within expansion cultures until MSCs approach the "Hayflick limit".[51] By adding special growth factors such as FGF to the basal medium, higher cumulative population doublings can be achieved.[52] Nevertheless, replicative aging is observed in these stem cell cultures, as indicated in Fig 38-1. Replicative aging is accompanied by reduced growth velocity, morphologic changes, enriched formation of stress fibers, and a shortening of telomeres (the "covers" at the end of the chromosomes), which become shorter by means of DNA replication.[51] The only known way of circumventing the Hayflick limit is by activation of telomerase to regenerate telomeres during DNA replication. Genetically engineered MSCs expressing human telomerase reverse transcriptase (hTERT, a catalytic subunit of telomerase) become immortalized and proliferate indefinitely.[53]

Attention should be paid to the fact that a few authors recently observed spontaneous transformation of MSCs in long-term culture associated with an altered karyotype, the expression of cancer-associated genes, and the expression of telomerase.[54,55] Furthermore, these MSCs were able to induce sarcoma formation.[56,57]

In expansion culture, attention to cell density is critical. MSCs must be passaged before reaching a confluent stage because contact inhibition reduces proliferative capacity within subsequent passages. Thus, MSCs need to be passaged upon reaching 60% to 70% confluency. Additionally, several laboratories have demonstrated that seeding densities severely affect the expansion potential of MSCs. Higher MSC proliferation can be attained with MSCs plated at low density (1-3 cells/cm²: 2000-fold expansion) in contrast to high density (12 cells/cm²: 60-fold expansion).[58] Thus, the fewer the cells/cm² that are seeded, the more the cells that can be harvested from a single TC-treated flask. It is optimal to produce cell numbers as high as possible within a short period of time in both clinical and nonclinical applications. The challenge is to gain sufficient numbers of cells at early passages with maintained MSC qualities but without intense laboratory efforts. One should keep in mind that seeding cells at very low densities and harvesting large amounts after one passage keeps passage numbers

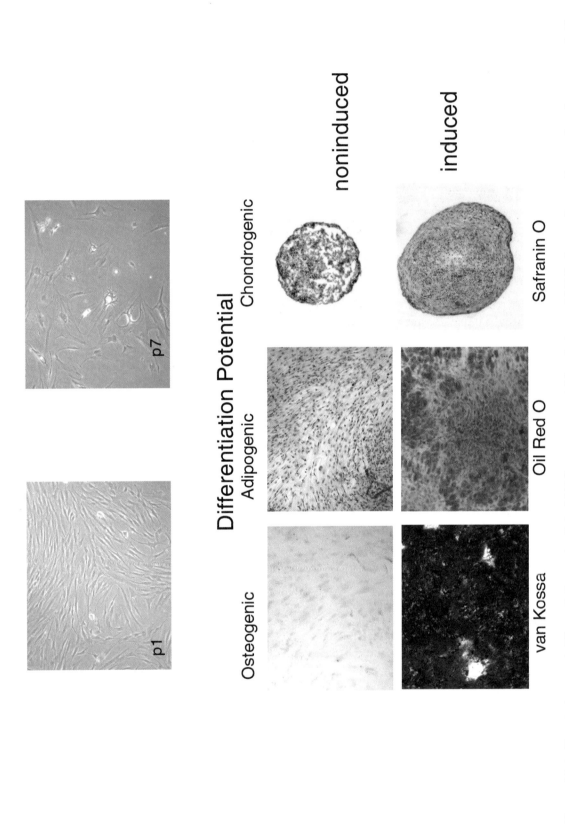

Figure 38-1. Morphology and differentiation potential of MSCs. *Upper panel:* Morphology of MSCs from adipose tissue at early passage (p1) and after prolonged passaging in culture (p7). Culture-induced senescence is indicated by a significantly prolonged growth rate and morphologic changes: spindle-shaped cells in low passage and a broad, flattened phenotype in late passage. *Lower panel:* Tri-lineage differentiation of MSCs from marrow. Both control and induced conditions are presented.

low, but still, individual cells undergo numerous cell doublings within this one passage. By adding growth factors, the life span can be prolonged and the differentiation capacity maintained.[59]

Clinical-Scale Isolation and Expansion

When planning for use of MSCs in clinical trials, current good manufacturing practice (cGMP) requirements must be considered. Marrow and UCB are already sources for obtaining stem cells for clinical applications, as addressed in detail in previous chapters. Procurement techniques for MSCs do not differ from those for HPCs up to the point where mononuclear cells are isolated and expanded in culture. Adipose tissue is an established source for autologous soft tissue augmentation used by aesthetic surgeons for years. Thus, isolation procedures can be regarded as noncritical in terms of the manufacturing process when experienced surgeons are performing the collection.

Because of the hypo-immunogenic nature and immunomodulatory capacities of these cells, described in detail later (see "Immunomodulatory Capacities"), MSCs have been used in both autologous and allogeneic settings. FBS is a reasonable supplement for research purposes but not for clinical application, as it poses the risk of either inducing immunologic reactions or transmitting xenogenic pathogens.[60-62] Although most of the current protocols use cGMP-grade FBS, in some countries, use of FBS is not permitted by regulatory authorities in the manufacturing process. Therefore, a variety of laboratories are focusing on the development of protocols to either diminish the FBS content or use alternative supplements or serum-free formulations.[63] Human serum or platelet-derived factors—formulated either as platelet lysate or platelet factor releasate—have demonstrated efficacy in generating MSCs with comparable characteristics to FBS MSCs.[64,65]

The next step toward a clinical-grade manufacturing process includes the use of culture devices allowing for large-scale closed system production. Some groups are using cell stack systems already in use for vaccine production.[32] Others have further optimized the process to a nearly closed system by using sterile connectors and tubing to enable aseptic liquid exchange and cell seeding/harvesting.[66]

Although protocols have not yet been standardized, the promise of clinical benefit from MSC therapies is causing a rapid increase in this translational research effort.

Characterization of MSCs In Vitro

Self-Renewal Potential

MSC frequencies and expansion potential are highly variable and dependent on donor characteristics such as age and disease status, as well as on the tissue source. The CFU-F assay can enumerate plating and colony formation efficacy. As indicated previously, MSC numbers can be significantly enhanced by optimizing culture conditions. Self-renewal can be tested by determining cell growth and viability at each subcultivation while controlling phenotype and differentiation potential. Various protocols exist to determine cell numbers and viability. The easiest method is to use a Neubauer hemacytometer and trypan blue as an exclusion dye to assess viability. To calculate the fold expansion of cells, the total number of cells at different time points is divided by the number of cells used to initiate each culture. To calculate cumulative population doublings, the population-doubling rate is determined at each passage by using the following formula: $x = [\log 10(N_H) - \log 10(N_I)]/\log 10(2)$, where N_I is the plated cell number and N_H is the cell number at harvest. Then the population doublings for each passage are calculated and added to the total of previous passages.[44]

Stemness

As indicated initially, scientists continue to debate whether MSCs should be regarded as stem cells or as stromal cells capable of multilineage differentiation. One way of detecting the "stemness" of MSCs is to transplant MSCs subcutaneously to demonstrate their ability to form bone, cartilage, adipose tissue, or hematopoietic stroma in vivo.[67] Some scientists regard the expression of certain genes—such as Octamer-4, Nanog, Rex-1, and SSEA-3 and -4 (stage-specific embryonic antigen), known to relate to stem cell phenotypes and associated with telomerase activity in embryonic stem cells—as indicative of a stem cell phenotype in MSCs as well.[68]

Immune Phenotype

As noted earlier, at present no unique antigenic marker, analogous to CD34 for hematopoietic stem cells, has been identified that allows a standardized prospective isolation of MSCs with predictable differentiation potential. Given that a cell surface marker exclusively defining MSCs has yet to be determined, the expression profile of culture-expanded MSCs consists of a variety of markers typical for other cell lineages. Thus, a combination of expressed and nonexpressed markers is currently used to define MSCs, and those that define hematopoietic lineages are of special importance. There is a consensus that culture-expanded MSCs express CD44, CD73 (SH-3, SH-4), CD90 (Thy-1), CD105 (SH-2, Endoglin), and HLA Class I antigens but lack the expression of CD14 (less than 2% positive cells within the MSC population; alternative CD11b), CD19 (alternative CD79a), CD34, CD45 (common leukocyte antigen), and HLA Class II antigens.[69,70] Surprisingly, there is little variation between populations and among cells derived from different sources (ie, marrow, UCB, etc) using antibodies to the markers listed above.

In-Vitro Differentiation

To promote the differentiation of MSCs along osteogenic, adipogenic, and chondrogenic pathways, the cells are subjected to inductive stimuli. Then, appropriate assays for evaluating the extent of differentiation must be conducted (Fig 38-1).[22]

Common osteogenic stimuli such as glycerophosphate and dexamethasone induce, in monolayered MSCs, the up-regulation of osteogenic markers (alkaline phosphatase, calcium mineralization, osteopontin, osteonectin, or other proteins), which can be assessed either by polymerase chain reaction or by immuno- or histochemical staining.[71,72]

To promote chondrogenic differentiation, MSCs are usually centrifuged to form a pellet or aggregate. The pellets are subsequently cultured in serum-free conditions supplemented with transforming-growth factor.[73,74] Typical markers expressed on these chondrocytes are glycosaminoglycans, collagen type II, and aggrecan.

Adipogenic differentiation is frequently induced by using 3-isobutyl-1-methyl-xanthine, insulin, dexamethasone, and indomethacin.[75] Differentiated cells are easily recognized with phase contrast microscopy by the appearance of lipid-filled vacuoles that can be stained with oil-red-o. Furthermore, the cells express peroxisome-proliferation-activated receptor gamma 2, lipase, and fatty acid binding proteins.

Various groups have reported the differentiation of MSCs within three-dimensional matrices and scaffolds to serve as tools in tissue-engineering approaches.[76] Within these settings, MSCs can predifferentiate into the respective lineage and can be transplanted within the scaffold to form solid tissue after grafting.

It is noteworthy that individual clones of MSCs exert heterogeneous differentiation potential. Some reports have demonstrated that only about one-third of clones are tripotential—capable of differentiating into bone, cartilage, and fat—suggesting that MSC preparations contain heterogeneous cells at different stages of their developmental commitment.[22,77] Extending the in-vitro differentiation into bone, cartilage, and fat, several publications indicate differentiation into hematopoietic stroma cells, muscular cells (smooth muscle as well as cardiomyocytes), and neuronal cells.[22,78-80] However, as indicated earlier, whether differentiation into nonmesodermal lineages is possible is at present controversial.

Homing and Migration

MSCs express the chemokine receptor CXCR-4 (receptor for stromal-derived factor-1 (SDF-1) and the receptor for hepatocyte growth factor (or scatter factor). These chemokines can therefore attract MSCs to specific tissue sites or stem cell niches.[81] MSCs have been shown to home specifically to sites of injury, including tumor tissue. In healthy animals, MSCs have been demonstrated to home to the marrow, but also to other tissues including cardiac muscle, teeth, and spleen, suggesting a mesenchymal-directed fate of engrafting cells.[82]

Immunomodulatory Capacities

Several groups address the immunologic properties of MSCs as part of their quality control testing to define MSCs. Numerous reports have demonstrated that MSCs do not induce an allogeneic immune response in mixed lymphocyte cultures but, rather, inhibit ongoing immunologic reactions by means of soluble or cell-contact-dependent mechanisms.[83]

MSCs are added to allogeneic peripheral blood MNCs, with T-cell proliferation assessed subsequently for induction of alloreactivity by comparing to T cells stimulated with allogeneic effector cells. To test immune-suppressive effects, MSCs are added either as third-party cells to mixed lymphocyte cultures containing alloreactive T cells or to mitogen-activated T cells, with proliferation inhibition then monitored.[84]

Hematopoietic Support

For hematopoiesis to occur, HPCs are reliant on the stromal microenvironment providing necessary cell-to-cell contacts as well as growth factors and cytokines. MSCs provide necessary signals for HPC maintenance and differentiation.[85] Whereas exogenous growth factors result in a boost of hematopoietic colony-forming cells within the first 2 to 3 weeks of cultivation, stromal layers, in general, maintain the more primitive progenitors. Stromal layers derived from MSCs have demonstrated the ability to maintain and, indeed, amplify colony-forming cells over a prolonged period of 16 weeks.[86] Early clinical reports suggest that cotransplanting MSCs can enhance HPC engraftment.[6,87]

Genomic Stability

Genomic stability is a major concern for the clinical application of MSCs. As mentioned above, a few publications have indicated spontaneous transformation of culture-expanded MSCs. Karyotype analyses could provide evidence of genetic stability or chromosomal abnormalities.[55,88] In addition, testing for telomerase activity is a simple assay, which could be considered as an additional test.[54] Chromosome loss or gain can be assessed by fluorescence in-situ hybridization and comparative genomic hybridization to further address chromosomal aberrations.[88,89] In general, to alleviate safety concerns, ex-vivo expansion of MSCs should be reduced to the minimum to generate adequate amounts of cells with maintained biologic capacity and genetic stability.

Clinical Potential

MSCs are attractive candidates for cellular therapies because of their qualities mentioned above—in summary:
1. Ease of isolation from a variety of tissues.
2. High expansion capacity with genetic stability in clinical-grade culture.
3. Multi-lineage differentiation potential.
4. Migration to sites of injury upon systemic administration.
   a. Production of trophic factors inducing endogenous repair.
   b. Differentiation into cells of injured tissues.
5. Integration of locally administered (predifferentiated) cells seeded onto scaffolds.
6. Stromal support for hematopoietic stem cells.
7. Immuno-privileged status and immunomodulatory capacities.
8. Transducibility with several vectors, allowing for gene therapy approaches.

Many animal transplantation studies have shown that MSCs are not only able to regenerate mesodermal tissues—such as intervertebral disc cartilage, articular cartilage, bone, myocytes, or cardiomyocytes—but also tissues from different embryonic germ layers, including neurons and epithelia in lung, skin, and intestine.[80,90-97] Beyond regenerative potential, the immune-modulatory capacities have drawn interest, with attention focused on the treatment of immune reactions, whether induced by transplantation-associated graft-vs-host-disease (GVHD) responses or autoimmune diseases.

Enhancement of Hematopoietic Engraftment

Marrow stroma offers an environment supporting hematopoiesis by providing cell-to-cell contacts and growth factors. Thus, several authors have tried to use MSCs to enhance HPC engraftment either by cotransplantation or by ex-vivo coculture to expand HPCs. Early studies testing the effect of cotransplanting MSCs to facilitate HPC transplantation have been carried out and have demonstrated safety and efficacy, initiating further studies.[6,87,98-101] In one early study, 1×10^6 to 50×10^6 autologous MSCs (expanded from 10-20 mL marrow aspirate) were intravenously infused without any toxicity.[102] Despite beneficial clinical effects, there was no evidence of donor chimerism, indicating that donor MSCs did not engraft.[103]

Immunomodulation

The first case report published in 2004 summarizing the effect of MSC-immunosuppressive activities described a boy who had been transplanted with allogeneic HPCs and was suffering from severe and treatment-resistant acute GVHD.[104] After the injection of haploidentical, culture-expanded MSCs from a third-party donor, the clinical symptoms improved rapidly. Additional patients have been treated successfully using either marrow or adipose-tissue–derived MSCs.[105-107] Accordingly, randomized trials have been initiated based on this encouraging initial experience.

In experimental settings, MSCs have been shown to ameliorate autoimmune and inflammatory reactions as well.[91,108,109] Although encouraging data have been published, safety issues are a major concern. MSCs cultured in FBS have been shown to elicit immune responses, at least against the serum component.[61] Furthermore, immune suppressive capacities have been shown to favor the growth of tumors in an animal model.[110]

Vehicles for Gene Therapy

MSCs are attractive targets for gene therapy and have been tested with a variety of vectors.[111] Gene therapy approaches are focused on one of two goals: either to correct inherited diseases or to target diseased, transformed tissues. In the first case, therapeutic genes must be introduced, and in the second case, anti-cancer agents are introduced. Accordingly, MSCs have been transduced with vectors expressing Factor VIII or Factor IX to provide a cure for hemophilic patients, and with bone morphogenetic proteins or collagen 1 in osteogenesis imperfecta (OI).[112-114] Because MSCs have been shown to home and engraft in tumor stroma, MSCs have been engineered to produce interferons.[115,116] Indeed, gene-modified MSCs inhibit metastatic cancer growth, suggesting their clinical potential in this setting as well.[116]

Tissue Regeneration/Tissue Engineering

One of the first examples of the clinical utility of MSCs has been in patients with OI.[5,117-119] In OI, a genetic defect minimizes the production of type I collagen, severely affecting bone stability. OI patients receiving allogeneic marrow transplants improved significantly, as noted by the production of normal collagen type I.[5] An induced acceleration of growth velocity, combined with reduced bone fracture frequencies during the first 6 months after infusion, was observed in another study employing culture-expanded MSCs.[118] MSCs have been transplanted with some clinical benefit in patients with inborn metabolic disorders such as metachromatic leukodystrophy and Hurler syndrome, as MSCs express a number of lysosomal enzymes.[120] In addition, MSCs have been used clinically to accelerate bone and cartilage formation when implanted onto a variety of matrices or engineered to produce growth factors.[7,121-124] In line with the intense research for cellular therapies to treat patients with myocardial infarction, MSCs have been employed here with some success as well. In most cases, volume-reduced mononuclear cells derived from marrow or UCB were used, but in a few cases, culture-expanded MSCs were applied.[125,126] Early clinical data indicate that MSCs, either directly or by inducing an anti-inflammatory milieu, can be used for tissue repair in toxic injury or fistulas in Crohn's disease.[127,128] Clinical results of patients with neurological disorders such as amyotrophic lateral sclerosis or spinal cord injury seem to be encouraging as well.[129-131] In addition, MSC applications to promote wound healing have demonstrated safety and efficacy in published pilot studies.[132,133]

Conclusion

In summary, the safety and, in some preliminary cases, efficacy of MSC-based therapies have been demonstrated. However, controlled trials of sufficient power using standardized production methods and quality control testing under cGMP conditions need to be conducted to further elucidate the potential of MSCs.

References/Resources

1. Caplan AI. Mesenchymal stem cells. J Orthop Res 1991; 9:641-50.
2. Fraser JK, Schreiber R, Strem B, et al. Plasticity of human adipose stem cells toward endothelial cells and cardiomyocytes. Nat Clin Pract Cardiovasc Med 2006;3:S33-7.

3. Liechty KW, Mackenzie TC, Shaaban AF, et al. Human mesenchymal stem cells engraft and demonstrate site-specific differentiation after in utero transplantation in sheep. Nat Med 2000;6:1282-6.

4. Giordano A, Galderisi U, Marino IR. From the laboratory bench to the patient's bedside: An update on clinical trials with mesenchymal stem cells. J Cell Physiol 2007; 211:27-35.

5. Horwitz EM, Prockop DJ, Fitzpatrick LA, et al. Transplantability and therapeutic effects of bone marrow-derived mesenchymal cells in children with osteogenesis imperfecta. Nat Med 1999;5:309-13.

6. Koc ON, Gerson SL, Cooper BW, et al. Rapid hematopoietic recovery after coinfusion of autologous-blood stem cells and culture-expanded marrow mesenchymal stem cells in advanced breast cancer patients receiving high-dose chemotherapy. J Clin Oncol 2000;18:307-16.

7. Carstens MH, Chin M, Ng T, Tom WK. Reconstruction of #7 facial cleft with distraction-assisted in situ osteogenesis (DISO): Role of recombinant human bone morphogenetic protein-2 with Helistat-activated collagen implant. J Craniofac Surg 2005;16:1023-32.

8. Baksh D, Song L, Tuan RS. Adult mesenchymal stem cells: Characterization, differentiation, and application in cell and gene therapy. J Cell Mol Med 2004;8:301-16.

9. Young HE, Mancini ML, Wright RP, et al. Mesenchymal stem cells reside within the connective tissues of many organs. Dev Dyn 1995;202:137-44.

10. da Silva ML, Chagastelles PC, Nardi NB. Mesenchymal stem cells reside in virtually all post-natal organs and tissues. J Cell Sci 2006;119:2204-13.

11. Sudo K, Kanno M, Miharada K, et al. Mesenchymal progenitors able to differentiate into osteogenic, chondrogenic, and/or adipogenic cells in vitro are present in most primary fibroblast-like cell populations. Stem Cells 2007;25:1610-17.

12. Phinney DG. Building a consensus regarding the nature and origin of mesenchymal stem cells. J Cell Biochem Suppl 2002;38:7-12.

13. Takashima Y, Era T, Nakao K, et al. Neuroepithelial cells supply an initial transient wave of MSC differentiation. Cell 2007;129:1377-88.

14. Friedenstein AJ, Gorskaja JF, Kulagina NN. Fibroblast precursors in normal and irradiated mouse hematopoietic organs. Exp Hematol 1976;4:267-74.

15. Krabbe C, Zimmer J, Meyer M. Neural transdifferentiation of mesenchymal stem cells—a critical review. APMIS 2005;113:831-44.

16. Dahlke MH, Popp FC, Larsen S, et al. Stem cell therapy of the liver—fusion or fiction? Liver Transpl 2004;10:471-9.

17. Tondreau T, Meuleman N, Delforge A, et al. Mesenchymal stem cells derived from CD133-positive cells in mobilized peripheral blood and cord blood: Proliferation, Oct4 expression, and plasticity. Stem Cells 2005;23:1105-12.

18. Jones EA, English A, Kinsey SE, et al. Optimization of a flow cytometry-based protocol for detection and phenotypic characterization of multipotent mesenchymal stromal cells from human bone marrow. Cytometry B Clin Cytom 2006;70:391-9.

19. Ebihara Y, Masuya M, Larue AC, et al. Hematopoietic origins of fibroblasts: II. In vitro studies of fibroblasts, CFU-F, and fibrocytes. Exp Hematol 2006;34:219-29.

20. Deschaseaux F, Gindraux F, Saadi R, et al. Direct selection of human bone marrow mesenchymal stem cells using an anti-CD49a antibody reveals their CD45med, low phenotype. Br J Haematol 2003;122:506-17.

21. Haynesworth SE, Baber MA, Caplan AI. Cell surface antigens on human marrow-derived mesenchymal cells are detected by monoclonal antibodies. Bone 1992;13:69-80.

22. Pittenger MF, Mackay AM, Beck SC, et al. Multilineage potential of adult human mesenchymal stem cells. Science 1999;284:143-7.

23. Dominici M, Le Blanc K, Mueller I, et al. Minimal criteria for defining multipotent mesenchymal stromal cells. The International Society for Cellular Therapy position statement. Cytotherapy 2006;8:315-17.

24. Ulloa-Montoya F, Kidder BL, Pauwelyn KA, et al. Comparative transcriptome analysis of embryonic and adult stem cells with extended and limited differentiation capacity. Genome Biol 2007;8:R163.

25. Kogler G, Sensken S, Airey JA, et al. A new human somatic stem cell from placental cord blood with intrinsic pluripotent differentiation potential. J Exp Med 2004;200:123-35.

26. Zipori D. The nature of stem cells: State rather than entity. Nat Rev Genet 2004;5:873-8.

27. Tondreau T, Lagneaux L, Dejeneffe M, et al. Isolation of BM mesenchymal stem cells by plastic adhesion or negative selection: Phenotype, proliferation kinetics and differentiation potential. Cytotherapy 2004;6:372-9.

28. Castro-Malaspina H, Gay RE, Resnick G, et al. Characterization of human bone marrow fibroblast colony-forming cells (CFU-F) and their progeny. Blood 1980;56:289-301.

29. Lennon DP, Haynesworth SE, Bruder SP, et al. Human and animal mesenchymal progenitor cells from bone marrow: Identification of serum for optimal selection and proliferation. In vitro Cell Dev Biol Anim 1996;32:602-11.

30. Lennon DP, Caplan AI. Isolation of human marrow-derived mesenchymal stem cells. Exp Hematol 2006;34:1604-5.

31. Kolf CM, Cho E, Tuan RS. Mesenchymal stromal cells. Biology of adult mesenchymal stem cells: Regulation of niche, self-renewal and differentiation (review). Arthritis Res Ther 2007;9:204.

32. Bartmann C, Rohde E, Schallmoser K, et al. Two steps to functional mesenchymal stromal cells for clinical application. Transfusion 2007;47:1426-35.

33. Lange C, Schroeder J, Stute N, et al. High-potential human mesenchymal stem cells. Stem Cells Dev 2005;14:70-80.

34. Jiang Y, Jahagirdar BN, Reinhardt RL, et al. Pluripotency of mesenchymal stem cells derived from adult marrow. Nature 2002;418:41-9.

35. Simmons PJ, Torok-Storb B. Identification of stromal cell precursors in human bone marrow by a novel monoclonal antibody, STRO-1. Blood 1991;78:55-62.

36. Quirici N, Soligo D, Bossolasco P, et al. Isolation of bone marrow mesenchymal stem cells by anti-nerve growth factor receptor antibodies. Exp Hematol 2002;30:783-91.

37. Aslan H, Zilberman Y, Kandel L, et al. Osteogenic differentiation of noncultured immunoisolated bone marrow-derived CD105+ cells. Stem Cells 2006;24:1728-37.

38. Gang EJ, Bosnakovski D, Figueiredo CA, et al. SSEA-4 identifies mesenchymal stem cells from bone marrow. Blood 2007;109:1743-51.

39. Gentry T, Foster S, Winstead L, et al. Simultaneous isolation of human BM hematopoietic, endothelial and mesenchymal progenitor cells by flow sorting based on aldehyde dehydrogenase activity: Implications for cell therapy. Cytotherapy 2007;9:259-74.

40. Jones EA, Kinsey SE, English A, et al. Isolation and characterization of bone marrow multipotential mesenchymal progenitor cells. Arthritis Rheum 2002;46:3349-60.

41. Gurevich O, Vexler A, Marx G, et al. Fibrin microbeads for isolating and growing bone marrow-derived progenitor cells capable of forming bone tissue. Tissue Eng 2002;8:661-72.

42. Guo KT, Schafer R, Paul A, et al. A new technique for the isolation and surface immobilization of mesenchymal stem cells from whole bone marrow using high-specific DNA aptamers. Stem Cells 2006;24:2220-31.

43. Bieback K, Kern S, Kluter H, Eichler H. Critical parameters for the isolation of mesenchymal stem cells from umbilical cord blood. Stem Cells 2004;22:625-34.

44. Kern S, Eichler H, Stoeve J, et al. Comparative analysis of mesenchymal stem cells from bone marrow, umbilical cord blood, or adipose tissue. Stem Cells 2006;24:1294-301.

45. Erices A, Conget P, Minguell JJ. Mesenchymal progenitor cells in human umbilical cord blood. Br J Haematol 2000;109:235-42.

46. Goodwin HS, Bicknese AR, Chien SN, et al. Multilineage differentiation activity by cells isolated from umbilical cord blood: Expression of bone, fat, and neural markers. Biol Blood Marrow Transplant 2001;7:581-8.

47. Lee OK, Kuo TK, Chen WM, et al. Isolation of multipotent mesenchymal stem cells from umbilical cord blood. Blood 2004;103:1669-75.

48. Parekkadan B, Sethu P, Van Poll D, et al. Osmotic selection of human mesenchymal stem/progenitor cells from umbilical cord blood. Tissue Eng 2007;13:2465-73.

49. Bjorntorp P, Karlsson M, Pertoft H, et al. Isolation and characterization of cells from rat adipose tissue developing into adipocytes. J Lipid Res 1978;19:316-24.

50. Zuk PA, Zhu M, Mizuno H, et al. Multilineage cells from human adipose tissue: Implications for cell-based therapies. Tissue Eng 2001;7:211-28.

51. Sethe S, Scutt A, Stolzing A. Aging of mesenchymal stem cells. Ageing Res Rev 2006;5:91-116.

52. Toyoda M, Takahashi H, Umezawa A. Ways for a mesenchymal stem cell to live on its own: Maintaining an undifferentiated state ex vivo. Int J Hematol 2007;86:1-4.

53. Abdallah BM, Haack-Sorensen M, Burns JS, et al. Maintenance of differentiation potential of human bone marrow mesenchymal stem cells immortalized by human telomerase reverse transcriptase gene despite [corrected] extensive proliferation. Biochem Biophys Res Commun 2005;326:527-38.

54. Rubio D, Garcia-Castro J, Martin MC, et al. Spontaneous human adult stem cell transformation. Cancer Res 2005;65:3035-9.

55. Wang Y, Huso DL, Harrington J, Kellner J, et al. Outgrowth of a transformed cell population derived from normal human BM mesenchymal stem cell culture. Cytotherapy 2005;7:509-19.

56. Riggi N, Cironi L, Provero P, et al. Development of Ewing's sarcoma from primary bone marrow-derived mesenchymal progenitor cells. Cancer Res 2005;65:11459-68.

57. Tolar J, Nauta AJ, Osborn MJ, et al. Sarcoma derived from cultured mesenchymal stem cells. Stem Cells 2007;25:371-9.

58. Colter DC, Class R, DiGirolamo CM, Prockop DJ. Rapid expansion of recycling stem cells in cultures of plastic-adherent cells from human bone marrow. Proc Natl Acad Sci U S A 2000;97:3213-18.

59. Bianchi G, Banfi A, Mastrogiacomo M, et al. Ex vivo enrichment of mesenchymal cell progenitors by fibroblast growth factor 2. Exp Cell Res 2003;287:98-105.

60. Spees JL, Gregory CA, Singh H, et al. Internalized antigens must be removed to prepare hypoimmunogenic mesenchymal stem cells for cell and gene therapy. Mol Ther 2004;9:747-56.

61. Sundin M, Ringden O, Sundberg B, et al. No alloantibodies against mesenchymal stromal cells, but presence of anti-fetal calf serum antibodies after transplantation in allogeneic hematopoietic stem cell recipients. Haematologica 2007;92:1208-15.

62. Halme DG, Kessler DA. FDA regulation of stem-cell-based therapies. N Engl J Med 2006;355:1730-5.

63. Mannello F, Tonti GA. Concise review: No breakthroughs for human mesenchymal and embryonic stem cell culture: conditioned medium, feeder layer, or feeder-free; medium with fetal calf serum, human serum, or enriched plasma; serum-free, serum replacement nonconditioned medium, or ad hoc formula? All that glitters is not gold! Stem Cells 2007;25:1603-9.

64. Doucet C, Ernou I, Zhang Y, et al. Platelet lysates promote mesenchymal stem cell expansion: A safety substitute for animal serum in cell-based therapy applications. J Cell Physiol 2005;205:228-36.

65. Kocaoemer A, Kern S, Kluter H, Bieback K. Human AB serum and thrombin-activated platelet-rich plasma are suitable alternatives to fetal calf serum for the expansion of mesenchymal stem cells from adipose tissue. Stem Cells 2007;25:1270-8.

66. Sensebe L, Bourin P, Douay L. Good manufacturing practices: Clinical-scale production of mesenchymal stem cells. In: Ho A, Hoffmann R, Zanjani E, eds. Stem cell transplantation: Biology, processing, and therapy.

Weinheim, Germany: Wiley-VCH Verlag GmbH and Co KgaA, 2006:91-105.

67. Friedenstein AJ. Stromal mechanisms of bone marrow: Cloning in vitro and retransplantation in vivo. Haematol Blood Transfus 1980;25:19-29.

68. Pochampally RR, Smith JR, Ylostalo J, Prockop DJ. Serum deprivation of human marrow stromal cells (hMSCs) selects for a subpopulation of early progenitor cells with enhanced expression of OCT-4 and other embryonic genes. Blood 2004;103:1647-52.

69. Majumdar MK, Thiede MA, Mosca JD, et al. Phenotypic and functional comparison of cultures of marrow-derived mesenchymal stem cells (MSCs) and stromal cells. J Cell Physiol 1998;176:57-66.

70. Gronthos S, Franklin DM, Leddy HA, et al. Surface protein characterization of human adipose tissue-derived stromal cells. J Cell Physiol 2001;189:54-63.

71. Marie PJ, Fromigue O. Osteogenic differentiation of human marrow-derived mesenchymal stem cells. Regen Med 2006;1:539-48.

72. Kratchmarova I, Blagoev B, Haack-Sorensen M, et al. Mechanism of divergent growth factor effects in mesenchymal stem cell differentiation. Science 2005;308:1472-7.

73. Djouad F, Mrugala D, Noel D, Jorgensen C. Engineered mesenchymal stem cells for cartilage repair. Regen Med 2006;1:529-37.

74. Guilak F, Awad HA, Fermor B, et al. Adipose-derived adult stem cells for cartilage tissue engineering. Biorheology 2004;41:389-99.

75. Gimble JM, Zvonic S, Floyd ZE, et al. Playing with bone and fat. J Cell Biochem 2006;98:251-66.

76. Bianco P, Robey PG. Stem cells in tissue engineering. Nature 2001;414:118-21.

77. Muraglia A, Cancedda R, Quarto R. Clonal mesenchymal progenitors from human bone marrow differentiate in vitro according to a hierarchical model. J Cell Sci 2000;113:1161-6.

78. Chan J, O'Donoghue K, Gavina M, et al. Galectin-1 induces skeletal muscle differentiation in human fetal mesenchymal stem cells and increases muscle regeneration. Stem Cells 2006;24:1879-91.

79. Behfar A, Terzic A. Derivation of a cardiopoietic population from human mesenchymal stem cells yields cardiac progeny. Nat Clin Pract Cardiovasc Med 2006;3:S78-82.

80. Zhao LR, Duan WM, Reyes M, et al. Human bone marrow stem cells exhibit neural phenotypes and ameliorate neurological deficits after grafting into the ischemic brain of rats. Exp Neurol 2002;174:11-20.

81. Son BR, Marquez-Curtis LA, Kucia M, et al. Migration of bone marrow and cord blood mesenchymal stem cells in vitro is regulated by stromal-derived factor-1-CXCR4 and hepatocyte growth factor-c-met axes and involves matrix metalloproteinases. Stem Cells 2006;24:1254-64.

82. Chamberlain G, Fox J, Ashton B, Middleton J. Concise review: Mesenchymal stem cells: Their phenotype, differentiation capacity, immunological features and potential for homing. Stem Cells 2007;25:2739-49.

83. Tyndall A, Walker UA, Cope A, et al. Immunomodulatory properties of mesenchymal stem cells: A review based on an interdisciplinary meeting held at the Kennedy Institute of Rheumatology Division, London, UK, 31 October 2005. Arthritis Res Ther 2007;9:301.

84. Le Blanc K, Tammik L, Sundberg B, et al. Mesenchymal stem cells inhibit and stimulate mixed lymphocyte cultures and mitogenic responses independently of the major histocompatibility complex. Scand J Immunol 2003;57:11-20.

85. Kilroy GE, Foster SJ, Wu X, et al. Cytokine profile of human adipose-derived stem cells: Expression of angiogenic, hematopoietic, and pro-inflammatory factors. J Cell Physiol 2007;212:702-9.

86. Robinson SN, Ng J, Niu T, et al. Superior ex vivo cord blood expansion following co-culture with bone marrow-derived mesenchymal stem cells. Bone Marrow Transplant 2006;37:359-66.

87. Lazarus HM, Koc ON, Devine SM, et al. Cotransplantation of HLA-identical sibling culture-expanded mesenchymal stem cells and hematopoietic stem cells in hematologic malignancy patients. Biol Blood Marrow Transplant 2005;11:389-98.

88. Bernardo ME, Avanzini MA, Perotti C, et al. Optimization of in vitro expansion of human multipotent mesenchymal stromal cells for cell-therapy approaches: Further insights in the search for a fetal calf serum substitute. J Cell Physiol 2007;211:121-30.

89. Takeuchi M, Takeuchi K, Kohara A, et al. Chromosomal instability in human mesenchymal stem cells immortalized with human papilloma virus E6, E7, and hTERT genes. In Vitro Cell Dev Biol Anim 2007;43:129-38.

90. Steck E, Bertram H, Abel R, et al. Induction of intervertebral disc-like cells from adult mesenchymal stem cells. Stem Cells 2005;23:403-11.

91. Augello A, Tasso R, Negrini SM, et al. Cell therapy using allogeneic bone marrow mesenchymal stem cells prevents tissue damage in collagen-induced arthritis. Arthritis Rheum 2007;56:1175-86.

92. Jager M, Degistirici O, Knipper A, et al. Bone healing and migration of cord blood-derived stem cells into a critical size femoral defect after xenotransplantation. J Bone Miner Res 2007;22:1224-33.

93. Gang EJ, Jeong JA, Hong SH, et al. Skeletal myogenic differentiation of mesenchymal stem cells isolated from human umbilical cord blood. Stem Cells 2004;22:617-24.

94. Strem BM, Zhu M, Alfonso Z, et al. Expression of cardiomyocytic markers on adipose tissue-derived cells in a murine model of acute myocardial injury. Cytotherapy 2005;7:282-91.

95. Dai Y, Li J, Li J, et al. Skin epithelial cells in mice from umbilical cord blood mesenchymal stem cells. Burns 2007;33:418-28.

96. Ortiz LA, Gambelli F, McBride C, et al. Mesenchymal stem cell engraftment in lung is enhanced in response to bleomycin exposure and ameliorates its fibrotic effects. Proc Natl Acad Sci U S A 2003;100:8407-11.

97. Komori M, Tsuji S, Tsujii M, et al. Efficiency of bone marrow-derived cells in regeneration of the stomach

after induction of ethanol-induced ulcers in rats. J Gastroenterol 2005;40:591-9.

98. Kim DW, Chung YJ, Kim TG, et al. Cotransplantation of third-party mesenchymal stromal cells can alleviate single-donor predominance and increase engraftment from double cord transplantation. Blood 2004;103:1941-8.

99. Le Blanc K, Samuelsson H, Gustafsson B, et al. Transplantation of mesenchymal stem cells to enhance engraftment of hematopoietic stem cells. Leukemia 2007; 21:1733-8.

100. Ball LM, Bernardo ME, Roelofs H, et al. Cotransplantation of ex vivo expanded mesenchymal stem cells accelerates lymphocyte recovery and may reduce the risk of graft failure in haploidentical hematopoietic stem cell transplantation. Blood 2007;110:2764-7.

101. Lee ST, Jang JH, Cheong JW, et al. Treatment of high-risk acute myelogenous leukaemia by myeloablative chemoradiotherapy followed by co-infusion of T cell-depleted haematopoietic stem cells and culture-expanded marrow mesenchymal stem cells from a related donor with one fully mismatched human leucocyte antigen haplotype. Br J Haematol 2002;118:1128-31.

102. Lazarus HM, Haynesworth SE, Gerson SL, et al. Ex vivo expansion and subsequent infusion of human bone marrow-derived stromal progenitor cells (mesenchymal progenitor cells): Implications for therapeutic use. Bone Marrow Transplant 1995;16:557-64.

103. Koc ON, Peters C, Aubourg P, et al. Bone marrow-derived mesenchymal stem cells remain host-derived despite successful hematopoietic engraftment after allogeneic transplantation in patients with lysosomal and peroxisomal storage diseases. Exp Hematol 1999;27:1675-81.

104. Le Blanc K, Rasmusson I, Sundberg B, et al. Treatment of severe acute graft-versus-host disease with third party haploidentical mesenchymal stem cells. Lancet 2004;363:1439-41.

105. Le Blanc K, Ringden O. Use of mesenchymal stem cells for the prevention of immune complications of hematopoietic stem cell transplantation (comment). Haematologica 2005;90:438.

106. Ringden O, Uzunel M, Rasmusson I, et al. Mesenchymal stem cells for treatment of therapy-resistant graft-versus-host disease. Transplantation 2006;81:1390-7.

107. Fang B, Song YP, Liao LM, et al. Treatment of severe therapy-resistant acute graft-versus-host disease with human adipose tissue-derived mesenchymal stem cells. Bone Marrow Transplant 2006;38:389-90.

108. Gerdoni E, Gallo B, Casazza S, et al. Mesenchymal stem cells effectively modulate pathogenic immune response in experimental autoimmune encephalomyelitis. Ann Neurol 2007;61:219-27.

109. Zappia E, Casazza S, Pedemonte E, et al. Mesenchymal stem cells ameliorate experimental autoimmune encephalomyelitis inducing T-cell anergy. Blood 2005;106:1755-61.

110. Djouad F, Plence P, Bony C, et al. Immunosuppressive effect of mesenchymal stem cells favors tumor growth in allogeneic animals. Blood 2003;102:3837-44.

111. Van Damme A, Vanden Driessche T, Collen D, Chuah MK. Bone marrow stromal cells as targets for gene therapy. Curr Gene Ther 2002;2:195-209.

112. Krebsbach PH, Zhang K, Malik AK, Kurachi K. Bone marrow stromal cells as a genetic platform for systemic delivery of therapeutic proteins in vivo: Human factor IX model. J Gene Med 2003;5:11-17.

113. Egermann M, Lill CA, Griesbeck K, et al. Effect of BMP-2 gene transfer on bone healing in sheep. Gene Ther 2006;13:1290-9.

114. Pochampally RR, Horwitz EM, DiGirolamo CM, et al. Correction of a mineralization defect by overexpression of a wild-type cDNA for COL1A1 in marrow stromal cells (MSCs) from a patient with osteogenesis imperfecta: A strategy for rescuing mutations that produce dominant-negative protein defects. Gene Ther 2005;12:1119-25.

115. Nakamizo A, Marini F, Amano T, et al. Human bone marrow-derived mesenchymal stem cells in the treatment of gliomas. Cancer Res 2005;65:3307-18.

116. Studeny M, Marini FC, Dembinski JL, et al. Mesenchymal stem cells: Potential precursors for tumor stroma and targeted-delivery vehicles for anticancer agents. J Natl Cancer Inst 2004;96:1593-603.

117. Horwitz EM, Prockop DJ, Gordon PL, et al. Clinical responses to bone marrow transplantation in children with severe osteogenesis imperfecta. Blood 2001;97:1227-31.

118. Horwitz EM, Gordon PL, Koo WK, et al. Isolated allogeneic bone marrow-derived mesenchymal cells engraft and stimulate growth in children with osteogenesis imperfecta: Implications for cell therapy of bone. Proc Natl Acad Sci U S A 2002;99:8932-7.

119. Le Blanc K, Gotherstrom C, Ringden O, et al. Fetal mesenchymal stem-cell engraftment in bone after in utero transplantation in a patient with severe osteogenesis imperfecta. Transplantation 2005;79:1607-14.

120. Koc ON, Day J, Nieder M, et al. Allogeneic mesenchymal stem cell infusion for treatment of metachromatic leukodystrophy (MLD) and Hurler syndrome (MPS-IH). Bone Marrow Transplant 2002;30:215-22.

121. Tilley S, Bolland BJ, Partridge K, et al. Taking tissue-engineering principles into theater: Augmentation of impacted allograft with human bone marrow stromal cells. Regen Med 2006;1:685-92.

122. Kuroda R, Ishida K, Matsumoto T, et al. Treatment of a full-thickness articular cartilage defect in the femoral condyle of an athlete with autologous bone-marrow stromal cells. Osteoarthritis Cartil 2007;15:226-31.

123. Yamada Y, Ueda M, Hibi H, Baba S. A novel approach to periodontal tissue regeneration with mesenchymal stem cells and platelet-rich plasma using tissue engineering technology: A clinical case report. Int J Periodontics Restorative Dent 2006;26:363-9.

124. Marcacci M, Kon E, Moukhachev V, et al. Stem cells associated with macroporous bioceramics for long bone repair: 6- to 7-year outcome of a pilot clinical study. Tissue Eng 2007;13:947-55.

125. Chen SL, Fang WW, Ye F, et al. Effect on left ventricular function of intracoronary transplantation of autologous bone marrow mesenchymal stem cell in patients with acute myocardial infarction. Am J Cardiol 2004;94:92-5.

126. No authors listed. A randomized, double-blind, placebo-controlled, dose-escalation study of intravenous adult human mesenchymal stem cells (provacel) following acute myocardial infarction (AMI) (abstract). Clin Cardiol 2007;30:364.

127. Ringdén O, Uzunel M, Sundberg B, et al. Tissue repair using allogeneic mesenchymal stem cells for hemorrhagic cystitis, pneumomediastinum and perforated colon. Leukemia 2007;21:2271-6.

128. Garcia-Olmo D, Garcia-Arranz M, Herreros D, et al. A phase I clinical trial of the treatment of Crohn's fistula by adipose mesenchymal stem cell transplantation. Dis Colon Rectum 2005;48:1416-23.

129. Kang KS, Kim SW, Oh YH, et al. A 37-year-old spinal cord-injured female patient, transplanted of multipotent stem cells from human UC blood, with improved sensory perception and mobility, both functionally and morphologically: A case study. Cytotherapy 2005;7:368-73.

130. Mazzini L, Mareschi K, Ferrero I, et al. Autologous mesenchymal stem cells: Clinical applications in amyotrophic lateral sclerosis. Neurol Res 2006;28:523-6.

131. Moviglia GA, Fernandez VR, Brizuela JA, et al. Combined protocol of cell therapy for chronic spinal cord injury. Report on the electrical and functional recovery of two patients. Cytotherapy 2006;8:202-9.

132. Bystrov AV, Polyaev YA, Pogodina MA, et al. Use of autologous bone marrow mesenchymal stem cells for healing of free full-thickness skin graft in a zone with pronounced hypoperfusion of soft tissues caused by arteriovenous shunting. Bull Exp Biol Med 2006;142:123-8.

133. Falanga V, Iwamoto S, Chartier M, et al. Autologous bone marrow-derived cultured mesenchymal stem cells delivered in a fibrin spray accelerate healing in murine and human cutaneous wounds. Tissue Eng 2007;13:1299-312.

Method 38-1. Isolating and Characterizing Mesenchymal Stem or Stromal Cells from Marrow

Description

A small volume of marrow (2-20 mL) is aspirated and processed to obtain mononuclear cells (MNCs). The cells are passaged and subjected to in-vitro characterization by expansion culture, flow cytometric analysis, and differentiation assays.

Note: The procedures in this chapter reflect standardized protocols performed in the authors' research laboratory and do not represent protocols designed for clinical manufacturing. All donors provided informed consent before cells or tissue were procured. Various modifications are possible, including avoiding use of media containing xenogeneic supplements.

Time for Procedure

1. Aspiration: 1 hour.
2. Isolation: 1 to 3 hours.
3. Primary culture: up to 14 days.
4. In-vitro characterization: up to 8 weeks.

Summary of Procedure

1. Marrow aspirate within a syringe containing heparin is transported to the processing laboratory and processed within a Class II biological safety cabinet (BSC).
2. The marrow aspirate is mixed with a complete culture medium and transferred into a tissue culture (TC)-treated flask.
3. MNCs are isolated by Ficoll gradient density centrifugation and transferred into a TC-treated flask.
4. Nonadherent cells are discarded on the following day.
5. A complete change of medium is performed twice a week.
6. Passaging of primary cells is performed once they reach approximately 60% to 70% confluency.

7. Characterization of culture-expanded cells is performed by flow cytometry and differentiation assays.

Equipment

1. BSC Class II.
2. Centrifuge.
3. CO_2 incubator.
4. Phase-contrast microscope.
5. Automatic cell counter.
6. Neubauer chamber for cell counting.
7. Flow cytometer.

Supplies and Reagents

1. 15-mL and 50-mL polypropylene tubes.
2. TC-treated flasks [eg, Nunclon Cell Factory (Thermo Fisher Scientific, Rochester, NY)].
3. Pasteur pipette.
4. Ficoll (GE Healthcare, Chalfont St Giles, United Kingdom) density gradient medium.
5. Phosphate-buffered saline (PBS).
6. PBS/EDTA.
7. Methanol.
8. Giemsa staining solution.
9. Complete medium: Dulbecco's modified eagle medium (DMEM)—low glucose, 10% fetal bovine serum (FBS), L-glutamine, antibiotics.
10. Trypsin/EDTA.
11. Adipogenic differentiation media and detection reagents.
12. Chondrogenic differentiation media and detection reagents.
13. Osteogenic differentiation media and detection reagents.
14. Flow cytometry reagents.

Procedure

A. *Mesenchymal Stromal Cell (MSC) Isolation*
   1. Place a small volume (100-200 μL) or $1 \times 10^5 - 5 \times 10^5$ MNCs/cm² of unprocessed

marrow into a TC-treated flask in complete medium after having removed a small aliquot for cell counting.

2. Discard the nonadherent cells after 3 days of incubation and add fresh complete medium every 3 to 4 days.

3. Examine culture for individual adherent fibroblastoid cells by phase-contrast microscopy after 3 to 5 days.

4. Passage cells after 10 to 14 days in primary culture when they have reached 60% to 70% confluency.

Alternative:

1. Eject the marrow sample from the syringe into a 50-mL polypropylene tube.

2. Remove a small aliquot for cell counting and for sterility testing.

3. Add an equal volume of PBS/EDTA to the marrow.

4. Dispense 10 mL of Ficoll into a 50-mL polypropylene tube and carefully layer 25 mL of diluted marrow aspirate on top.

5. Centrifuge 30 minutes at 430 *g*.

6. Carefully harvest the buffy coat interface using a Pasteur pipette, place the buffy coat interface into a new 50-mL polypropylene tube, and fill the tube with PBS/EDTA.

7. Centrifuge 10 minutes at 430 *g*.

8. Wash the buffy coat with PBS/EDTA 2 to 3 times until the supernatant is clear.

9. Suspend the pellet in 10 mL complete medium and remove a small aliquot for cell counting.

10. Add 1 to 5×10^5 of MNCs/cm^2 into a TC-treated flask in complete medium.

11. Discard the nonadherent cells after 3 days of incubation and add fresh complete medium every 3 to 4 days.

12. Examine culture for individual adherent fibroblastoid cells by phase-contrast microscopy after 3 to 5 days.

13. Passage cells after 10 to 14 days in primary culture, when they have reached 60% to 70% confluency.

B. *Passaging*

1. Discard the used culture medium completely.

2. Rinse the cell layer once with prewarmed PBS.

3. Add trypsin/EDTA to completely wet the monolayer and incubate at 37 C for 5 minutes.

4. Add complete medium to neutralize the trypsin and remove a small aliquot for cell counting.

5. Replate the cells as passage +1 cells at 200 cells/cm^2 in complete medium.

C. *Cryopreservation*

1. Store early-passage cells for further analyses in the vapor phase of liquid nitrogen (LN$_2$). Individual protocols should be developed, but 1×10^6 MSCs are often frozen in complete medium containing 10% dimethyl sulfoxide (DMSO).

   a. Mix cells with the cryoprotectant medium.

   b. Equilibrate cells for a few minutes.

   c. Transfer cells into a freezing container that allows for a 1-C/minute cooling rate.

2. For long-term storage, transfer cells to LN$_2$ containers and store in the vapor phase.

D. *Quality Control*

1. CFU-F assay: The CFU-F assay can be performed with primary and all subsequent cultures to assess precursor frequency.

   a. Plate primary MNCs as replicates at serial dilutions (eg, 5×10^6, 1×10^6, 2×10^5, to be optimized according to the individual conditions) into six-well plates or T25 TC-treated flasks in complete medium and incubate for 14 days.

   b. Stain by removing medium, fixing the monolayer with methanol (5 minutes at room temperature), and then staining with Giemsa solution.

   c. Enumerate CFU-F colonies macroscopically.

   d. Ensure that there is a linear relationship between the colony number and the dilution step.

2. After the primary culture, seeding concentrations may need to be adapted.

a. Morphology and phenotype:
   - Cultures should be continuously monitored to check phenotypic alterations or contaminants.
   - MSCs appear as spindle-shaped fibroblastoid cells.
   - As MSCs reach a senescent stage, their shape becomes flatter, with the occurrence of stress fibers.
b. Self-renewal: Cell counting and viability testing are performed with each subculture.
   - To calculate fold expansion of cells, the total number of cells at different time points is divided by the number of cells used to initiate each culture.
   - To calculate cumulative population doublings, the population doubling rate is determined at each passage by using the following formula:
     $X = [\log10(N_H) - \log10(N_1)]/\log10(2)$ where N_1 is the plated cell number and N_H is the cell number at harvest.
c. Flow cytometry: Both at early and at late passages, the immune phenotype should be addressed. At subculture, about 10^5 MSCs per flow cytometry tube are stained with the appropriate antibodies to detect the MSC phenotype as well as possible contamination with hematopoietic cells.
d. Differentiation assays: At early passages, the differentiation potential of each culture is evaluated.

- The appropriate number of MSCs is seeded into well plates or chamber slides in complete medium.
- Upon reaching a subconfluent (osteogenesis) or postconfluent (adipogenesis) stage, half of the cultures are subjected to the inducing conditions.
- The other half of the cultures is maintained in complete medium to serve as a negative control.
- After three weeks with biweekly change of medium, the cultures are stained using appropriate protocols to detect osteogenic differentiation (eg, van Kossa stain) or adipogenic differentiation (eg, oil-red-o stain).
- For chondrogenic differentiation, cells are centrifuged and incubated as a pellet in chondrogenic supplements. For control, a pellet can be maintained in complete medium.
- After 3 to 4 weeks, cryosections can be stained with safranin-o.

3. Further assays can be performed for quality control of MSCs. In-process, sterility controls are recommended, including mycoplasma testing. It has recently become more common to perform karyotype analyses to check for chromosomal abnormalities. Depending on the final goal, some groups address the immunomodulatory capacities or test differentiation into other lineages.

Method 38-2. Isolating and Characterizing Mesenchymal Stem or Stromal Cells from Cord Blood

Description

Umbilical cord blood (UCB) is collected into a sterile bag containing citrate-phosphate-dextrose (CPD) anticoagulant. The UCB is processed to obtain mononuclear cells (MNCs), which are cultured, harvested, and characterized.

Note: The procedures in this chapter reflect standardized protocols performed in the authors' research laboratory and do not represent protocols designed for clinical manufacturing. All donors provided informed consent before cells or tissue were procured. Various modifications are possible, including avoiding use of media containing xenogeneic supplements.

Time for Procedure

1. UCB harvest: up to 30 minutes.
2. Isolation: 1 to 3 hours.
3. Primary culture: up to 4 weeks.
4. In-vitro characterization: up to 8 weeks.

Summary of Procedure

1. UCB is collected into a bag containing CPD anticoagulant.
2. The UCB is then transported to the processing laboratory and processed within a biological safety cabinet (BSC).
3. MNCs are isolated by Ficoll (GE Healthcare, Chalfont St Giles, United Kingdom) density gradient centrifugation and transferred to a tissue culture (TC)-treated flask.
4. After 1 day of culture, nonadherent cells are discarded.
5. The medium is changed completely twice a week.
6. Primary cells are passaged once they approximate 60% to 70% confluency.
7. Culture-expanded cells are characterized by flow cytometry and differentiation assays.

Equipment

1. UCB collection bag containing CPD.
2. Class II BSC.
3. Centrifuge.
4. CO_2 incubator.
5. Phase-contrast microscope.
6. Equipment for manual or automated cell counting.
7. Flow cytometer.

Supplies and Reagents

1. 15-mL and 50-mL polypropylene tubes.
2. TC-treated flasks.
3. Pasteur pipette.
4. Ficoll.
5. Phosphate-buffered saline (PBS)/EDTA.
6. Pure fetal bovine serum (FBS).
7. FBS-precoated plastic flask for primary culture to improve adherence kinetics of myeloid cells:
   a. Add a volume of FBS sufficient to wet the whole bottom of the culture flask.
   b. Incubate the flask for 30 minutes.
   c. Remove all FBS.
8. Complete medium: Dulbecco's modified eagle medium (DMEM)—low glucose, 10% FBS, antibiotics, L-glutamine.
9. Trypsin/EDTA.
10. Flow cytometry reagents.

Procedure

A.   UCB Collection
(As described previously; see Chapter 24 describing UCB collection techniques for details.)

B.   Mesenchymal Stromal Cell (MSC) Isolation
   1. Using a syringe, transfer 25 mL of UCB from the collection bag to a 50-mL polypropylene tube.
   2. Add 25 mL of PBS/EDTA.

3. Remove a small aliquot for cell counting.
4. Remove a small aliquot for sterility testing.
5. Add 10 mL of Ficoll into a 50-mL polypropylene tube and carefully layer 25 mL of diluted UCB on top.
6. Centrifuge 30 minutes at 430 *g*.
7. Using a Pasteur pipette, carefully transfer the buffy coat interface into a new 50-mL polypropylene tube, and fill the tube with PBS/EDTA.
8. Centrifuge 10 minutes at 430 *g*.
9. Wash with PBS/EDTA two to three times until the supernatant is clear.
10. Suspend the pellet in 10 mL complete medium and remove a small aliquot for cell counting.
11. Transfer all MNCs into a T225-cm^2 FBS-precoated, cell-culture-treated, plastic flask in complete medium.
12. Discard the nonadherent cells after 1 to 3 days of incubation, and add fresh complete medium every 3 to 4 days.
13. Examine culture for presence of individual adherent fibroblastoid cells by phase-contrast microscopy after 14 to 30 days. Passage cells when they have reached 60% to 70% confluency in primary culture.
14. If no colonies of fibroblastoid cells appear within 4 to 6 weeks, discard the culture.

C. *Passaging*
   1. Discard the used culture medium.
   2. Rinse the cell layer once with prewarmed PBS.
   3. Add trypsin/EDTA to completely wet the monolayer and incubate at 37 C for 5 minutes.
   4. Add complete medium to neutralize the trypsin and remove a small aliquot of the cell suspension for cell counting.
   5. Replate cells as in passage #1: 700-1000 cells/cm^2 in complete medium.

Method 38-3. Isolating and Characterizing Mesenchymal Stem or Stromal Cells from Adipose Tissue

Description

Adipose tissue contains mature adipocytes as well as stromal vascular components, including mesenchymal stromal cells (MSCs) from adipose tissue. The tissue is washed and digested, after which time the resulting cells are separated by centrifugation. The pelleted cells are cultured overnight and washed, and the remaining adherent cells passaged upon reaching a subconfluent stage. The adipose tissue MSCs are then characterized using the techniques described for marrow MSCs (Method 38-1).

Note: The procedures in this chapter reflect standardized protocols performed in the authors' research laboratory and do not represent protocols designed for clinical manufacturing. All donors provided informed consent before cells or tissue were procured. Various modifications are possible, including avoiding use of media containing xenogeneic supplements.

Time for Procedure

1. Isolation: 3 to 5 hours.
2. Primary culture: up to 14 days.
3. In-vitro characterization: up to 8 weeks.

Summary of Procedure

1. Lipoaspiration is performed by the appropriate technique, and the lipoaspirate is transported to the processing laboratory and processed within a biological safety cabinet (BSC).
2. The lipoaspirate is rigorously washed and digested with collagenase for 30 minutes at 37 C with gentle agitation.
3. The cell suspension is centrifuged to separate mature adipocytes (supernatant) and stromal vascular fraction cells (pellet).
4. The pellet is resuspended in complete medium and cultured overnight in a tissue culture (TC)-treated flask.
5. Primary cells are passaged once they approximate 60% to 70% confluency.
6. Culture-expanded cells are characterized by flow cytometry and differentiation assays.

Equipment

1. Class II BSC.
2. Centrifuge.
3. CO_2 incubator.
4. Phase-contrast microscope.
5. Cell-counting equipment.
6. Flow cytometer.

Supplies and Reagents

1. 15-mL and 50-mL polypropylene tubes.
2. TC-treated flasks.
3. Sterile phosphate-buffered saline (PBS).
4. Collagenase type 1: 0.075% in PBS.
5. Complete medium: Dulbecco's modified eagle medium (DMEM)—low glucose, 10% FBS, L-glutamine, antibiotics.
6. Trypsin/EDTA.
7. Flow cytometry reagents.

Procedure

1. Transfer 25 mL of lipoaspirate tissue to a 50-mL polypropylene tube.
2. Add 25 mL of sterile PBS.
3. Centrifuge 10 minutes at 430 *g*.
4. Repeat the washing step until cellular debris and erythrocytes are removed.
5. With gentle agitation, digest washed lipoaspirates with 0.075% collagenase for 30 minutes at 37 C.
6. Inactivate the collagenase with an equal volume of DMEM/10% FBS.
7. Centrifuge at 1200 *g* for 10 minutes to obtain the stromal vascular fraction as a pellet.
8. Suspend the pellet in 10 mL complete medium, and filter it through a 100-μm nylon mesh filter to remove cellular debris.

9. Centrifuge at 1200 *g* for 10 minutes.
10. Resuspend cells in complete medium and transfer them into a TC-treated flask.
11. After overnight culture, discard the nonadherent cells by extensive washing.
12. Incubate the remaining adherent cells, and add fresh complete medium every 3 to 4 days.
13. Examine individual adherent fibroblastoid cells by phase-contrast microscopy after 3 to 5 days.
14. Passage cells after 10 to 14 days in primary culture when they have reached 60% to 70% confluency.

In: Areman EM, Loper K, eds
Cellular Therapy: Principles, Methods, and Regulations
Bethesda, MD: AABB, 2009

◆◆◆ **39** ◆◆◆

Generation and Characterization of Human Dendritic Cells for Therapy

Theresa L. Whiteside, PhD

ACTIVE IMMUNOTHERAPY WITH EX-VIVO-manipulated dendritic cells (DCs) has been widely used in a variety of human diseases. However, the generation of therapeutic DC products remains a challenge, and the quality of such products is often not uniform.

Description

DCs are antigen-presenting cells (APCs) that recognize, process, and present foreign antigens to T cells, a process that represents an effector arm of the immune system.[1] Immature DCs (iDCs) are responsible for the capture and internalization of antigens via receptor- and nonreceptor-mediated mechanisms, and mature DCs (mDCs) have the task of antigen presentation to T cells.[2,3] To date, two peripheral blood subsets of DCs have been described that are distinguishable by their ability to express CD11c: The CD11c+ subset represents myeloid-derived DCs (type 1 DCs or DC1), whereas the CD11c– DCs, which express high levels of CD123 [interleukin-3 (IL-3) receptor], are known as lymphoid-derived DCs (type 2 DCs or DC2).[1] DC1 prime Th1 responses, whereas DC2 support the development of Th2 immune responses.[1] DCs currently used for vaccine-based therapies are myeloid-derived cells that are obtained in large numbers from cultures of peripheral blood monocytes or marrow progenitors (CD34+) in the presence of such cytokines as IL-4 and granulocyte/macrophage colony-stimulating factor (GM-CSF).

Antigen processing and presentation to cognate T cells are the main functions of DCs. Antigens taken up by iDCs are first processed in the endoplasmic reticulum. A complex array of intracellular molecules, called antigen-processing machinery (APM) components, reduces the internalized antigens to peptides that are subsequently loaded into the HLA molecules and expressed on the DC surface as a trimolecular complex of the peptide/major histocompatibility complex (MHC) Class I heavy chain/$\beta2$ microglobulin.[4] These complexes are recognized by peptide-specific T cells, which need to

---

Theresa L. Whiteside, PhD, Professor of Pathology, Immunology, and Otolaryngology, and Director, Immunologic Monitoring and Cellular Products Laboratory, Hillman Cancer Center, Pittsburgh, Pennsylvania

The author has disclosed no conflicts of interest.

receive T-cell receptor (TCR)-mediated (signal 1), costimulatory (signal 2), and cytokine-mediated (signal 3) activation stimuli to initiate an effective immune response.[5] Through their ability to deliver all three signals to cognate T cells, DCs can prime as well as induce memory responses.[1-3] This unique ability of DCs is harnessed in antitumor vaccines, which use ex-vivo-cultured autologous DCs to stimulate tumor-specific response in immunized subjects.[2-3]

Different culture methods for therapeutic-grade DCs have been introduced, and there is no standardized process that is currently applied.[6] Production methods vary from manual techniques to semiautomated functionally closed systems for monocyte isolation, cell culture, and final product formulation. The DC phenotype and function are manipulated in vitro by the use of cytokines for DC culture and maturation. It is possible to generate low- or high-stimulatory and tolerogenic DCs, depending on the growth and maturation conditions used. Therefore, the quality of antigen-loaded DCs has to be carefully assessed before the product is released for clinical use. However, a substantial patient-to-patient variability in starting material makes it difficult to ensure batch uniformity and functional consistency. Because the production process is long and complex, procedural or technical differences between facilities are likely to further decrease product consistency. For these reasons, a central manufacturing site for DC production is more likely to provide optimal quality final products.[6]

To date, the methodology for culture and characterization of therapeutic DCs has not been standardized and continues to evolve. The method of generating DCs from monocytes, which are obtained from leukapheresis products, is the least invasive and most widely used today. One such procedure is described in Method 39-1. It results in DC purity in the range of 50% to 95%. The procedure consists of several steps, as follows:

1. Isolation of peripheral blood monocytes from a leukapheresis product by elutriation.
2. Culture of monocytes in the presence of cytokines to generate iDCs.
3. Maturation of iDCs in a cytokine cocktail to yield mDCs.
4. Pulsing or loading of mDCs with peptides.

5. Characterization of the DC-based product and its release for therapy.

Summary of Procedure

DC generation from monocytes requires prolonged incubation with cytokines.[7] The length, complexity, and variations in the DC generation process among different manufacturing facilities create a valid concern about the quality and consistency of the final product. DC characteristics, and presumably their in-vivo performance, can be affected by differences in a manufacturing process. For example, the generation of stimulatory DCs vis-a-vis tolerogenic DCs is determined by cytokines used in culture media and/or different amounts of time in culture.[8] Culture of monocytes in flasks vs Aastrom cartridges (Aastrom Biosciences, Ann Arbor, MI) will necessitate different methods of harvest that might influence DC functionally. Maturation of DCs in different cytokine cocktails and the length of the maturation period will tend to alter DC activation. The antigen loading process, which is critically dependent on the type of the antigen payload, is a very important step that will likely determine DC performance in vivo. The number of vaccines to be made from one lot of DCs will also be an important variable in the process. Thus, several critical steps in the DC generation process exist, and the quality of therapeutic products will depend on rigorous quality control being implemented at each step of this process.

Overall, the procedure involves culture of monocytes recovered by elutriation from a leukapheresis collection in the presence of media plus cytokines able to support monocyte differentiation into iDCs. The medium is supplemented with IL-4 and GM-CSF, the two cytokines that are essential for iDC generation.[7] iDCs that meet the defined criteria for viability, purity, and sterility, including a negative test for mycoplasma, are harvested and matured to mDCs by further culture in the presence of a cytokine mix, which may vary in composition, depending on the DC subtype desired.[9] Pulsing of mDCs with defined preparations of immunogenic peptides follows.

In the event undefined antigens such as proteins, live or apoptotic tumor cells, cell lines, cell lysates, or tumor-DC fusions are used as payload instead of peptides, antigen uptake and processing by iDCs are required. These antigens are introduced to iDCs before the maturation process to allow for processing and presentation of the resulting peptides on the DC surface. Following antigen loading and processing during DC maturation, mDCs are harvested and tested as a final product.

References/Resources

1. Liu YJ. Dendritic cell subsets and lineages and their functions in innate and adaptive immunity. Cell 2001; 106:259-62.
2. Whiteside TL, Odoux C. Dendritic cell biology and cancer therapy. Cancer Immunol Immunother 2004;53:240-8.
3. Osada T, Clay TM, Woo GY, et al. Dendritic cell-based immunotherapy. Int Rev Immunol 2006;25:377-413.
4. Whiteside TL, Stanson J, Shurin MR, Ferrone S. Antigen-processing machinery in human dendritic cells: Up-regulation by maturation and down-regulation by tumor cells. J Immunol 2004;173:1526-34.
5. Stager S, Kaye PM. CD8+ T-cell priming regulated by cytokines of the innate immune system. Trends Mol Med 2004;10:366-71.
6. Nicolette C, Healey D, Tcherepanova I, et al. Dendritic cells for active immunotherapy: Optimizing design and manufacture in order to develop commercially and clinically viable products. Vaccine 2007;25(Suppl 2):B1-3.
7. Sallusto F, Lanzavecchia A. Efficient presentation of soluble antigen by cultured human dendritic cells is maintained by granulocyte/macrophage colony-stimulating factor plus interleukin 4 and downregulated by tumor necrosis factor alpha. J Exp Med 1994;179:1109-18.
8. Rutella S, Danese S, Leone G. Tolerogenic dendritic cells: Cytokine modulation comes of age. Blood 2006;108: 1435-40.
9. Wesa A, Kalinski P, Kirkwood JM, et al. Polarized type-1 dendritic cells (DC1) producing high levels of IL-12 family members rescue patient TH1-type antimelanoma CD4+ T cell responses in vitro. J Immunother 1997;30: 75-82.
10. Butterfield L, Gooding W, Whiteside TL. Development of a potency assay for human dendritic cells: IL-12p70 production. J Immunother 2008;31:89-100.
11. Lutz MB, Schuler G. Immature, semi-mature and fully mature dendritic cells: Which signals induce tolerance or immunity? Trends Immunol 2002;23:445-9.

Method 39-1. Generating and Characterizing Human Dendritic Cells for Cellular Therapy

Time for Procedure

The time needed to generate a dendritic cell (DC) product and accomplish its characterization varies, depending on the DC origin, type of DC required for therapy, maturation conditions, and antigen loading. The total time from leukapheresis to a DC vaccine release is 7 to 10 days. The total time is divided into individual steps of DC preparation as follows:

1. Leukapheresis processing by elutriation to recover the monocyte fraction: 3.5 hours.
2. Culture of recovered monocytes in a cartridge or flasks in the presence of interleukin-4 (IL-4) and granulocyte/macrophage colony-stimulating factor (GM-CSF) to obtain immature DCs (iDCs): 5 to 6 days.
3. iDC harvest and phenotyping: 5 to 6 hours.
4. iDC maturation in a cytokine cocktail: 24 to 48 hours.
5. Mature DC (mDC) loading with peptides and their phenotypic characterization: 6 hours.
6. Final testing to meet the release criteria: 4 hours.

Summary of Procedure

The procedure involves a leukapheresis collection, recovery of monocytes by elutriation, and culture of the monocytes in the presence of media containing cytokines able to support monocyte differentiation into iDCs. The medium is supplemented with IL-4 and GM-CSF, the two cytokines essential for iDC generation. iDCs meeting the defined criteria for viability, purity, and sterility, including a negative test for mycoplasma, are harvested and matured to mDCs by further culture in the presence of a cytokine mixture, which may vary in composition, depending on the DC subtype desired. Pulsing of mDCs follows with defined preparations of immunogenic peptides.

Note: In the event undefined antigens such as proteins, live or apoptotic tumor cells, cell lines, cell lysates, or tumor-DC fusions are used as payload instead of peptides, uptake and antigen processing by iDCs are required. These antigens are introduced to iDCs before the maturation process, which takes from 24 to 48 hours, to allow for processing and presentation of the resulting peptides on the DC surface. Following antigen loading and processing during DC maturation, mDCs are harvested and tested as a final product.

Equipment

1. Elutriator (Elutra, CaridianBCT, Lakewood, CO).
2. Aastrom Replicell System (cartridges, incubators, media exchange system, tubing, computer; Aastrom Biosciences, Ann Arbor, MI).
3. Inverted microscope.
4. Hemacytometer.
5. Brightfield microscope.
6. Table-top centrifuge.
7. CO_2 incubator.
8. Controlled-rate freezer.
9. Flow cytometer.
10. Pipetman.
11. Sterile connecting device (TSCD, Terumo, Somerset, NJ)
12. Tubing sealer.

Supplies and Reagents

1. Sterile T-162 flasks with canted neck and vented cap.
2. Sterile conical centrifuge tubes.
3. Sterile polystyrene pipettes.
4. Sterile plastic syringes.
5. Sterile 20-gauge needles.
6. Aspiration flask.
7. Sterile cryovials.

8. Bottles for sterility sampling.
9. CellGro DC medium (CellGenix, Freiburg, Germany).
10. AIM V medium (Invitrogen Corp, Carlsbad, CA) modified, no antibiotics.
11. Sterile saline, preservative free.
12. TrypLE Select (Invitrogen).
13. Human serum albumin, pharmaceutical grade.
14. Recombinant human IL-4.
15. Recombinant human GM-CSF.
16. DC maturation cocktail of cytokines—eg, IL-1β, IL-6, tumor necrosis factor alpha (TNF-α), prostaglandin E$_2$ (PGE$_2$), interferon-γ (IFN-γ), IFN-α, Poly I:C.
17. Peptides or antigens for DC pulsing.
18. Mycoplasma/endotoxin testing reagents.
19. Labeled antibodies for DC phenotyping.

Procedure

1. The leukapheresis product (usually autologous) is delivered to the manufacturing facility.
2. The leukapheresis product is elutriated on the Elutra to yield a monocyte fraction, which usually contains 70% to 85% of viable CD14+CD3– cells.
3. The recovered cells are harvested, washed, and counted. Cell viability is assessed by trypan blue dye exclusion, and the percentage of CD3–/CD14+ monocytes is assessed by flow cytometry.
4. Monocytes are placed either in a plastic cartridge (Aastrom) at the cell concentration of 0.5×10^9 to 2.5×10^9 cells/cartridge or in tissue culture flasks at 0.5 to 1.0×10^6 cells/mL. Cells are incubated in the culture medium supplemented with 1×10^5 IU/mL of IL-4 and 1×10^5 IU/mL of GM-CSF (both clinical grade) and are cultured for 5 to 6 days in an atmosphere of 5% CO$_2$ in air at 37 C. The medium for DC generation may vary, depending on the laboratory, but antibiotic-free AIM V or CellGro DC medium (CellGenix) are commonly used. The cell concentration, the type of container or vessel used for DC culture, and the type of medium selected are the crucial factors in the process. For large-scale cGMP manufacturing, a closed, computer-assisted system is preferred for DC generation so that the medium can be automatically exchanged as needed.

Note: Small-scale cultures in flasks or wells of plastic plates will require replacement of half of the medium with fresh medium on day 3.

5. Two days before iDC harvest, the cells are sampled for 14-day sterility and mycoplasma tests.
6. Following 5- or 6-day culture, iDCs are harvested by centrifugation. As DCs tend to adhere to plastic, their recovery from culture vessels can be greatly increased by the use of TrypLE Select. Viability and numbers of iDCs are determined.
7. The phenotype of the generated iDCs is determined by flow cytometry to indicate the percentage of harvested cells that are CD14–, CD11c+, HLA-DR+, CD86+, and CD80+. Lymphocyte contamination should be less than 10% (CD3+, CD19+, CD56/CD16+).
8. iDCs are incubated in the cytokine mixture for 24 to 48 hours to obtain mDCs, which are defined by phenotype as HLA-DR+CD86+, CD83+, CD80+CCR7+ cells. The ability of mDCs to present peptides to cognate T cells is much greater than that of iDCs. However, this ability will vary, depending on the content of the maturation cocktail. Cocktails containing IFN-γ, IFN-α, and Poly I:C, which are used to produce "αDC1," are more effective than those containing TNF-α, IL-1β, and IL-6 used to generate "conventional DCs." The αDC1 type of DCs is more effective in activating T cells than conventional DCs.
9. mDCs are pulsed with defined peptides (2-4 hours at 37 C) used at the concentration of 1 to 10 ng/mL, washed, and harvested for final testing.
10. Testing of the final DC product to meet release criteria includes the following:
   a. Sterility: free from bacteria, fungi (14-day culture), mycoplasma, and endotoxin; negative Gram's stain.
   b. Viability: >75% by the trypan blue dye exclusion or propidium iodide/7-amino-actinomycin D (PI/7AAD) staining and flow cytometry.
   c. Purity: >75% by flow cytometry for CD40, CD80, CD83, CD86, CD11c/CD123, CD25, HLA-DR.
   d. Maturation: >50% up-regulated expression of CD83 and CCR7 by flow cytometry.

e. Potency: as indicated by IL-12p70 production in a coculture assay.

f. Stability: resistance to freezing/storage by viability and functional assays.

11. A vaccine lot is cryopreserved in aliquots for future vaccinations using a controlled-rate device. Final release testing is obligatory following thawing and manipulation of the cryopreserved final DC product.

Anticipated Results

The final therapeutic product (ie, the DC-based vaccine) is expected to be sterile, mycoplasma and endotoxin free, and to contain at least 75% DCs as defined by the phenotype. The DC viability should be >75%. DCs are expected to be matured (>50% based on expression of CD83 and CCR7 surface markers) and peptide pulsed or antigen loaded, as defined in the relevant standard operating procedure. DCs are expected to produce IL-12p70 upon CD40L cross-linking at levels appropriate for the DC type. Specifically, DC1 generally produce significantly more IL-12p70 than conventional DCs. Finally, the DC product needs to be stable at room temperature for a defined period of time and amenable to cryopreservation without an appreciable loss of function.

The type of antigen for DC loading, the conditions for DC culture and maturation steps, as well as the DC activation process and the DCs' ability to produce IL-12p70 are the key variables in the DC production process. Any factor may affect the properties of the final DC vaccine, but perhaps DC maturation is the most critical step for generating DC-based immunotherapy products. Appropriately matured DCs should be superior to iDCs in the induction of immunologic responses in vivo. An approximation of the in-vivo function can be modeled in vitro when antigen-specific T cells are available. Antigen-pulsed mDCs coincubated with these T cells in enzyme-linked immunosorbent spot (ELISPOT) assays will induce IFN-γ production. A strongly reactive DC-based vaccine will induce IFN-γ secretion by multiple antigen-specific T cells in such ELISPOT assays.

The use of mDCs in vaccines is also critical for avoiding the induction of regulatory T cells. Dosing with iDCs can lead to immune suppression rather than immune activation.

Note

The Aastrom device is not commercially available; however, the procedure can also be performed using tissue culture-treated flasks.

References/Resources

1. Liu YJ. Dendritic cell subsets and lineages and their functions in innate and adaptive immunity. Cell 2001; 106:259-62.

2. Whiteside TL, Odoux C. Dendritic cell biology and cancer therapy. Cancer Immunol Immunother 2004;53:240-8.

3. Osada T, Clay TM, Woo GY, et al. Dendritic cell-based immunotherapy. Int Rev Immunol 2006;25:377-413.

4. Whiteside TL, Stanson J, Shurin MR, Ferrone S. Antigen-processing machinery in human dendritic cells: Up-regulation by maturation and down-regulation by tumor cells. J Immunol 2004;173:1526-34.

5. Stager S, Kaye PM. CD8+ T-cell priming regulated by cytokines of the innate immune system. Trends Mol Med 2004;10:366-71.

6. Sallusto F, Lanzavecchia A. Efficient presentation of soluble antigen by cultured human dendritic cells is maintained by granulocyte/macrophage colony-stimulating factor plus interleukin 4 and downregulated by tumor necrosis factor alpha. J Exp Med 1994;179:1109-18.

7. Rutella S, Danese S, Leone G. Tolerogenic dendritic cells: Cytokine modulation comes of age. Blood 2006;108: 1435-40.

8. Wesa A, Kalinski P, Kirkwood JM, et al. Polarized type-1 dendritic cells (DC1) producing high levels of IL-12 family members rescue patient TH1-type antimelanoma CD4+ T cell responses in vitro. J Immunother 1997;30: 75-82.

In: Areman EM, Loper K, eds
Cellular Therapy: Principles, Methods, and Regulations
Bethesda, MD: AABB, 2009

◆ ◆ ◆   **40**   ◆ ◆ ◆

Pancreatic Islet Cells

*Elina Linetsky, MSc, MT; Aisha Khan, MS, MBA; and
Camillo Ricordi, MD*

DIABETES MELLITUS (DM) POSES A SIG-nificant public health challenge in the United States and around the world. It is increasing in prevalence and, at the present time, affects almost 20 million people in the United States.[1] DM is considered to be the sixth leading cause of death in the United States and is a major morbidity hazard[2,3] because of its associated complications. Presently, the disease lowers average life expectancy by about 15 years, increases cardiovascular disease (CVD) risk by about two- to fourfold, and is the main cause of kidney failure, lower limb amputations, and adult-onset blindness. DM is a costly disease: The estimated total attributable costs in 2002 were approximately $132 billion.[1]

DM manifests itself in two forms.[4] Type 2 DM, or non-insulin-dependent DM (NIDDM), until recently was characterized by an adult onset, but this picture is rapidly changing. The occurrence of type 2 DM, with its associated complications is the most common form of the disease and is on the rise in the United States, where it accounts for 90% to 95% of all diabetes cases. It is characterized by both resistance to insulin action and impaired insulin secretion.

Type 1 DM, or insulin-dependent DM (IDDM), has an early childhood or young adulthood onset, although it can be diagnosed at any age. It is characterized by an absolute deficiency in insulin secretion caused by an autoimmune destruction of insulin-producing cells in the pancreas, the pancreatic β-cells. This type of DM accounts for approximately 5% to 10% of all diabetes cases. Although autoimmune in nature, other factors that are thought to contribute to the development of type 1 DM are genetic and environmental.[5] It is the autoimmune component of type 1 DM that is responsible for the progressive destruction of insulin-producing β-cells in the pancreas.

Until recently, the only available treatment for type 1 DM was the administration of exogenous insulin. However, the Diabetes Control and Complications Trial (DCCT)[6] demonstrated that insulin replacement therapy—although able to delay the

Elina Linetsky, MSc, MT, Director, Quality Assurance/Regulatory Affairs, Cell Transplant Center, Diabetes Research Institute and Wallace H. Coulter Center, University of Miami Miller School of Medicine; Aisha Khan, MS, MBA, Director of Operations, cGMP Cell Processing Facility, Cell Transplant Center, Diabetes Research Institute, University of Miami Miller School of Medicine; and Camillo Ricordi, MD, Scientific Director, Diabetes Research Institute, University of Miami Miller School of Medicine, Miami, Florida

The authors have disclosed no conflicts of interest.

occurrence of DM-associated complications—did not result in the complete abrogation of their development. Thus, the need for alternative or additional therapies has been apparent for some time. Endocrine replacement, achieved either through transplant of a whole pancreas[7] or allogeneic islet cells[7,8] has been under investigation for quite some time. There is little doubt that pancreas transplants, especially when performed simultaneously with kidney transplants, have shown more favorable metabolic control compared to islet transplantation.[7] Eighty percent of the patients receiving simultaneous kidney-pancreas transplants demonstrate good graft function and insulin independence at 1 year following surgery, with 50% of the recipients maintaining their euglycemia at 5 years.[8] However, the relative ease and simplicity of islet transplantation, safety of the surgical procedure required to implant the graft, and lack of transplant-associated morbidity and mortality are all factors that contribute favorably toward a wider application of allogeneic islet cell transplantation.

As a result of considerable improvements made to the islet isolation process to optimize the method itself, the reagents used during the procedure, and the quantity and quality of the islet preparations, islet transplantation became a reality in the 1990s. Unfortunately, following the initial enthusiasm, the International Islet Transplant Registry[9] reported that only 10% of the patients receiving allogeneic islet grafts during this period could maintain insulin independence at ≥1 year following transplantation. The publication of the results of the Edmonton Protocol in 2000[10] and continued improvement in clinical outcomes reported by a number of centers[10-14] clearly demonstrated that allogeneic islet transplantation had the potential to become a viable therapy for patients with severe forms of type 1 DM. However, despite significant improvements in the islet isolation process in the last two decades,[15,16] continued success reported in the clinical outcomes of allogeneic islet transplantation,[10-13] and the availability of new immunosuppressive regimens,[10-13] notable challenges to transplanting allogeneic islet cells remain.

Before allogeneic islet cells can be marketed as a bona fide treatment for patients with type 1 DM, several critical issues must be addressed:

- Isolation of a maximum number of high-quality islet cells from the exocrine tissue, which composes 98% to 99% of the pancreas.
- Overcoming immune rejection, which is quite difficult to monitor, given a very small volume of the transplanted tissue and limited ability to characterize the process.
- Prevention of recurrence of autoimmunity, demonstrated to have successful outcomes in murine models.[5]
- Induction of immune tolerance, which could potentially alleviate the need for lifelong immunosuppressive regimens presently required to keep the islet allograft acquiescent.
- Development of more refined immunosuppressive regimens that are less toxic to the patient, as well as the graft.

Since the automated method for human islet cell isolation was developed,[17] the process has undergone a number of progressive modifications for optimization. The purpose of this chapter is to provide a historical perspective of the development of the islet isolation procedure and to offer a description of the latest methods used to isolate human pancreatic islet cells.

Historical Perspective

In 1922, the Canadian physician Frederic Banting discovered that the pancreas generated a "sugar-producing substance"[18] called insulin. Since then, scientists have been interested in how this hormone is released. Initial attempts to isolate islet cells from a donor pancreas were not consistent and involved a severely disruptive mechanical component.[19,20] While trying to investigate whether glucose can stimulate insulin release in vitro, Moskalewski[19] was able to isolate islet cells from the guinea pig by combining a mechanical disruption of the pancreas with an enzymatic digestion. Noting that Moskalewski did not report any damage to the islet cells as a consequence of their exposure to the collagenase enzyme, Lacy et al[20] proceeded to isolate islet cells from the rat pancreas, disrupting the acinar tissue by distending the common bile duct with Hank's Balanced Salt Solution (HBSS). Although the islets were separated from the acinar tissue using both mechanical disruption and enzymatic digestion, Lacy[20] demonstrated that a good majority of the islet cells could be purified by centrifugation on discontinuous sucrose gradients. However, because of differences in size, structure, cellular content, and their attachment to the surrounding tissue, islets found in large animals differ from those found in small animals such as rats, mice, and guinea pigs.[17,20] Because of these factors, procedures developed for isolation of islets from rodent species were found to be ineffective when applied to large animals and humans.

Through numerous modifications made to the islet isolation method developed earlier, novel procedures for the mass isolation of human islets were developed. A method for large-scale isolation of canine islets, using an enzymatic perfusion of the pancreatic duct,[21,22] involved the exposure of the collagenous framework of the pancreas to the enzymatic action before the digestion step with collagenase, thereby significantly increasing the resulting islet cell yield. This technique was encouraging because it involved a series of culture stages following the ductal perfusion of the pancreas with collagenase, avoiding any mechanical chopping. Kuhn et al[23] continued using the intraductal perfusion of the canine pancreas, while retaining the partially digested tissue using Velcro strips in the digestion tubes. Although neither purity nor viability of the islet cells was discussed, a yield of 80,000 islet cells per pancreas was reported. Ricordi et al[24] developed a method for mass isolation of intact, viable porcine islets, using both enzymatic digestion and mechanical disruption with a tissue macerator, followed by filtration of the digested tissue and purification on Ficoll (GE Healthcare, Piscataway, NJ) gradients. This method resulted in highly purified and functional cells, with average yields of 80,000 islets per splenic lobe of the porcine pancreas.[24]

The human islet isolation procedure required further modifications in order to improve isolation yield,[25,26] purification efficiency, and quality of the preparation, mainly because of different dissociation rates of the human pancreas. Gray et al[25] reported a technique that employed perfusion of the human pancreas through the pancreatic duct, incubation at 37 C to digest the organ, and teasing the pancreas apart after cutting it into several small pieces. In this procedure, islet cells were purified from the exocrine tissue using discontinuous Ficoll gradients,[25] resulting in improved isolation yield and islet purity of approximately 10% to 40%. The

end result was a simple and quick technique that avoided any mechanical trauma and consequent detrimental effect on islet cell viability. Scharp et al[26] demonstrated that distention of the pancreas by injection of collagenase solution through the pancreatic duct, subsequent digestion at 37 C, and liberation of islets through a tissue macerator further improved the yield from 150,000 to 250,000 islets per pancreas. However, using an elutriator to purify the islets from the exocrine tissue resulted in low purity of the preparation—20% to 25% islets.[26] These islet preparations, which would now be considered crude, were used for pilot clinical studies with encouraging results. Functional activity of the islet cells was demonstrated in several patients for 2 to 3 months by stimulated plasma C-peptide levels and a 60% to 90% decrease in insulin requirements.

Although these clinical studies with crude islet preparations were encouraging, the need for more purified preparations was apparent. Further efforts reported by Scharp[26] resulted in significantly improved purity of 60% to 90% islets when the digest was purified using Ficoll or Percoll (GE Healthcare, Piscataway, NJ) gradients. The best purification was achieved when Ficoll was used. The islets were reported to maintain their morphologic appearance and functionality during the 7-day culture following the isolation process. Other studies followed.

Subsequently, allotransplantation of human pancreatic cells became a reality, although questions related to the cause of graft failure remained. These questions had much to do with the inability to isolate adequate numbers of functional islet cells from a human deceased heart-beating donor. One of the persistent problems with the methods developed for human islet isolation was the common necessity to use a mechanical, and often significantly traumatic, component to dissociate the digested tissue. Methods included chopping, teasing, and passaging of the tissue through different-sized needles or a macerator. All of these methods resulted in fragmentation and even destruction of the islet cells. In addition, the decision to transfer from the digestion to the tissue disruption phase was subjective and based on visual evaluation of the digestion process. This approach would result in both over- and underdigestion of tissue.[17] The automated method[17] allowed for continuous release of large numbers of islet cells during the digestion phase, preventing overdigestion. This method had a minimal traumatic effect on the islets, releasing large numbers of liberated islets while it protected them from any further enzymatic action. The digestion process was allowed to proceed until only a fibrous network of ducts and vessels of the pancreas remained.

The Ricordi method, which used the entire organ, resulted in the isolation of a larger number of islet cells. Since the introduction of this method in 1986, several modifications to the procedure have been introduced to optimize both the quantity and quality of islet preparations. The next section of this chapter provides a discussion of the most recent methodology used to isolate human pancreatic islet cells from deceased heart-beating donors. Factors that profoundly influence the islet yield will be discussed.

Donor Selection

Allogeneic islet cells are isolated from a pancreas procured from a deceased heart-beating donor. There is a paucity of historical evidence regarding the contribution of donor variables toward the islet cell yield and clinical transplant outcome.[28] Each human islet isolation is different and unique as a result of a number of donor factors. Donor variables include age, cause of death, body mass index (BMI), condition and size of the organ, and the time between the cross-clamp and the start of processing. In addition, when current good tissue practice (cGTP) is taken into account, each donor differs in terms of medical, clinical, and social histories and must be qualified according to these standards before tissue from the organ can be used for further manufacture. Furthermore, each transplant center involved in human islet cell isolation deals with a large number of organ procurement organizations (OPOs) around the country, each with its own practices for organ procurement and preservation.

Islet Isolation

To isolate human pancreatic islets, the authors use a modified version of the "automated method,"[17]

which has undergone a number of progressive improvements in the last two decades since it was first reported. Method 40-1 provides a detailed description of this procedure. Figure 40-1 diagrams the isolation setup. Once the organ is accepted and received in the processing laboratory, it is cleaned, cannulated, and distended with an enzymatic solution. Tissue such as fat and lymph nodes is removed to maximize the efficiency of the perfusion and digestion process (see Fig 40-2). Procedures for enzyme solution preparation follow in Methods 40-2 and 40-3. A sufficient intraductal perfusion of the pancreas is crucial for a successful islet isolation result. It ensures an even distribution of collagenase throughout different portions of the gland, resulting in a better dissociation of the organ. In the case of unsatisfactory perfusion, a series of evenly distributed collagenase injections into the parenchyma using a disposable syringe and needle should increase the islet yield. Alternatively, the organ can be distended manually, using a 60-mL disposable syringe attached to the cannula.

The optimal mixture of enzymes required for human islet isolation is of critical importance and has a significant impact on the islet isolation outcome. One critical development in the 1990s that contributed to the standardization of the reagents and process was the availability of Liberase (Roche, Indianapolis, IN), a purified enzyme blend. Compared to collagenases used previously (eg, collagenase P, Sigma Type X, Sigma Type V), Liberase seemed to demonstrate consistent lot-to-lot reproducibility because of the quality control (QC) of raw reagents used in the fermentation of the *Clostridia histolyticum* bacteria. However, despite notable improvements in both quantity and quality of human islet preparations, it became clear over time that Liberase was still associated with lot-to-lot variability, mainly because of the relative contents of its components, collagenase Type I and Type II, as well as Thermolysin protease.[16] To complicate matters even further, bovine brain-derived raw material was used during the early stages of the Liberase manufacture. The fact that bovine brain-derived materials have potential to transmit prions causing transmissible spongiform encephalopathies (TSEs) became a serious concern and resulted in Liberase being withdrawn from the market.

For the past several years, another enzyme blend available from Nordmark, SERVA collagenase NB 1

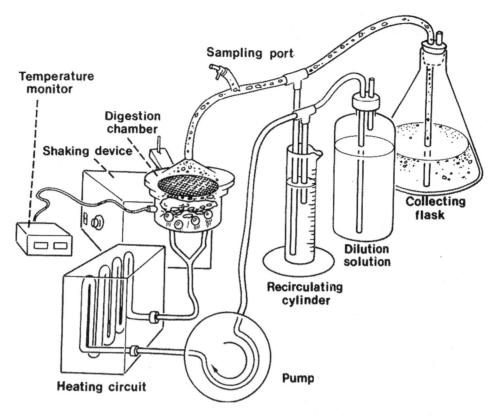

Figure 40-1. A schematic representation of human islet isolation setup using the automated method, with a 500-mL or 600-mL Ricordi chamber (Biorep Technologies, Miami, FL). The pancreas is digested during a continuous digestion process, while the free islets are salvaged from further exposure to enzymatic action by the continuous flow afforded by the process. (Reprinted with permission from Ricordi.)

(premium grade; SERVA Electrophoresis, Heidelberg, Germany), blended with separately packaged neutral protease (NP), has been used by several European and US groups that report positive results.[16] Despite extensive islet isolation data available for SERVA collagenase, questions such as optimal concentration of both collagenase and NP, calcium concentration in the enzyme buffer, temperature, and duration of the digestion step, as well as the use of such additives as protease inhibitors, DNase, and heparin, are issues that continue to be addressed.

Islet cells are isolated from the exocrine component of the pancreas during the continuous digestion process, which takes approximately 30 to 60 minutes. The latest modifications to the islet isolation procedure described in this chapter, compared to the original report,[17] are 1) the Ricordi (Biorep Technologies, Miami, FL) digestion chamber made of plastic (see Fig 40-3), 2) the use of the perfusion

apparatus, and 3) the Ricordi isolator, equipped with a peristaltic pump action, a heating and a cooling system, and the capacity to measure pressure, pH, and temperature. The use of a mechanical shaker leads to the standardization of the oscillation amplitude and rate during the digestion phase. The intensity of shaking varies according to the age of the donor. Pancreata from young donors require gentle shaking movement, whereas the organs from older donors are treated more vigorously. Although experienced operators can easily distinguish islet cells from exocrine tissue, lymph nodes, ducts, and ganglia under the light microscope, the use of diphenyl-thiocarbazone (DTZ), a stain specific to the zinc in the insulin granules of islet cells, is strongly recommended (see Fig 40-4; also, see Section VIII). As a general rule, when most of the islet cells are free from the surrounding exocrine tissue and a significant amount of tissue is observed in the sample, a switch from the digestion/recircula-

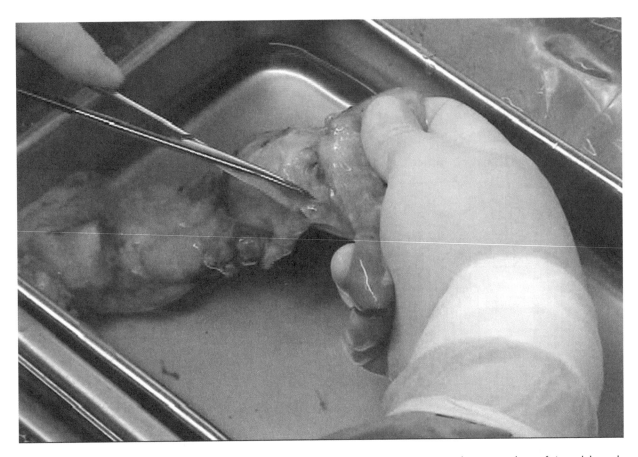

Figure 40-2. In the preparation of the pancreas for perfusion, all the excess tissue such as fat and lymph nodes is removed to maximize the efficiency of the perfusion and digestion process.

tion phase to the dilution/collection phase should be made. If signs of overdigestion appear, the decision to switch should be made immediately, regardless of how many islets are observed to be embedded. This decision has a critical effect on the outcome of the isolation process. When making a decision to switch, several factors should be taken into consideration: the number of free islets in the sample, degree of overdigestion, morphologic appearance of both islets and exocrine tissue (islets should have intact borders), and amount and size of the exocrine tissue.

When the digestion phase is nearing completion, preparations should be made for the dilution/collection phase to collect the digested tissue. During this phase of the isolation process, the goal is to stop enzymatic action by switching to a lower temperature and sufficiently diluting the digest with fresh media. The total dilution phase lasts approximately 30 to 50 minutes and continues until islets

are no longer detected in the sample. The digest containing both islet and exocrine tissue is concentrated by progressive centrifugation and collected in University of Wisconsin (UW) organ transport solution.

Islet Purification

It is critical that the purification step be performed while keeping the digest and the gradients at low temperatures (4-15 C). This procedure is necessary because some of the components that make up gradient solutions might be toxic to the islet cells at room temperature, where islets are metabolically active. The source for potential islet toxicity can be twofold: from the gradient itself, as a result of osmolar shock, and from the inclusion of impurities such as endotoxin—a result of limitations of commercial processing. Therefore, it is beneficial to

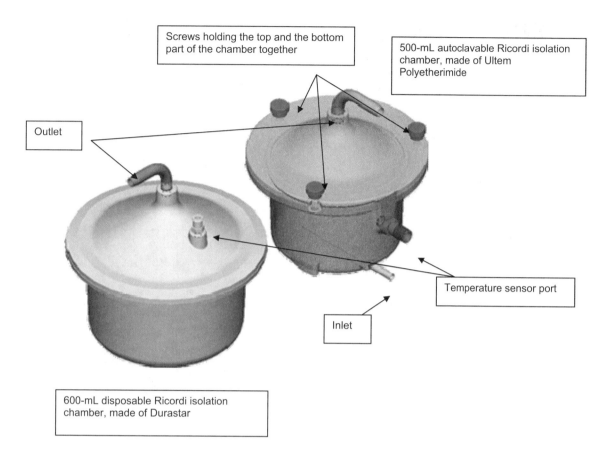

Figure 40-3. Schematic representation of a 600-mL and a 500-mL Ricordi isolation chamber. The 500-mL chamber is made of a reusable or autoclavable chamber material, Ultem (GE Healthcare, Chalfont St Giles, United Kingdom) polyetherimide—a tough, rigid, biocompatible plastic of superior thermostatic strength. The 600-mL disposable chamber is made of Durastar (Eastman Chemical Company, Kingsport, TN)—a clear, tough, and chemically resistant material.

keep the islet tissue at a low temperature, which reduces its metabolic activity.

Density-dependent, or isopycnic separation, is achieved when cells end up at the density within the gradient equal to the density of the gradient, as a consequence of time and force. Over time, isopycnic density centrifugation, while remaining the most accepted method for purification of islet cells, has undergone many modifications regarding the type of gradient and the density layers used. Progressive changes introduced over time have led to the optimization of the 1) purity of the islet preparation, 2) recovery of islet cells from the digest, and 3) viability of purified islet cells. In addition to Ficoll, many investigators used Percoll, albumin, dextran, and others.[26,32] The use of Ficoll- and Percoll-based purification gradients[26] and the COBE

2991 cell processor (CaridianBCT, Lakewood, CO)[32] resulted in a much more effective method of islet purification. Over time it became clear[33] that in addition to the density differences between the islet and the exocrine components, other factors, such as osmolality, high glucose content, and viscosity of the purification solution, were all critical components of the purification process. In the late 1990s, a gradient less hypertonic than others, Optiprep (Nycomed/Axis-Shield PoC, Oslo, Norway), was introduced. This gradient isolated islets of high purity and viability[34] and, in addition, good islet cell recovery was observed.

At the time of writing, Eurocollins (Mediatech, Indianapolis, IN)-Ficoll continuous gradients with densities of 1.100 and 1.077 are commonly used. The digested pancreatic tissue is top-loaded using a

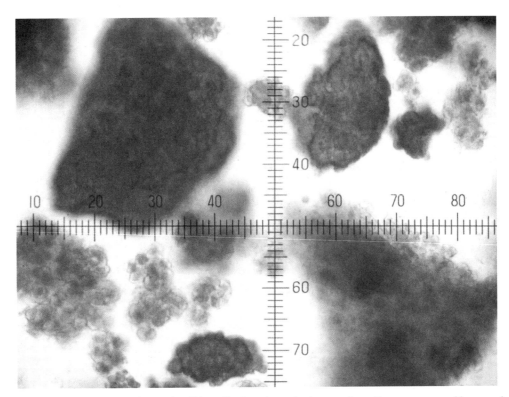

Figure 40-4. Sample removed from the Ricordi chamber during a digestion process. Human islets (red) stained with diphenyl-thiocarbazone (DTZ) are easily distinguishable from the exocrine tissue which appears light brown.

peristaltic pump connected to a COBE 2991 cell processor. It is critical to ensure a complete resuspension of the pelleted digest in the lighter gradient layer, following a 30-minute incubation in 100 mL of UW solution, to preserve and improve the density differences between the islets and acinar tissue. An uneven dispersion of the tissue in the density gradient would result in decreased purity of the islet preparation and low post-purification recovery of islet cells. The digest should be gently resuspended by slow hand mixing, avoiding any sudden movements that can result in fragmentation of the islet cells. It is critical to be careful not to overload the COBE bag, which has a finite volume of 600 mL. No more than 25 mL of pelleted digest should be loaded into each bag to achieve the best possible purification results.

To form a proper continuous gradient, constant mixing during gradient recombination is recommended. For this purpose, a stirring plate can be used. As the gradients are being recombined, they can be slowly loaded into the COBE bag, using a speed of 15-20 mL/minute.

Care should be taken not to allow the gradient maker to become empty to prevent air from entering the system. Once the gradients are loaded in the COBE bag, the digest is added to the gradient maker and slowly loaded into the COBE bag. Once the tissue has entered the COBE bag, 20 mL of HBSS is then loaded in the system.

Because the human islet isolation procedure yields a large number of islet cells, the authors recommend using large, 175-cm^2, untreated (to prevent cell adherence), tissue culture flasks. A concentration of approximately 20,000 islet equivalents (IEQ) in 30 mL of culture medium is preferred. Compensation for the purity of the islet preparation is recommended during culture, such that the number of islets placed into the culture is decreased (from 20,000 IEQ) as the purity decreases.

After isolation and purification, allogeneic islets are typically cultured for up to 2 days. Culture methods differ with institutional practices. A brief description of one such method is included in Method 40-1.

Acknowledgment

Methods 40-2 and 40-3 were submitted by A. N. Balamurugan, PhD, Assistant Professor of Surgery and Director, Islet Core, Diabetes Institute for Immunology and Transplantation, University of Minnesota, Minneapolis, Minnesota.

References/Resources

1. All about diabetes. Alexandria, VA: American Diabetes Association, 2009. [Available at http://www.diabetes.org/about-diabetes.jsp (accessed March 30, 2009).]
2. US Department of Health and Human Services. Healthy people 2010: Objectives for improving health. Diabetes 2000;5:2-40.
3. Zimmet P, Shaw J. Diabetes on six continents—ethnic and geographic differences: Views on the culture. In Raz I, Skyler J, Shafrir E, eds. Diabetes: From research to diagnosis and treatment. London, UK: Taylor and Francis Group, 2003:1-10.
4. Centers for Disease Control and Prevention. National diabetes fact sheet: General information and national estimates on diabetes in the United States (rev ed). Atlanta, GA: CDC, 2003.
5. Bottino R, Trucco M. Multifaceted therapeutic approaches for a multigenic disease. Diabetes 2005;54: S79-86.
6. The Diabetes Control and Complications Trial Research Group. The effect of intensive treatment of diabetes on the development and progression of long-term complications of insulin-dependent diabetes mellitus. N Engl J Med 1993;329:977-86.
7. Robertson RP. Islet transplantation as a treatment for diabetes: A work in progress. N Engl J Med 2004;350: 694-705.
8. Weir G, Bonner-Weir S. Scientific and political impediments to successful islet transplantation. Diabetes 1997; 16:1217-56.
9. Hering BJ. Insulin independence following islet transplantation in man: A comparison of different recipient categories. International Islet Transplant Registry Newsletter 7 1996;6:5-19.
10. Shapiro AM, Lakey JR, Ryan EA, et al. Islet transplantation in seven patients with type 1 diabetes mellitus using glucocorticoid-free immunosuppressive regimen. N Engl J Med 2000;323:230-8.
11. Froud T, Ricordi C, Baidal DA, et al. Islet transplantation in type 1 diabetes mellitus using cultured islet and steroid-free immunosuppression: Miami experience. Am J Transplant 2005;5:2037-46.
12. Markmann JF, Deng S, Huang X, et al. Insulin independence following isolated islet transplantation and single islet infusions. Ann Surg 2003;237:741-9.
13. Hirshberg B, Rother KI, Digon BJ III, et al. Benefits and risks of solitary islet transplantation for type 1 diabetes using steroid-sparing immunosuppression: The National Institutes of Health experience. Diabetes Care 2003;26: 3288-95.
14. Shapiro AM, Ricordi C, Hering B. Edmonton's islet success has indeed been replicated elsewhere (letter). Lancet 2003;362:1242.
15. Linetsky E, Bottino R, Lehman R, et al. Improved human islet isolation using a new enzyme blend, Liberase. Diabetes 1997;46:1120-3.
16. Bucher P, Mathe A, Morel P, et al. Assessment of a novel two-component enzyme preparation for human islet isolation and transplantation. Transplantation 2005;79: 91-7.
17. Ricordi C, Lacy PE, Finke EH, et al. Automated method for isolation of human pancreatic islets. Diabetes 1988; 37:413-20.
18. Preface. In: Ricordi C. One century of transplantation for diabetes: Pancreatic cell transplantation. Austin, TX: RG Landes Company, 1992.
19. Moskalewski S. Isolation and culture of the islets of Langerhans of the guinea pig. Gen Comp Endocrin 1965; 5:342-53.
20. Lacy P, Kostianovsky M. Method for the isolation of intact islets of Langerhans from the rat pancreas. Diabetes 1965;16:35-9.
21. Horaguchi A, Merrell RC. Preparation of viable islet cells from dogs by a new method. Diabetes 1981;30:455-8.
22. Noel J, Rabinobitch A, Olson L, et al. A method for large-scale, high-yield isolation of canine pancreatic islets of Langerhans. Metabolism 1982;31:184-7.
23. Kuhn F, Schultz HJ, Lorentz D, et al. Morphological investigations in human islets of Langerhans isolated by the Velcro-technic. Biomed Biochim Acta 1985;44:149-53.
24. Ricordi C, Finke EH, Lacy PE. A method for the mass isolation of islets from the adult pig pancreas. Diabetes 1986;35:649-53.
25. Gray DWR, McShane P, Gant A, et al. A method for isolation of islets of Langerhans from the human pancreas. Diabetes 1984;33:1055-61.
26. Scharp DW, Lacy PE, Finke E, et al. Low-temperature culture of human islets isolated by the distention method and purified with Ficoll or Percoll gradients. Surgery 1987;5:869-79.
27. Alejandro R, Mintz DH, Latif Z, et al. Islet cell transplantation in type 1 diabetes mellitus. Transplant Proc 1987; 19:2359-61.
28. Ricordi C. Islet cell transplantation: Beyond the paradigms. Diabetes Metab Rev 1996;12:361-72.
29. Lindall A, Steffes M, Sorensen R. Immunoassayable insulin content of subcellular fractions of rat islets. Endocrinology 1969;85:218-23.
30. Ashcroft SJH, Bassett JM, Randle PK. Isolation of human pancreatic islets capable of releasing insulin and metabolizing glucose in vitro. Lancet 1971;1:888-9.
31. Ballinger WF, Lacy PE. Transplantation of intact pancreatic islets in rats. Surgery 1972;72:175-86.
32. Lake SP, Bassett PD, Larkins A, et al. Large scale purification of human islets utilizing discontinuous albumin

gradient on IBM 2991 cell processor. Diabetes 1989;38: 143-5.

33. Ricordi C. The automated method for islet isolation. In: Ricordi C, ed. Pancreatic islet cell transplantation:1882-1992, one century of transplantation for diabetes. Austin, TX: RG Landes Company, 1992:99-112.

34. Van der Burg MPM, Graham JM. Iodixanol density gradient preparation in University of Wisconsin solution for porcine islet purification. Scientific WorldJournal 2003; 3:1154-9.

35. Ricordi C. Quantitative and qualitative standards for islet isolation assessment in humans and large animals. Pancreas 1991;2:242-4.

Method 40-1. Isolating Human Islet Cells

Description

This method describes the process of islet cell isolation from human pancreata for clinical transplantation or research purposes.

Note: Islet isolation is a complex and cumbersome procedure. A detailed description of the process is beyond the scope of this text. Therefore, an abbreviated method follows. The media preparation methods were provided by a different facility than the one that provided this method.

Time for Procedure

From 5 to 6 hours.

Summary of Procedure

A human islet isolation procedure consists of several different processes: 1) pancreas cleaning and cannulation, 2) perfusion and distention, 3) digestion and recirculation, 4) dilution and collection, 5) purification using density gradients, and 6) islet enumeration and culture. The overall goal of islet isolation is to dislodge islet cells (islets of Langerhans) from the exocrine tissue through the breakup of the pancreatic connective tissue, using enzymatic and mechanical action. The end result of this process is the purified islet cell product. This procedure must be performed under strict aseptic conditions.

Equipment

A. *Sterile Nondisposables*
   1. Balance/scale.
   2. Sterile prepack as described in facility-specific standard operating procedures (SOPs).
   3. Sterile Ricordi chamber pack [containing a 500-mL or 600-mL Ricordi chamber (Biorep Technologies, Miami, FL)].
   4. Sterile perfusion tray (with disposable perfusion tubing set).
   5. Sterile 250-mL isolation chamber with lid, rubber ring, and screen (use only if pancreas is <20 g).
   6. Sterile 530-mm screen.
   7. Sterile 380-mm screen (if donor is <24 years old).
   8. Sampling port.
   9. Plastic-covered hammer/mallet.
   10. Racks for 250-mL conicals.
   11. Racks for 50-mL conicals.
   12. Sterile cable ties.
   13. Marbles, sterilized.

B. *Other Equipment*
   1. 1 Perfusion machine.
   2. 3 Portable pipette-aids (pipettors).
   3. 1 sterile Drummond pipette with capillary tubes, 100 μL.
   4. 1 heated waterbath (45 C).
   5. 2 or more refrigerated floor centrifuges.
   6. 37-C CO_2 incubator (standard 5% CO_2).
   7. 22-C CO_2 incubator (standard 5% CO_2).
   8. Inverted light microscope.
   9. 1 Ricordi isolator (Biorep Technologies, Miami, FL).
   10. 2 peristaltic pump drives with pump heads.
   11. 1 Monotherm temperature monitor (Mallinckrodt Medical, Athlone, Ireland) with attached temperature sensor holders (for backup).
   12. 1 top-loading balance.
   13. 1 analytical balance.
   14. 1 Sebra heat-sealer (Sebra, Tuscon, AZ).
   15. Laboratory timers.
   16. 4 biological safety cabinets (BSCs).
   17. 2 COBE 2991 cell washers with four tubing clamps (two on each machine); (CaridianBCT, Lakewood, CO).
   18. Central vacuum system.
   19. 1 circulating chiller (ethanol) for 4 C.
   20. 1 circulating chiller (ethanol) for 30 C.
   21. 4 stirrer plates.

Disposables (or Equivalents)

1. 6 × 1 L frozen sterile water (injection).
2. 10 × 1 L cold sterile water (irrigation).
3. Sterile tissue culture (TC)-treated flasks, vented: T-175 and T-75 nontreated tissue suspension flasks.
4. Sterile tissue culture bags (gas permeable).
5. Sterile 50-cc conical tubes.
6. Sterile 10 × 35 counting and petri dishes and 100 × 15 petri dishes.
7. Sterility test containers: follow facility-specific SOP for contaminant and sterility testing for islet cell products.
8. Sterile 15-mL conical tubes.
9. Vacuum collection flask with two associated sterile tubing sets.
10. Sterile disposable half sheets.
11. Sterile disposable gowning supplies, masks, and face shields.
12. pH strips and/or pH meter.
13. Absorbent sheets.
14. Pump tubing (size 16 and size 17, sterilized, 5 feet each).

Reagents and Media

1. Hank's Balanced Salt Solution (HBSS): 1 L, for enzyme preparation.
2. Reconstituted Liberase (Roche, Indianapolis, IN)/collagenase with additives, or equivalent (eg, SERVA reagent).
3. Ancef [(cefazolin) SmithKline Beecham, Philadelphia, PA].
4. ViaSpan UW Belzer's solution (DuPont Pharmaceuticals, Wilmington, DE).
5. Custodiol HTK solution (Essential Pharmaceuticals, Newtown, PA).
6. Glucose solution (Eurocollins, Mediatech, Indianapolis, IN).
7. Human serum albumin (HSA) 25% (fatty-acid-free HSA).
8. Additive #1 (Fluka, Sigma Aldrich, St Louis, MO).
9. RPMI-1640 medium (1000 mL) for dilution: 8-10 L.
10. RPMI-1640 (1000 mL) for washing: 3-5 L.
11. Culture medium: Miami Media #1A (CMRL-1066 based), 1-4 L, depending on how many islets are cultured.
12. Shipping medium (facility specific): 1-4 L, depending on how many islets are shipped.
13. Continuous density gradients: 1.100, 1.077.
14. Discontinuous density gradients: 1.037, 1.096, 1.108 (Mediatech).
15. Stock Ficoll solution.
16. HBSS with phenol red: 1 L, for priming the chamber.
17. Dithizone solution: 50 mg in a final volume of 30 mL.
18. Reagent-grade alcohol.
19. P-Phase II [Mediatech; availability may be limited to Clinical Islet Consortium (CIT) trials].
20. H-Phase II (Mediatech; availability may be limited to CIT trials).
21. Pentastarch 10%.
22. CMRL 1066 supplemented.
23. Optiprep (Nycomed/Axis-Shield PoC, Oslo, Norway).
24. H-HD stock solution (Mediatech).
25. CMRL 1066 (Invitrogen, Carlsbad, CA, or equivalent).
26. H/P phase I solution (Mediatech).
27. DNAse [Pulmozyme (dornase alpha), Genentech, South San Francisco, CA).

Procedure

A. *Pancreas Cleaning and Cannulation*
   Note: Before bringing the pancreas container into the clean room, verify infectious disease screening and testing results and proper labeling.
   1. Using sterile technique, open the pancreas container in the BSC and remove 5 to 6 mL of the preservation solution for sterility (sample #1) testing.
      Note: The same preservation medium should be used for pancreas cleaning and cannulation as was used during shipment.
   2. Move the pancreas to a sterile surgical dissection pan containing preservation solution. Ensure that the organ is completely submerged in the solution at all times during the cleaning process. Remove the spleen, if it is attached to the pancreas, and place it in a container with preservation medium. Remove the duodenum as described below:

a. Visualize the edge of the pancreas connected to the duodenum.

b. While holding the duodenum away from the pancreas, cut the connective tissue between pancreas and duodenum.

c. Locate and clamp the pancreatic duct, which exits proximally to the head of the pancreas, using two hemostat clamps: one proximal to the pancreas and the other proximal to the duodenum, to ensure that the contents of the duodenum are contained after the duct is cut. Cut the duct between the two clamps.

d. In case of a cut or a leak from the duodenum, clamp it immediately and dip the pancreas in a 10% Betadine solution (Purdue Products, Stamford, CT) for 5 seconds. Rinse the organ with HBSS twice and remove the duodenum from the pan as quickly as possible. When finished cleaning, rinse once more in HBSS (see Step 5).

3. Examine the pancreas and document the amount of surface and infiltrating fat, presence of edema, presence of blood, and texture of the pancreas.

4. Dip the pancreas in a "Betadine dip solution" for 5 seconds.

5. Rinse twice with HBSS, transfer to a new container of HBSS, and rinse again.

6. Change gloves while the pancreas is in HBSS.

7. Remove the original dissection pan and all the instruments from the BSC, and replace it with a clean pan and a second set of sterile instruments.

8. Return the pancreas to a new pan pre-filled with cold preservation solution.

9. If more cleaning is required, using sterile surgical scissors and forceps, remove fat and connective tissue. Do not trim the pancreas too closely, as leaks may develop.

Note: Fat floats, whereas pancreatic tissue does not.

10. Once the pancreas is free of any excess fat, use a scalpel to cut it at the neck, just below the head, in a single nonstop motion.

11. Locate the main pancreatic duct, in preparation for the cannulation of the head and body/tail portions of the pancreas.

12. Cannulate the pancreatic duct of both the head and body/tail sections of the organ.

13. Secure the catheters in the duct of the head and the body/tail.

14. Once both catheters are in place and tied, rinse the pancreas with plain HBSS and place the head and body/tail of the pancreas inside a sterile Nalgene jar (Thermo Fisher Scientific, Rochester, NY). Close the jar before removing it from the BSC.

15. Weigh the Nalgene jar and record the weight.

16. Aseptically, place the jar with the pancreas back in the BSC.

17. The pancreas is now ready to be distended or perfused. At the completion of the perfusion phase, weigh the empty Nalgene jar, cannula, nonpancreatic tissue removed, and clamps, if any were used.

B. *Pancreas Distention or Perfusion*

1. The pancreas may be distended using either of two methods:
   a. Cold perfusion technique using a perfusion apparatus (Step 2).
   b. Manual distention technique (Step 3).

2. Cold perfusion technique:
   a. Prime the perfusion circuit with HBSS. After confirming that there are no leaks or loose connections, empty the perfusion circuit and drain the HBSS solution.
   b. Add cold enzyme to the enzyme chamber and refill the perfusion circuit, removing all air bubbles.
   c. Connect the stopcock and perfusion tubing to the cannula (in the head and body/tail sections). Distend the pancreas for 4 minutes at 80 mm Hg, followed by another 6 minutes at 180 mm Hg.
   d. If leaks from the pancreas are detected, use sterile hemostats to

clamp off the area in order to prevent the enzyme from leaking out.

e. Monitor and document the temperature before and during the perfusion.

f. After 10 minutes of cold perfusion, stop the perfusion machine and remove the cannula and suture, which should be weighed before discarding.

g. Proceed to Step 4.

3. Manual distention technique: Distend the pancreas using a syringe, as described below:

a. Distend the head of the pancreas with approximately 150 mL of the collagenase solution, using a 60-cc syringe connected to the catheter. Slowly, push on the syringe barrel to force the enzyme solution into the pancreas. Avoid creating any bubbles. If there are no leaks or cuts in the pancreas, it will slowly inflate.

b. When leaks are observed, use sterile hemostats to clamp off the area, preventing the enzyme from leaking out.

c. Distend the tail of the pancreas using approximately 200 mL of the enzyme solution.

4. After perfusion or manual distention, weigh excised tissue, suture, and cannula to determine the true weight of the pancreas. Calculate the "trimmed" weight of the pancreas and record.

5. Cut the pancreas into seven to nine pieces and place it in the Ricordi digestion chamber. Alternatively, the head and tail of the pancreas can be placed in the chamber without being cut.

6. Refer to Table 40-1-1 to determine the number of marbles to be placed in the digestion chamber. Add enough enzyme solution to reach the level of the screen.

7. Place the screen in its groove and close the digestion chamber. Ensure that the chamber is sealed properly so that leaks do not develop.

8. Refer to Table 40-1-1, below, for the circuit volume required for different chamber sizes.

C. *Pancreas Digestion*

1. Phase 1 of the digestion phase begins when the distended pancreas, along with the marbles, is placed inside the digestion chamber, which is filled with the collagenase solution. Before the chamber is securely tightened, the screen and an O-ring are placed in their respective grooves. These are located under the top, conical part of the chamber (lid).

2. Enzyme recirculation is carried out in a 250-mL conical tube. Add no more than 50 mL of collagenase/HBSS solution at a time until no more enzyme solution is available. The total volume in the 250-mL conical tube should not exceed 100 mL.

3. Start pumping HBSS through the system to complete the circuit (because 350 mL of the enzyme solution is not sufficient) at a rate of 200 to 300 mL/minute while the circuit is filling. Add enough HBSS to the recirculation container to fill the cir-

Table 40-1-1. Digestion Chamber Contents and Flow Rates

Chamber Size (mL)	Amount of Enzyme to Be Used (g)	Number of Marbles Required	Volume of Enzyme Required (mL)	Flow Rate at Digestion (mL/minute)	Flow Rate at Dilution (mL/minute)
125	125	3	88	38	75
250	250	4	175	75	150
500	500	7	350	150	225
600	600	8	400	150	200-300

cuit completely and to eliminate the air from the circuit. The chamber must be filled through the bottom inlet, using size 16 tubing connected to the port at the bottom of the chamber.

4. When using the Ricordi Isolator, set the heater at 37 C and the cooler at 4 C. When manually shaking the chamber, place a heating coil in the waterbath and check the temperature.

5. As soon as the circuit is complete and if no air bubbles are observed in the system, adjust the pump speed (flow rate), according to Table 40-1-1. Begin recording the temperature in the chamber. The desired rate of heating is 2 C/minute until 37 C is reached (the time required to reach 37 C is approximately 5-8 minutes).

6. Begin shaking and start timing the digestion process.

7. If shaking by hand, gently mix the digestion chamber in order to mix its contents. If using the Ricordi Isolator, secure the chamber in the arm of the shaker.

8. Adjust the intensity of the shaking based on the age of the donor. Pancreata from young donors require more gentle shaking than organs from older donors.

9. During digestion, the temperature should not increase above or drop below 37 C. After the temperature in the chamber has reached 37 C, the digestion should continue for about 10-15 minutes.

10. After about 6-8 minutes of digestion or when tissue starts to accumulate in the 250-mL conical tube with the recirculating digest, take a 1-mL sample of the digest, place it in a 10 × 35 mm culture dish, and add a few drops of DTZ stain. Mix the sample to center the tissue in the culture dish, and observe it under a microscope.

11. During the digestion, take samples every 1-2 minutes; during the dilution phase, take samples every 5 minutes, depending on the amount of tissue left in the chamber. As the amount of tissue decreases, samples can be taken less frequently.

12. Record the start time of the digestion, digestion chamber temperature, and flow rate. As the digestion proceeds, fat cells are normally seen first, followed by ascinar and, later, an occasional islet.

13. Prepare for the dilution phase by preparing dilution and collection containers (1-L Erlenmeyer flasks). This step should be done in advance, while the digestion phase is still in progress.

14. Be cautious when making the decision to switch to the dilution/collection phase. Prolonged exposure to heat and enzymatic action can damage the islets. The decision to switch should be made:
    a. When most islets in the sample are free of the surrounding acinar tissue and have intact borders.
    b. When an increased amount of acinar is liberated from the digestion chamber, with the acinar component becoming finer—ie, smaller.

15. Use Tables 40-1-2 and 40-1-3 as a guide for switching to the dilution/collection phase. Document the time and temperature of the switch and other applicable observations.

16. When the digestion is judged complete, switch to the dilution phase of the islet isolation process.

17. Prepare collection containers in the following manner and keep them at 4 to 8 C before use:
    a. First collection container: 400 mL of RPMI-1640, 200 mL of 25% HSA, 200 units insulin (final concentration = 0.2 units/mL), and 10,000 units heparin (final concentration = 10 units/mL).
    b. Second collection container: 400 mL of RPMI-1640, 200 mL of 25% HSA, 200 units insulin (final concentration = 0.2 units/mL), and 10,000 units heparin (final concentration = 10 units/mL).
    c. Third collection container: 500 mL of RPMI-1640, 100 mL of 25% HSA, 200 units insulin (final concentration = 0.2 units/mL), and 10,000

Table 40-1-2. Timing of Switch to Dilution/Collection Phase

Factors	Ranges for Switching
Amount of acinar tissue Estimate the amount of tissue by centering the sample in the culture dish: • 6 = tissue covers the entire visual field at 40 ×power • 3 = tissue covers about one-half of the visual field • 0 = no tissue	3-6
Acinar tissue cluster diameter Estimate the diameter range of acinar tissue clusters observed in the sample (50-100, 50-300, 50-500 µm)	50 µm to 500 µm
Number of islets Estimate the number of islets in the sample (a rough visual count: 1-20, 30-50, etc)	>30 islets
Percentage of free islets Estimate the percentage of free islets (free islets vs the total number of islets in the sample: 25%, 50%, 90%, etc)	>50%
Percentage of overdigested (fragmented) islets Estimate the percentage of islets that are fragmented (fragmented islets vs the total number of islets in the sample: 10%, 15%, 50%, etc)	<25%
Quality of islets Grade the quality of the islets in the sample based on the criteria in Table 40-1-3 **Note:** Islet quality grade is not a criterion to switch but is a retrospective qualification of the islet quality at switch time.	

Table 40-1-3. Grading Islet Quality

Parameter	0 Points	1 Point	2 Points
Shape (3D)	flat/planar	in between	spherical
Border (2D)	irregular	in between	well rounded
Integrity	fragmented	in between	solid/compact
Single cells	many	a few	almost none
Diameter	all <100 µm	a few >200 µm	>10% >200 µm

• 9 to 10 points = A = outstanding-looking islets
• 7 to 8 points = B = good-looking islets
• 4 to 6 points = C = fair-looking islets
• 2 to 3 points = D = poor-looking islets
• 0 to 1 point = F = very poor-looking islets

units heparin (final concentration = 10 units/mL).

d. Fourth collection container: 500 mL of RPMI-1640, 100 mL of 25% HSA, 200 units insulin (final concentration = 0.2 units/mL), and 10,000 units heparin (final concentration = 10 units/mL).

e. If necessary, fill any additional collection containers with a sufficient volume of 25% HSA to provide a final concentration of 1.5%.

D. Dilution/Collection Phase

1. Immediately after the switch, remove the heating coil from the waterbath or adjust the Ricordi Isolator heater to 30 C, place the cooling coil in the cooling chamber, turn off the pump, and stop shaking the chamber. Simultaneously, place the end of the size-16 tubing into the dilution container with 3 L of dilution solution (RPMI-1640) and the end of the size-17 tubing into the first collection container with 400 mL of dilution solution and 200 mL of HSA to neutralize the effect of the enzyme.

2. Adjust the pump speed to provide faster flow of the dilution media according to Table 40-1-1 (225 mL/minute).

3. Begin shaking the chamber again.

4. During the dilution, the digest is no longer recirculated, but, rather, a fresh room-temperature dilution solution is introduced into the Ricordi chamber while its contents are collected in a collection container.

5. Pour the digest from the 250-mL conical tube into the collection container and rinse the conical tube with dilution media. Mix the contents of the collection container gently while collecting the first 250 mL of the digest.

6. Continue collecting the digest, making sure there is enough dilution solution in the dilution flask, until the dilution phase is complete.

7. When the first four collection containers are filled, the digest can be collected in 2-L flasks prefilled with 120 mL of 25%

HSA (or 1-L flask with 60 mL of 25% HSA).

Note: Ensure proper mixing of tissue and HSA during collection.

8. After the digest is collected, the tissue is washed and concentrated by centrifugation with progressive collection of the tissue pellets. Tissue recombination is performed in 250-mL conical tubes by the following method:

a. Decant the supernatant with a single smooth motion, making sure that the tissue pellet is visible at all times and is not dispersed. Leave a small amount of supernatant (approximately 5-10 mL) in the conical tube to resuspend the pellet.

b. Detach the pellets from the bottom of the conical tubes and combine in one conical tube. Gently resuspend the tissue in a small volume of supernatant left for this purpose. Avoid using a pipette unless absolutely necessary.

c. Centrifuge at $140 \times g$ for 3 to 4 minutes at 4 C.

d. Perform another wash by repeating the three steps above.

9. The dilution phase must continue *until islets are no longer detected in a sample.*

10. If, at any time during the dilution phase, tissue clumping is observed, treat the cells with DNAse as described below:

a. Resuspend the tissue with wash medium and bring it up to 200 mL.

b. Add 100 μL of DNAse.

c. Mix the collected tissue in the conical tube by gently inverting it a few times.

d. Filter the contents of the conical tube into another conical tube using an 800-μm sieve placed inside a plastic funnel.

e. Rinse the sieve a few times with dilution solution to make sure that no islets remain on the screen.

f. Centrifuge the conical tube at $140 \times g$ for 1 minute at 4 C.

g. After centrifugation, aspirate the supernatant and resuspend the tissue in fresh dilution solution.

11. When dilution is complete, weigh and record the weight of the undigested tissue. Do not subtract the weight of the undigested pancreas from the total weight of the pancreas.

12. After the second wash, resuspend the tissue in UW solution for continuous gradients or Eurocollins for discontinuous gradients. If the volume of the final pellet exceeds 25 mL, then bring the volume up to 200 mL with UW or 180 mL with Eurocollins. Using a positive displacement pipette, take two 100-μL samples for the prepurification count.

13. Incubate the digested tissue in the appropriate solution (UW solution for continuous gradients or Eurocollins for discontinuous gradients) in a sterile, closed, flat-bottom jar. Place the jar in a sterile ice bath.

    Note: If there is a large amount of tissue, the preparation may need to be divided into several aliquots for incubation and purification. Approximately 20-25 mL of tissue is processed during each COBE run, with either continuous or discontinuous gradients.

E. *Setup of the COBE 2991 Cell Processor for Purification*
1. Turn on the COBE 2991 and prime according to the operator's manual.
2. Open the Plexiglas cover by removing the metal latch. Remove the locking glass bowl cover, Plexiglas cover, and the underlying foam ring from the bowl area.
3. Place the COBE centrifuge bag inside the bowl according to the manufacturer's instructions.
4. Close the sliding Plexiglas cover and place the metal latch over the four posts and the rotating seal.
5. Turn the locking rod down to a locking position.
6. Place the tubing into the valve slots on the COBE, but *outside* the pinch valves, using the color coding to determine the tubing position.

7. Clamp or seal the yellow, purple, and blue tubing. Red and green tubing remains open or unclamped.
8. For continuous gradients:
   a. Connect one end of the size-16 tubing to the COBE line (pink color) and the other end to the port of the gradient maker.
   b. Connect both beakers of the gradient maker with size-17 tubing and clamp the tubing.
   c. Put a magnetic stirrer in the beaker of the gradient maker.
   d. Label seven 250-mL conical tubes with a layer number and COBE run number and fill each with 175 mL of wash solution.
9. For discontinuous gradients:
   a. Connect one end of the size-16 tubing to the pink tubing with the other end remaining in the 250-mL conical tube.
   b. Prepare the syringe/bag setup as follows:
      • In the BSC, set up a 60-cc wide-mouth syringe in a ring stand clamp, and remove its plunger.
      • Attach a sterile piece of silicone tubing (inside diameter = 6.4 mm) to the tip of the syringe. Connect the other end of the silicone tubing to the nonspiked end of the COBE coupler. Use the COBE coupler to spike the side port of the 600-mL transfer bag, and tie a loose knot in the tubing of the transfer bag.

F. *Islet Purification*
1. Continuous density gradients:
   a. Load 150 mL of 1.100 gradient at a speed of 300 mL/minute. While loading, the COBE must remain static. Check the COBE settings to ensure that:
      • SUPER OUT is "0."
      • SUPER OUT VOLUME is "Max."
      • RPM is "2400."
   b. Remove air from the COBE:
      • Press the START button.
      • Remove the tubing from the pump.
      • Press SUPER OUT.

- Increase the SUPER OUT VOLUME to the maximum and monitor flow.
- When fluid reaches the gradient maker, clamp the tube and press STOP.

c. Reattach the tubing to the pump and place 120 mL of 1.100 gradient in the front beaker of the gradient maker.

d. Place 130 mL of 1.077 gradient in the rear beaker and start the COBE.

e. Begin mixing gradients by starting the magnetic stirrer. Open the port between 1.100 and 1.077 gradient beakers.

f. Start the pump and load the gradients into the COBE bag at a speed of 50 mL/minute. Make sure not to disturb the gradients while loading to allow for proper layering of the gradients.

g. Slowly, tilt the 1.077 gradient beaker until the chamber is completely empty, to prevent air from entering the line, as the solution moves toward the outlet.

h. Close the connection between the 1.077- and 1.100-gradient beakers of the gradient maker to prevent air from entering the line.

i. Gradually, tilt the 1.100-gradient beaker before completely voiding it to prevent air from entering the line as the solution descends toward the outlet.

j. Before completely voiding the 1.100-gradient beaker, when the outlet is immersed in the final 1 to 2 mL of the gradient solution, gently add the cell suspension into the chamber.

k. Start loading the cell suspension into the COBE bag at a speed of 20 mL/minute. The pump can be stopped or slowed as necessary to prevent tissue backup. Larger tissue volumes may require slower speeds.

l. Gradually tilt the beaker holding the tissue before completely voiding it to prevent air from entering the line as

the cell suspension descends toward the outlet.

m. Load 20 mL of HBSS (with phenol red). Allow approximately 1 inch of air to enter the line before loading another 20 mL of HBSS.

n. Allow the HBSS to enter the COBE bag and simultaneously clamp the line between the COBE and the pump.

o. Release the air as follows:
- Clamp all open tubing.
- Remove the tubing from the peristaltic pump.
- Press SUPER OUT.
- Very slowly remove the clamp from the tubing leading to the gradient maker.

p. Allow the COBE to centrifuge in SUPER OUT mode for 5 minutes at 2400 rpm.
   Note: SUPER OUT speed must be set at 0.

q. Adjust SUPER OUT rate to 80 to 100 mL/minute. Collect and discard the first 100 mL collected. This fraction contains membrane balls.

r. Collect 50 mL of consecutive fractions in each of the seven 250-mL conical tubes prefilled with 175 mL of wash solution.

s. Islets are collected on the basis of their purity level:
- Purest islets in tubes labeled #1 through 3.
- Less pure islets in tubes labeled #4 and 5.
- Least pure islets in tubes labeled #6 and 7.

t. Using a 24-well plate, take 0.1- to 0.3-mL samples from each of the seven conical tubes for purity determination, mixing each sample with a few drops of DTZ stain.

u. Centrifuge the conical tubes at $280 \times g$ for 3 to 4 minutes at 4 C.

v. Using a vacuum pump, remove the supernatant and combine islet cells of similar purities (Table 40-1-4). Refill the tubes containing recombined islets with fresh wash medium and centrifuge at $140 \times g$ for 3 to 4 minutes at 4 C.

- Seal and cut the tubing leading to the COBE bag and remove the bag from the machine.
- Connect the COBE coupler to the port of the COBE bag and remove a sample of ~5 mL of the pellet. Stain the sample with DTZ and observe it under the microscope to determine whether any islets remain in the pellet. If a significant number of free islets are observed (>60,000 IEQ), collect the entire pellet in a 250-mL conical tube, wash it twice with the washing solution, and proceed to Step 2.

2. Rescue using discontinuous density gradients:
   a. The semiautomated method using the COBE 2991 cell processor is used for discontinuous gradient purification of islet tissue. Eurocollins-Ficoll gradients are used, with densities of 1.108, 1.096, and 1.037, prepared as 75-mL aliquots.
   b. When significant numbers of islets remain in the less pure layers and/or the pellet, rescue purification may be necessary to salvage unpurified islets.
   c. Combine layers with large tissue volumes and/or purities less than 40% with the pellet, and wash them twice (at $140 \times g$ and 4 C for 3 to 4 minutes each time) to remove any traces of Ficoll.

d. The purification procedure should be performed while maintaining tissue and purification gradients at 4 to 10 C. The discontinuous gradients are composed of Ficoll powder (Ficoll DL-400) dissolved in Eurocollins solution. Therefore, they are hyperosmolar, high in glucose, and highly viscous. These solutions can be damaging to metabolically active islets.

e. No more than 20 mL of tissue should be loaded on a single rescue gradient. After the tissue is well resuspended, the suspension is divided into two or more 250-mL conical tubes, depending on the tissue volume (eg, if the total digest pellet is 35 to 40 mL, divide it equally between two conical tubes).

f. Resuspend the tissue in 300 mL of stock Ficoll solution (1.132 density). First, resuspend the tissue in the 50 mL of stock Ficoll, then slowly add another 150 mL of Ficoll, and continue to resuspend the tissue, not leaving any clumps.

g. Prepare the syringe/bag setup in the BSC as follows:
   - Place a wide-mouth syringe in a ring stand and remove the syringe plunger.
   - Connect the syringe to the side port of a sterile 600-mL transfer bag using a COBE coupler and size-17 tubing splice.
   - Make a loose knot in the tubing of the bag.

Table 40-1-4. Combining Islet Cells

Purity	Combine or Separate?
80% to 100% (volume <2 mL)	Can be combined together
50% to 79% (volume <3 mL)	Can be combined together
30% to 49%	Can be combined together
Below 30%	Culture separately

h. Load the first 200 mL of the Ficoll-tissue suspension into the 600-mL transfer bag, using a 60-cc wide-mouth syringe. Allow the tissue to flow into the transfer bag by gravity, without applying any pressure.

i. Rinse the conical tube that contains the tissue with Ficoll stock solution, using another 100 mL of stock Ficoll. The plunger may be used to force the stock Ficoll into the bag once all of the tissue has passed through. Tighten the loose knot in the bag line and/or heat-seal the line.

j. Remove the transfer bag with the tissue from the BSC and hang it on the side of the COBE cell processor. Spike the transfer bag with the COBE tubing, using a central port. Clamp all COBE bag tubing lines using hemostats.

k. Load the COBE bag into the COBE machine as described above.

l. Unclamp the line attached to the transfer bag so that the tissue flows from the transfer bag into the COBE bag in the centrifuge bowl.

m. While tissue is loading, fill four conical tubes with 125 mL of wash solution to collect purified islet fractions. Label the tubes as follows: "Hanks," "1," "2," "3."

n. At the same time, prepare a peristaltic pump, feeding sterile size-16 silicone tubing through it, so that one end of the tube is resting in the 1.108 gradient, while the other is connected to the COBE tubing.

o. Once the tissue is in the COBE bag, clamp the tubing attached to the transfer bag, and unclamp the tubing attached to the size-16 silicone tubing placed in the 1.108 gradient. Start the pump, and pump the 1.108 gradient up to the T-junction of the COBE tubing attached to the COBE bag.

p. When the solution reaches the T-junction, stop the pump and clamp the COBE tubing connected to the silicone tube. Unclamp the tubing

line connected to the transfer bag and remove the air in the centrifuge bag as follows:

• Set the COBE speed to 2000 rpm. The speed should be maintained at this setting throughout the whole procedure.

• Hit the START button.

• When the centrifuge reaches 2000 rpm, push the SUPER OUT button.

• Immediately adjust the SUPER OUT rate to 150 mL/minute. At this time, the solution will be pushed up through the COBE tubing toward the T-junction.

• Clamp the tubing connected to the transfer bag as the solution reaches the T-junction and simultaneously press the STOP/RESET button.

• When the machine stops, reset the SUPER OUT rate to "0" and press the START button again.

q. When the COBE has attained the desired speed, unclamp the COBE tubing connected to the size-16 silicone tubing, start the pump, and begin pumping the density gradient solutions at a rate of approximately 90 mL/minute. This step is accomplished by placing a free end of size-16 silicone tubing in a bottle or conical tube containing a density gradient and moving the tubing to the next designated container when the previous gradient solution has been loaded into the COBE bag. When moving size-16 silicone tubing from one gradient to another, the pump should be stopped to avoid introducing air into the COBE processor. Discontinuous gradients should be loaded in the following order:

• Load 75 mL of 1.108-density gradient on top of the 300-mL Ficoll suspension containing the pellet and other unpurified tissue.

• Load 75 mL of 1.096-density gradient on top of the 1.108 layer.

- Load 75 mL of 1.037-density gradient on top of the 1.096 density layer.
- Load 50 mL of HBSS (with phenol red) until the fluid/air interface reaches midway down the tubing leading to the rotating seal. HBSS with phenol red removes proteins deposited on the rotating seal and allows improved visibility of different layers during tissue collection.

r. After all the gradients are loaded and the rotating seal is rinsed with HBSS, turn off the pump, clamp the tubing connected to the size-16 silicone tube, adjust the SUPER OUT rate to 0, open the pump head, and completely release the tubing from the pump head. Press SUPER OUT, immediately opening the tube leading to the transfer bag to relieve the excess pressure. Reclamp the tubing. Allow the COBE to spin for 3 minutes.

s. During the COBE 3-minute centrifugation, four fractions become visible and are collected:
- The first layer has a volume of 100 to 125 mL. Collect this layer in the conical tube labeled "Hanks." When the layer reaches the inside metal rim, wait 3 seconds, press HOLD, and move the tubing to the next conical tube labeled "1."
- When 75 mL are collected or the layer reaches the inside metal rim, wait 3 seconds, press HOLD, and then move the tubing to the next conical tube labeled "2."
- When 75 mL are collected or the layer reaches the inside metal rim, wait 3 seconds, press HOLD, and transfer the tubing to the conical tube labeled "3."
- Collect 100 mL of fraction "3" and press STOP/RESET.

t. Take a sample of ~0.1 to 0.3 mL from each fraction collected, stain with DTZ, and observe the samples under the microscope to determine the purity of each layer.

u. Discard the "Hanks" fraction after confirming that it does not contain islets, and keep the fractions labeled "1," "2," and "3."

v. Centrifuge the tubes at $280 \times g$ for 3 to 4 minutes at 4 C (first wash).

w. Subsequent washes (rescued islets should be washed at least twice), using washing media, should be centrifuged at $140 \times g$ for 3 to 4 minutes at 4 C.

x. Determine which tubes can be combined and take counting samples for each layer.

y. Culture the islet layers that are <40% pure and have low tissue volume.

G. Islet Cell Enumeration

Determine the islet count, islet purity, and percentage of trapped or embedded islets (see Section VIII).

H. Islet Cell Culture

1. If clumping is observed before or during the culture, treat the cells with DNAse.
2. Label each flask with the identification number, purity, date, in-process label, the number of islets cultured, and the fraction number.
3. Culture the islets in supplemented CMRL1066 for 24 to 48 hours before transplantation.
   a. "Pure" islets (70% to 100%) are cultured overnight at 37 C, with 95% air and 5% CO_2. Following the initial incubation, pure islets are transferred to 22 C, with 95% air and 5% CO_2, for the remaining 24 to 48 hours.
   b. Islets of lower purities (<70%) are cultured at 22 C, with 95% air and 5% CO_2, for the entire duration of culture.
4. The concentration at which the islets should be cultured is approximately 20,000 IEQ per 30 mL medium, in a 175-cm² TC-treated flask. Cell culture in flasks allows for the detection of contamination before transplantation. The num-

ber of culture flask required is based on purity and is determined as follows:

a. For preparations with purity >70%:
- IEQ per flask = 20,000 × (purity/100)
- Number of flasks needed* = total IEQ ÷ (IEQ per flask × % purity)

*Round up to next whole number

> **Example:** 500,000 IEQ isolated with 90% purity:
> - IEQ per flask = 20,000 × (90/100) = 18,000
> - **Number of flasks required** 500,000 ÷ (20,000 × 0.09) = **27.8 Therefore, 28 flasks are needed.**

b. For preparations with purity ≤70%:
- IEQ per flask = 20,000 × (purity/100)
- Number of flasks required* = [Total IEQ ÷ (IEQ per flask × purity/100)] + [(total packed volume/0.1 mL)/2]

*Round up to next whole number

> **Example:** 100,000 IEQ isolated with 70% purity and a total packed volume of 2.5mL
> - IEQ per flask = 20,000 × (70/100) = 14,000
> - **Number of flasks required** = [100,000 ÷ 14,000] + [(2.5 mL/0.1 mL)/2] = [7.14] + [(12.5)] = **19.6 Therefore, 20 flasks are needed.**

> **Note:** Some facilities adjust culture parameters for purity ≤70% as in this example and others adjust culture conditions such as incubation time and/or temperature.

5. Add enough culture medium to the beaker containing the islets that the number of islets to be cultured per flask is resuspended in 10 mL of medium (eg, if five flasks are to be cultured, the pellet should be resuspended in a total volume of 50 mL of culture medium).

6. When transferring resuspended islets to culture flasks, follow these steps:
   a. Gently resuspend the islet cells by using a wide-mouth 10-mL pipette.
   b. Aliquot 2 mL of islet cell suspension from a 100-mL beaker containing the resuspended islets, and transfer it into a culture flask. Repeat the process five times. The total volume transferred into each tissue-culture flask should be 10 mL.
   c. Do not allow the islet cells to settle at any time. Ensure that the cells are well resuspended by continuous mixing.
      Note: Even distribution of islets during culture plays a very important role in islet viability and recovery.
7. Add enough supplemented CMRL 1066 medium to each flask to total 30 mL.
8. Cap all flasks and place in the 37-C or 22-C CO_2 incubator (depending on the islet purity), with the T-neck up to prevent leakage.

I. *Media Change*
1. Inspect all flasks after the first 24 hours of culture.
2. After inspection, place all the flasks in the BSC, tilt each flask at a 45-degree angle, and allow islet cells to settle for 2 to 3 minutes.
3. Aseptically remove 20 mL of culture medium and replace it with fresh supplemented CMRL 1066.
4. Return all flasks to the 22-C CO_2 incubator for another 24 to 48 hours.

References/Resources

1. London AJM, James RFL, Bell PRF. Islet purification. In: Ricordi C, ed. Pancreatic islet cell transplantation:1882-1992, one century of transplantation for diabetes. Austin, TX: RG Landes Company, 1992:113-23.
2. Ricordi C, Rastellini C. Automated method for pancreatic islet separation. In: Ricordi C, ed. Methods in cell transplantation. Austin, TX: RG Landes Company, 1995: 433-8.

Method 40-2. Preparing Pancreatic Digestion Media: SERVA Enzyme Preparation

Description

This method describes how to prepare the enzyme solution for digestion of human pancreatic tissue.

Equipment

1. Biological safety cabinet.
2. Sterile media bottle (500 mL).
3. Bottle top filter (500-mL, 0.22-μm cellulose acetate filter).
4. Cooling block or (if block is unavailable) sterile, wet ice slush.
5. 25-mL sterile serologic pipette.

Supplies

1. Hank's Balanced Salt Solution (HBSS) 1× + 10 units/mL heparin: ~345 mL.
2. Sterile water for injection: 10 mL.
3. 1 M 4-(2-hydroxyethyl)-1-piperazineethane-sulfonic acid (HEPES): 35 mL.
4. $CaCl_2$ anhydrous [molecular weight (MW) = 110.99]: 0.39 g; or $CaCl_2.2H_2O$ (MW = 147.02): 0.52 g.
5. Collagenase NB 1, good manufacturing practice (GMP) grade, lyophilized (SERVA): see Procedure (C) below to calculate quantity.
6. Neutral protease NB, GMP grade, lyophilized (SERVA): see Procedure D below to calculate quantity.

Procedure

A. *Collagenase NB 1 Reconstitution*
1. *About 45 minutes before perfusion,* add 10 mL of HBSS, 1× + heparin to one vial of collagenase NB 1.
2. Let collagenase dissolve at 2 to 8 C (about 30 minutes). Swirl gently and occasionally.

B. *Calcium Chloride, 11 mM*
1. Add 0.39 g $CaCl_2$ (or 0.52 g $CaCl_2.2H_2O$) to a 50-mL sterile conical tube.
2. Add 35 mL of 1 M HEPES to the 50-mL conical tube and mix to dissolve.
3. Filter the $CaCl_2$ solution through a 0.22-μm filter into a sterile 500-mL bottle.

C. *Collagenase NB-1*
1. Calculate the volume of collagenase NB-1 solution to use in order to have 1600 units:

$$\frac{1600 \text{ collagenase units}}{\text{collagenase units/vial}} \times 10 \text{ mL} = \underline{\quad} \text{ mL of collagenase needed}$$

2. Add the calculated volume of dissolved collagenase NB-1 (1600 units) to the sterile 500-mL bottle.

D. *Reconstituting Neutral Protease NB Just Before Use*
1. Add 10 mL of sterile water for injection to one vial of neutral protease NB and mix to dissolve.
2. Calculate the volume of neutral protease NB solution to use in order to have 200 units:

$$\frac{200 \text{ neutral protease NB units}}{\text{neutral protease units/vial}} \times 10 \text{ mL} = \underline{\quad} \text{ mL of neutral protease NB needed}$$

3. Add the calculated volume of dissolved neutral protease NB (200 units), or the entire 10 mL if there are less than 200 units/vial, to the sterile 500-mL bottle immediately before the start of perfusion.
4. Add enough HBSS, 1× + heparin to the 500-mL bottle to bring the volume to 350 mL. Swirl gently to mix.

5. Label the bottle with the following:
   - "Enzyme Solution."
   - "Store at 2 C to 8 C."
   - Date and time prepared.
   - Expiration date and time (one-half hour after preparation).
   - Initials of the person who prepared the solution.

Quality Control

1. If the final islet preparation is reported to be contaminated, the sample of prepared enzyme should be cultured for bacterial and fungal contamination. The extent of contamination and the likelihood of it affecting transplanted islets should be determined, and appropriate corrective actions should be taken.

2. Certificates of analysis should be retained for all preparations, and the enzyme should be used only if it meets the release criteria.

3. Lot numbers and expiration dates of all media should be checked and recorded.

References/Resources

1. Package insert. SERVA collagenase and NP. Heidelberg, Germany: Nordmark/SERVA.

2. Standards for tissue banking. 12th ed. McLean, VA: American Association of Tissue Banks, 2008.

Method 40-3. Preparing Pancreatic Digestion Enzyme: Collagenase and Thermolysin

Description

This method describes how to prepare collagenase and Thermolysin to digest human pancreatic tissue.

Equipment

1. Biological safety cabinet.
2. Sterile media bottle (500 mL).
3. Bottle top filter (500-mL, 0.22-μm cellulose acetate filter).
4. Cooling block or (if block is unavailable) sterile wet ice slush.
5. 25-mL sterile serologic pipette.

Supplies

1. Collagenase and Thermolysin purified enzyme blend (Roche, Indianapolis, IN).
2. Perfusion solution: 350 mL (Mediatech, Indianapolis, IN; #99-781-CV).

Procedure

1. Place the cooling block or (if necessary) sterile ice slush inside the flow hood and keep the perfusion solution on ice.
2. Remove enzymes (collagenase and Thermolysin) from the –70-C freezer and place on ice. Climatize for approximately 2 to 5 minutes and reconstitute with the cold perfusion solution (30-50 mL). Gently swirl the bottle every 5 minutes for 30 to 45 minutes, visually inspecting the solution to be sure all the enzyme is dissolved. (Be careful not to promote foaming.)
3. When the enzyme is dissolved, pre-wet the sterile cellulose acetate filter with a 30- to 50-mL aliquot of cold perfusion solution. Keep the bottle and top filter on ice during filtering.

4. Pour the enzyme solution onto the filter and rinse the enzyme bottles a minimum of three times with the cold perfusion solution (30-50 mL each time). Pour these rinses also onto the filter slowly, and then pour additional perfusion solution through the sterile filter (to be sure all enzyme is rinsed through), until the total volume of the collagenase enzyme preparation is approximately 350 mL.
5. Label the bottle with the words "Enzyme Solution" and the date, and keep it in the cooling block or on ice until required. Use it within 2 hours of final preparation.
6. Aseptically transfer a 1- to 5-cc sample from the bottle into a sterile tube, label it appropriately, and date and save it in the refrigerator for bacterial and fungal cultures if they are indicated.

Quality Control

1. If the final islet preparation is reported to be contaminated, the sample of prepared enzyme should be cultured for bacterial and fungal contamination. The extent of contamination and the likelihood of it affecting transplanted islets should be determined, and appropriate corrective actions should be taken.
2. Certificates of analysis should be retained for all preparations, and the enzyme should be used only if it meets the release criteria.
3. Lot numbers and expiration dates of all media should be checked and recorded.

References/Resources

1. Package insert. Roche collagenase, Thermolysin: Purified enzyme blend for human islet isolation. Indianapolis, IN: Roche Diagnostics Corporation.
2. Standards for tissue banking. 12th ed. McLean, VA: American Association of Tissue Banks, 2008.

In: Areman EM, Loper K, eds
Cellular Therapy: Principles, Methods, and Regulations
Bethesda, MD: AABB, 2009

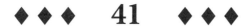

Biorepositories

Kathy Loper, MHS, MT(ASCP), and Melissa Croskell, MT(ASCP)

OWING TO THEIR ABILITY TO FREEZE, store, and effectively track human products, cellular therapy (CT) laboratories may be asked to assist with or manage biorepositories. The term *biorepository* most often refers to the physical entity that stores biospecimens that are intended for research purposes. The specimens may be tissue, urine, blood, or other human material, including white blood cells. The nearly limitless list of sources of specimens includes biopsies, blood samples, tissue, bone, skin, organs, gametes, or waste material such as nail clippings or placenta. Portions or aliquots of a biospecimen are referred to as *samples*. The *biospecimen resource* is the collection of specimens, their associated data, the physical entity where the samples are stored, and all of the relevant processes and procedures. These libraries of samples and their associated data vary widely in their size, material, and purpose. However, their usefulness may be limited by several parameters, including collection methods and subsequent handling, the quality of the associated data, and ethical and legal policies. The lack of standardization in this field has, at times, resulted in decreased efficiency of research and unreliable conclusions.

Introduction

Biomolecular technology has experienced unprecedented advances in recent years. These advances in analytical tools have increased the power and precision associated with cancer research, diagnosis, and treatment—accelerating the drive toward personalized medicine. In this rush of technology and information, the human specimens, serving as analytical sources, have emerged as a critical resource for these new technology platforms, for both basic and translational research. These samples are often the source for molecular data used to detect cancer and develop therapies. The reliability of these platforms depends on the quality and integrity of the source biospecimens. The increased need for quality and increasing collaborative efforts among researchers have led to a move toward standardization.

Kathy Loper, MHS, MT(ASCP), Director, Cellular Therapies, AABB, Bethesda, Maryland; Melissa Croskell, MT(ASCP), Manager of Regulatory Compliance, Department of Pathology and Laboratory Services, and BMT Program Quality Manager, The Children's Hospital–Aurora, Aurora, Colorado

The authors have disclosed no conflicts of interest.

History

The National Cancer Institute (NCI) has been performing due diligence in this arena since 2002 in its efforts to understand the state of its funded biospecimen resources and the quality of the samples used in its cancer research initiatives. What began as a series of community forums has expanded to several publications, including the *National Biospecimen Network Blueprint and Case Studies of Existing Human Tissue Repositories,* numerous working committees, and, most recently, the *NCI Best Practices for Biospecimen Resources.*[1] The NCI formed the Office of Biorepositories and Biospecimen Research (OBBR) to address these and other related issues, including informed consent and privacy protection of patients who may decide to donate their unused samples to research projects.

These developments have not been confined to the United States. The International Society for Biological and Environmental Repositories (ISBER) was formed in 2000 to provide information and guidance on the safe and effective management of specimen collections. As stated on ISBER's website, "Careful management ensures the collections are available for study as new biomarkers emerge and more sensitive measurement technologies become pertinent."[2] The organization published a consensus document of its own best practices.[3] The European Blood and Marrow Transplantation (EBMT) and European School of Hematology (ESH) have held biobanking conferences, as have many individual countries, in efforts to understand the scale and nature of the biospecimen resources and to establish standardization. Great Britain and Norway plan to cooperate on biobank-based research into attention deficit hyperactivity disorder (ADHD), autism, schizophrenia, and diabetes. Samples from between 200,000 and 300,000 individuals are estimated for this project. An additional 500,000 volunteers will participate in a British lifestyles database, which includes blood and urine samples for research on heart disease. Japan, Estonia, Mexico, and Sweden all have their own plans and banks.[4]

There are already some success stories from research on samples from biorepositories. The development of trastuzumab (Herceptin, Genentech, South San Francisco, CA) for treating breast cancer is one such story. Human epidermal growth factor receptor 2 (EGFR-2) normally controls aspects of cell growth and division. The compound was shown in tumor samples (from the NCI Cooperative Breast Cancer Tissue Resource) to be amplified in 20% to 30% of breast cancer cases. The development of an antibody to this receptor (Herceptin) as a therapeutic treatment might not have succeeded if it had been tested on the general breast cancer patient population. The biospecimens, however, pointed researchers toward a targeted, highly effective therapy for a subpopulation of breast cancer patients. Secondly, Gleevec (Novartis, East Hanover, NJ) was originally developed for the treatment of a form of leukemia by targeting the BCR-ABL protein. After conducting molecular profiling studies on biospecimens collected from different tumor types, investigators discovered that a mutant form of KIT, a protein related to BCR-ABL, is responsible for the progression of a rare but deadly type of cancer, gastrointestinal stromal tumors (GIST). This led to the hypothesis that Gleevec could be used to treat GIST, and subsequent clinical trials confirmed the effectiveness of this new indication for Gleevec.[5]

Technical Points to Consider

Most of the best practices deal with principles, rather than procedures, that should be in place. Table 41-1 describes some items for consideration in technical and operational practice in biorepositories. The list will look familiar to most CT professionals because it contains many quality system essentials.

Other considerations that are outside the scope of this text include the following:

1. The collection and management of clinical data.
2. Bioinformatic support.
3. Quality assurance (QA) and quality control (QC) policies.
4. Standard operating procedure (SOP) manual for all procedures and policies.
5. Biosafety practices.
6. Electronic data management and tracking (including validation).
7. Ethical and legal policies.

Table 41-1. Technical and Operational Considerations

Task	Considerations
Identify samples to be collected.	Prioritize the samples based on the purpose and type of research. Diversity and demographics should be appropriate for the research goals.
Define collection and processing methods.	Minimize the time interval for each step. Collect critical data relating to the collection and processing steps. For tissues, decrease the temperature as soon as possible. Optimal processing times vary according to the source of the sample. The processing methods should be selected to preserve the greatest number of analytes, unless the protocol specifies a specific agent.
Employ qualified personnel.	Personnel should be aware of their purpose, goals, and role in the project. They should be qualified and trained according to SOP. For surgical and biopsy specimens, a pathologist should determine which portion of the sample is necessary for diagnosis and which can be banked. Patient care should not be compromised.
Store samples appropriately.	Standardized protocols and storage conditions should be used. Avoid unnecessary thawing and refreezing. Inventory tracking and sample retrieval procedures should be in place. Sample type, anticipated length of storage, study goals, temperature, and humidity controls should be considered. For large-scale studies, whole blood, rather than fractionated, is cost effective. Storage vessels and containers including the vial size and number of each, volume, and container closures should be considered. Labeling and printing systems should be appropriate to both the duration of storage and temperature conditions. Each sample should contain a unique identifier on the label. The inventory system should include the specific location of each sample in each position in the freezer, including shelf, box location, etc. Continuous monitoring and backup storage should be in place.
Create unique identifiers for specimens.	The identifier should be tied to all other data relating to specimens, including consent and confidentiality.
Use effective shipping procedures.	SOPs should be in place. Consider the climate at both the shipping and receiving locations. Use tested, qualified shipping containers and materials. The number of biospecimens may affect the temperature of the shipped package. Documentation of the shipment should include the confirmation of receipt, tracking number, description and quantity of samples, condition upon arrival, study name or details, investigator's name, and recipient's signature. ISBER recommendations and IATA regulations may apply. International regulations may also apply for international shipments. Consult OSHA for toxic and hazardous substance labeling. Shipping staff should be trained appropriately.

SOP = standard operating procedure; ISBER = International Society for Biological and Environmental Repositories; IATA = International Air Transport Association; OSHA = Occupational Safety and Health Administration.

8. Custodianship.
9. Informed consent.
10. Privacy protection.
11. Access to data by other researchers and the public.
12. Intellectual property and resource sharing.
13. Research review board oversight.

Data Management

Data management considerations include the following:
1. Ability to expand data analysis capability.
2. The need to share samples and data between disparate organizations.
3. Security needs.
4. Data integrity—manual logs vs electronic logs.
5. Access privileges.
6. Maintenance and backup.
7. Training and ease of use.
8. Validation—system and entry testing.

The NCI has developed a prototype database that is a stand-alone system but also permits the integration of other researchers' data. The bioinformatics component of Biomedical Informatics Grid (caBIG, NCI, Bethesda, MD) is in its fifth year at the time of this printing and includes two free, open software tools, as well as an option for external connection. All of these data could serve as fertile ground for private-sector computer giants who are expected to propose solutions to tackle the large amounts of data that have yet to be collected. Most of the technologies to manage these samples exist, and software developers may soon take advantage of the opportunities biorepositories present.

Ethical and Legal Issues

The data associated with biospecimens are often clinical, demographic, and, therefore, private in nature. Information gathering is best viewed as a process, rather than as a single document—although documentation is critical to the process. It is imperative that donors provide informed consent for their donations, receive appropriate information on the study, and understand how their information will be protected.[6] In the United States, the Health Insurance Portability and Accountability Act (HIPAA) aims to standardize electronic data exchanged in health-care transactions, specify security requirements for stored or exchanged protected health information, and establish privacy regulations for protected health information. This last category places many requirements on the collection and transmission of the clinical annotations on biospecimens for research. (It is the data or information, rather than the tissues themselves, that are subject to HIPAA.) A number of HIPAA regulations ease the burden on research. "The Common Rule" is the section of the *Code of Federal Regulations* governing patient protection for research conducted with federal funds and the sites that conduct research that is supported with federal funds. Thus, the code effectively applies to every US academic medical center. The code delineates requirements for conducting ethically sound research using federal funds—requirements such as informed consent, institutional review boards (IRBs), deidentifying samples, etc.

Experts debate the terms "ownership" and "custodianship," with a trend toward using the latter in relation to biospecimens—clarifying that the research community's role toward these samples is more that of steward than owner. Intellectual property, conflicts of interest, and the development of new therapies should all be addressed in the consent process, and each institution may have specific language requirements regarding these issues. Ownership in the event of investigator relocation has been debated and is the subject of at least one court case. Gifting rules and the relinquishment of ownership laws often apply at the state level. The court dockets list several cases, including *Tilousi vs The Arizona Board of Regents,* in which Havasupai Tribe members donated blood for a diabetes study, but the samples were used to study schizophrenia and population genetics. The plaintiffs stated they would not have donated the samples had they known the intent of the studies.[7]

The Patient Perspective

Numerous studies and surveys have shown that most patients intend for all qualified researchers to have open access to their samples when donated for a particular purpose, rather than that access be limited to an individual researcher. The privilege of custodianship carries a responsibility to honor donors' wishes. Collaborative efforts to share specimens and their related data at both national and international levels support donors' wishes for wide access to samples.

Current Status

The NCI has developed the cancer caBIG to create infrastructure that will facilitate the exchange of data and access to programs among cancer investigators. Information tools to support the collection, annotation, storage, and dissemination of high-quality specimens are also in the final stages of development. In addition, the project includes guidance on uniform, nonredundant sample nomenclature; tracking procedures; and informatics systems to support queries. These tools will be publicly available to all biospecimen resources. A self-evaluation process or tool is also planned to allow individual researchers to monitor and improve the quality management systems of individual biobanks. Finally, the NCI has launched the Biospecimen Research Network (BRN) to generate data for evidence-based methodologies. The BRN will examine such items as how DNA, RNA, and protein analyses are affected by individual preacquisition and postacquisition variables. To the extent that SOPs are developed, the focus should be on preserving—to the greatest degree possible—the quality of the analytes of interest. All of these tools, including the data search, will be Web based.

The Future

The diversity of biological samples that could potentially be banked is almost limitless, but the resources for banking them are not. Individual biorepositories will need to determine what materials they should bank and for what purposes. Validated systems for data and inventory management must be developed and maintained. Although operating and maintaining biorepositories involve many challenges, biorepositories provide opportunities for the discovery of new therapies and diagnostic assays.

References/Resources

1. National Cancer Institute. OBBR: Office of Biorepositories and Biospecimen Research. Bethesda, MD: Office of Biorepositories and Biospecimen Research, 2009. [Available at http://biospecimens.cancer.gov/index.asp (accessed April 1, 2009).]

2. International Society for Biological and Environmental Repositories. About ISBER. Bethesda, MD: ISBER, 2009. [Available at http://www.isber.org/aboutisber.html (accessed April 1, 2009).]

3. Aamodt R, Anouna A, Baird P, et al. Best practices for repositories I: Collection, storage, and retrieval of human biological materials for research. Cell Preserv Technol 2005;3:5-48.

4. Medicine's new central bankers. Economist Technology Quarterly 2005;18-19.

5. National Cancer Institute. FAQs—NCI and biorepositories. Are there examples of how well-characterized biospecimens can accelerate cancer research? Bethesda, MD: Office of Biorepositories and Biospecimen Research. [Available at http://biospecimens.cancer.gov/patientcorner/faq.asp (accessed April 1, 2009).]

6. Eiseman E, Bloom G, Brower J, et al. Case studies of existing human tissue repositories: "Best practices" for a biospecimen resource for the genomic and proteomic era. Santa Monica, CA: RAND, 2003.

7. Tilousi vs The Arizona Board of Regents (No. 04-CV-1290-PCT-FJM). [See http://www.whoownsyourbody.org/havasupai-arizona.pdf (accessed April 1, 2009).]

In: Areman EM, Loper K, eds
Cellular Therapy: Principles, Methods, and Regulations
Bethesda, MD: AABB, 2009

◆◆◆ 42 ◆◆◆

Regenerative Medicine Approaches for Cellular and Tissue Therapies

Bryan Tillman, MD, PhD; Jennifer L. Olson, PhD; and James J. Yoo, MD, PhD

THE FIELD OF REGENERATIVE MEDICINE encompasses many scientific and medical disciplines, such as tissue engineering, stem cells, and cloning. It focuses primarily on developing biological substitutes that could restore and maintain normal cell, tissue, and organ function. Regenerative medicine strategies include the use of biomaterials, which depend on the body's natural ability to use the material as a scaffold on which to regenerate functional tissue, and the use of matrices combined with cells to form functional tissues and organs when introduced into the living host.

Biomaterials used in regenerative medicine may serve as cell carriers, provide structural support for tissue formation, or deliver macromolecules to target locations. Biomaterials can be fabricated from synthetic materials, naturally derived substances, or both, and they can be configured into liquid, gel, or solid forms, depending on the specific needs. Biomaterials alone or combined with cells can be introduced into the host via injection or implantation. Cells used in regenerative medicine can be derived from autologous, allogeneic, or xenogeneic sources, and cells at various developmental stages, from embryonic stem cells (ESCs) to fully differentiated somatic cells, are being used. This chapter presents some of the investigative approaches aimed at improving, replacing, or restoring normal tissue function using regenerative medicine strategies.

Components of Regenerative Medicine

Biomaterials

Biomaterials are an essential component of regenerative medicine, and they can be used alone or with cells, depending on the therapeutic goals. Biomaterials are designed to replicate the biological and physico-mechanical functions of the native

Bryan Tillman, MD, PhD, Clinical Fellow, Department of Vascular and Endovascular Surgery, Wake Forest University School of Medicine; Jennifer L. Olson, PhD, Medical Writer, Wake Forest Institute for Regenerative Medicine, Wake Forest University School of Medicine; James J. Yoo, MD, PhD, Associate Professor, Wake Forest Institute for Regenerative Medicine, Wake Forest University School of Medicine, Winston-Salem, North Carolina

The authors have disclosed no conflicts of interest.

extracellular matrix (ECM) found in tissues in the body by serving as an artificial ECM. Biomaterials provide a three-dimensional environment for the cells to attach and form new tissues with appropriate structure and function. Because the majority of mammalian cell types are anchorage-dependent, biomaterials provide a cell-adhesion substrate that can deliver cells to specific sites in the body with adequate loading efficiency.

Biomaterials can also provide structural support against in-vivo forces so that the predefined three-dimensional structure is maintained during tissue development. Furthermore, bioactive signals, such as cell-adhesion peptides and growth factors, can be incorporated along with cells to help regulate cellular function.[1] Cell behavior in the newly formed tissue can be regulated by multiple interactions of the cells with their microenvironment, including interactions with cell-adhesion ligands and with soluble growth factors.[2] Some materials are designed to carry these factors into the body and release them at a specified rate to assist the cells in the organizational process.

The ideal biomaterial should be biodegradable and bioresorbable to support the replacement of normal tissue only as long as necessary and with minimal inflammation. Materials that are incompatible with the body's microenvironment are destined for an inflammatory or foreign-body response that eventually leads to graft failure. Commonly used biomaterials in regenerative medicine include 1) naturally derived materials (eg, collagen and alginate),[3,4] 2) acellular tissue matrices (eg, bladder submucosa and small intestinal submucosa),[5-8] and 3) synthetic polymers [eg, polyglycolic acid (PGA), polylactic acid (PLA), and poly(lactic-co-glycolic acid) (PLGA)].[9-11] These classes of biomaterials have been tested for their biocompatibility.[12,13] However, their utility depends on various factors, such as the type and function of target application, because each biomaterial has its innate properties. Naturally derived materials and acellular tissue matrices have the potential advantage of biological recognition. However, synthetic polymers can be prepared reproducibly on a large scale with controlled properties such as strength, degradation rate, and microstructure.

Cells

One limitation of cell-based tissue-engineering techniques has been the difficulty of growing specific cell types in large quantities. Even in the case of organs, such as the liver, that have a high regenerative capacity in vivo, in-vitro expansion of cells derived from these organs proved to be difficult. However, the discovery of privileged sites for committed precursor cells in specific organs and extensive study of the conditions that promote precursor cell maintenance and differentiation within these sites have begun to overcome some of the limitations associated with cell expansion in vitro.

Urothelial cells that are present in the bladder, for instance, have been grown in culture in the past, but with only limited success. However, several novel culture protocols have been developed over the past two decades that allow the maintenance of precursor cells in an undifferentiated state. Because these cells can remain in the growth phase, the ability to expand urothelial cultures is vastly improved.[14-17] These studies suggest that it may be possible to collect autologous urothelial cells from human bladders, expand them in culture, and return them to the donor in sufficient quantities for reconstructive purposes.[14,16-20] In addition to urothelial cells, methods to induce the in-vitro expansion of a variety of primary human cells have been developed, making the use of autologous cells for clinical applications a real possibility, though there are still hurdles to overcome.

Use of autologous cells has been the preferred source for regenerative medicine therapies because of the lack of immunologic problems, such as rejection and prolonged immunosuppressive treatments. However, there are instances where autologous cells are unavailable because of extensive damage or total loss of the tissue to be regenerated. Other cell sources, such as allogeneic and xenogeneic cells, have been proposed for regenerative medicine therapies. However, these cells have been frequently encapsulated in microspheres to protect them from host immune cells.

Stem and progenitor cells have been an attractive cell source for these situations. Stem cells can be derived from different stages of development and they are able to undergo self-renewal that can result in large quantities of undifferentiated cells. Moreover, these cells have the ability to differentiate into many specialized cell types.[21-23] For example, human ESCs can develop into cells comprising all three embryonic germ layers in vitro.[24] Skin and neurons have been formed, indicating ectodermal differentiation.[25-27] Blood, cardiac, cartilage, endothelial, and muscle cells have been produced, indicating mesodermal differentiation.[28-30] Finally, pancreatic cells and other cell types have been formed, indicating endodermal differentiation.[31] Other stem cell sources that have been proposed and used for regenerative medicine therapies include fetal and amniotic fluid, umbilical cord blood, and adult stem cells.[32-39]

Nuclear transfer, or cloning, can serve as another source of pluripotent "stem" cells that could possibly be used for regenerative medicine therapies. Two types of cloning procedures exist—reproductive cloning and therapeutic cloning. Banned in most countries for human applications, reproductive cloning is used to generate an embryo that has identical genetic material to its cell source. This embryo is then implanted into the uterus of a pseudopregnant female to give rise to an infant that is a clone of the donor. Although therapeutic cloning also produces an embryo that is genetically identical to the donor nucleus, this process is used to generate blastocysts that are explanted and grown in culture, rather than in utero, to produce embryonic stem cell lines. These autologous stem cells have the potential to become almost any type of cell in the adult body, and thus they would be useful in tissue and organ replacement applications.[40] Therefore, therapeutic cloning, which has also been called somatic cell nuclear transfer, may provide an alternative source of transplantable cells that are identical to the patient's own cells.[41]

Regenerative Medicine Therapies

Many therapeutic approaches have been employed in regenerative medicine with the goal of developing systems that lead to restoration of damaged tissues and organs. In recent years, interest in cell-based therapies has grown because of the potential of creating functional cell-tissue-organs that may complement or give alternatives to existing therapies. Cell-based investigations have been pursued in many tissue and organ systems to develop solutions to various disease conditions. Although many

of these investigations are at the development stage, some of the therapies have reached patients. This section describes some of the regenerative medicine therapies that address specific disease conditions.

Cellular Therapy

Injectable Chondrocytes

Vesicoureteral reflux (VUR), a condition in which urine flows backward from the bladder into the ureter and kidney, and stress urinary incontinence are two urologic conditions that can result from dysfunction of a specific sphincter muscle. When severe, these conditions are repaired surgically. However, cell-based therapies for both VUR and incontinence would be an important alternative to surgical repair of these conditions. Ideally, such a therapy would be easily administered by injection and well tolerated by the patient. The injectable therapy should be nonantigenic, nonmigratory, volume stable, and safe for human use. In addition, it should be able to carry cells and serve as a matrix in vivo.

Toward this goal, long-term studies were conducted to determine the effects of injectable chondrocytes for the treatment of VUR in vivo.[42] Chondrocytes were chosen because the use of autologous cartilage for the treatment of VUR in humans would satisfy all of the requirements for an ideal injectable cell-based therapy. Chondrocytes derived from an ear biopsy can be readily grown and expanded in culture. Neocartilage formation can be achieved in vitro and in vivo using chondrocytes cultured on synthetic biodegradable polymers. In the VUR experiments, chondrocytes were suspended in an alginate matrix and injected around the vesicoureteral sphincter. In time, normal cartilage replaced the alginate as the alginate slowly degraded. This system was then adapted for the treatment of vesicoureteral reflux in a porcine model.[43] These studies show that chondrocytes can be easily harvested and combined with alginate in vitro, that the suspension can be easily injected cystoscopically, and that the elastic cartilage tissue formed is able to correct VUR without any evidence of obstruction.

Two multicenter human clinical trials were conducted using this engineered chondrocyte technology in the setting of VUR and urinary incontinence. Patients with VUR were treated at 10 centers throughout the United States. The patients had a cure rate similar to those of patients treated with other injectable substances. Cartilage formation was not noted in patients with treatment failure. Patients who were cured probably have a biocompatible region of engineered autologous tissue present.[44] Secondly, patients with urinary incontinence were treated endoscopically with injected chondrocytes at three different medical centers. Phase 1 trials showed an approximate success rate of 80% at 3 and 12 months postoperatively.[45]

Injectable Muscle Cells

The potential for injectable, cultured myoblasts in the treatment of stress urinary incontinence was suggested several years ago.[46,47] In one study, labeled myoblasts were directly injected into the proximal urethra and lateral bladder walls with a microsyringe in an open surgical procedure. Tissue harvested up to 35 days after injection contained the labeled myoblasts, as well as evidence of differentiation into regenerative myofibers. This study showed that a significant portion of the injected myoblast population survived and remained in vivo. Similar techniques of sphincter-derived muscle cells have been used for the treatment of urinary incontinence in a porcine model.[48] Based on this preclinical data, human trials were initiated. A recent study by Mitterberger et al[49] demonstrated successful use of cultured autologous skeletal myoblasts for the treatment of stress urinary incontinence.

The use of injectable muscle precursor cells has also been investigated for use in the treatment of urinary incontinence from irreversible urethral sphincter injury or developmental defects. Muscle precursor cells are the quiescent satellite cells found in each myofiber that can proliferate to form myoblasts and, eventually, myotubes and new muscle tissue. Intrinsic muscle precursor cells have been shown to play an active role in the regeneration of injured, striated, urethral sphincter.[50] In a subsequent study, autologous muscle precursor cells were injected into a rat model of urethral sphincter injury, and both replacement of mature myotubes and restoration of functional motor units were noted in the regenerating sphincter muscle tissue.[51] This study was the first demonstration of the replacement of both sphincter muscle tissue and its innervation by the injection of muscle precursor cells. This result suggests the possibility that muscle precursor cells may be a minimally invasive solution for urinary incontinence in patients with irreversible urinary sphincter muscle injury or insufficiency.

Degenerative muscle diseases such as Duchenne's muscular dystrophy have devastating effects on quality of life. To date, these genetic disorders have no suitable treatment. Early enthusiasm for gene therapy interventions has been tempered by issues of vector toxicity and inadequate gene transfer to target muscle cells in vivo. However, natural mechanisms of muscle repair have suggested that cell-based therapy could take advantage of natural homing mechanisms to direct cells to the proper location. Experiments using the *mdx* mouse model, in which the dystrophin gene is mutated, indicate that injection of normal muscle precursors and dermal fibroblasts into skeletal muscle can lead to the increased expression of dystrophin and improved functional outcomes.[52] However, this treatment option requires further studies before it can be widely applied in the clinic.

Cellular Therapies for Heart Disease

In the United States, more than 5 million people currently live with some form of heart disease, and many more are diagnosed each year. Although many medications have been developed to assist the ailing heart, the treatment for end-stage heart failure still remains transplantation. Unfortunately, as with other organs, donor hearts are in short supply, and even when a transplant can be performed, the patient must endure the side effects created by lifelong immunosuppression. Thus, alternatives are desperately needed, and the development of novel methods to regenerate or replace damaged heart muscle using tissue engineering and regenerative medicine techniques presents an attractive option.

An assortment of cell types has been investigated for their potential to regenerate damaged myocardium. Various cell sources, including skeletal muscle cells, marrow stem cells (both mesenchymal and hematopoietic), amniotic fluid stem cells, and embryonic stem cells, have been used for this purpose.[53-56] Currently, the most common method of introducing these cells into the heart is via injection of a cell suspension. In this technique, cells are suspended in a biocompatible matrix that can range from simple normal saline to complex, yet biocompatible, hydrogels, depending on the type of injection to be performed. Cells are either injected into the damaged area of the heart itself, or they are injected into the coronary circulation with the hope that they will home to the damaged area, take up residence there, and begin to repair the tissue.[57] However, injectable therapies have been shown to be relatively inefficient, and cell loss is quite substantial.[57,58] Newer methods of tissue engineering include the development of engineered "patches," which are composed of cells adhered to a biomaterial that can theoretically be used to replace the damaged area of the heart. These techniques have promise but require further research into the optimal cell types and biomaterials for this purpose before they can be used extensively in the clinic.[59]

The methods described above could be used only in cases where a relatively small section of heart muscle was damaged. In cases where a large area or even the whole heart has become nonfunctional, a more radical approach may be required. In these situations, the use of a bioartificial heart would be ideal, because rejection would be avoided and the problems associated with a mechanical heart (such as thromboembolus formation) would be eliminated. To this end, Ott et al[60] recently developed a novel heart construct in vitro using decellularized cadaveric hearts. The group reseeded the tissue scaffold that remained after a specialized decellularization process with various types of cells that make up a heart (cardiomyocytes, smooth muscle cells, endothelial cells, and fibrocytes), and they cultured the resulting construct in a bioreactor system designed to mimic physiologic conditions. As a result, this group was able to produce a construct that could generate pump function on its own,[60] suggesting that production of bioartificial hearts may one day be possible.

Tissue Therapy

It is evident that injectable cell-based therapies will likely become important clinical solutions for many disorders in the future. However, some very extensive disease conditions may require complete replacement of tissues or entire organs. In such instances, implantable tissues may be required to repair damage and restore tissue and organ function.

Urethra

Various biomaterials without cells, such as PGA and acellular collagen-based matrices from the small intestine and bladder, have been used experimentally in animal models for the regeneration of urethral tissue.[5,61-64] Some of these biomaterials, such as collagen-based tissue matrices, have also been combined with autologous cells for urethral reconstruction. In one experimental study, collagen matrices derived from urinary bladders have been used to repair rabbit urethral defects in a patch. Histologic examination showed complete epithelialization and progressive vessel and muscle infiltration, and the animals were able to void through the neo-urethras.[5] These results were confirmed in clinical studies of patients with a hypospadias (a congenital malformation in which the urethral opening appears on the bottom of the penile shaft, rather than at the end, and which requires reconstruction) and urethral stricture disease.[65,66] A collagen matrix obtained from cadaveric bladders was used as an onlay patch for urethral repair in these patients. Patent, functional neo-urethras were noted in these patients up to 7 years later. The use of this type of matrix appears to be beneficial and obviates the need for obtaining autologous grafts, thus decreasing operative time and eliminating donor site morbidity. However, these techniques may not be ideal for large urethral defects requiring tubularized urethral repair. In such instances, a collagen matrix configured in a tubular form can be seeded with autologous cells for damaged tissue repair.[67]

Bladder

Currently, bowel segments are commonly used as tissues for bladder replacement or repair. However, bowel tissue is not ideal for bladder reconstruction because of many associated problems. Engineered autologous tissues have been proposed as an alternate material for diseased bladders. The success of cell transplantation strategies for bladder reconstruction depends on the ability to use donor tissue efficiently and to provide the right conditions for long-term survival, differentiation, and growth.

Bladder cells (urothelial and muscle cells) can be expanded in vitro, seeded onto polymer scaffolds, and allowed to attach and form sheets of cells.[68] These principles were applied in the creation of tissue-engineered bladders in an animal model that required a subtotal cystectomy with subsequent replacement with a tissue-engineered organ in beagles.[69] This study showed that it is possible to tissue-engineer bladders that are anatomically and functionally normal.

A clinical experience involving engineered bladder tissue for reconstruction was conducted using 1) a collagen scaffold seeded with cells with or without omentum coverage or 2) a combined PGA-collagen scaffold seeded with cells and omental coverage. The patients reconstructed with the engineered bladder tissue created with the PGA-collagen cell-seeded scaffolds showed increased compliance, decreased end-filling pressures, increased capacities, and longer dry periods.[70] The successful outcome of this study has led to an FDA-approved Phase II multicenter clinical study.

Kidney

Renal failure is a devastating condition that requires renal transplantation.[71,72] However, availability of kidneys for transplantation is severely limited as a result of the current donor shortage. Augmentation of renal function with engineered kidney cells may be a potential option. Previous efforts have been directed toward the development of extracorporeal renal support systems made of biologic and synthetic components,[73-78] and these ex-vivo renal replacement devices are known to be life-sustaining. However, there would be obvious benefits for patients with end-stage kidney disease if these devices could be implanted for long-term use without the need for an extracorporeal perfusion circuit or immunosuppressive drugs.

The principles of both tissue engineering and therapeutic cloning have been used to produce genetically identical renal tissue in a bovine model.[79] Bovine skin fibroblasts from adult Holstein steers were obtained from the ear, and single nuclei were isolated and microinjected into the perivitelline space of donor enucleated oocytes (nuclear transfer). The resulting blastocysts were implanted into progestin-synchronized recipients to allow for further in-vivo growth. After 12 weeks,

cloned renal cells were culture-expanded in vitro and seeded onto scaffolds consisting of three collagen-coated cylindrical polycarbonate membranes, followed by transplantation into the same steer from which the genetic material originated. In this study the implants formed tissue that produced a urine-like fluid and consisted of kidney structures that were confirmed with immunohistochemistry and molecular analyses. This study showed that cells derived from nuclear transfer can be successfully harvested, expanded in culture, and transplanted in vivo using biodegradable scaffolds. On the scaffolds, single suspended cells can organize into tissue structures that are genetically identical to those of the host. In another study, Sagrinati et al have described a population of CD24+CD133+ multipotent resident renal progenitor cells.[80] These cells, when injected alone, were able to engraft into kidneys recovering from renal failure. The cells, which continue to reside in the Bowman's capsule well into adulthood, may be harnessed for renal repair therapy.

Blood Vessels

Nearly 8 to 12 million Americans are affected by vascular disease each year. Currently, xenogenic or synthetic materials have been used as replacement blood vessels for complex cardiovascular lesions. However, these materials typically lack growth potential and may place the recipient at risk for complications such as stenosis, thromboembolization, or infection.[81] To solve this problem, tissue-engineered vascular grafts have been constructed using autologous cells and biodegradable scaffolds. These grafts have been applied in dog and sheep models.[82-85] The key advantage of using these autografts is that the scaffolding slowly degrades in vivo, allowing new tissue to form without the long-term presence of foreign material. Translation of these techniques from the laboratory to the clinical setting has begun. Autologous vascular cells have been harvested, expanded, and seeded onto a biodegradable scaffold.[84] The resultant autologous construct was used to replace a stenosed pulmonary artery that had been previously repaired using traditional methods. Seven months after implantation, no evidence of graft occlusion or aneurysmal changes was noted in the recipient.

Liver

The liver can sustain a variety of insults, including viral infection, alcohol abuse, surgical resection of tumors, and acute drug-induced hepatic failure. The current therapy for liver failure is liver transplantation. However, this therapy is limited by the shortage of donors and the need for lifelong immunosuppressive therapy. Cell transplantation has been proposed as a potential solution for liver failure because the liver has enormous regenerative potential in vivo. That fact suggests that, in the right environment, it may be possible to expand liver cells in vitro in sufficient quantities for tissue engineering.[86] Many approaches have been tried, including development of specialized media, coculture with other cell types, identification of growth factors that proliferate these cells, and culture on three-dimensional scaffolds within bioreactors.[86]

Extracorporeal bioartificial liver devices that use porcine hepatocytes have been designed and applied. These devices are designed to filter and purify the patient's blood as the patient's own liver would, and the blood is returned to the patient in a manner similar to kidney dialysis. Another cell-based approach—the injection of liver cell suspensions in vivo—has been performed in animal models. Intraportal hepatocyte injection has also been used in patients with Crigler-Najjar syndrome, type 1[87]; however, complications such as portal vein thrombosis and pulmonary embolism are major concerns, especially when large cell numbers are used.[88] Finally, stem cells, oval progenitor cells, and mature hepatocytes have been seeded onto liver-shaped biocompatible matrices to engineer artificial, implantable livers. Although these livers have been tested in various animal models,[89,90] the transplantation efficiency, as well as the functionality of these constructs, must be improved substantially before the technology can be moved into the clinic.

Summary

Regenerative medicine efforts are currently under experimentation for virtually every type of tissue and organ within the human body. Much of the effort expended to engineer tissues has occurred within the last decade. Regenerative medicine techniques require a cell-culture facility designed for human application. This innovative branch of science incorporates the fields of tissue engineering, cell biology, nuclear transfer, and materials science. Therefore, regenerative medicine requires personnel who have mastered the techniques of cell harvest, culture, expansion, transplantation, and polymer design, which are essential for the successful application of these technologies. Various tissues are at different stages of development: Some are already being used clinically, a few are in preclinical trials, and some are in the discovery stage. Recent progress suggests that engineered tissues may have an expanded clinical applicability in the future and may represent a viable therapeutic option for those who require tissue replacement or repair.

References/Resources

1. Kim BS, Mooney DJ. Development of biocompatible synthetic extracellular matrices for tissue engineering. Trends Biotechnol 1998;16:224-30.

2. Hynes RO. Integrins: Versatility, modulation, and signaling in cell adhesion. Cell 1992;69:11-25.

3. Silver FH, Pins G. Cell growth on collagen: A review of tissue engineering using scaffolds containing extracellular matrix. J Long Term Eff Med Implants 1992;2:67-80.

4. Smidsrod O, Skjak-Braek G. Alginate as immobilization matrix for cells. Trends Biotechnol 1990;8:71-8.

5. Chen F, Yoo JJ, Atala A. Acellular collagen matrix as a possible "off the shelf" biomaterial for urethral repair. Urology 1999;54:407-10.

6. Dahms SE, Piechota HJ, Dahiya R, et al. Composition and biomechanical properties of the bladder acellular matrix graft: Comparative analysis in rat, pig and human. Br J Urol, 1998;82:411-9.

7. Piechota HJ, Dahms SE, Nunes LS, et al. In vitro functional properties of the rat bladder regenerated by the bladder acellular matrix graft. J Urol 1998;159:1717-24.

8. Yoo JJ, Ming J, Oberpenning F, Atala A. Bladder augmentation using allogenic bladder submucosa seeded with cells. Urology 1998;51:221-5.

9. Gilding D. Biodegradable polymers. In: Williams D, ed. Biocompatibility of clinical implant materials. Boca Raton, FL: CRC Press, 1981:209-32.

10. Ishaug SL, Yaszemski MJ, Bizios R, Mikos AG. Osteoblast function on synthetic biodegradable polymers. J Biomed Mater Res 1994;28:1445-53.

11. Mikos AG, Lyman MD, Freed LE, Langer R. Wetting of poly(L-lactic acid) and poly(DL-lactic-co-glycolic acid) foams for tissue culture. Biomaterials 1994;15:55-8.

12. Pariente JL, Kim BS, Atala A. In vitro biocompatibility assessment of naturally derived and synthetic biomaterials using normal human urothelial cells. J Biomed Mater Res 2001;55:33-9.

13. Pariente JL, Kim BS, Atala A. In vitro biocompatibility evaluation of naturally derived and synthetic biomaterials using normal human bladder smooth muscle cells. J Urol 2002;167:1867-71.

14. Cilento BG, Freeman MR, Schneck FX, et al. Phenotypic and cytogenetic characterization of human bladder urothelia expanded in vitro. J Urol 1994;152:665-70.

15. Scriven SD, Booth C, Thomas DF, et al. Reconstitution of human urothelium from monolayer cultures. J Urol 1997;158:1147-52.

16. Liebert M, Hubbel A, Chung M, et al. Expression of mal is associated with urothelial differentiation in vitro: Identification by differential display reverse-transcriptase polymerase chain reaction. Differentiation 1997;61:177-85.

17. Puthenveettil JA, Burger MS, Reznikoff CA. Replicative senescence in human uroepithelial cells. Adv Exp Med Biol 1999;462:83-91.

18. Freeman MR, Yoo JJ, Raab G, et al. Heparin-binding EGF-like growth factor is an autocrine growth factor for human urothelial cells and is synthesized by epithelial and smooth muscle cells in the human bladder. J Clin Invest 1997;99:1028-36.

19. Nguyen HT, Park JM, Peters CA, et al. Cell-specific activation of the HB-EGF and ErbB1 genes by stretch in primary human bladder cells. In Vitro Cell Dev Biol Anim 1999;35:371-5.

20. Liebert M, Wedemeyer G, Abruzzo LV, et al. Stimulated urothelial cells produce cytokines and express an activated cell surface antigenic phenotype. Sem Urol 1991;9:124-30.

21. Brivanlou AH, Gage FH, Jaenisch R, et al. Stem cells: Setting standards for human embryonic stem cells (see comment). Science 2003;300:913-6.

22. Reubinoff BE, Pera MF, Fong CY, et al. Embryonic stem cell lines from human blastocysts: Somatic differentiation in vitro [see comment; erratum appears in Nat Biotechnol 2000;18:559]. Nat Biotechnol 2000;18:399-404.

23. Thomson JA, Itskovitz-Eldor J, Shapiro S, et al. Embryonic stem cell lines derived from human blastocysts [see comment; erratum appears in Science 1998;282:1827]. Science 1998;282:1145-7.

24. Itskovitz-Eldor J, Schuldiner M, Karsenti D, et al. Differentiation of human embryonic stem cells into embryoid bodies compromising the three embryonic germ layers. Mol Med 2000;6:88-95.

25. Reubinoff BE, Itsykson P, Turetsky T, et al. Neural progenitors from human embryonic stem cells (see comment). Nat Biotechnol 2001;19:1134-40.

26. Schuldiner M, Eiges R, Eden A, et al. Induced neuronal differentiation of human embryonic stem cells. Brain Res 2001;913:201-5.

27. Schuldiner M, Yanuka O, Itskovitz-Eldor J, et al. Effects of eight growth factors on the differentiation of cells derived from human embryonic stem cells. Proc Natl Acad Sci U S A 2000;97:11307-12.

28. Kaufman DS, Hanson ET, Lewis RL, et al. Hematopoietic colony-forming cells derived from human embryonic stem cells. Proc Natl Acad Sci U S A 2001;98:10716-21.

29. Kehat I, Kenyagin-Karsenti D, Snir M, et al. Human embryonic stem cells can differentiate into myocytes with structural and functional properties of cardiomyocytes (see comment). J Clin Invest 2001;108:407-14.

30. Levenberg S, Golub JS, Amit M, et al. Endothelial cells derived from human embryonic stem cells. Proc Natl Acad Sci U S A 2002;99:4391-6.

31. Assady S, Maor G, Amit M, et al. Insulin production by human embryonic stem cells. Diabetes 2001;50:1691-7.

32. Delo DM, De Coppi P, Bartsch G Jr, Atala A. Amniotic fluid and placental stem cells. Methods Enzymol 2006;419:426-38.

33. De Coppi P, Bartsch G Jr, Siddiqui MM, et al. Isolation of amniotic stem cell lines with potential for therapy (see comment). Nat Biotechnol 2007;25:100-6.

34. Guillot PV, O'Donoghue K, Kurata H, Fisk NM. Fetal stem cells: Betwixt and between. Semin Reprod Med 2006;24:340-7.

35. Broxmeyer HE, Srour E, Orschell C, et al. Cord blood stem and progenitor cells. Methods Enzymol 2006;419:439-73.

36. Becker C, Jakse G. Stem cells for regeneration of urological structures (see comment). Eur Urol 2007;51:1217-28.

37. Humphreys BD, Duffield JD, Bonventre JV. Renal stem cells in recovery from acute kidney injury. Minerva Urol Nefrol 2006;58:13-21.

38. Burke ZD, Thowfeequ S, Peran M, Tosh D. Stem cells in the adult pancreas and liver. Biochem J 2007;404:169-78.

39. Nern C, Momma S. The realized niche of adult neural stem cells. Stem Cell Rev 2006;2:233-40.

40. Hochedlinger K, Rideout WM, Kyba M, et al. Nuclear transplantation, embryonic stem cells and the potential for cell therapy. Hematol J 2004;5:S114-7.

41. Lanza RP, Cibelli JB, West MD. Prospects for the use of nuclear transfer in human transplantation. Nat Biotechnol 1999;17:1171-4.

42. Atala A, Cima LG, Kim W, et al. Injectable alginate seeded with chondrocytes as a potential treatment for vesicoureteral reflux. J Urol 1993;150:745-7.

43. Atala A, Kim W, Paige KT, et al. Endoscopic treatment of vesicoureteral reflux with a chondrocyte-alginate suspension. J Urol 1994;152:641-4.

44. Diamond DA, Caldamone AA. Endoscopic correction of vesicoureteral reflux in children using autologous chondrocytes: Preliminary results. J Urol 1999;162:1185-8.

45. Bent AE, Tutrone RT, McLennan MT, et al. Treatment of intrinsic sphincter deficiency using autologous ear chondrocytes as a bulking agent. Neurourol Urodyn 2001;20:157-65.

46. Yokoyama T, Huard J, Chancellor MB. Myoblast therapy for stress urinary incontinence and bladder dysfunction. World J Urol 2000;18:56-61.

47. Chancellor MB, Yokoyama T, Tirney S, et al. Preliminary results of myoblast injection into the urethra and bladder wall: A possible method for the treatment of stress urinary incontinence and impaired detrusor contractility. Neurourol Urodyn 2000;19:279-87.

48. Strasser H, Berjukow S, Marksteiner R, et al. Stem cell therapy for urinary stress incontinence. Exp Gerontol 2004;39:1259-65.

49. Mitterberger M, Marksteiner R, Margreiter E, et al. Autologous myoblasts and fibroblasts for female stress incontinence: A 1-year follow-up in 123 patients. BJU Int 2007;100:1081-5.

50. Yiou R, Lefaucheur JP, Atala A. The regeneration process of the striated urethral sphincter involves activation of intrinsic satellite cells. Anat Embryol 2003;206:429-35.

51. Yiou R, Yoo JJ, Atala A. Restoration of functional motor units in a rat model of sphincter injury by muscle precursor cell autografts. Transplantation 2003;76:1053-60.

52. Torrente Y, Tremblay JP, Pisati F, et al. Intraarterial injection of muscle-derived CD34(+)Sca-1(+) stem cells restores dystrophin in mdx mice. J Cell Biol 2001;152:335-48.

53. Dai W, Field LJ, Rubart M, et al. Survival and maturation of human embryonic stem cell-derived cardiomyocytes in rat hearts. J Mol Cellular Cardiol 2007;43:504-16.

54. Dai W, Kloner RA. Myocardial regeneration by human amniotic fluid stem cells: Challenges to be overcome (comment). J Mol Cell Cardiol 2007;42:730-2.

55. Laflamme MA, Murry CE. Regenerating the heart. Nat Biotechnol 2005;23:845-56.

56. Laflamme MA, Gold J, Xu C, et al. Formation of human myocardium in the rat heart from human embryonic stem cells. Am J Pathol 2005;167:663-71.

57. Hofmann M, Wollert KC, Meyer GP, et al. Monitoring of bone marrow cell homing into the infarcted human myocardium. Circulation 2005;111:2198-202.

58. Grossman PM, Han Z, Palasis M, et al. Incomplete retention after direct myocardial injection. Catheter Cardiovasc Interv 2002;55:392-7.

59. Jawad H, Ali NN, Lyon AR, et al. Myocardial tissue engineering: A review. J Tissue Eng Regen Med 2007;1:327-42.

60. Ott HC, Matthiesen TS, Goh SK, et al. Perfusion-decellularized matrix: Using nature's platform to engineer a bioartificial heart. Nat Med 2008;14:213-21.

61. Atala A, Vacanti JP, Peters CA, et al. Formation of urothelial structures in vivo from dissociated cells attached to biodegradable polymer scaffolds in vitro. J Urol 1992;148:658-62.

62. Olsen L, Bowald S, Busch C, et al. Urethral reconstruction with a new synthetic absorbable device. An experimental study. Scand J Urol Nephrol 1992;26:323-6.

63. Kropp BP, Ludlow JK, Spicer D, et al. Rabbit urethral regeneration using small intestinal submucosa onlay grafts. Urol 1998;52:138-42.

64. Sievert KD, Bakircioglu ME, Nunes L, et al. Homologous acellular matrix graft for urethral reconstruction in the rabbit: Histological and functional evaluation. J Urol 2000;163:1958-65.

65. Atala A, Guzman L, Retik AB. A novel inert collagen matrix for hypospadias repair. J Urol 1999;162:1148-51.

66. El-Kassaby AW, Retik AB, Yoo JJ, Atala A. Urethral stricture repair with an off-the-shelf collagen matrix. J Urol 2003;169:170-3.

67. De Filippo RE, Yoo JJ, Atala A. Urethral replacement using cell seeded tubularized collagen matrices. J Urol 2002;168:1789-93.

68. Atala A, Freeman MR, Vacanti JP, et al. Implantation in vivo and retrieval of artificial structures consisting of rabbit and human urothelium and human bladder muscle. J Urol 1993;150:608-12.

69. Oberpenning F, Meng J, Yoo JJ, Atala A. De novo reconstitution of a functional mammalian urinary bladder by tissue engineering (see comment). Nat Biotechnol 1999;17:149-55.

70. Atala A, Bauer SB, Soker S, et al. Tissue-engineered autologous bladders for patients needing cystoplasty (see comment). Lancet 2006;367:1241-6.

71. Sarnak MJ, Levey AS. Cardiovascular disease and chronic renal disease: A new paradigm. Am J Kidney Dis 2000;35:S117-31.

72. Zeier M. Risk of mortality in patients with end-stage renal disease: The role of malnutrition and possible therapeutic implications. Horm Res 2002;58:30-4.

73. Amiel GE, Atala A. Current and future modalities for functional renal replacement. Urol Clin North Am 1999;26:235-46.

74. Aebischer P, Ip TK, Panol G, Galletti PM. The bioartificial kidney: Progress towards an ultrafiltration device with renal epithelial cells processing. Life Support Syst 1987;5:159-68.

75. Amiel GE, Yoo JJ, Atala A. Renal therapy using tissue-engineered constructs and gene delivery. World J Urol 2000;18:71-9.

76. Humes HD, Buffington DA, MacKay SM, et al. Replacement of renal function in uremic animals with a tissue-engineered kidney (see comment). Nat Biotechnol 1999;17:451-5.

77. Ip TK, Aebischer P, Galletti PM. Cellular control of membrane permeability: Implications for a bioartificial renal tubule. ASAIO Trans 1988;34:351-5.

78. Joki T, Machluf M, Atala A, et al. Continuous release of endostatin from microencapsulated engineered cells for tumor therapy (see comment). Nat Biotechnol 2001;19:35-9.

79. Lanza RP, Chung HY, Yoo JJ, et al. Generation of histocompatible tissues using nuclear transplantation (see comment). Nat Biotechnol 2002;20:689-96.

80. Sagrinati C, Netti GS, Mazzinghi B, et al. Isolation and characterization of multipotent progenitor cells from the Bowman's capsule of adult human kidneys. J Am Soc Nephrol 2006;17:2443-56.

81. Conte MS. Molecular engineering of vein bypass grafts. J Vasc Surg 2007;45:A74-81.

82. Watanabe M, Shin'oka T, Tohyama S, et al. Tissue-engineered vascular autograft: Inferior vena cava replacement in a dog model. Tissue Eng 2001;7:429-39.

83. Shinoka T, Breuer CK, Tanel RE, et al. Tissue engineering heart valves: Valve leaflet replacement study in a lamb model. Ann Thorac Surg 1995;60:S513-6.

84. Shin'oka T, Imai Y, Ikada Y. Transplantation of a tissue-engineered pulmonary artery. N Engl J Med 2001;344:532-3.

85. Shinoka T, Shum-Tim D, Ma PX, et al. Creation of viable pulmonary artery autografts through tissue engineering. J Thorac Cardiovasc Surg 1998;115:536-46.

86. Bhandari RN, Riccalton LA, Lewis AL, et al. Liver tissue engineering: A role for co-culture systems in modifying hepatocyte function and viability. Tissue Eng 2001;7: 345-57.

87. Fox IJ, Chowdhury JR, Kaufman SS, et al. Treatment of the Crigler-Najjar syndrome type I with hepatocyte transplantation (see comment). N Engl J Med 1998;338: 1422-6.

88. Nieto JA, Escandon J, Betancor C, et al. Evidence that temporary complete occlusion of splenic vessels prevents massive embolization and sudden death associated with intrasplenic hepatocellular transplantation. Transplantation 1989;47:449-50.

89. Kaufmann PM, Kneser U, Fiegel HC, et al. Long-term hepatocyte transplantation using three-dimensional matrices. Transplant Proc 1999;31:1928-9.

90. Gilbert JC, Takada T, Stein JE, et al. Cell transplantation of genetically altered cells on biodegradable polymer scaffolds in syngeneic rats. Transplantation 1993;56:423-7.

Assessment and Characterization of Cellular Therapy Products

♦ ♦ ♦

IN THE 1980s, CELLULAR THERAPY (CT) PRODucts were primarily marrow grafts collected and transplanted with little or no manipulation. The assessment and characterization of those products consisted of volume determination and the total nucleated cell count, usually performed by a manual technique. The number of nucleated cells per mL of marrow, multiplied by the volume collected and divided by the weight of the recipient, determined the administered dose of the marrow product. Cell types and subtypes were not identified, characterized, or enumerated. Cell-counting procedures were rarely, if ever, validated, and substances such as fat and fibrin often interfered with obtaining an accurate count. Sometimes a smear of the marrow was stained and examined microscopically to calculate the mononuclear cell population, within which could be found the small number of hematopoietic stem cells expected to engraft.

As the field of CT has progressed, studies examining functions of a variety of cell populations have led to the development of unique treatments targeted at an expanding number and variety of conditions. Novel methods for the selection and depletion of cells with specific phenotypic or morphologic characteristics, or both, have been and continue to be developed. Manual and automated techniques are used for culturing and expanding targeted cell populations in oncology and regenerative medicine. This wide array of products and processes requires an even wider set of valid assays to demonstrate that the CT products indeed contain the purported therapeutic agent and that various quality and safety specifications have been met. This section describes tests and assay systems for enumerating and characterizing CT products as well as for evaluating their quality and safety.

Section Editors: Ellen Areman, MS, SBB(ASCP), Senior Consultant, Biologics Consulting Group, Inc, Alexandria, Virginia, and Lynn O'Donnell, PhD, Director, Cell Therapy Laboratory, OSU James Cancer Hospital and Solove Research Institute, Columbus, Ohio

The editors have disclosed no conflicts of interest.

Current State of the Field

Manufacturers of cellular products that are regulated as biological drugs by the US Food and Drug Administration (FDA) are required to comply with the relevant sections of the US Code of Federal Regulations (CFR), which include the current good manufacturing practice (cGMP) for pharmaceuticals (21 CFR, Parts 210 and 211), general biologics standards (21 CFR 610), and portions of the regulations governing human cells, tissues, and cellular and tissue-based products (HCT/Ps; 21 CFR 1271). These regulations describe and define the characteristics a biological product manufacturer must assess for the FDA to license the product. Investigational products are subject to many of the same requirements, although the assays used for characterization may be undergoing development and refinement along with the product. By the time clinical trials have been completed and the product is ready for licensure, all relevant release tests must be in place and validated for use with the cellular product formulation the manufacturer intends to market. According to cGMP, licensed biologics must undergo testing at the final stage of the manufacturing process to confirm they meet the release criteria specified in the product license. The product cannot be distributed unless it falls within predetermined limits for safety, purity, potency, and identity. Manufacturers of cellular products distributed in the United States that are not classified as biological drugs are still required by the FDA to provide assurance that the product does not expose the recipient to communicable or infectious diseases under current good tissue practice (cGTP) regulations.

In addition to FDA requirements, professional organizations such as AABB and the Foundation for the Accreditation of Cellular Therapy require that CT products manufactured by accredited CT establishments be tested for safety and quality. Furthermore, because a large percentage of administered CT products are from either autologous or allogeneic directed donations, real clinical decisions are made based on product testing. The dose of a particular cell type contained in a product may determine whether another collection is needed from an allogeneic donor or whether the recipient can proceed to transplant. The failure of an investigational CT product to meet specifications may mean the recipient cannot remain on a clinical protocol and must seek other treatment options, if any are available.

To demonstrate that CT products meet requirements, appropriate assays must be performed. Scientists in academia and industry are constantly working to develop test systems that can accurately and reproducibly evaluate and characterize the wide array of CT products both during their manufacture and at the completion of the manufacturing process.

Section Overview

The methods described in this section are representative of the field as it exists. But along with the rapid discovery and development of new CT products and "designer" cellular treatments, new methods for evaluating their safety, purity, and potency must also be designed and developed.

To expect any test method to yield accurate and reliable results, the laboratory must first demonstrate that the method is appropriate for use with the type and volume of product sample that will be used in actual laboratory practice. This section begins with a discussion of approaches to validation that should clarify some of the issues to consider when planning implementation of a new test method or system. The remainder of the section describes methods for characterizing and assessing the safety and quality of CT products:

- **Quantitation and Enumeration.** Clinical trials to determine safe and effective doses of CT products depend on accurate measurements of the cell populations under study. Being able to calculate the recovery or removal of different cell populations is critical for product development and quality control.
- **Viability.** A reliable viability assay can provide assurance that the cells have not been damaged during collection, processing, shipping, or storage. Combining cell phenotyping with viability analysis using flow cytometry can also demonstrate the survival or removal of individual populations of viable cells.
- **Function and Potency.** Few, if any, assays can directly measure the therapeutic effect of a CT preparation in vitro. Therefore, tests measuring

the level of a biological or functional activity must be used as surrogates for in-vivo effects. Often a combination of tests is needed to provide a reliable measure of the potency of a CT product. Functional tests are commonly used for investigational CT products but may also be used in response to deviations in manufacturing or poor viability test results.

- **Microbial Contamination.** To reduce the risk of a contaminated product reaching a patient, all CT products are tested for microbial contamination using routine culture techniques that detect a wide range of bacteria and fungi. Additional testing for clinically relevant contaminants such as *Mycoplasma* or endotoxin from gram-negative pathogens may also be required.

- **Characterization and Identity.** In addition to enumerating specific therapeutic cells in a CT product, identifying other cell populations contained in a heterogeneous mixture is often important. Changes in surface and intracellular markers during cell culture, expansion, or other manufacturing steps can provide evidence that the process is performing as expected. For allogeneic CT products, identification of donor and recipient HLA and ABO types provides critical information for the selection of appropriate donors to minimize graft-vs-host disease as well as for appropriate processing methods to prevent acute reactions caused by ABO incompatibility. The ABO or HLA type may also be used to confirm the identity of a CT product, thus providing assurance that the source of the product is the donor of record, the correct product has been selected for administration, and no mix-ups occurred during manufacture.

Future Directions

Along with continual development of more sophisticated cellular therapies must come the sustained development of more accurate and reproducible test systems for assessing all aspects in the production of cellular products. Cellular products collected from different individuals will have different characteristics regardless of the consistent manner in which they are collected and processed. Even with meticulous cell selection methods, a cell suspension will not be completely pure but will contain a number and variety of less-desirable cells. Cells that appear identical in phenotype and morphology may function at different levels of activity. These differences can be seen not only among different donors but also among cell collections from the same donor at different times. In addition, products for CT cannot be produced in large batches of identical units from which a percentage can be tested as representative of the batch. Frequently, a lot or batch is at most a few bags or vials of cells collected and processed for a specific individual recipient. Although heterogeneity and inconsistency of CT products are expected, that fact places a great part of the responsibility for release of a safe and effective product in the hands of the laboratories performing assessment and characterization of those products.

In: Areman EM, Loper K, eds
Cellular Therapy: Principles, Methods, and Regulations
Bethesda, MD: AABB, 2009

◆◆◆   43   ◆◆◆

Validation of Test Methods

Nina K. Garlie, PhD

PROCESS IMPROVEMENT IS A SUBSTANTIAL goal in any cellular therapy (CT) laboratory. As new technologies emerge, existing technologies improve, or new information about the biology and mechanism of action of CT products becomes available, new or alternative test methods may offer advantages over existing test methods. New tests are often needed to characterize new CT products that may require unique functional assays or phenotypic markers. Regulatory agencies and clinical trial sponsors may also require the use of specific test methods.

Test method validation is required when bringing new tests online, whether the test is an alternative for an existing method or entirely new. Validation is always a balance among costs, risks, and technical possibilities. Some of the questions to be answered are the following:

- Which biologic properties should be measured?
- Is a test available that correlates as well (or better) with clinical outcomes?
- Can a better way be devised to demonstrate a test outcome?

- Is a real-time test available that will provide a high degree of confidence that the sample will meet release criteria?
- Is a more sensitive test, a quicker test, or a less expensive test available?

Good manufacturing practice (GMP) regulations require facilities to establish procedures to ensure the fitness for use of methods that generate data supporting regulated product testing.[1] However, GMP regulations do not provide definitive guidance for the qualification of test methods. The Food and Drug Administration (FDA) defines methods validation as "the process of demonstrating that analytical procedures are suitable for their intended use"[2] and as "establishing documented evidence which provides a high degree of assurance that a specific process will consistently produce a product meeting its predetermined specifications and quality attributes."[3] Therefore, the intended purpose of the method and the outcomes (specifications/attributes) must be clearly defined at the outset of the validation.

Nina K. Garlie, PhD, Research Scientist and Director, William Schuett Cellular Laboratory Immunotherapy Program, Aurora St Luke's Medical Center, Milwaukee, Wisconsin

The author has disclosed no conflicts of interest.

It is also important to clarify the difference between validation and verification. *Validation* is restricted to the demonstration of suitability of a method for its intended purpose, whereas *verification* of methods involves demonstration that the conditions under which the method is to be performed will be appropriate for the method.[4] For example, if a stain is used to distinguish nonviable cells from viable cells, a variety of specifications will apply to the stain, such as formulation, concentration, and temperature. Testing that ensures conformance to these specifications is verification. If the dye stains all cells including viable cells during use, however, then it would fail validation. It may have met all the material specifications (verification), but it did not work as a vital stain (validation).

The goal of finding a validation scheme that is applicable to all test method validations may be efficient but not realistic. For instance, trying to demonstrate comparability between two methods by parallel testing is logical and efficient. Testing the final product by the standard method and by the alternate method to directly compare and show equivalent (or superior) results by the alternate is reasonable. However, in some situations this approach cannot be used. One example is in testing a new sterility method, where the normal test result is "negative" or "no growth." Performing the number of parallel tests required to statistically distinguish failure rates between the two methods would be impractical. Instead it might be necessary to devise a validation plan in which test samples are seeded with a known number and variety of microorganisms to demonstrate the new method's ability to detect contamination at a level comparable to that of the standard method. In addition, results obtained during validation may necessitate changes to the validation plan. For example, the original validation study design may require parallel testing of existing and new methods using reference standards such as cell populations with known CD34 content. If the existing method of CD34 enumeration does not involve quality control using the reference standards, the results using the existing method may be consistently "out of range" of the manufacturer's specifications for the reference standards. Because little benefit accrues from comparing the two methods in this manner, another approach must be taken to evaluate equivalence.

Validation of a test method requires studies to ensure that the method can be performed in a manner that is accurate, specific, reproducible, and precise over the expected range of use. Method validation may include assessment of the parameters discussed in the following paragraphs; however, evaluating every analytical performance parameter is not always necessary. The type of method and intended use dictate which parameters need to be investigated.

Performance Parameters

Precision

Precision of a method is the measure of its degree of repeatability under normal conditions. Three different measures of precision should be performed when possible: repeatability, intermediate precision, and reproducibility. Precision should be determined over the expected range of samples to be assayed, and the conditions used during the validation should be clearly stated. To assess precision of a method, reference standards are routinely used to eliminate the variability that is found in heterogeneous test samples. Documentation in support of precision studies should include standard deviation, relative standard deviation, coefficient of variation, and confidence interval.

- *Repeatability* is the most common measure of precision and refers to the results achieved by the method when operating in the same assay run or over a short time interval under the same conditions (ie, intra-assay precision). Repeatability should be assessed using a minimum of nine determinations covering the specified range for the procedure (eg, three concentrations/three replicates each), or a minimum of six determinations at 100% of the test concentration.
- *Intermediate precision*, or *ruggedness* in USP chapter <1225>,[5] pertains to the effect of random events on results from within-laboratory variations such as differing equipment, analysts, days, or sample sources.
- *Reproducibility* refers to the results of collaborative studies between laboratories. These should be performed when possible and feasible, for example, by having a laboratory experienced with the test method analyze duplicate samples.

The stability of test samples may be critical, especially if samples must be shipped between laboratories.

Accuracy

Accuracy is a determination of how close the measured value is to the true value or to an accepted reference value. Accuracy may be defined as the true value plus error, where error may contain systematic error (bias) and imprecision of measurement. Accuracy should be assessed using a minimum of nine determinations over a minimum of three concentration levels covering the specified range (eg, three concentrations and three replicates each of the total analytical procedure).

Sensitivity and Specificity

The terms sensitivity and specificity have different meanings depending on whether the test is being used for screening or quantitative purposes. For screening tests, sensitivity refers to the proportion of positive reference test samples that are detected as positive with the screening test. Specificity then refers to the proportion of negative reference test samples that are shown to be negative with the screening test.

For quantitative tests, sensitivity refers to the smallest concentration of a substance that can be reliably measured by a given analytical method (see more on limit of detection and limit of quantitation below). Specificity then refers to the ability to measure accurately and specifically the article of interest in the presence of much higher quantities of similar but not identical articles. Specificity can be demonstrated by the ability to discriminate between compounds of closely related structures or by comparison to known reference materials. One concern in testing alternative methods is the possibility of decreased sensitivity of the alternative method. The new test must detect every problem that the standard test would have found. The new method should not allow a product to pass that the standard method would have failed.

Limit of Detection

The *limit of detection* (LOD) is defined as the lowest concentration of material in a sample that can be detected above background noise (determined from 10 independent blank controls). The LOD is typically set as the mean of the blank plus two to three times the standard deviation (SD) of the blank, followed by conversion of the test readout units (eg, fluorescence) to the result units (eg, concentration). Accuracy, precision, and linearity are not considered at this level. LOD is a limit test that specifies whether or not the amount of material in a sample is above or below a certain value. For example, if the LOD for a material is 3 ng, then a sample containing 3 ng of material would elicit a signal discernible above background noise. Stating that the sample contains at least 3 ng of material would be appropriate, whereas stating that the sample contains an exact amount of material would not.

Limit of Quantitation

The *limit of quantitation* (LOQ) is loosely defined as the minimum quantity of material in a sample that elicits a signal within the linear range of data (ie, the lowest end of the range). It requires acceptable precision and accuracy under the stated operational conditions of the method. Therefore, the LOQ is significantly more demanding to establish than the LOD. Several methods for determining the LOQ, or other closely related values such as the biological limit of detection (BLD), have been described.[6] The analytical method and its intended use dictate the preferred method for establishing the LOQ. LOQ may be established as the mean of the blank plus 5 times the SD of the blank. BLD is defined as the LOD plus two to three times the interassay SD (between runs) of a spiked reference sample at a concentration near the LOD. Because precision and accuracy are worse at the low end of the linear range, the LOQ is a compromise between the concentration and the required precision and accuracy. That is, as the LOQ concentration decreases, the imprecision of the test increases. If better precision is required, a higher concentration must ultimately be reported for LOQ.

Linearity

Linearity refers to the ability of the method to elicit results that are directly proportional to the quantity of article contained in the sample being analyzed within a given range. Linearity is generally reported as the variance of the slope of the regression line.

Range

Range is the interval between the upper and lower levels of sample material (inclusive), which have been demonstrated to be determined with the required precision, accuracy, and linearity using the method as written. The range is normally expressed in the same units as the test results obtained by the method.

Robustness

Robustness is directly related to the conditions under which a validated method is shown to be suitable. It is a measure of the capacity of a method to remain unaffected by small and deliberate variations in analytical conditions, such as incubation times, incubation temperatures, sample preparation and storage conditions, buffer pH, and buffer and reagent expiration times. Robustness should be considered early in the development of a method. If method suitability is susceptible to variations in analytical conditions, these parameters should be adequately controlled and a precautionary statement should be included in the method documentation to ensure that the validity of the method is maintained whenever it is used.

Conclusion

In addition to evaluating test performance using the measures described above, the techniques used for validating alternative methods may include calibration using reference standards or reference materials, comparison of results achieved with other methods, interlaboratory comparisons, systematic assessment of the results, assessment of the uncertainty of the results based on scientific understanding of the theoretical principles of the method, and evaluation of practical experience and logistical issues. Sometimes, the most precise and accurate assay may take too long or cost too much to be practical. As method development proceeds, regular review is required to verify that the needs of the CT facility are still being met. Validation of

methods is absolutely necessary not only to comply with regulations but also to reach process improvement goals. A complete set of validated methods for all aspects of the CT facility will improve the consistency, accuracy, and overall quality of the data that are generated and the cellular products produced.

References/Resources

1. Code of federal regulations. Title 21, CFR Part 211.160. Current good manufacturing practice for finished pharmaceuticals; laboratory controls; general requirements. Washington, DC: US Government Printing Office, 2009 (revised annually).

2. Food and Drug Administration, Guidance for industry: Analytical procedures and methods validation; chemistry, manufacturing, and controls documentation (draft guidance). (August 2000) Rockville, MD: Center for Drug Evaluation and Research, Center for Biologics Evaluation and Research, 2000. [Available at http://www.fda.gov/cder/guidance/2396dft.htm (accessed April 8, 2009).]

3. Food and Drug Administration. Guideline on general principles of process validation. (May 1987) Rockville, MD: Center for Drug Evaluation and Research, 1987. [Available at http://www.fda.gov/cder/guidance/pv.htm (accessed April 8, 2009).]

4. International Conference on Harmonisation of Technical Requirements for Registration of Pharmaceuticals for Human Use. (November 2005) ICH harmonised tripartite guideline. Validation of analytical procedures: Text and methodology. Q2(R1). (October 27, 1994; updated November 2005) Geneva, Switzerland: ICH, 2005.

5. USP <1225>. Validation of compendial methods. In: USP 29-NF 24. Rockville, MD: United States Pharmacopeial Convention, 2006.

6. Stamey TA. Lower limits of detection, biological detection limits, functional sensitivity, or residual cancer detection limit? Sensitivity reports on prostate-specific antigen assays mislead clinicians. Clin Chem 1996;42: 849-52.

7. Food and Drug Administration. Guidance for industry: Validation of growth-based rapid microbiological methods for sterility testing of cellular and gene therapy products (draft guidance). (February 2008) Rockville, MD: Center for Drug Evaluation and Research, Center for Biologics Evaluation and Research, 2008. [Available at http://www.fda.gov/cber/gdlns/stercgtp.htm (accessed April 8, 2009).]

Appendix 43-1. Sample Validation Form

Title:
Purpose: __Prospective___ Retrospective___ Revalidation
Process Parameters and Outcomes
Process parameters:
Outcomes:
Procedure
Study procedure:
Required reagents:
Required supplies:
Required equipment:
Summary of procedure:
Titles of required SOPs:
Titles and locations of necessary manuals:
Validation study forms required:
System Description
Expected results or function:
Critical control points:

Target Replicates

The following number of replicates (runs, etc) should be run for each parameter, unless otherwise directed.

Parameter	Number of Replicates
Test kit sensitivity	
Inhibiting substances (for each medium to be tested)	
Dilution to remove inhibition	
Responsibilities	**Responsible Personnel**
Equipment installation qualification	
Performance qualification	
Study plan author	
Study plan approval	
Data review	
Final approval and implementation	

Results

Inclusive dates of study:

Work forms:

Raw data:

Statistical analysis:

Graphs:

Data summary:

Summary Evaluation

Overall description of study results:

Additional comparison to external labs:

Summary:

This process is considered:___ validated___ not validated

If not validated, give reason:

Further instruction, if disapproved:

Implementation Plan	Responsible Personnel	Date
SOP implementation or modification		__/__/__
Work form creation or modification		__/__/__
Personnel notification		__/__/__
Personnel training		__/__/__
Effective dates		__/__/__

Authorization	Signature	Date
Study plan author		__/__/__
	Title:	Date
Study plan approval		__/__/__
	Title:	Date
Data review		__/__/__
	Title:	Date
Final approval and implementation		__/__/__
	Title:	Date

SOP = standard operating procedure.

Method 43-1. Validating Test Methods

Description

Developing a new test method may be initiated for many reasons. New test methods must be validated before use to ensure that the test is suitable for the intended use as well as to meet regulations and standards. This procedure describes a framework for developing and executing validation plans. However, every validation must be individually designed with consideration for the particular test method and its intended use, as well as the phase of development of the cellular therapy product and available resources.

Time for Procedure

The time required to validate a test method may range from part of a day to months or even years. This wide variation is caused by many factors, such as the complexity of the test method and the validation plan, the resources required and available to complete the validation, and the challenges encountered during validation.

Summary of Procedure

1. Write a complete validation plan.
2. Submit the validation plan for appropriate approvals.
3. Perform the validation.
4. Summarize and evaluate the results.
5. Submit validation results for appropriate approvals.
6. Implement the validated test method.

Procedure

1. Write a complete validation plan. Use a template that includes the following elements. See Appendix 43-1 for an example.
   a. Write a descriptive title and describe the reason the validation is being performed.
   b. Define the expectations for the validation, including acceptable results of various parameters to be evaluated. For example, if the precision and accuracy of an existing test method are known, the new test method should exhibit equal or better performance.
   c. Write the step-by-step procedures to be followed during the validation. Include a listing of all required supplies and equipment.
   d. Describe the system being validated, including the anticipated results, function, intended use of the test method, and critical controls.
   e. Define the target number of replicates to be performed for each parameter being evaluated. It is recommended that a minimum of three replicates be compared for each parameter; however, the more results, the better the comparison. The number of replicate runs should be sufficient to demonstrate reproducibility and provide an accurate measure of variability among successive runs. A statistical package should be used for comparing the data using linear regression, thereby calculating any bias.
   f. Define the responsibilities of personnel involved in the validation. Personnel may be identified by either job title or by name. If they are defined by job title, validation records should clearly indicate who performed various parts of the validation.
2. Submit the validation plan for appropriate approvals. Typically, a laboratory director, a medical director, or both must approve the plan before beginning the validation. Quality assurance staff may also be required to approve the validation plan.
3. Perform the validation. Thoroughly document performance of the validation and all results. Any changes to the validation plan must be approved by the appropriate personnel.
   a. Ensure that the testing equipment is properly installed and calibrated.

b. Establish repeatability during a single assay run or over a short period of time from a minimum of nine determinations covering the specified range of the procedure—for example, three concentration levels tested with three replicates each. Alternatively, repeatability can be determined from a minimum of six determinations at 100% of the test or target concentration.

c. To establish ruggedness, perform the test at different times and under different conditions. Record random variables throughout the validation, such as dates and times, analysts, equipment identifiers, sample type and age, and reagent lot. Evaluate the effects of the individual variables, with no less than three determinations for each potential variable performed.

d. Establish accuracy by collecting data from a minimum of nine determinations over a minimum of three concentration levels covering the specified range (eg, three concentrations, three replicates each). The specified range of values should be useful for the specific method applied. Use of an appropriate reference material is critical (ie, purchased standards or samples established with a high degree of certainty using the current "gold standard").

e. For screening tests, determine the number of samples that test positive or negative with the method being validated and a reference method (ie, the gold standard). Calculate the sensitivity and specificity of the new method as shown in Table 43-1-1.

f. For quantitative tests, determine the LOD and LOQ by testing a sample blank (eg, assay buffer) during a single assay run or over a short period of time from 10 to 20 replicates. If desired, also test reference material or spiked samples at concentrations near the LOD. Determine the SD of each sample and calculate the LOD and LOQ.

g. To determine the analytic specificity, evaluate the extent that an assay detects only a specific substance vs closely related substances (eg, interleukin-12 p40 rather than p70; human interferon-gamma rather than mouse interferon-gamma; insulin rather than proinsulin).

h. Evaluate the robustness of the test system by determining the effect of deliberate changes on test accuracy, precision, and other factors. Conditions to be tested should represent normal conditions that are likely to be encountered and that can be controlled through specifications in the assay protocol.

4. Summarize and evaluate results as completely as possible. Graph data to aid in interpretation and apply appropriate statistical methods.

5. Submit validation results for appropriate approvals. The same individuals responsible for approving the validation plan should review and approve validation results.

6. Implement the validated test method. Notify customers of the changes in the test method and any impacts they may have.

Table 43-1-1. Parameters for Qualitative Screening Tests

Test Outcome	Condition		Predictive Value
	True	**False**	
Positive	True positive	False positive	Positive predictive value = TP / (TP + FP)
Negative	False negative	True negative	Negative predictive value = TN / (TN + FN)
	Sensitivity = TP / (TP + FN)	**Specificity =** TN / (FP + TN)	

TP = true positive; FP = false positive; FN = false negative; TN = true negative.

Note: In many cases, it is helpful to seek input from customers throughout the validation.

Notes

See a sample validation form in Appendix 43-1.

Anticipated Results

Method is validated and can be implemented in the facility.

In: Areman EM, Loper K, eds
Cellular Therapy: Principles, Methods, and Regulations
Bethesda, MD: AABB, 2009

♦♦♦ **44** ♦♦♦

Cell Counts and Differentials of Cellular Therapy Products

Carolyn A. Keever-Taylor, PhD

DETERMINATION OF THE TOTAL NUMBER of nucleated cells (NCs) or white blood cells (WBCs) in hematopoietic progenitor cell (HPC) and other cellular therapy (CT) products can provide valuable information about product quality at the time of collection, during and after processing, and at infusion. For marrow and umbilical cord blood (UCB) products (HPC-M and HPC-C), this information serves as an indicator of HPC content because approximately 0.5% to 1% of the WBCs express CD34, an HPC phenotypic marker. HPCs from apheresis (HPC-A) products contain a more variable percentage of CD34+ cells, making the WBC content alone less relevant as a surrogate for progenitor cells. However, the WBC count combined with the product differential usually reflects the quality of the collection. Monitoring the number of WBCs, and in some cases WBC subsets, after critical steps in processing [buffy coat preparation, mononuclear cell (MNC) preparation, cell enrichment or cell depletion, etc] can provide rapid evidence that the desired endpoints have been achieved.[1] For some products, the WBC count itself

may be one of the product release criteria, or it may be a component of the calculation and assessment of the cell dose (eg, CD34+ cells/kg, CD3+ cells/kg) that is one of the release criteria. In any case, a reliable assay method for WBC counting is critical to evaluation of a CT product.

Electronic hematology analyzers are widely used in clinical laboratories for the performance of WBC counts. The precision (reproducibility) of a hematology analyzer is superior to that of manual cell-counting methods because larger numbers of cells can be counted and fewer sample manipulations are required. However, hematology analyzers are designed for assessing nonmobilized peripheral blood collected in EDTA anticoagulants. HPC products, especially HPC-M, have unique characteristics that may affect the accuracy of cell counts performed on these hematology analyzers. Therefore, the laboratory must properly validate the assay and have good control systems in place. The use of a hematology analyzer to differentially assess WBC subsets is even more problematic for both HPC-M and HPC-A products. This chapter dis-

Carolyn A. Keever-Taylor, PhD, Director, BMT Processing Laboratories, and Professor of Medicine, Division of Neoplastic Diseases, Medical College of Wisconsin, Milwaukee, Wisconsin

The author has disclosed no conflict of interest.

cusses expected results and methodologic approaches to ensure the accuracy of WBC counts and differentials performed on HPC products.

Marrow HPC Products

Although mobilized peripheral blood (PB), or HPC-A, has become the HPC product of choice for many transplant centers, HPC-M may be preferred in some situations. The autologous or allogeneic donor may fail to mobilize, certain ex-vivo procedures may require a marrow cell source, a marrow concentrate may be preferable for some pediatric patients, or a donor may prefer to donate marrow rather than undergo growth factor mobilization followed by apheresis.[2] The physical composition of marrow harvested for clinical transplant differs from PB in that it contains substantial populations of stromal elements, including bone spicules, mesenchymal stromal cells, fibroblasts, and fat. The procedure for harvesting marrow from within the bone may result in a given product also containing considerable PB and cell aggregates. By its nature, the cellular composition of marrow is greatly enriched for immature blood elements, including nucleated red blood cells (NRBCs), megakaryocytes, and myeloid and lymphoid precursors that are not normally found in PB. Marrow may also contain hemolyzed red cells as a result of the trauma of the harvest or the use of anticoagulants that are not isotonic. Additional variation is introduced by components of the medium into which marrow is harvested (ie, tissue culture medium, saline, isotonic electrolyte solutions) and in the source and concentration of anticoagulant [ie, heparin, acid (or anticoagulant)-citrate-dextrose, or both].

Marrow Nucleated Cell Counts

Several of the differences between marrow and nonmobilized PB can affect the accuracy of WBC counts performed by hematology analyzers. The collection medium may inhibit the lysis of red cells within the analyzer, resulting in overestimation of cell numbers, or cell aggregates or small clots that are not trapped by the harvest filters may block tubing, resulting in lower counts. The author's experience as well as that of others indicates that the amount of fat in the collected marrow has the most influence on the accuracy of the WBC count when using a hematology analyzer.[3,4] All marrow harvests contain fat in varying amounts. Higher fat content is associated with older donor age and with multiple chemotherapy treatment courses.[4-6] Approaches that have been taken to minimize the effect of fat on the WBC count assay include use of manual cell-counting methods and removal of fat from the sample before analysis.[3] To take advantage of the higher accuracy of the hematology analyzer, the author's laboratory explored two methods of removing fat from marrow product samples before counting. Because fat is insoluble in water, it rises to the surface when centrifugal force is applied to the sample. Either all or only the topmost part of the plasma/fat layer can be removed and the volume replaced with saline before counting. The data in Table 44-1 compare these two approaches and indicate that removal and replacement of the top portion of plasma alone is as efficient as removal and replacement of the entire plasma layer in correcting the hematology analyzer WBC counts. Processing steps that include plasma removal generally reduce fat content adequately to preclude the necessity for a saline replacement procedure for WBC sample aliquots taken during or after processing. The procedure described in Method 44-1 is used for partial plasma removal from marrow samples.

The contribution of NRBCs to the WBC count of marrow or UCB has long been a concern because both products have a high concentration of these cells. Flow-cytometry-based hematology analyzers such as the CELL-DYNA4000 (Abbott Diagnostics, Santa Clara, CA) and the XE-2100 and XE-5000 (Sysmex Corp, Kobe, Japan) are able to separately distinguish and enumerate NRBCs.[7,8] However, many CT facilities use less-sophisticated electrical-impedance-based analyzers that include NRBCs in the WBC count. Some laboratories correct the WBC count based on the percentage of NRBCs detected on manual blood smears, but for UCB products, NRBC content correlates with the number of CD34+ cells and with the rate of myeloid engraftment, suggesting that excluding NRBCs will not improve the value of the WBC count in predicting product quality.[9]

The CT facility is often called upon to provide estimates to the marrow collection team of the volume of marrow required to reach a predetermined

Table 44-1. Effect of Complete or Partial Plasma/Fat Removal on Marrow Nucleated Cell Counts

Experiment	Cells/mL × 10⁶ (Percentage Difference from Manual)					
	Analyzer,* Fat In[†]	Manual,[‡] Fat In	Analyzer, Partial[§]	Manual, Partial	Analyzer, Complete[‖]	Manual, Complete
Exp 1	22.6	20.3	20.1	20.3	20.6	20.4
Exp 2	19.7	17.5	17.4	17.4	17.7	17.5
Exp 3	20.5	17.6	17.1	17.5	17.6	17.7
Mean	20.9 (9.6%)	18.5	18.2 (1.1%)	18.4	18.6 (0.8%)	18.5
Standard deviation	±1.2	±1.3	±1.3	±1.3	±1.4	±1.3
p value[‖]		0.001		0.092		0.252

*Counts were performed using an impedance-based hematology analyzer (Coulter AC•T diff 2, Beckman Coulter, Fullerton, CA).
[†]Counts were performed without removal of fat.
[‡]Counts were performed by a manual method.
[§]Counts were performed after removal of the fatty layer and replacement by saline.
[‖]Counts were performed after removal of the complete plasma layer and replacement by saline.
[¶]Paired students T test.

total cell harvest goal. The laboratory may also be asked to provide cell counts at intervals during the harvest to monitor progress toward the harvest goal. In both cases, establishing the expected range of WBC/mL appropriate for the donor undergoing harvest is important. The WBC/mL of marrow from a healthy donor depends on several variables, including the following: 1) donor age, with younger donors having a more cellular marrow[6]; 2) the volume collected in each individual aspiration, with larger volume aspirates drawing in more PB and thus diluting the number of marrow cells[10]; and 3)

the total volume of the collected product. Analysis of data from 1496 HPC-M products processed in the author's laboratory confirmed the effect of donor age on marrow cellularity previously reported by Buckner et al[6] (see Table 44-2) and the effect of the total volume of collected marrow (see Table 44-3) on the WBC/mL in the final product. The effect of harvest volume was seen within each donor age group, with the highest cell counts in the <11 years age group when <500 mL of total product was harvested, and the lowest cell counts in the >60 years age group, with the largest harvest vol-

Table 44-2. Effect of Donor Age on Marrow Cellularity

Measure	Donor Age (Years) and Cells/mL × 10⁷						
	<11	11-20	21-30	31-40	41-50	51-60	>60
Mean	3.19	2.42	2.73	2.59	2.45	2.27	2.15
Standard deviation	±1.26	±0.84	±1.06	±0.87	±1.02	±0.78	±0.07
N	107	94	262	491	372	157	13

Table 44-3. Effect of Marrow Product Volume on Cellularity

Measure	Marrow Product Volume in mL (Cells/mL $\times 10^7$)					
	<501	501-800	801-1100	1101-1400	1401-1700	>1700
Mean	3.34	2.91	2.60	2.43	2.28	2.09
Standard deviation	±1.41	±1.04	±0.88	±0.83	±0.68	±0.59
N	179	222	293	339	292	171

umes (>1700 mL) (data not shown). These volume-based differences likely reflect donor age (smaller volumes are typically harvested from younger donors) as well as the volume of each aspirate because, with larger target harvest volumes, individual aspirate volume also tends to be larger (C Taylor, unpublished observations).

Marrow Differentials

Monitoring subsets of WBCs during processing provides useful information to the cell-processing laboratory. Hematology analyzers that use the electrical-impedance method of direct current are able to identify three major subsets of WBCs, classified as 1) lymphocytes, 2) a midsize population that includes mostly monocytes along with basophils and eosinophils, and 3) granulocytes. This degree of differential is sufficient to monitor products during processing steps that involve enrichment of the MNC fraction (lymphocytes and monocytes) or specific depletion of marrow lymphocytes or lymphocyte subsets. Unfortunately, the ability of impedance-based analyzers to correctly distinguish even these three major populations in marrow is poor compared to PB. This weakness is in part because of the presence of NRBCs, which are classified as lymphocytes by most analyzer software, and because of large populations of immature myeloid cells that may share characteristics of lymphocytes. Manual differentials determined by blood smear examination can be a reliable method if performed by qualified staff.[11] However, analysis by flow cytometry using an antibody panel that includes an antibody to CD45 (an antigen present on all human hematopoietic cells except red cells, platelets, and their precursors) is more specific than a manual differential and is more accurate than the use of standard hematology analyzers in identifying WBC subsets.[12,13] One such flow-cytometry-based method using anti-CD45 together with anti-CD14 to distinguish mature lymphocytes (bright CD45+, CD14–) and mature monocytes (bright CD45+, CD14+) within normal and abnormal whole blood samples was found to correlate closely with blood smear examination.[12] Figure 44-1 illustrates this method applied to whole blood, marrow, and a mobilized apheresis product.

The author's facility assessed lymphocyte and monocyte populations in marrow before and after processing by density gradient separation using both a flow cytometer and an impedance-based hematology analyzer (Coulter AC·T diff 2, Beckman Coulter, Fullerton, CA). With whole marrow, agreement for lymphocyte content between the two methods was poor: more than 50% more cells were classified as lymphocytes by the hematology analyzer, likely reflecting that instrument's assessment of NRBCs as lymphocytes (Table 44-4). Likewise, significantly more cells were classified as monocytes by the hematology analyzer (39% more than by flow cytometry), possibly because of the inclusion of basophils and eosinophils in this population. In marrow, the light-density cell fraction is largely depleted of red cells, NRBCs, and mature granulocytes but contains a large population of immature lymphocytes and myeloid cells in addition to mature lymphocytes and monocytes. Even in the less heterogeneous marrow MNC fraction, discrepancies occurred in the correct identification of lymphocytes by the hematology analyzer. These differences, which may have reflected the presence of immature lymphocytes, were of less magnitude (23% higher) than for the unseparated marrow suspension. Indeed, no significant difference (p

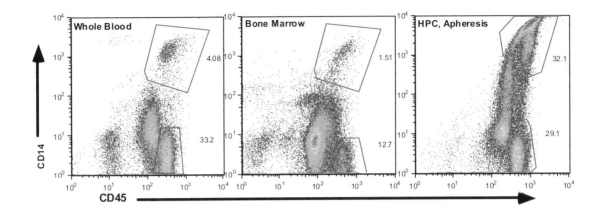

Figure 44-1. Flow-cytometry differential using CD45 together with CD14 to identify lymphocytes (bright CD45+, CD14–) and monocytes (bright CD45+, CD14+).

>0.5) existed between the percentage of monocytes detected by the two methods for marrow MNC products, likely because of depletion of mature eosinophils and basophils. Therefore, either flow-cytometry-based methods or manual differentials should be used for monitoring lymphocytes during marrow processing.

Apheresis HPC Products

HPC-A has increasingly become a preferred HPC source for both autologous and allogeneic transplantation since the pioneering observations of Siena et al.[14] They reported that CD34+ cells could be found in the circulation following chemother-

apy and that CD34+ cell content could be enhanced further by in-vivo treatment with recombinant hematopoietic growth factors. Unlike HPC-M, HPC-A consists exclusively of hematopoietic cells, lacks fat that can interfere with cell counts, and contains relatively few of the NRBCs that so seriously affect marrow differentials performed by hematology analyzers. However, the mobilized population may contain large numbers of immature myeloid cells that can affect the measurement of WBC counts and differentials.

HPC-A WBC Counts

Assessment of WBCs in apheresis products usually requires sample dilution to reduce the cell counts to

Table 44-4. Flow-Cytometry Differential Compared to Hematology-Analyzer Marrow

	Flow Cytometer		Hematology Analyzer	
	Lymphocytes	Monocytes	Lymphocytes	Monocytes
Whole marrow* mean	16.1%	3.3%	34.1%	5.4%
Whole marrow standard deviation	±9.0%	±1.4%	±7.3%	±2.5%
p value‡	0.0000	0.0000		
Marrow mononuclear cells† mean	38.1%	5.8%	49.7%	6.7%
Marrow mononuclear cells standard deviation	±16.2%	±2.2%	±12.7%	±2.7%
p value‡	0.0000	0.0564		

*n = 49.
†Density-gradient-prepared marrow mononuclear cells (n = 32).
‡Paired students T-test.

within the linear range of the hematology analyzer. HPC-A from healthy allogeneic donors ($3.3 \times 10^8 \pm 1.4 \times 10^8$/mL; n = 117) are in general more cellular than products from autologous donors who have previously undergone myelotoxic therapy ($1.9 \times 10^8 \pm 1.0 \times 10^8$/mL; n = 107). The high cellular content of HPC-A products requires extra care during sampling to ensure that a representative sample for WBC assessment is obtained. With care in sampling (see "Sampling and Determination of Product Volume" below) and in preparing extra dilutions required for counting, WBC assessment of HPC-A products using a hematology analyzer can produce results as reliable as those obtained from normal PB samples.

Mobilized Peripheral Blood Differentials

Although the MNC content together with colony-forming units of peripheral blood stem cells were reported to correlate with the rate of engraftment,[15] CD34+ cell content as determined by flow cytometry was subsequently found to be a superior and more reproducible predictor of engraftment kinetics.[16] Nevertheless, assessment of HPC-A MNC content is valuable for predicting both post-thaw

recovery of cryopreserved products and potential for adverse reactions at infusion. Viable cell recovery after thawing is directly correlated with total MNC content, as shown from the author's experience in Fig 44-2. Cryopreserved products with a high percentage of granulocytes (and, correspondingly, a low percentage of MNCs) not only thaw poorly but also are associated with adverse reactions after infusion, both with and without removal of dimethyl sulfoxide before infusion.[18,19] Products collected by the author's program have shown an inverse relationship between the percentage of product MNCs and the number of cells collected, whereas MNC content has shown no correlation with the absolute number of CD34+ cells collected (data not shown). Therefore, monitoring apheresis collections to maximize MNC content can reduce laboratory workload (fewer bags need to be frozen), increase available freezer storage space, improve post-thaw cell recovery, and reduce the likelihood of infusion reactions. For these reasons, HPC-A MNC content can be considered a monitor of product quality and should routinely be tested for quality assurance purposes.

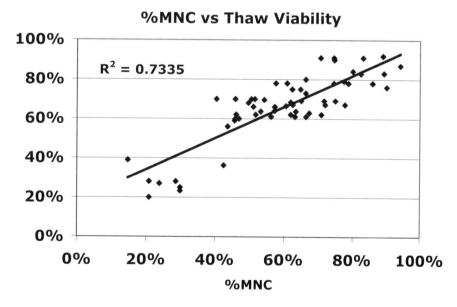

Figure 44-2. Correlation of post-thawing cell viability with mononuclear cell (MNC) content. MNC content was determined by flow cytometry, and thaw viability was assessed by trypan blue dye exclusion in the laboratory after dimethyl sulfoxide removal using a dextran/albumin thawing procedure.[17] Data are from 64 products frozen and thawed at the Medical College of Wisconsin.

Despite the absence of significant numbers of NRBCs in HPC-A products, the author has found that an impedance-based hematology analyzer consistently overestimates the percentage of lymphocytes in HPC-A compared to the flow-cytometry differential standard (p <0.0000 by paired students T test; n = 91; see Table 44-5). In contrast to marrow, where more cells were classified as monocytes by the hematology analyzer, fewer HPC-A cells were identified as monocytes compared to the flow-cytometry differential (Table 44-5). The overall MNC content (lymphocytes plus monocytes) determined by the hematology analyzer, although significantly different by the paired students T test, showed only a 12% difference compared to the flow-cytometry method. Therefore, although differences from the true value exist, the hematology analyzer appears to provide useful information regarding the overall MNC content of HPA-A products.

For facilities without access to hematology analyzers able to perform a differential or to perform a flow-cytometry-based differential, HPC-A product differentials may be performed by manual methods with appropriate modification.[11,12] Because HPC-A products contain approximately one-tenth the number of red cells in whole blood or whole marrow, standard methods of slide preparation may result in poor dispersion or physical disruption of the cells. More consistent slide preparation results may be obtained using a cytocentrifuge to apply the sample. Product samples that are held for a period of time before slide preparation, especially if the collection contains a high percentage of myeloid cells, are more susceptible to disruption during slide preparation. These issues together with the increased time and technical expertise required to perform manual differentials make the flow cytometry or hematology analyzer methods (for total MNC) preferable to manual methods. Because nearly all processing facilities assess CD34+ cell content using flow cytometry, the addition of a test sample containing anti-CD45 and anti-CD14 may be the most accurate method for determining product MNC content when a flow-cytometry-based hematology analyzer is not available.

Sampling and Determination of Product Volume

Regardless of the product type, CT product NC counts and differentials require representative sampling, whereas determination of the total NC content requires an accurate assessment of product volume. As noted in Table 44-3, the collection volume of marrow products may vary over a wide range to more than 1700 mL. In contrast, the collected volume of HPC-A is more consistent, with differences usually dependent on factors such as the apheresis instrument used and the number of blood volumes processed rather than on donor or product variability. Marrow products may be received into the laboratory in multiple bags collected over the course of the harvest procedure. Each bag must be sampled and tested separately because the cells per mL in each bag will likely vary. In all cases, the product must be well mixed before sampling. If product bags are overfilled, an event that occasionally occurs, adequate mixing may not be possible by inversion of the bag. In such cases, the product should be aseptically transferred to a

Table 44-5. Flow-Cytometry Differential Compared to Hematology Analyzer for HPC-A*

Statistical Value	Flow Cytometer			Hematology Analyzer		
	Ly	Mo	MNC	Ly	Mo	MNC
Mean	28.5%	35.3%	63.8%	35.7%	23.2%	58.9%
Standard deviation	±17.5%	±14.2%	±21.1%	±14.6%	±11.2%	±20.8%
p value†	0.0000	0.0000	0.0000			

*Data are from 91 HPC-A products processed at the Medical College of Wisconsin.
†Paired students T test.
Ly = lymphocytes; Mo = monocytes; MNC = mononuclear cells (lymphocytes and monocytes).

new, larger bag to allow adequate mixing before sampling. The product bag should be inverted a sufficient number of times (6-10) to ensure the product is well mixed, especially for apheresis products that are highly cellular. A minimum of a 1-mL sample should be removed from each product bag to permit repeat testing. Product present in attached tubing should not be used as a representative sample unless the bag was well mixed before the cells were introduced into the tubing. Clearing sampling ports of cells before removing the sample for counting is also important. NC counts and differentials should be performed as soon after sampling as possible, preferably within 24 hours. Product samples should not be stored at refrigerator temperatures to avoid granulocyte aggregates that might result in artificially low counts.

Product volume may be determined by direct measurement if products are transferred by syringe from one container to another. Most often, however, product volume is determined by weight. The initial product weight is probably best determined by weighing the product in the bag at receipt, transferring the product to a new bag, and then subtracting the tare weight of the original bag with its attached tubing and ports. If products do not require transfer before processing or infusion, however, the laboratory should determine the weight of empty bags of like size and source and subtract the standard bag weight before determining the product volume. Care must be taken to include the weight of any attached tubing, ports, and connectors.

The correlation of product weight to volume is a function of the specific gravity of the product. The specific gravity of blood is affected by the red cell content of the product. The correlation of volume to weight for whole blood products with a packed red cell mass of approximately 40% is 1 mL = 1.058 g, with the volume calculated by dividing the weight by 1.058.[20] The hematocrit of whole marrow is similar to that of whole blood, so the same conversion factor is typically used. HPC apheresis products contain fewer red cells, with a typical hematocrit of approximately 5%. The author's own validation studies comparing weighed volume with measured volume have shown that a conversion factor of 1 mL = 1.030 grams provides the closest correlation of weighed to measured volume. This conversion factor of 1.030 is typically used for

platelets and plasma products in the blood bank.[20] However, in many laboratories where multiple CT processing steps are performed, weight and volume are often used interchangeably. Because specific gravity of the product can change with each processing step, a different conversion factor would be needed for each in-process cell count, increasing the probability of calculation errors. Because of all the variables described above, it is doubtful that a cell count based on weight is much less accurate than one based on a calculated volume. Whenever feasible, a direct measure of product volume is preferred.

Instrument and Equipment Quality Control

All instrumentation (flow cytometers, hematology analyzers) and equipment (scales, centrifuges, pipettes) used for the assessment of WBC counts and product differentials must be properly qualified, maintained, and calibrated. Control cells should be tested each day of use (or more often if recommended), and the laboratory testing should participate in the appropriate external proficiency studies for the tests that are performed.

Summary

Accurate determination of the NC count and assessment of product differential to at least the level of lymphocytes, monocytes, and granulocytes depend on a number of variables unique to HPC products as compared to PB. Representative sampling and accurate volume determination are essential for the assessment of WBC content for all products. WBC counts of HPC-M products are greatly affected by the presence of fat, which should be removed from the sample aliquot for a more accurate count. The expected cellularity of HPC-M products is a function of both donor age and the volume of marrow that has been collected. Differentials for unmanipulated marrow are best performed using a flow cytometer or a flow-cytometry-based hematology analyzer, whereas impedance-based hematology analyzers provide a better estimate of MNC content of light-density cell-enriched HPC-M products. The WBC count of

HPC-A products requires an extra dilution step but can be accurately assessed using an impedance-based hematology analyzer. Although the flow cytometer provides a better estimate of lymphocytes and monocytes in HPC-A products, the hematology analyzer gives a good estimate of total MNC and can be used as a measure of product quality.

References/Resources

1. Lasky L, Johnson N. Quality assurance in marrow processing. In: Areman E, Deeg H, Sacher R, eds. Bone marrow and stem cell processing: A manual of current techniques. Philadelphia: FA Davis, 1992:386-443.

2. Urbano-Ispizua A. Risk assessment in haematopoietic stem cell transplantation: Stem cell source. Best Pract Res Clin Haematol 2007;20:265-80.

3. Bentley SA, Taylor MA, Killian DE, et al. Correction of bone marrow nucleated cell counts for the presence of fat particles. Am J Clin Pathol 1995;104:60-4.

4. Read E, Carter C, Cullis H. Bone marrow cell counting: Methodological issues. In: Gee A, ed. Bone marrow processing and purging: A practical guide. Boca Raton, FL: CRC Press, 2000:107-19.

5. Hartsock RJ, Smith EB, Petty CS. Normal variations with aging of the amount of hematopoietic tissue in bone marrow from the anterior iliac crest: A study made from 177 cases of sudden death examined by necropsy. Am J Clin Pathol 1965;43:326-31.

6. Buckner CD, Clift RA, Sanders JE, et al. Marrow harvesting from normal donors. Blood 1984;64:630-4.

7. Mori Y, Mizukami T, Hamaguchi Y, et al. Automation of bone marrow aspirate examination using the XE-2100 automated hematology analyzer. Cytometry 2004;58:25-31.

8. Yamamura R, Yamamura R, Hino M, et al. Automated bone marrow analysis using the CD4000 automated haematology analyser. J Autom Methods Manag Chem 2000;22:89-92.

9. Stevens CE, Gladstone J, Taylor PE, et al. Placental/umbilical cord blood for unrelated-donor bone marrow reconstitution: Relevance of nucleated red blood cells. Blood 2002;100:2662-4.

10. Dresch C, Faille A, Poirier O, et al. The cellular composition of the granulocyte series in the normal human bone marrow according to the volume of the sample. J Clin Pathol 1974;27:106-8.

11. Gulati GL, Hyun BH. Blood smear examination. Hematol Oncol Clin North Am 1994;8:631-50.

12. Hubl W, Hauptlorenz S, Tlustos L, et al. Precision and accuracy of monocyte counting. Comparison of two hematology analyzers, the manual differential and flow cytometry. Am J Clin Pathol 1995;103:167-70.

13. Kim M, Kim J, Lim J, et al. Use of an automated hematology analyzer and flow cytometry to assess bone marrow cellularity and differential cell count. Ann Clin Lab Sci 2004;34:307-13.

14. Siena S, Bregni M, Brando B, et al. Circulation of CD34+ hematopoietic stem cells in the peripheral blood of high-dose cyclophosphamide-treated patients: Enhancement by intravenous recombinant human granulocyte-macrophage colony-stimulating factor. Blood 1989;74:1905-14.

15. To LB, Shepperd KM, Haylock DN, et al. Single high doses of cyclophosphamide enable the collection of high numbers of hemopoietic stem cells from the peripheral blood. Exp Hematol 1990;18:442-7.

16. Ketterer N, Salles G, Raba M, et al. High CD34(+) cell counts decrease hematologic toxicity of autologous peripheral blood progenitor cell transplantation. Blood 1998;91:3148-55.

17. Rubinstein P, Dobrila L, Rosenfield RE, et al. Processing and cryopreservation of placental/umbilical cord blood for unrelated bone marrow reconstitution. Proc Natl Acad Sci U S A 1995;92:10119-22.

18. Milone G, Mercurio S, Strano A, et al. Adverse events after infusions of cryopreserved hematopoietic stem cells depend on non-mononuclear cells in the infused suspension and patient age. Cytotherapy 2007;9:348-55.

19. Calmels B, Lemarie C, Esterni B, et al. Occurrence and severity of adverse events after autologous hematopoietic progenitor cell infusion are related to the amount of granulocytes in the apheresis product. Transfusion 2007;47:1268-75.

20. Trudnowski RJ, Rico RC. Specific gravity of blood and plasma at 4 and 37 degrees C. Clin Chem 1974;20:615-6.

Method 44-1. Partial Plasma Removal from Marrow Samples

Description

Fat in collected marrow can negatively affect the accuracy of the white cell (WBC) count when using a hematology analyzer. All marrow harvests contain fat in varying amounts. Partial removal of plasma and replacement with a saline solution results in a more accurate WBC count.

Time for Procedure

Approximately 10 minutes.

Summary of Procedure

After a marrow sample is centrifuged, a portion of the plasma/fat layer is removed and replaced with a saline solution. The WBC count is performed on this sample.

Procedure

1. Remove a 2.0-mL sample from the well-mixed marrow product and transfer to a 12×75-cm tube.

2. Cap the tube and centrifuge at 220 *g* for 5 minutes.
3. On the outside of the tube, mark the topmost liquid layer with a marker, remove the cap, and from the top of the tube aspirate sufficient volume to remove the visible fatty layer (approximately 0.2 mL).
4. Replace any removed liquid with saline, phosphate-buffered saline, or another isotonic solution suitable for the suspension of marrow cells.
5. Cap the tube, and mix the sample well.
6. Perform a WBC count using a hematology analyzer.

Anticipated Results

An accurate WBC count should be obtained with this method.

In: Areman EM, Loper K, eds
Cellular Therapy: Principles, Methods, and Regulations
Bethesda, MD: AABB, 2009

◆◆◆ **45** ◆◆◆

Enumeration of CD34+ Cells by Flow Cytometry

*D. Robert Sutherland, MSc, and
Michael Keeney, FIMLS, FCSMLS(D)*

THE PIONEERING STUDIES OF THOMAS ET al in the late 1950s first established that a cellular component of syngeneic marrow was capable of regenerating multilineage hematopoiesis in cancer patients receiving supralethal doses of radiation.[1,2] The marrow cells responsible for engraftment, termed hematopoietic progenitor cells (HPCs), were also found in low numbers in the peripheral circulation as assessed by colony-forming cell assays.[3] In the mid-1980s, monoclonal antibodies to a molecule called CD34 were developed, and CD34 was found to represent the first documented cell-surface antigen whose expression within the hematopoietic system is restricted to

stem and progenitor cells of all lineages.[4,5] The subsequent availability of an increasing number of CD34 antibodies that could be conjugated with bright fluorochromes without loss of specific binding capabilities led to the development of simple, single-color, flow-cytometric assays to assess graft adequacy.[6] More-sophisticated multiparameter flow assays could accurately enumerate rare CD34+ cells and also perform a qualitative (ie, CD34+ cell subset) assessment of an HPC product or assess the level of T-lymphocyte contamination in a CD34+ cell-selected product in the allotransplant setting. Accurate enumeration of CD34+ cells can provide crucial clinical information to the transplant physi-

D. Robert Sutherland, MSc, Professor, Department of Medicine, University of Toronto, and Technical Director, Clinical Flow Cytometry, University Health Network/Toronto General Hospital, Toronto, Ontario, Canada; and Michael Keeney, FIMLS, FCSMLS(D), Coordinator, Hematology/Flow Cytometry, and Associate Scientist, Lawson Health Research Institute, London Health Sciences Centre, London, Ontario, Canada

D. R. Sutherland has disclosed no conflicts of interest. M. Keeney has disclosed a consulting relationship with Beckman Coulter, Inc.

cian. Currently, flow cytometry is the only methodology capable of rapidly measuring this most clinically useful surrogate marker of graft adequacy in all sources of HPCs.

CD34+ Cell Enumeration Using Multiparameter Cytometry and Sequential Boolean Gating: The ISHAGE Protocol

Although a number of simple, flow-cytometric assays were developed beginning in 1989,[6] a standardized protocol to enumerate CD34+ cells in the HPC transplant setting that was flexible, robust, and accurate did not emerge until about 1995.[7] Earlier methods had not taken into account the structural characteristics of the mucin-like CD34 molecule, the physical composition of the three broad classes of epitopes, and the unanticipated constraints imposed by different conjugates; neither had they taken full advantage of the "composite phenotype" and light-scattering characteristics of bona fide CD34+ cells[5] (see below). To eliminate nonleukocytes and debris from the analysis and generate a much more stable denominator against which to measure CD34+ cells, CD45 was used as a counter stain. Note was also taken of the observation that primitive blast cells, which exhibit light-scattering properties that are generally similar to lymphocytes, express lower levels of CD45 on their surfaces, thus providing a means of delineating lymphocytes from normal blast cells using this surface marker.[8] Just as lymphocytes, monocytes, and granulocytes form discrete clusters on CD45 staining vs side-scatter analysis, so do CD34+ cells.[7,9]

Thus, a sensitive and accurate multiparameter flow methodology was devised that used the maximum information available—ie, four parameters: forward and side light scatter and the intensities of CD34 and CD45 staining.[7] As shown in Fig 45-1 and Fig 45-2, plots 1 through 4, these four parameters were combined in a sequential Boolean gating strategy that could be used on a variety of sources of HPCs. Only basic software was required for data analysis, and the methodology was deployable on a range of cytometers. This method subsequently

formed the basis of a clinical guideline established in association with the International Society of Hematotherapy and Graft Engineering (ISHAGE) for CD34+ cell quantitation in peripheral blood (PB) and PB stem cell products.[9] (ISHAGE was subsequently renamed the International Society for Cellular Therapy.)

By incorporating a known number of fluorescent counting beads in the flow-cytometric analysis and by assessing the ratio between the number of beads and CD34+ cells counted, an absolute CD34+ cell count could be generated using a flow cytometer alone[10] ("single-platform" methodology), thus eliminating the need for a hematology analyzer (Fig 45-1, plot 7, and Fig 45-2, plot 5). Simple ammonium-chloride-based red cell lysis without washing (lyse-no-wash) sample processing was used. Finally, the inclusion of the viability dye 7-amino-actinomycin D (7-AAD) allowed the exclusion of dead cells and the enumeration of viable CD34+ cells[10] (Fig 45-1, plot 5, Fig 45-2, plot 8, and Fig 45-3, plot 9).

Several commercial kits have been developed based on the single-platform, viable CD34 ISHAGE protocol, the first of which was the Stem-Kit from Beckman Coulter (Fullerton, CA). The Stem-Kit performs equally well on a variety of flow cytometers from both Beckman Coulter (Fig 45-1) and BD Biosciences (San Jose, CA; Fig 45-2), using a wide variety of sources of HPCs. Dako (Glostrup, Denmark) produced the CD34 Count Kit, which contains CD45/CD34, 7-AAD, an ammonium-chloride-based lysing agent, and fluorescent counting beads for use in conjunction with an ISHAGE gating protocol. BD Biosciences markets Trucount tubes that contain a known number of freeze-dried fluorescent counting beads as a stand-alone product as well as all analyte-specific reagents (ASRs) necessary to perform the enumeration of viable CD34+ cells (CD45FITC, CD34PE, PharmLyse, and Via-Probe) using single-platform ISHAGE methodologies.[11] As detailed below and elsewhere,[12] some modifications to the original single-platform method[10] are required because of the small size of the beads. An example of a Trucount-based method incorporating the latest modifications is presented in Fig 45-4.

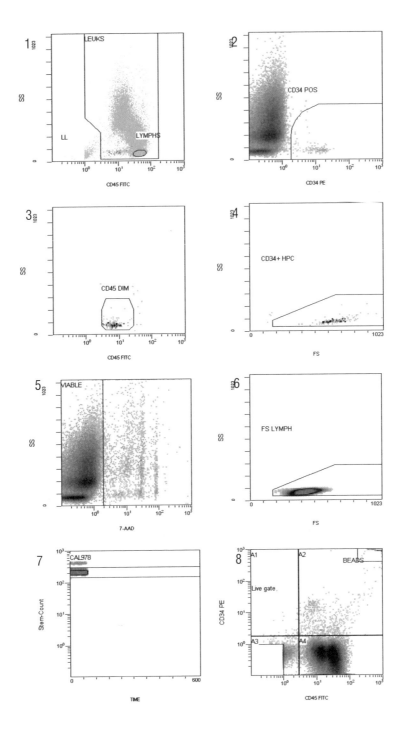

Figure 45-1. Enumeration of viable CD34+ cells with Stem-Kit and Automated Stem-CXP software analysis on a Beckman Coulter FC 500 (Beckman Coulter, Fullerton, CA). Fresh apheresis sample diluted 1/10 with PBS/ 1% bovine serum albumin. Plot 1 is all CD45+ leukocytes, gated on 7-amino-actinomycin D-negative (viable) events from plot 5. Plots 2-4 are sequentially Boolean gated from plot 1. Plot 6 is gated on lymphocytes from plot 1 to allow the discriminator to be set on forward scatter. Plot 7 is gated on singlet Stem-Count fluorospheres (FL3) vs time. Plot 8 shows fluorospheres captured in the top right-hand corner and a "live gate" in the bottom left corner, which is used to exclude debris from the listmode file, particularly important in cord blood, peripheral blood, or marrow files. The leukocyte count was 18.3×10^9/L; viable CD34+ percent and absolute count were 0.19% and 37/µL, respectively (from plot 4). The sample was 97.4% viable (from plot 5).

(Continued)

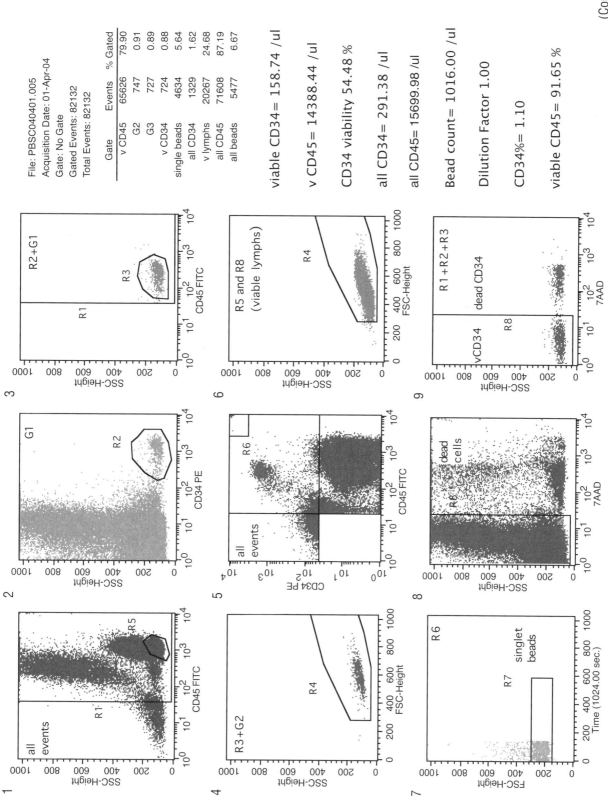

Figure 45-2. Enumeration of viable CD34+ cells with Stem-Kit on a BD Biosciences (San Jose, CA) FACSCalibur cytometer equipped with CellQuest. An apheresis sample that had been stored overnight at room temperature was stained with the Stem-Kit reagent set. Viable CD34+ cells were identified using Boolean gating and regions R1 through R4 (plots 1-4), including only viable (7-AAD-negative) cells from region R8 (plot 8). Viable lymphocytes from region R5 (plot 1) and R8 are displayed on plot 6 and the duplicate blast-lymphocyte region R4 adjusted to include the smallest viable lymphocytes. Duplicate gating region R4 on plot 4 self-adjusts accordingly. Plot 5 shows the position of a "live" gate in the bottom left corner, which excludes debris resulting from lyse-no-wash sample processing of peripheral blood, cord blood, and marrow sample types. The number of CD34+ cells in region R4 is compared with the total number of singlet beads counted in the same listmode file. In the example shown, total beads are gated in region R6 on plot 5 and displayed on plot 7 (time vs forward scatter). Singlet beads are then delineated and enumerated in gating region R7. Sample analysis was performed using CellQuest Pro (BD Biosciences) software with semiautomated expression editors. For earlier versions of CellQuest, the absolute number of viable (v)CD34+ cells/μL is calculated as follows:

$$\frac{\text{Number of CD34+ cells}}{\text{Number of singlet beads}} \times \text{bead concentration} \times \text{DF}$$

In the formula, the number of CD34+ cells is determined from logical gate G4 (vCD34 in gate stats = R1 + R2 + R3 + R4 + R8), the bead concentration is specified by the manufacturer, DF is the sample dilution factor, and the singlet bead count is determined from plot 7 (singlet beads in gate stats = R6 + R7). Plot 9 shows total CD34+ cells (viable and nonviable) from gating regions R1 + R2 + R3 only and shows viable cells on-scale in about the first decade of fluorescence. This plot is useful when samples with poor viability are to be analyzed because it is easier to set region R8 on this plot vs plot 8. Additionally, it shows that the fluorescence compensation between photomultiplier tube (PMT) 2 (CD34PE) and PMT 3 (7-AAD) is optimally set.

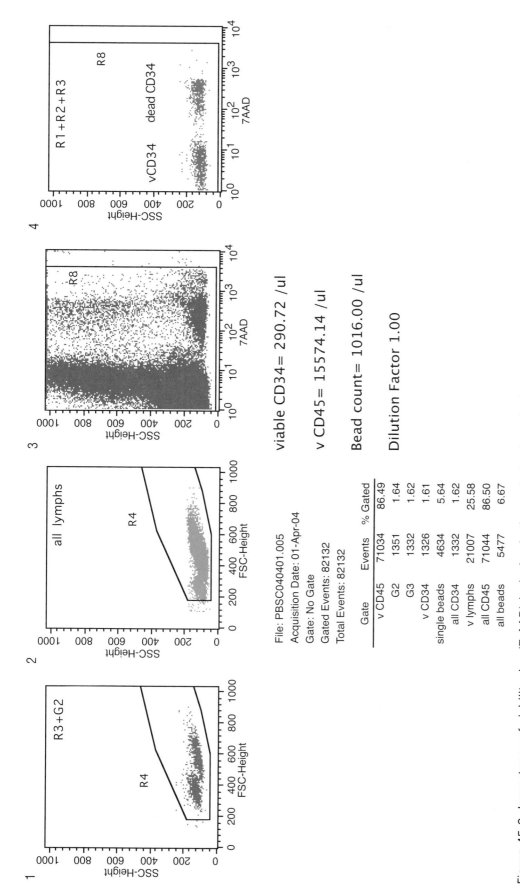

File: PBSC040401.005
Acquisition Date: 01-Apr-04
Gate: No Gate
Gated Events: 82132
Total Events: 82132

viable CD34= 290.72 /ul

v CD45= 15574.14 /ul

Bead count= 1016.00 /ul

Dilution Factor 1.00

Gate	Events	% Gated
v CD45	71034	86.49
G2	1351	1.64
G3	1332	1.62
v CD34	1326	1.61
single beads	4634	5.64
all CD34	1332	1.62
v lymphs	21007	25.58
all CD45	71044	86.50
all beads	5477	6.67

Figure 45-3. Importance of viability dye (7-AAD) inclusion in the analysis of nonfresh samples. Analysis of the same sample as Fig 45-2, except that viability discrimination with 7-AAD has not been applied. When gating region R8 is expanded to include both viable and nonviable cells (plots 3 and 4), and region R4 is moved to include both live and dead lymphocytes (plot 2), both dead and live CD34+ cells cluster within the duplicate lymph-blast region R4 on plot 1. Both the absolute CD34 and CD45 counts are significantly increased vs the values obtained in Fig 45-2. Note the extra population of both CD34+ cells (plot 1) and lymphocytes (plot 2) with reduced forward-angle light scatter; these are the dead cells.

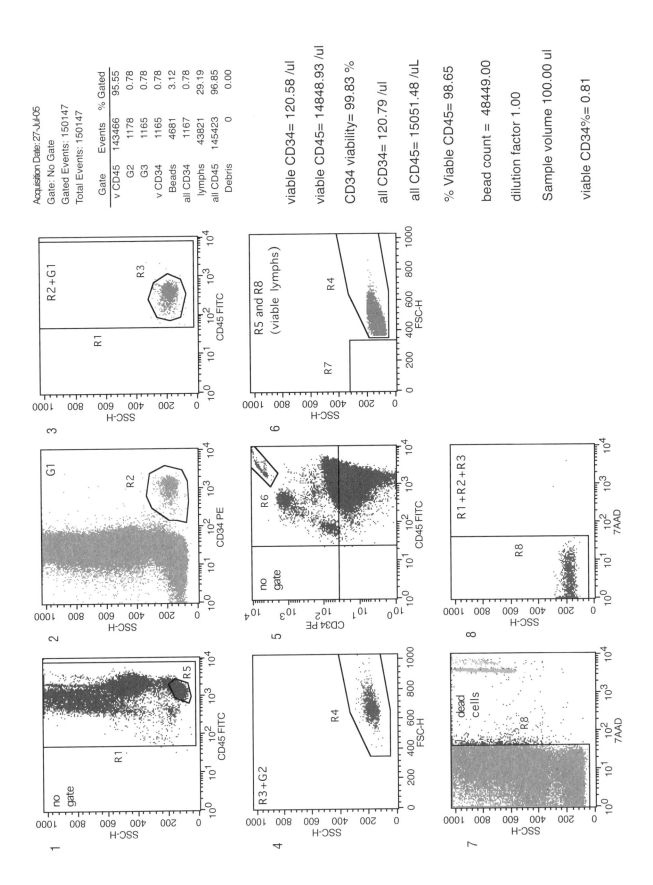

Figure 45-4. Absolute viable CD34+ cell enumeration with the ISHAGE single-platform protocol using Trucount tube (BD Biosciences, San Jose, CA); analysis of a fresh apheresis sample stained with CD45 FITC, CD34 PE, and 7-amino-actinomycin D in a Trucount tube. After 20 minutes, sample lysed with ammonium chloride for 10 minutes at room temperature and listmode data acquired on FACSCalibur cytometer (BD Biosciences). A threshold was established on FL1 (CD45 FITC), and an exclusion gate (R7) was established on plot 6 (instead of plot 5) to prevent the inclusion of debris in the listmode file as described in the text. All Trucount beads were detected in region R6, which has been modified to capture the smaller Trucount beads. Sample analysis was performed using CellQuest Pro software version 5.2 (BD Biosciences), using semiautomated editors.

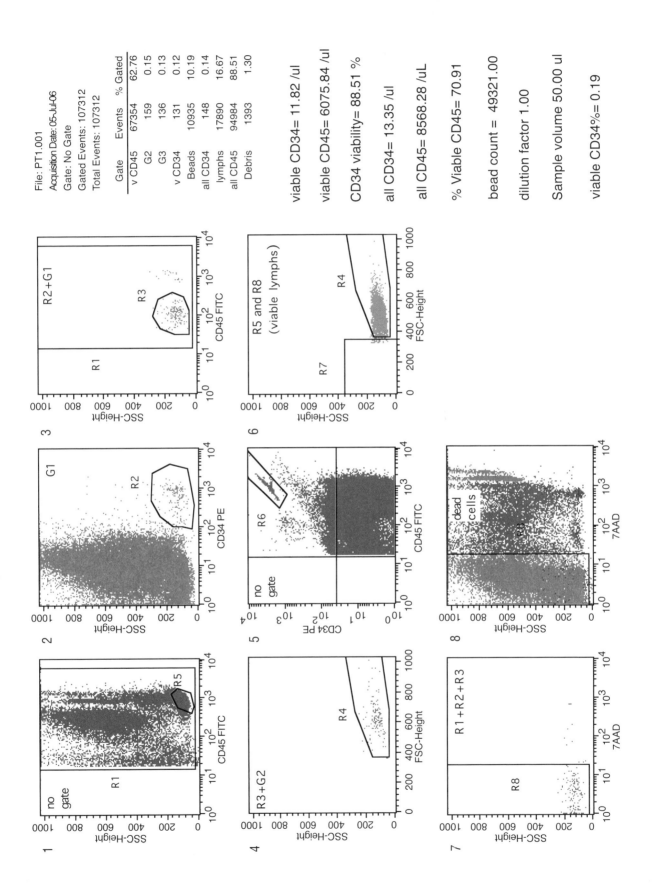

File: PT1.001
Acquistion Date: 05-Jul-06
Gate: No Gate
Gated Events: 107312
Total Events: 107312

Gate	Events	% Gated
v CD45	67354	62.76
G2	159	0.15
G3	136	0.13
v CD34	131	0.12
Beads	10935	10.19
all CD34	148	0.14
lymphs	17890	16.67
all CD45	94984	88.51
Debris	1393	1.30

viable CD34= 11.82 /ul

viable CD45= 6075.84 /ul

CD34 viability= 88.51 %

all CD34= 13.35 /ul

all CD45= 8568.28 /uL

% Viable CD45= 70.91

bead count = 49321.00

dilution factor 1.00

Sample volume 50.00 ul

viable CD34%= 0.19

Figure 45-5. Absolute viable CD34+ cell enumeration with the ISHAGE single-platform protocol using Trucount tubes (BD Biosciences, San Jose, CA) on a post-thawed cord blood sample. A frozen cord blood sample was thawed and processed as described by Keeney and Sutherland[12] and stained with CD45 FITC, CD34 PE, and 7-amino-actinomycin D immediately after thawing in a Trucount tube. After 15 minutes at room temperature, the sample was diluted with 1 mL of PBS/1% bovine serum albumin (ammonium chloride lysis is not required or recommended for post-thaw samples), and data were acquired on FACSCalibur cytometer using CellQuest Pro software (BD Biosciences) as described for Fig 45-4.

Critical Issues in CD34+ Cell Enumeration

CD34 Antigen: Structural Considerations and Choice of Antibody Conjugates

The CD34 antigen is a heavily glycosylated mucin-like structure with an apparent molecular mass of 110 kDa, with the polypeptide moiety accounting for about 40 kDa.[5,13] Such structural characteristics have important implications for the choice of an appropriate CD34 antibody clone for flow-based enumeration techniques. Epitopes recognized by CD34 monoclonal antibody (mAb) can be categorized in three classes, depending on their sensitivity to neuraminidase and glycoprotease.[5,13]

Class I epitopes are sensitive to both enzymes, and they generate inconsistent data on clinical samples because of their dependency for their efficient binding on carbohydrate moieties and terminal sialic acids, which are present only on some forms of the CD34 molecule. CD34 mAbs that detect Class II epitopes (sensitive to glycoprotease) and Class III epitopes (insensitive to both enzymes) detect all glycoforms of CD34 and detect similar if not identical numbers of CD34+ cells in a wide variety of normal and abnormal samples.

Commercially produced phycoerythrin (PE) conjugates of Class II (QBEnd10) and Class III (8G12, 581, and Birma K3) antibodies can be used with confidence. If fluorescein isothiocyanate (FITC) conjugates of CD34 antibodies have to be used, Class III reagents are recommended because they detect similar, if not identical, numbers of CD34+ cells as their PE-conjugated versions in parallel analyses of clinical samples using the ISHAGE protocol. Because of electrical charge constraints, however, FITC conjugates of the Class II CD34 antibody QBEnd10 should not be used.[9,12,13]

Various other CD34 antibody conjugates, including peridinium chlorophyll protein (PerCP), PE-coupled cyanin 5 (PE:Cy5), and allophycocyanin reagents, have been tested in two-, three-, and four-color combinations. However, some of these conjugates are not suitable for all applications and instrument platforms; they should be exhaustively evaluated alongside currently validated reagents before introduction into the clinical laboratory. Overall, selecting an appropriate CD34 antibody clone that retains high specificity and avidity of binding after conjugation to the designated fluorochrome is critically important.

CD45 Antigen: Structural Considerations and Choice of Fluorochromes

In multiparameter analyses such as the ISHAGE protocols that use CD45 antibodies to identify total nucleated white cells, it is important to use pan-CD45 antibodies that detect not just all isoforms but also all glycoforms of CD45.[9,12,14] The antibodies J33, HLE-1, and T29/33 can be used with confidence. Although other pan-CD45 antibodies can be used, the selected conjugate should be carefully evaluated and properly titrated before routine use in clinical protocols.

Counting Statistics of Rare-Event Detection

CD34+ cell enumeration by flow cytometry is an example of rare-event analysis, for which Poisson statistics apply:

$$SD = \sqrt{\text{target events counted}},$$

where SD is the standard deviation, and $\sqrt{}$ is the square root (of the target events).

Therefore, to ensure a coefficient of variation no higher than 10%, at least 100 CD34+ cells need to be collected in the listmode file. In other words, the lower the frequency of the target population, the larger the data file needs to be to satisfy Poisson statistics. Rare-event analysis also requires that the flow cytometer be rigorously cleaned and maintained, properly set up, and compensated for multiparameter analysis.

Use of Isotype or Isoclonic Controls

A key issue of how to distinguish specific staining of rare events from nonspecific staining of perhaps a greater number of events was problematic for early, less-sophisticated flow methodologies that used isotype-matched controls.[6] However, negative reagent controls are of limited use in the enumeration of CD34+ cells. Some isotype controls stain more cells nonspecifically than are specifically stained by the CD34 conjugate.[15] Isoclonic controls stain nothing, either specifically or nonspecifically,[10] and are not recommended.[15] Modern CD34+ cell enumeration methods such as the ISHAGE protocols use a multiparameter approach and a Boolean gating strategy to distinguish specific from nonspecific staining and have dispensed with redundant "negative antibody controls" entirely.[12,14] Stem-Kit (Beckman Coulter) contains an isoclonic control and, because this kit is approved by the Food and Drug Administration, should be run as recommended. However, if the laboratory chooses to validate the kit without the control, this would satisfy regulatory bodies and reduce the three-tube test to a two-tube test.

Positive Reagent Controls and Proficiency Testing

Although localized proficiency-testing schemes can be designed around the use of fresh mobilized PB or fresh apheresis samples, shipping the samples in such a manner that cellular viability is maintained is of critical importance. For sending out larger samples in large proficiency-testing schemes, fresh material generally cannot be obtained, so stabilized cell preparations have been developed to fulfill this role. Commercially available, stabilized whole blood samples or CD34+ cell lines can be used to validate CD34 and CD45 conjugates and new antibody lots. A positive control sample containing an assayed concentration of CD34+ cells should be run each day the CD34 enumeration assay is performed on patient or donor material. Some licensing authorities (eg, College of American Pathologists) require that two levels of control be performed each day, one of which should be at or near the level that clinical decisions are made to proceed to collect the patient by apheresis. One disadvantage of using stabilized controls is the cells are nonviable and as such are all stained by viability dyes. Furthermore, such cells exhibit different light-scatter characteristics from those of fresh samples, and routine instrument settings may need to be optimized for their accurate analysis. Finally, although having stabilized controls available in the 5 to 10 cells/μL range would be desirable, to mimic the levels at which clinical decisions are made at many institutions, such low levels of CD34+ cells can be problematic to identify in stabilized samples. Furthermore, unless the "low range" control is at least 10 to 15 cells/μL, complying with the requirement to collect at least 100 CD34+ cells within the time frame during which the fluorescent counting beads will remain in suspension can be difficult.

Challenging Sample Types

Marrow samples are, with the possible exception of post-thawed cord blood samples, the most difficult source of CD34+ cells to enumerate accurately. Marrow CD34+ cells are markedly more heterogeneous in terms of their qualitative composition, range, and quantity of stem/progenitor types. For example, a wide range of CD34+/CD10+/CD19+ pre-B cells are present in marrow samples but play no (claimed) role in the reconstitution of hematopoiesis after transplantation. Furthermore, automated software can be easily fooled by the increased debris, platelet aggregates, and nucleated red cells encountered in such samples.

An example of the analysis of a post-thawed cord blood sample performed using the single-platform assay is shown in Fig 45-5. This sample was processed, frozen, and thawed using the methodology of Rubinstein et al.[16] After staining 50 μL of the post-thawed sample for 15 minutes at room temperature in a Trucount tube, it was diluted with 1 mL of phosphate-buffered saline (PBS) and immediately acquired. Lysing agents such as ammonium chloride are not necessary on post-thawed samples because red cells lyse during thaw.

Another difficult sample type to analyze can be post-CD34+ cell selected samples. Some CD34+ cell selection devices can cause aggregation of the CD34+ cells after elution from the column (see Fig 2B in reference 12).[12] Although this problem can be minimized by diluting the CD34+ cells into ice-cold PBS supplemented with 1% albumin immediately upon elution, remaining aggregates can scatter outside the standardized blast-lymph region (region R4 in Figs 45-2 and 45-4), thus rendering impossible the accurate enumeration of CD34+ cells.

References/Resources

1. Thomas ED, Lochte HL Jr, Lu JF, et al. Intravenous infusion of bone marrow in patients receiving radiation and chemotherapy. N Eng J Med 1957;257:491.
2. Thomas ED, Lochte HL Jr, Cannon JH, et al. Supralethal whole body irradiation and isologous marrow transplantation in man. J Clin Invest 1959;38:1709.
3. McCreadie KB, Hersh EM, Freireich EJ. Cells capable of colony formation in the peripheral blood of man. Science 1971;171:293.

4. Berenson RJ, Andrews RG, Bensinger WI, et al. Antigen CD34-positive marrow cells engraft lethally irradiated baboons. J Clin Invest 1988;81:951.

5. Sutherland DR, Keating A. The CD34 antigen: Structure, biology and potential clinical applications. J Hematother 1992;1:115.

6. Siena S, Bregni M, Brando B, et al. Circulation of CD34+ hematopoietic stem cells in the peripheral blood of high-dose cyclophosphamide-treated patients: Enhancement by intravenous recombinant human granulocyte-macrophage colony-stimulating factor. Blood 1989;74:1905-14.

7. Sutherland DR, Keating A, Nayar R, et al. Sensitive detection and enumeration of CD34+ cells in peripheral and cord blood by flow cytometry. Exp Hematol 1994;22:1003-10.

8. Borowitz MJ, Guenther KL, Schults KE, et al. Immunophenotyping of acute leukemia by flow cytometry: Use of CD45 and right angle light scatter to gate on leukemic blasts in three color analysis. Am J Clin Pathol 1993;100:534-40.

9. Sutherland DR, Anderson L, Keeney M, et al. The ISHAGE guidelines for CD34+ cell determination by flow cytometry. J Hematother 1996;3:213.

10. Keeney M, Chin-Yee I, Weir K, et al. Single platform flow cytometric absolute CD34+ cell counts based on the ISHAGE guidelines. Cytometry 1998;34:61-70.

11. Brocklebank AM, Sparrow RL. Enumeration of CD34+ cells in cord blood: A variation on a single-platform flow cytometric method based on the ISHAGE gating strategy. Cytometry 2001;46:254.

12. Keeney M, Sutherland DR. Current methods for identification of hematopoietic stem and progenitor cells in the clinical laboratory. In: Keren DF, McCoy JP Jr, Carey JL, eds. Flow cytometry in clinical diagnosis. 4th ed. Chicago: ASCP Press, 2007:1-24.

13. Lanza R, Healy L, Sutherland DR. Structural and functional features of the CD34 antigen: An update. J Biol Regul Homeost Agents 2001;15:1-13.

14. Sutherland DR, Keeney M, Gratama JW. Enumeration of CD34+ hematopoietic stem and progenitor cells. In: Robinson JR, Darzynkiewicz Z, Dean PN, et al, eds. Current protocols in cytometry. New York: John Wiley and Sons, 2003:1-23(Unit 6.4).

15. Keeney M, Chin-Yee I, Gratama JW, Sutherland DR. Perspectives: Isotype controls in the analysis of lymphocytes and CD34+ stem/progenitor cells by flow cytometry—time to let go! Cytometry 1998;34:280-3.

16. Rubinstein P, Dobrila L, Rosenfield RE, et al. Processing and cryopreservation of placental/umbilical cord blood for unrelated bone marrow reconstitution. Proc Natl Acad Sci U S A 1995;92:10119-22.

Method 45-1. Flow Cytometric Enumeration of CD34+ Hematopoietic Progenitor Cells According to ISHAGE Protocol

Description

The ISHAGE (International Society of Hematotherapy and Graft Engineering, subsequently renamed the International Society for Cellular Therapy) protocol uses CD34 and CD45 staining together with a sequential Boolean gating strategy to delineate and enumerate bona fide CD34+ cells from nonspecifically stained events.[1,2] By incorporating a known number of fluorescent counting beads in the analysis and by assessing the ratio between the number of beads and CD34+ cells counted, an absolute CD34+ cell count can be generated using a flow cytometer alone ("single-platform methodology"), thus eliminating the need for a hematology analyzer.[3-5] Simple ammonium-chloride-based lyse-no-wash sample processing is used. Finally, the inclusion of the viability dye 7-aminoactinomycin D (7-AAD) allows the exclusion of dead cells and the enumeration of viable (v)CD34+ cells.[3]

Time for Procedure

The time required for sample preparation, staining, acquisition, and analysis is 35-40 minutes.

Summary of Procedure

1. Create analysis/acquisition template on flow cytometer.
2. Stain samples.
3. Perform flow acquisition and analysis.

Equipment

1. Electronic pipettor capable of reverse pipetting.
2. Flow cytometer.
3. Vortex mixer.

Supplies and Reagents

1. Phosphate-buffered saline (PBS), 1% (w/v) human serum albumin.

2. Red cell lysis buffer (eg, PharmLyse, BD Biosciences, San Jose, CA).
3. Anti-CD34-PE (eg, clone 581, Beckman Coulter, Fullerton, CA; clone HPCA-2, BD BioSciences) or validated equivalent.
4. Anti-CD45-FITC (clone J33, Beckman Coulter) or anti-CD45-PerCP (clone 2D1, BD Biosciences) or validated equivalent.
5. 7-AAD.
6. Fluorescent beads for single-platform assay (eg, Flow-Count Fluorospheres, Beckman Coulter).
7. 12 × 75-mm polystyrene tubes.
   Note: If Trucount tubes (BD Biosciences) are used, fluorescent beads are pre-aliquoted in 12 × 75 mm tubes.
8. Pipette tips.

Procedure

1. Create acquisition/analysis template on flow cytometer.
   Note: Beckman Coulter has developed a reagent and software package that contains all necessary components for preparation and automated instrument setup and compensation as well as automated data acquisition and analysis of samples. This reagent/software was developed for both the Coulter XL (StemOne) and, more recently, FC500 instruments (StemCXP) (see Fig 45-1). BD Biosciences CellQuest software (version 4.0 and above) contains expression editors that can automate the analysis phase of the process regardless of counting beads used (see Figs 45-2 through 45-5). The following protocol setup shows how to create the protocol for analysis on BD instruments. More information on templates for Beckman

Coulter instruments is found in the "Notes" section.

a. Create the following bivariate histograms (dot plots):
    - Plot 1: CD45-FITC (FL1) vs side scatter (SS).
    - Plot 2: CD34-PE (FL2) vs SS.
    - Plot 3: CD45-FITC (FL1) vs SS.
    - Plot 4: Forward scatter (FS) vs SS.
    - Plot 5: CD45-FITC (FL1) vs CD34-PE (FL2).
    - Plot 6: FS vs SS.
    - Plot 7: Time vs FS (for BD FACS instruments if Flow-Count beads are used). (If Trucount tubes are used, this plot is not required. See below for specific modifications required for the Trucount-tube-based assay shown in Fig 45-4.)
    - Plot 8: 7-AAD vs SS.
    - Plot 9 (optional): 7-AAD vs SS (for R1 + R2 + R3). This plot is useful for analysis of thawed samples and some fresh samples containing significant numbers of dead/apoptotic cells. Figure 45-3 shows the value of such an approach using the same listmode file as used in Fig 45-2 without viability discrimination (only plots 4, 6, 8, and 9 are shown).

b. Create gating regions and logical gates: In the following description, specific terminology for gating regions (eg, R1) and logical gates (eg, G1) is for BD Biosciences FACS instruments.
    - Logical gate setup for BD template using Flow-Count fluorospheres (Figs 45-2 to 45-5):
        – Gate 1 (vCD45): R1 and R8.
        – Gate 2: R2 and G1.
        – Gate 3: R3 and G2.
        – Gate 4 (vCD34): R4 and G3.
        – Gate 5 (singlet beads): R6 and R7.
        – Gate 6 (all CD34): R1 and R2 and R3.
        – Gate 7 (v lymphs): R5 and R8.
        – Gate 8 (all CD45): R1 and not R6.
        – Gate 9 (all beads): R6.
    - Plot 1 (leukocyte gate): Display all events. Draw a rectangular region (R1) to include all CD45 events (from dim to bright) and to exclude debris, platelets, and unlysed erythrocytes, which are all CD45–. The counting beads are found in the brightest FL1, FL2, and FL3 channels and also exhibit very high SS. Because the gate statistics are obtained from events in plot 1, it is critical that region R1 includes the highest FL1 and SS channels.
    - Plot 2 (total CD34 gate): Display events from the leukocyte gate (gate G1 = R1). Draw an amorphous polygon region (R2) to include all CD34+ events.
    - Plot 3 (CD34+ blast gate): Display events that fulfill the criteria of both preceding gates (Regions R1 and R2; G2 = R2 and G1). Draw an amorphous polygon region (R3) to include only those events that form a cluster with low to intermediate SS and dim CD45 expression.
    - Plot 4 (lymph-blast gate): Display events that fulfill the criteria of all three preceding gates (Regions R1, R2, and R3, G3 = R3 and G2). Draw an amorphous polygon region (R4) to include only those events that form a cluster with low to intermediate SS and low to intermediate FS. Set logical gate G4 = R4 and G3. The lymph-blast gate serves to exclude platelets and debris that may show weak nonspecific binding of CD34 and CD45. Its optimal positioning and lower boundaries are set as described in plot 6.
    - Plot 5: Display ungated data. Draw a quad-stat region to establish the lower limit of CD45 expression by the CD34+ events. On plot 5, draw a small rectangular region (R6) to include the brightest events that fall in the highest FL1 and FL2 channels. Although not readily visible, all of the Flow-Count beads (singlets and aggregates) are contained in this region. A rectangular region is established before listmode data acquisition to exclude CD34–/CD45– debris. This is particularly useful for any sample containing high red cell content, and much debris can be thereby excluded from acquisition.

- Plot 6 (duplicate lymph-blast gate): On plot 1, draw an amorphous polygon region (R5) to include the lymphocytes (bright CD45, low SS) to create a lymphocyte gate. Display the events from this region on plot 6 gated on G7 (logical gate G7 = R5 and R8). Copy region R4 from plot 4 into plot 6 (creating the duplicate lymph-blast gate), and adjust the position of the duplicate so that the smallest lymphocytes from region R5 are just included. The original region R4 on plot 4 will automatically move to the same position as that on plot 6.
- Plot 7 (bead gate): Display events from R6 on plot 7 (time vs FS). If beads are not visible, lower FS threshold until all singlet beads can be acquired. Set region R7 to include only singlet beads. Set logical gate G5 = R6 and R7.
- Plot 8: Draw a rectangular region (R8) to include only living (7-AAD–) cells. Display data from region (R8) on plots 1-4 and 6 (see logical gates above). Plot 5 should remain ungated.
- Plot 9 (optional, see Fig 45-3): Duplicate rectangular region (R8) and display data from regions R1, R2, and R3 only. This plot shows all CD34+ cells regardless of viability and is useful for the accurate placement of the viability gate R8 in thawed samples (see Fig 45-5) or other samples containing large proportions of nonviable cells. The detection of the viable cells on-scale in the first decade or so of fluorescence also confirms the appropriate instrument setup and compensation between the PE and 7-AAD channels of the cytometer.

c. Make specific modifications required for Trucount-tube-based protocols (Figs 45-4 and 45-5):

- Because of the very small size of Trucount beads, a threshold is set in the FL1 channel rather than on FS. With an appropriately set FL1 threshold (see plot 1, Figs 45-4 and 45-5), much of the CD34–/CD45– debris is excluded from listmode file acquisition. However, some small debris is usually stained by CD45 FITC, and to exclude it, a small, rectangular exclusion gate (region R7) is established on plot 6. Although this debris can be removed during analysis, excluding it during acquisition and further optimizing it if necessary during analysis is most advantageous, as was performed for the data file shown in Figs 45-4 and 45-5. This modification greatly increases the accuracy of the absolute CD45+ cell count. The latter, when compared to the absolute white cell count derived from a hematology analyzer, represents an important quality assurance characteristic of the methodology, especially if only a single tube is stained.

- Trucount beads are gated on plot 5 within an amorphous region R6. Because the assayed bead content of Trucount tubes is determined on all beads (singlets and aggregates), it is not necessary to further analyze the events therein. Logical gate setup for BD Trucount analysis template (Fig 45-4):
  - Gate 1 (vCD45): not R7 and R1 and R8.
  - Gate 2: R2 and G1.
  - Gate 3: R3 and G2.
  - Gate 4 (vCD34): R4 and G3.
  - Gate 5 (beads): R6 .
  - Gate 6 (all CD34): R1 and R2 and R3.
  - Gate 7 (v lymphs): R5 and R8.
  - Gate 8 (all CD45): R1 and not R6 and not R7.
  - Gate 9 (debris): R7.

2. Stain samples.
   a. If necessary, dilute specimen with PBS containing 1% serum albumin to obtain a total nucleated cell count of 10 to 20×10^9/L.
   b. To a 12×75-mm test tube (or Trucount tube), add CD45 FITC/CD34PE (appropriately titrated) and 7-AAD (final concentration = 1 μg/mL).
   c. Accurately pipette 100 μL of well-mixed specimen into the very bottom of the tube and mix. This step requires the use of positive displacement techniques or electronic pipettors with reverse pipetting capabilities.

d. Incubate tubes at room temperature for 20 minutes, protected from the light.

e. Add 2 mL of freshly diluted (1:10) ammonium chloride lysing solution at room temperature and vortex to mix.

> **Note:** When thawed samples are stained, this step is not necessary. PBS can be used instead, and after addition of the beads (step h), the sample can be acquired immediately.

f. Incubate 10 minutes at room temperature, protected from the light.

g. Following incubation, keep samples on melting ice and protected from the light until flow acquisition is performed, for a maximum of 60 minutes.

h. Immediately before analysis, accurately pipette 100 µL of properly suspended Flow-Count Fluorospheres to the tube using the same pipette as above. (This step not required if Trucount tubes are used.)

i. Cap tube and gently mix by inversion. Immediately proceed to flow acquisition.

3. Perform flow acquisition and analysis.

a. Once fluorescent beads are added, acquisition should take place immediately.

b. A minimum of 75,000 CD45+ events should be collected, with a minimum of 100 CD34+ cells to maintain a coefficient variable of 10%.

Anticipated Results

The lower limit of sensitivity is partially determined by the number of CD34+ events collected. The method is sensitive at least to a level of 5 CD34+ cells per µL. Increasing the total number of CD34+ events collected will allow for accuracy below this value.

Notes

There are specific issues with Flow-Count beads on Beckman Coulter vs BD FACS instruments. On Beckman Coulter instruments, the FS threshold is set just below the smallest lymphocytes. On BD FACS series instruments, a similar setting would exclude the Flow-Count beads from acquisition. Thus, the FS has to be reduced to a point below where singlet Flow-Count beads are detected on the FS vs time plot (plot 7).

References/Resources

1. Sutherland DR, Keating A, Nayar R, et al. Sensitive detection and enumeration of CD34+ cells in peripheral and cord blood by flow cytometry. Exp Hematol 1994;22:1003-10.

2. Sutherland DR, Anderson L, Keeney M, et al. The ISHAGE Guidelines for CD34+ cell determination by flow cytometry. J Hematother 1996;3:213.

3. Keeney M, Chin-Yee I, Weir K, et al. Single platform flow cytometric absolute CD34+ cell counts based on the ISHAGE guidelines. Cytometry 1998;34:61-70.

4. Brocklebank AM, Sparrow RL. Enumeration of CD34+ cells in cord blood: A variation on a single-platform flow cytometric method based on the ISHAGE gating strategy. Cytometry 2001;46:254.

5. Keeney M, Sutherland DR. Current methods for identification of hematopoietic stem and progenitor cells in the clinical laboratory. In: Keren DF, McCoy JP Jr, Carey JL, eds. Flow cytometry in clinical diagnosis. 4th ed. Chicago: ASCP Press, 2007:1-24.

In: Areman EM, Loper K, eds
Cellular Therapy: Principles, Methods, and Regulations
Bethesda, MD: AABB, 2009

♦ ♦ ♦   **46**   ♦ ♦ ♦

Pancreatic Islet Characterization

Elina Linetsky, MSc, MT

ACCURATE AND RELIABLE METHODS FOR enumeration of human islet cells are important. Otherwise, any comparison of research and clinical results, as well as the correct estimation of islet cells in a given preparation, is impossible. In a human preparation, where islet cell yields are too high to count directly, a reproducible technique for the assessment of islet cell yield had to be developed. Even though experienced operators can easily distinguish islet cells from exocrine tissue, lymph nodes, ducts, and ganglia under the light microscope, the use of dithizone (DTZ), a stain specific to the zinc in the insulin granules of islet cells, causes islet cells to stain with a characteristic red color (see Fig 46-1), making them easily distinguishable from the exocrine tissue, which appears light brown.

Islet cell preparations are complex mixtures of cells and raise several challenges for enumeration and determination of clinically relevant cell doses. Islets are clusters of multiple cell types that vary in size, ranging from very small particles of <50 μm in diameter to clusters that exceed 350 μm. Islets are not flat but, in fact, have a three-dimensional structure and can vary in shape as well as size. Islet volume is approximately proportional to the cube of its radius. Some of these challenges were addressed through development of a consensus on islet enumeration reached during the Second Congress on Pancreas and Islet Transplantation.[1] In addition to recommendations for islet number and volume, other considerations were offered for avoiding sampling error and performing additional tests for islet purity, morphology, viability, and function.

One of the most important elements of this consensus was the establishment of a standardized measure of islet mass, the islet equivalent (IEQ). To account for the large variation in islet size, the IEQ determination normalizes counts to a "standard" spherical islet with a diameter of 150 μm. Stained islets are counted according to size on an inverted microscope with a calibrated ocular micrometer. Diameter increments of 50 μm are used, without taking particles smaller than 50 μm into consideration because their contribution to the total volume of the preparation is insignificant. The number of islets in each size group is then multiplied by standard factors to determine the IEQ. Table 46-1 shows the mean islet volume and relative conversion factor for each diameter class.[1]

Elina Linetsky, MSc, MT, Director, Quality Assurance/Regulatory Affairs, Cell Transplant Center, Diabetes Research Institute and Wallace H. Coulter Center, University of Miami Miller School of Medicine, Miami, Florida

The author has disclosed no conflicts of interest.

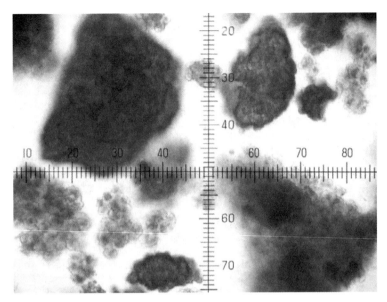

Figure 46-1. Sample removed from the Ricordi chamber during a pancreas digestion process. Human islets (red) stained with DTZ are easily distinguishable from the exocrine tissue, which appears light brown.

The sampling technique represents another critical element in the determination of the islet number. Because islet cells settle rapidly in any container, care must be taken to properly resuspend the islet preparation before sampling to ensure collection of a representative sample. Samples can be collected and placed in 10×35-mm culture dishes using any commercially available positive displacement pipette, sterilized before use. To calculate the IEQ in the islet product, all the islets in a given sample must be counted. Accurately recording the volume of sample taken and the volume of the islet product at the time of sampling is also critical. To minimize variability and counting errors between operators, as well as in the sampling technique, it is recommended to collect at least two 100-μL samples after the suspension of the preparation. The number and size of samples may be adjusted depending on the stage of the process being evaluated and the number of islets in the sample. For example, on a high-yield islet preparation, four separate 50-μL samples may be much easier to enumerate than two 100-μL samples or one 200-μL sample.

Acknowledgments

Methods 46-1 and 46-2 were submitted by Lynn O'Donnell, PhD, Director, Cell Therapy Laboratory, OSU James Cancer Hospital and Solove Research Institute, Columbus, Ohio.

Table 46-1. Mean Islet Volume in Each Diameter Class

Islet Diameter Range (μm)	Mean Volume	Conversion Factor*
50-100	294,525	n / 6.00
101-150	1,145,373	n / 1.50
151-200	2,977,968	n × 1.7
201-250	6,185,010	n × 3.5
251-300	11,159,198	n × 6.3
301-350	18,293,231	n × 10.4
>350	27,979,808	n × 15.8

*Relative conversion factor into an equivalent number of islet cells with a diameter of 150 μm.

Reference/Resource

1. Ricordi C. Quantitative and qualitative standards for islet isolation assessment in humans and large animals. Pancreas 1991;6:242-4.

Method 46-1. Enumerating Pancreatic Islets by Dithizone Staining

Description

To distinguish islets from other cell clusters, isolated islet products are stained with a solution of diphenyl thiocarbazone (dithizone, or DTZ). DTZ is a zinc chelating agent that selectively stains islets a red color, making them distinguishable from the other cell types. Stained islets are counted on an inverted microscope with an ocular micrometer according to size. Islet equivalents are a measure of islet mass, which accounts for the large variation in islet size by normalizing counts to a standard spherical islet with a diameter of 150 μm. The number of islets in each size group is multiplied by standard factors to determine IEQ. The numbers of acinar/exocrine tissue clusters and mantled islets (ie, still attached to exocrine tissue) are counted to establish islet purity and percentage of free islets, respectively. Islet quality is assessed by assigning point values to specific parameters or traits.

Time for Procedure

Samples stain in only 2 to 5 minutes. Depending on the number of islets and replicate samples and the experience of the operator, the entire procedure can be completed in 10 to 30 minutes.

Summary of Procedure

1. Prepare the DTZ stain.
2. Stain the sample with DTZ.
3. Enumerate the islets.
4. Calculate IEQ in the islet product.

Equipment

1. Phase-contrast microscope: inverted stage, with ocular micrometer with 50-μm divisions.
2. Eight-position hematology differential counter.

Supplies and Reagents

1. DTZ.
2. Dimethyl sulfoxide (DMSO).

3. Hanks' Balanced Salt Solution (HBSS), without phenol red.
4. 35-mm petri dishes.
5. Conical tubes.
6. 0.2-μm nylon filters.
7. Aluminum foil.

Procedure

1. Prepare DTZ stain.
   a. Transfer 0.1 g DTZ to a 250-mL conical tube, and dissolve in 20 mL DMSO. Vortex vigorously to dissolve DTZ.
   b. Dilute with 30 mL HBSS, and filter using a 0.2-μm bottle-top filter. Following filtration, an additional 50 mL HBSS is added for a final volume of 100 mL.
2. Stain sample with DTZ.
   a. In a 35-mm dish, add DTZ to the sample.
   b. Let sample stain for 2 to 5 minutes.
   c. Scan sample at low magnification (eg, 40×).
   d. Scan the entire surface of the dish on low magnification, ensuring that islets are evenly distributed and not clustered at the edges or center of the petri dish.
   e. If the islets in the sample are too numerous to count, obtain a smaller sample or dilute. If diluting, the volume of the stained sample must be known to calculate the dilution factor.
3. Enumerate the islets.
   a. Switch to high magnification (eg, 100×).
      Note: The ocular micrometer must be calibrated for *each* objective lens.
   b. Use the stage controls to maneuver the field to an outer edge of the petri dish.
   c. Using the ocular micrometer, estimate the size of each islet larger than 50 μm in the field. Assign each islet to a size group (ie, 50-100 μm, 101-150 μm … >350 μm) and use the eight-position differential counter to tally the size groups. For islets with one

axis that is significantly longer than the other, estimate the average of the two axes.

d. Using the stage controls in a single direction, move to a new field and continue enumerating islets in the next field.

e. Enumerate the entire petri dish. Be careful not to count clusters more than once, skip areas of the plate, or cause repositioning of the islets during enumeration.

f. Determine the percentage of free islets by performing a second scan of the dish to count the number of free islets and the number of mantled islets (ie, still attached to or embedded in exocrine tissue). Again, only include islets larger than 50 μm in the count. The entire dish does *not* need to be counted, but a minimum of 100 islets must be enumerated.

g. Determine islet purity by performing a third scan of the dish to count the number of islets larger than 50 μm and the number of acinar (or exocrine) tissue clusters larger than 50 μm (unstained, gray, or brown). The entire dish does *not* need to be counted, but a minimum of 100 acinar clusters or islets must be enumerated.

h. Determine islet quality by evaluating five categories: spherical shape, smooth/intact border, single cells, size distribution, and overall level of fragmentation. Points are assigned to each category, as shown in Table 46-1-1. Assign a score for each category and tally the points (0-10 points).

4. Calculate IEQ in the islet product.

a. Multiply the islet count of each size group by the appropriate IEQ factor; then total all size groups to obtain the IEQ counted.

b. Divide the IEQ counted by the sample volume to obtain IEQ/mL; then multiply by the product volume to obtain the total IEQ in the product. If dilution of the sample was performed, also include the dilution factor in the calculation.

Anticipated Results

1. Islet enumeration is associated with a high level of variability because of the subjective nature of the assay and the wide variation in islet sizes and samples. For release testing of islet products, duplicate samples are enumerated, and the results must be within 25% of each other.

2. Islet purity and IEQ dose per kg recipient weight are typically release specifications for islet products, as specified in the clinical protocol and the investigational new drug application. An IEQ dose of at least 4000 IEQ/kg and an islet purity of at least 30% are typical release criteria for these products.

Notes

1. DTZ solution should be prepared freshly, before each isolation procedure. Some facilities will store DTZ for up to 1 year at −20 C, then before use, thaw completely in a 37 C waterbath, and vortex vigorously.

2. Although the necessary calculations to estimate the islet number and IEQ in a given preparation can be obtained manually, it is convenient to build a simple spreadsheet that can perform the required calculations. This results in significant time savings during the islet isolation procedure and eliminates mathematical errors when performing manual calculations.

Table 46-1-1. Point Assignments for Assessing Islet Quality

Category	0 Points	1 Point	2 Points
Spherical shape	Few	Some	Most
Smooth/intact border	Few	Some	Most
Single cells	Many	A few	None
Size distribution	All <100 μm	A few >200 μm	At least 10% >200 μm
Overall fragmentation	Significant	Moderate	Minimal

3. To calculate the islet content of the islet product, accurately recording the volume of sample taken and the volume of the islet product at the time of sampling is critical.

Reference/Resource

1. Ricordi C. Quantitative and qualitative standards for islet isolation assessment in humans and large animals. Pancreas 1991;6:242-4.

Method 46-2. Determining Pancreatic Islet Function by Insulin Release

Description

Release of insulin in response to elevated glucose levels is a critical biologic function of islets and is expected to correlate with the in-vivo mechanism of action and the clinical efficacy of transplanted islets. Measurement of this ability of isolated islets serves as a functional assay, but results do not always correlate with clinical outcome, thus limiting the ability to use insulin release as a stand-alone true measure of islet potency.

The assay involves two separate processes. First, islets undergo static incubation with "high" (16.7-mM) or "low" (1.67-mM) glucose concentrations. Functional islets should secrete higher levels of insulin when challenged with higher concentrations of glucose. Supernatant is collected, and insulin released by the islets is measured using an enzyme-linked immunosorbent assay (ELISA) kit for human insulin. Insulin concentrations are determined by extrapolating from a standard curve. The stimulation index (SI) is calculated as the proportion of insulin released at high glucose concentration divided by insulin released at low glucose concentration.

Time for Procedure

Glucose stimulation takes approximately 2 hours. Insulin ELISA takes approximately 1 hour.

Summary of Procedure

1. Prepare the reagents.
2. Perform glucose stimulation of islet preparation.
3. Perform the insulin ELISA.

Equipment

1. Humidified incubator: 37 C, 5.0% CO_2.
2. Inverted microscope.
3. Waterbath (37 C).
4. Centrifuge.
5. Microplate shaker and reader.
6. Pipettors.

Supplies and Reagents

1. RPMI-1640 (Gibco, Grand Island, NY), without glucose and sodium bicarbonate, without phenol red.
2. D(+) glucose.
3. 1 M HEPES buffer.
4. Bovine serum albumin (BSA).
5. Human insulin ELISA kit containing a 96-well microplate coated with mouse monoclonal anti-insulin, insulin calibrators, monoclonal anti-insulin conjugated to horseradish peroxidase, diluent, wash buffer, substrate (peroxide and 3,3′-5,5′-tetramethyl-benzidine), stop solution.
6. 0.2-μm filter units.
7. 60-mm petri dish.
8. 1.5-mL microcentrifuge tubes.

Procedure

1. Prepare the reagents.
   a. Prepare base medium—RPMI-1640, 25-mM HEPES, 0.1% (w/v) BSA—and ensure that the pH is approximately 7.2. Sterile-filter, label, and store at 2 to 8 C.
   b. Prepare "high" glucose medium· Dissolve 0.30 g D(+) glucose in 100 mL base medium (300 mg/dL = 16.7 mM final concentration). Sterile-filter, label, and store at 2 to 8 C.
   c. Prepare "low" glucose medium: Dilute 10 mL high glucose medium with 90 mL base medium (30 mg/dL = 1.67 mM final concentration). Sterile-filter, label, and store at 2 to 8 C.
   d. Prepare ELISA kit reagents per the manufacturer's instructions.
2. Perform glucose stimulation of islet preparation.
   a. Prefill a 60-mm petri dish with 10 mL of low glucose medium and transfer the sam-

ple containing approximately 200 islets to the dish.

b. Cover the dish and incubate at 37 C for 30 minutes to condition the cells before stimulation.

c. Label five 15-mL conical tubes "LOW" and five 15-mL conical tubes "HIGH."

d. Prefill each "LOW" tube with 0.5 mL low glucose medium and each "HIGH" tube with 0.5 mL high glucose medium.

e. At the end of the 30-minute incubation, swirl the petri dish to center the islets. Using the inverted microscope, handpick five islets using a 10-μL manual pipettor and transfer to a prefilled conical tube. Keep the tube caps loose to allow diffusion of air.

f. Repeat until islets are transferred to each conical tube. Alternate "LOW" and "HIGH" tubes so that incubation times are approximately the same for each series.

g. Incubate the tubes in a waterbath at 37 C for 1 hour, shaking tubes by hand periodically.

h. After incubation, vortex the tubes gently and centrifuge at 1400 rpm at room temperature, brake *on*, for 3 minutes.

i. Remove 200 μL of supernatant from each "LOW" tube and pool in a microcentrifuge tube. Repeat for "HIGH" tubes.

j. Store at or below –20 C until the ELISA is performed.

3. Perform insulin ELISA.

a. Remove "LOW" and "HIGH" glucose samples from the freezer and thaw at room temperature. Vortex samples briefly before use.

b. Perform the ELISA assay according to manufacturer's instructions. Assay insulin calibrators in duplicate and "LOW" and "HIGH" glucose samples in triplicate.

c. Construct a calibration curve from the average absorbance readings of the insulin.

d. Average the absorbance readings of the "HIGH" and "LOW" glucose samples by manual extrapolation or by entering the values into the linear regression equation from a computer-generated calibration curve.

e. Calculate the SI by dividing the insulin concentration of the "HIGH" glucose samples by the insulin concentration of the "LOW" glucose samples.

Anticipated Results

High-quality islets exhibit SI of 5 or higher, but preparations with SI of 1 to 2 are acceptable and functional in vivo.

Note

To avoid biasing the results, avoid selecting exceptionally large or small islets.

Reference/Resource

1. Bottino R, Balamurugan AN, Bertera S, et al. Preservation of human islet cell functional mass by anti-oxidative action of a novel SOP mimic compound. Diabetes 2002; 51:2561-7.

In: Areman EM, Loper K, eds
Cellular Therapy: Principles, Methods, and Regulations
Bethesda, MD: AABB, 2009

◆◆◆   *47*   ◆◆◆

Assessment of Viability and Apoptosis in Cellular Therapy Products

Nicholas Greco, PhD, and Lynn O'Donnell, PhD

MOST CELLULAR THERAPIES RELY ON living cells to achieve some biologic or therapeutic effect. Thus, testing cellular therapy (CT) products to determine the proportion of living and dead cells is an important first step in determining the functional capacity and, ultimately, potency of the product. Cells undergoing necrotic cell death typically swell rapidly, lose membrane integrity, shut down metabolic activity, and release their cytoplasmic contents into the surrounding medium. One of the earliest assays of cell viability, the chromium release assay, is based on cells taking up radioactive chromium that is released as the cell membrane loses integrity; it is still used extensively as a cytotoxicity assay. This assay has been replaced as a measure of viability by the current "gold standard" assay of membrane integrity: microscopic examination of cells stained with trypan blue. Viable cells prevent trypan blue from crossing the intact cell membrane and appear colorless under a light microscope, whereas the damaged cell membranes of nonviable cells allow the stain into the cells, coloring them blue.[1] A procedure for trypan blue viability determination is presented in Method 47-1. Although the trypan blue staining method is simple and inexpensive, it is also subjective.

The development of several fluorescent dyes has led to improved methods for viability determination that are still based on membrane integrity but allow simultaneous staining of viable and nonviable cells. One alternate method using the fluorescent dyes acridine orange and propidium iodide is presented in Method 47-2. This method has been shown to result in reduced variability, better linearity, improved ease of scoring because of reduced background, longer stability of stained cells, and improved correlation with clonogenic assays.[2]

Additional targets for assessing cells undergoing necrotic cell death include measures of basic metabolic pathways such as adenosine triphosphate (ATP) production and reducing equivalents. Furthermore, some enumeration assays include viability assessment as part of the determination, such as flow-cytometry-based assays that apply gating

Nicholas Greco, PhD, Senior Research Associate, Department of Medicine, Case Western Reserve University, and Director of Laboratory Operations, Cleveland Cord Blood Center, Cleveland, Ohio; Lynn O'Donnell, PhD, Director, Cell Therapy Laboratory, OSU James Cancer Hospital and Solove Research Institute, Columbus, Ohio

The authors have disclosed no conflicts of interest.

strategies to exclude nonviable cells. Aspects of viability determination for some of these methods are covered elsewhere in this section.

In addition to necrotic cell death, cells may undergo a distinct process referred to as programmed cell death, or *apoptosis*. Assessing apoptosis has recently been discussed as an alternative measure of cell viability for CT products. Apoptosis involves complex interdependent and independent pathways that can vary among different cells. These pathways involve cell surface receptors, mitochondrial components, transcription factors, and numerous proteases and protease inhibitors. Initiation of apoptosis pathways is important for the development of organisms, cellular differentiation, homeostasis, and removal of harmful (cancerous, autoreactive, or infected) cells. Important for the purposes of this section, apoptosis also facilitates the elimination of cells damaged by irradiation, toxic drugs, and lack of survival signals as well as those damaged as a consequence of phlebotomy, cryopreservation, or other manipulations.[3] Methods have been developed to measure apoptosis by evaluating changes in protein synthesis, membrane permeability, mitochondrial membrane polarization, orientation of phosphatidylserine in the cell membrane, and DNA fragmentation and other nuclear changes. Measurements using several apoptotic markers may define the progression of apoptosis and therefore differentiate the occurrence of early vs late apoptotic events.[4,5] Although discussion of the numerous apoptosis assays is beyond the scope of this chapter, a method is presented that has been used to simultaneously measure CD34+ cells with various apoptotic markers using a single-platform flow-cytometric assay with the International Society of Hematotherapy and Graft Engineering (ISHAGE) gating strategy (Method 47-3).[6] This method can be easily modified to analyze other populations of cells undergoing apoptosis.

Acknowledgments

Method 47-2 was submitted by David H. McKenna, Jr, MD, Scientific and Medical Director, Molecular and Cellular Therapeutics, University of Minnesota Medical Center, St Paul, Minnesota.

References/Resources

1. Tennant JR. Evaluation of the trypan blue technique for determination of cell viability. Transplantation 1964;2:685-94.
2. Mascotti K, McCullough J, Burger SR. HPC viability measurement: Trypan blue versus acridine orange and propidium iodide. Transfusion 2000;40:693-6.
3. Baust JM, Vogel MJ, Van Buskirk R, Baust JG. A molecular basis of cryopreservation failure and its modulation to improve cell survival. Cell Transplant 2001;10:561-71.
4. Schuurhuis GJ, Muijen MM, Oberink JW, et al. Large populations of non-clonogenic early apoptotic CD34-positive cells are present in frozen-thawed peripheral blood stem cell transplants. Bone Marrow Transplant 2001;27:487-98.
5. de Boer F, Drager AM, Pinedo HM, et al. Early apoptosis largely accounts for functional impairment of CD34+ cells in frozen-thawed stem cell grafts. J Hematother Stem Cell Res 2002;11:951-63.
6. Greco NJ, Seetharaman S, Kurtz J, et al. Evaluation of the reactivity of apoptosis markers before and after cryopreservation in cord blood CD34+ cells. Stem Cells Dev 2006;15:124-35.

Method 47-1. Determining Cellular Viability Using Trypan Blue

Description

Viability determination by trypan blue dye exclusion is based on the principle that nonviable cells have membrane damage that permits certain dyes to enter the cell by passive diffusion, whereas viable cells can exclude the dye from entering the cell. Cells are mixed with trypan blue dye and are examined microscopically. Viable cells are impermeable to trypan blue dye and appear clear, well rounded, and refractile. Nonviable (dead) cells cannot exclude the trypan blue dye, and the cell interior has a blue appearance. The percent viability is calculated by dividing the number of unstained (viable) cells counted by the total number of cells (stained and unstained) counted.

Time for Procedure

Viability measurement takes approximately 10 to 15 minutes, including time for sample preparation.

Summary of Procedure

1. Prepare the trypan blue working solution. Label the container and store at room temperature.
2. Prepare the sample by thawing and/or diluting as appropriate.
3. Perform viability measurement.

Equipment

1. Phase-contrast microscope.
2. Neubauer hemacytometer and coverslip.
3. Manual pipettor.

Supplies and Reagents

1. 12×15-mm and 17×100-mm polystyrene tubes.
2. 50-mL conical centrifuge tubes.
3. Disposable serologic pipettes.
4. Pipette tips.
5. 0.2-micron sterile filter unit, 50- or 115-mL.
6. 0.4% trypan blue stock solution.

7. Dulbecco's phosphate-buffered saline (DPBS).

Procedure

1. Prepare and filter 0.04% trypan blue working solution and store at room temperature.
2. Prepare sample by thawing and/or diluting cell suspension according to facility procedure.
   a. Dilute cell suspension in a 12×75-mm or 17×100-mm tube using DPBS as diluent. Dilute to an appropriate concentration for microscopic viewing, typically 0.5 to 2×10^6 cells/mL. Mix gently but thoroughly.
3. Perform viability measurement.
   a. Mix 0.5 mL of the cell suspension and 0.5 mL of the 0.04% trypan blue working solution in a fresh 12×75-mm polystyrene tube. Allow the cell suspension to stand at room temperature for 2 to 3 minutes.
   b. Load the stained cell suspension into a Neubauer hemacytometer, using a manual pipettor and pipette tip. Allow to settle for approximately 1 minute. Do not overfill.
   c. Place the hemacytometer on the stage of a phase-contrast microscope and view the cells using the 10× objective. Locate the counting grid and adjust the scope to ensure that the field is lit with appropriate contrast for discrimination of light blue, dark blue, and unstained cells.
   d. Count all cells in the four corner squares of the grid. Distinguish between viable cells, which will appear clear, well rounded, and refractile, and nonviable cells, which will be stained blue and have a flattened appearance.
   Note: Include both light blue and dark blue cells in the nonviable count.
   Note: Do not include red cells when counting. Red cells can be distinguished by their smaller size compared to white cells. They may also

appear wrinkled or crenated and may have a greenish cast.

e. Calculate and record percent viability:

$$\frac{\text{Viable cells counted}}{\text{Total cells counted}} \times 100 = \% \text{ viability}$$

Anticipated Results

As a general guideline, viability of fresh cell products should be >90%; viability of thawed cell products should be >70%.

Notes

1. Solutions of 0.4% trypan blue are available from several chemical supply companies.

Sigma catalog #T8154 is sterile filtered and cell culture tested.

2. Trypan blue is classified as a probable carcinogen and an irritant (eyes, skin, respiratory). Proper precautions must be taken during use, and fluid-resistant lab coats and disposable gloves must be worn at a minimum. Refer to the manufacturer's material safety data sheet.

Reference/Resource

1. Tennant JR. Evaluation of the trypan blue technique for determination of cell viability. Transplantation 1964;2: 685-94.

Method 47-2. Determining Viability by Fluorescence Microscopy Using Acridine Orange and Propidium Iodide

Description

This method for determining cell viability uses two reagents, acridine orange (AO) and propidium iodide (PI), allowing for simultaneous visualization of both live and dead cells. Both AO and PI are fluorescent dyes that interact with nucleic acids. AO is a viable cell membrane-permeable dye that intercalates with DNA and fluoresces green (excitation wavelength = 500 nm; emission wavelength = 526 nm). PI, on the other hand, is permeable only to nonviable cells, intercalating with DNA and fluorescing orange (excitation wavelength = 536 nm; emission wavelength = 617 nm).

Time for Procedure

Viability measurement takes approximately 5 to 10 minutes.

Summary of Procedure

1. Prepare stock solutions.
2. Prepare AO/PI solution.
3. Perform viability measurement.

Equipment

1. Fluorescence microscope with appropriate filters (see wavelengths above).
2. Neubauer hemacytometer and coverslip.
3. Differential counter/laboratory hematology analyzer.
4. Manual pipettor and pipette aid.
5. Biological safety cabinet (BSC).

Supplies and Reagents

1. 12 × 75-mm polystyrene tubes.
2. Sterile serologic pipettes of various sizes.
3. Manual pipettor with pipette tips.
4. Lint-free wipes.
5. Acridine orange.
6. Propidium iodide.
7. Sterile water.
8. Dulbecco's phosphate-buffered saline (DPBS).

Procedure

1. Prepare stock solutions (see notes on safety in the "Notes" section):
   a. Prepare a 1-mM AO stock solution by diluting 41.0 mg AO to 100 mL with sterile water. Label container with solution name, date prepared, and initials.
   b. Prepare a 0.5-mg/mL PI stock solution by diluting 50 mg PI to 100 mL with sterile DPBS. Label container with solution name, date prepared, and initials.
2. Prepare AO/PI solution.
   a. In a BSC, prepare AO/PI solution by combining the following reagents in an appropriate sterile container:
      • 1.0 mL of 1-mM AO stock solution.
      • 2.0 mL of 0.5-mg/ml PI stock solution.
      • 47 mL DPBS.
   b. Label the container with ingredient names, date prepared, expiration date, and initials. Store at 2 to 8 C, protected from light (wrapped in foil if necessary). The AO/PI solution is stable up to 1 year under proper storage conditions.
3. Perform viability measurement.
   a. Make a 1:15 or 1:20 dilution of cell suspension to AO/PI solution in a 12 × 75-mm tube. Mix gently but thoroughly.
      Example: Add 190 μL of AO/PI solution to a tube. Add 10 μL cell suspension to the tube. Mix.
   b. Load the stained cell suspension into a Neubauer hemacytometer, using a microliter or manual pipettor. Allow 30 seconds for the cells to settle. Do not overfill.
   c. Count cells under fluorescence. Viable cells will appear green. Dead cells will appear orange. Count a total of at least 100 cells;

200 cells may be counted to obtain an adequate representation of cells and may be required for certain protocols. Also, note that it may be necessary to adjust the ratio of cell suspension to AO/PI solution if too few or too many cells are present to obtain an adequate representation.

d. Calculate and record percent viability:

$$\frac{\text{Viable cells counted}}{\text{Total cells counted}} \times 100 = \% \text{ viability}$$

Anticipated Results

As a general guideline, viability of fresh cell products should be >90%; viability of thawed cell products should be >70%.

Notes

1. The powder form of PI is toxic and may cause heritable genetic damage. The powder form of AO is harmful by inhalation and skin or eye contact. It is a possible mutagen. Refer to the material safety data sheets for both AO and PI when preparing the stock solutions.

2. When a new batch of AO/PI reagent is made, validate the solution before use by performing a viability measurement on three samples in duplicate (ie, perform one viability using the current solution and a second viability using the new solution). The viabilities for the current and new solutions must agree within 10% for each of the three samples.

3. AO/PI staining can also be used to stain multicell clusters such as pancreatic islets by estimating the percentage of individual islet clusters that contains viable green cells, then averaging the individual islet viabilities.

References/Resources

1. Mascotti K, McCullough J, Burger SR. HPC viability measurement: Trypan blue versus acridine orange and propidium iodide. Transfusion 2000;40:693-6.
2. Bank HL. Assessment of islet cell viability using fluorescent dyes. Diabetologia 1987;30:812-6.

Method 47-3. Assessing Viability by Measuring Apoptotic Cells Using Flow Cytometry

Description

An alternative to microscopic determination of viability is the use of flow cytometry to enumerate the number of cells that are nonviable or apoptotic. Antibodies to phenotypic markers, such as CD34 and CD45, are used to fluorescently label the cells of interest. This single-platform procedure uses fluorescent beads to determine the absolute cell number by mixing a known volume of sample with a known volume of beads. To eliminate cell loss, the method uses a lyse-no-wash procedure. 7-aminoactinomycin-D (7-AAD) is used to identify nonviable (necrotic) cells.

Additional antibodies and reagents are then used to identify cells at various stages of apoptosis. These apoptotic markers may more accurately define functional cells present in the cellular therapy product:

- **Annexin V** is a Ca^{2+}-dependent protein with a high affinity for phosphatidylserine. The assay measures the translocation of membrane phosphatidylserine from the inner to the outer leaflet of the plasma membrane.
- **APO2.7 antibody** is a protein confined to the mitochondrial membrane that can be detected during apoptosis following disruption of the mitochondrial membrane and fusion with the plasma membrane.
- **Tetramethyl rhodamine ethyl ester (TMRE)** is a cell-permeable cationic dye that has a strong fluorescent signal that accumulates inside the mitochondria of healthy cells in proportion to the membrane potential, which results in a high fluorescence intensity. In apoptotic cells, where the mitochondrial membrane potential is compromised, TMRE is not accumulated in the mitochondria, resulting in decreased fluorescence.
- **SYTO16** is a vital nucleic acid dye that labels viable cells with high-fluorescence intensity. During apoptosis, nuclear changes such as the breakdown of the nuclear membrane and DNA fragmentation result in decreased fluorescence.

Time for Procedure

The time required for sample preparation, flow cytometry staining, acquisition, and analysis is 2 to 3 hours.

Summary of Procedure

1. Prepare fresh or cryopreserved samples.
2. Incubate samples with fluorescently tagged apoptosis reagents, phenotypic markers, apoptotic markers, and a known volume of fluorescent beads.
3. Analyze stained samples by flow cytometry for the cell population of interest.

Equipment

1. Waterbath at 37 C.
2. Centrifuge.
3. Flow cytometer.
4. Cell counter/hematology analyzer.
5. Manual pipettor.

Supplies and Reagents

1. Thaw medium: 10% dextran, 5% human serum albumin (HSA) in Normosol-R (Hospira, Lake Forest, IL).
2. Flow cytometry buffer: Phosphate-buffered saline, 0.02% (w/v) NaN_3, 0.5% (w/v) HSA.
3. Red cell lysis buffer (eg, PharMLyse, BD Biosciences, San Jose, CA).
4. Annexin-binding buffer (10×, Beckman Coulter Immunotech, Fullerton, CA).
5. Anti-CD34-PE (eg, HPCA-2 clone, Becton Dickenson, Franklin Lakes, NJ) or validated alternative.
6. Anti-CD45-FITC or anti-CD45-PerCP (eg, clone 581, Becton Dickenson) or validated alternative.

7. 7-AAD.
8. Anti-APO2.7 (clone 2.7A6A3, Immunotech).
9. Annexin-V-FITC (Immunotech).
10. TMRE, 100 nM (Molecular Probes, Eugene, OR).
11. SYTO16 (Molecular Probes).
12. Verapamil (10 μM, Sigma-Aldrich, St Louis, MO).
13. Fluorescent beads for single-platform assay.
14. 12×75-mm polystyrene tubes.
15. Pipette tips.

Procedure

1. Prepare fresh or cryopreserved samples.
   a. Thaw cryopreserved samples rapidly in a waterbath at 37 C and dilute 1:2 with thaw medium (final concentrations = 5% dextran, 2.5% HSA).
   b. Lyse a 100-μL aliquot of thawed or fresh sample by adding 1 mL of 1× red cell lysis buffer. Incubate for 15 minutes at room temperature.
   c. Centrifuge (5 minutes, $100 \times g$, room temperature) and resuspend cells in 200 μL flow buffer or, for annexin staining, in 200 μL 1× annexin-binding buffer.
   d. Obtain a nucleated cell count and dilute samples to a desired cell number of 5×10^5 cells per 200 μL flow buffer or annexin-binding buffer.
2. Incubate samples with fluorescently tagged apoptosis reagents, phenotypic markers, apoptotic markers, and a known volume of fluorescent beads. SYTO16 and annexin-V reagents must be incubated with cells before adding antibodies.
   a. To assess SYTO16 staining, add the ATP-binding cassette inhibitor verapamil to a final concentration of 10 μM and SYTO16 to a final concentration of 5 nM. Incubate at 37 C for 45 minutes. Dilute the sample with 1 mL flow buffer, centrifuge (5 minutes, $100 \times g$, room temperature), and suspend the sample in 200 μL flow buffer.
   b. To assess annexin-V binding, add annexin-V-FITC according to manufacturer's instructions and incubate at room temperature for 15 minutes. Dilute sample with 1 mL 1× annexin-binding buffer, centrifuge

(5 minutes, $100 \times g$, room temperature), and suspend sample in 200 μL 1× annexin-binding buffer.
   c. Label cells with appropriate phenotypic markers (eg, anti-CD34 and anti-CD45). Use antibodies conjugated to the appropriate fluorochromes according to manufacturer's instructions and existing procedures. If a different cell population is to be analyzed, the appropriate antibodies and fluorochromes may be substituted.
      • Add 7-AAD according to manufacturer's instructions and/or existing procedures.
      • Add APO2.7 antibody according to manufacturer's instructions.
      • Add TMRE at a final concentration of 100 nM.
   d. For single-platform counting, add fluorescent beads according to the manufacturer's instructions. The remaining markers of necrotic and apoptotic cell death are added as described below.
   e. Incubate all tubes in the dark at room temperature for 15 minutes.
3. Analyze stained samples by flow cytometry for the cell population of interest.
   a. To obtain statistically sufficient events, flow cytometry operators should collect >100 gated CD34+ cells. Flow cytometry file sizes may be reduced by excluding from storage the majority of CD45– and/or CD34– events.
   b. Cells showing markers of necrotic or apoptotic cell death can be excluded from sequential gating for phenotypic markers, and the absolute number of viable nonapoptotic cells can then be determined using fluorescent beads. This practice is now routinely done for 7-AAD+ cells. The appropriate "nonviable" populations to be excluded for the assays described above are 7-AAD+, SYTO16low, TMRElow, annexin+, or APO2.7+ cells (Fig 47-3-1). For example, event markers are set on the created histogram of viable APO2.7low cells in the first decade. Sequential gating strategies are then used to determine the proportion of CD34+ cells that are APO2.7 negative and hence viable (Fig 47-3-2).

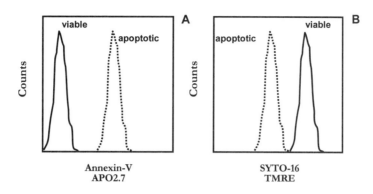

Figure 47-3-1. Flow cytometry histograms showing the labeling of viable and apoptotic cells with several diverse apoptotic reagents.

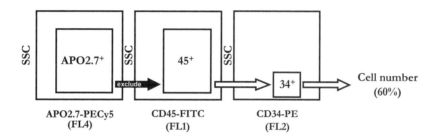

Figure 47-3-2. Proposed flow cytometry gating strategy to enumerate viable CD34+ cells after labeling with apoptotic markers.[6] This example shows the exclusion of nonviable APO2.7+ cells on a plot of side scatter (SSC) vs FL1 events from sequential Boolean gating of an SSC vs CD45+ dot plot and SSC vs CD34+ dot plot.

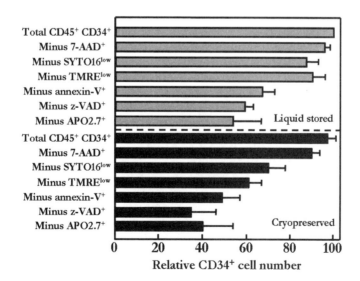

Figure 47-3-3. Comparison of the absolute number of CD34+ cells of liquid stored and cryopreserved/thawed cord blood samples.[6]

Anticipated Results

Use of this method is expected to result in decreased absolute counts of the cells of interest (eg, CD34+ cells) if cells expressing markers of apoptotic or necrotic cell death are present and therefore excluded from enumeration (Fig 47-3-3). Exclusion of early apoptotic cells (APO2.7+ or annexin-V+ cells) should result in lower absolute counts than exclusion of late apoptotic cells, as measured by SYTO16 and TMRE. The highest absolute counts are expected when only necrotic cells (7-AAD+ cells) are excluded.

Notes

1. Unlike SYTO16, which requires incubation at 37 C for 45 minutes, and annexin-V, which requires a specified Ca^{2+}-binding buffer, the APO2.7 antibody and TMRE may be incubated in an identical manner at the same time as the CD34 and CD45 antibodies.

2. Negative controls should be included to set voltage settings and gates:
   - Unstained cells for 7-AAD and for SYTO16.
   - Either unstained cells or, because annexin-V does not bind in the absence of the Ca^{2+}-containing annexin-binding buffer, cells labeled with annexin-V in flow buffer.
   - Cells labeled with appropriate isotype antibody for APO2.7.
   - The initial cell populations of gated CD34+ cells are used to define the apoptotic (TMRE^{low}) and nonapoptotic (TMRE^{high}) cells.

References/Resources

1. Baust JM, Vogel MJ, Van Buskirk R, Baust JG. A molecular basis of cryopreservation failure and its modulation to improve cell survival. Cell Transplant 2001;10:561-71.
2. Schuurhuis GJ, Muijen MM, Oberink JW, et al. Large populations of non-clonogenic early apoptotic CD34-positive cells are present in frozen-thawed peripheral blood stem cell transplants. Bone Marrow Transplant 2001;27:487-98.
3. de Boer F, Drager AM, Pinedo HM, et al. Early apoptosis largely accounts for functional impairment of CD34+ cells in frozen-thawed stem cell grafts. J Hematother Stem Cell Res 2002;11:951-63.
4. Keeney M, Brown W, Gratama J, et al. Single platform enumeration of viable CD34^{pos} cells. J Biol Regul Homeost Agents 2003;17:247-53.
5. Greco NJ, Seetharaman S, Kurtz J, et al. Evaluation of the reactivity of apoptosis markers before and after cryopreservation in cord blood CD34+ cells. Stem Cells Dev 2006;15:124-35.

In: Areman EM, Loper K, eds
Cellular Therapy: Principles, Methods, and Regulations
Bethesda, MD: AABB, 2009

◆◆◆ **48** ◆◆◆

Colony-Forming Cell Assays for Determining Potency of Cellular Therapy Products

Emer Clarke, PhD

COLONY-FORMING CELL (CFC) ASSAYS HAVE been used to understand the complex system of hematopoiesis for over 40 years. Hematopoietic progenitor cells (HPCs) represent a small fraction of the cells present in adult marrow, mobilized and unmobilized peripheral blood, and umbilical cord blood. These rare stem and progenitor cells are responsible for the development of the hematopoietic system and produce a heterogeneous pool of lineage-committed progenitors that can be detected in vitro using CFC assays. Although the frequency of CFCs varies somewhat among normal donors, in patients with hematologic diseases, CFCs often differ significantly in number and size from those of normal donors. Furthermore, the relative frequency of CFCs differs among human tissues, with lower numbers of CFCs in peripheral blood compared to marrow. When cultured in a semisolid methylcellulose-based medium supplemented with appropriate nutrients and growth factors, HPCs proliferate and differentiate to produce colonies of maturing cells. The CFCs may then be classified (depending on the morphologic characteristics of the colonies and the types of cells within them) and enumerated in situ by light microscopy.

The data generated from CFC assays (ie, the number and type of colonies present in the cultures) provide valuable information to physicians and researchers for various purposes. These assays have been useful in the identification of stimulatory molecules, including cytokines and, more recently, chemokines, as well as in the qualification of many growth factors. In addition, CFC assays have been used as a supportive diagnostic test for myeloproliferative disorders and various forms of leukemia.[1,2] Their greatest clinical utility, however, has been to quantify the HPC content of cellular products destined for transplantation. CFC assays may be initiated from a number of primary cell sources, including marrow, umbilical cord blood, peripheral blood, and mobilized peripheral blood stem cells, as well as from populations derived from these sources and further enriched for HPCs, such as those expressing the CD34 and CD133 antigens.

Emer Clarke, PhD, Chief Scientific Officer, ReachBio, LLC, Seattle, Washington

The author has disclosed no conflicts of interest.

Although often considered to be subjective, microscopic enumeration and classification of CFCs remains the only direct method to identify progenitors. Colony identification and quantification data generated from testing multiple individuals within single centers may well report coefficients of variation (CVs) below 10%; however, in national proficiency-testing programs, the CVs for the various progenitors have been shown to be considerably higher. This finding may explain, in part, why some groups have seen correlations between the progenitor content and engraftment,[3,4] whereas others have found no such associations.[5,6] Nonetheless, consensus exists within the transplantation community that cell samples that fail to support the growth of CFCs are suggestive of an inferior product. The CFC assays may therefore be used as a qualitative potency test in some institutions (eg, growth or no growth) or as a more quantifiable, high-content one in others (eg, relative numbers and types of colonies in different samples). Such potency tests have remained the benchmark method to assess the viability and functionality of cellular products, especially following ex-vivo manipulations such as cryopreservation, red cell depletion, T-cell depletion, CD34+ cell enrichment, and the like.

Another complaint often made about CFC assays is the training time required to become proficient at recognizing and counting the colonies, as well as the time it takes even a trained individual to evaluate the samples. Many clinical institutions have longed for an automated counting system to decrease staff training time as well as to reduce the variability of technologists' CFC counts. However, many hurdles must still be overcome in the development of such automation, including accurate recognition of diverse colony morphologies, low contrast of myeloid colonies relative to background, efficient scanning through all planes of the three-dimensional culture, and the meniscus effect of the growth matrix within a dish or well. Until such time as a rapid and accurate automated system becomes available, the CFC assay will require extensive training and good procedures to ensure that optimal information from the assay can be realized.

References/Resources

1. Eaves AC, Barnet MJ, Ponchio L, et al. Differences between normal and CML stem cells: Potential targets for clinical exploitation. Stem Cells 1998;16(Suppl 1):77-83(discussion 89).
2. Nissen-Drury C, Tichelli A, Meyer-Monard S. Human hematopoietic colonies in health and disease. Basel, Switzerland: S Kagler Medical and Scientific Publishers, 2005.
3. Bacigalupo A, Piaggio G, Podesta M, et al. Influence of marrow CFU-GM on engraftment and survival after allogeneic bone marrow transplantation. Bone Marrow Transplant 1995;15:221-6.
4. Cancelas JA, Querol S, Canals C, et al. Peripheral blood CD34+ cell immunomagnetic selection in breast cancer patients: Effect on hematopoietic progenitor content and hematologic recovery after high-dose chemotherapy and autotransplantation. Transfusion 1998;38:1063-70.
5. Torres A, Alonso MC, Gomez-Villagran JL, et al. No influence of number of donor CFU-GM on granulocyte recovery in bone marrow transplantation for acute leukemia. Blut 1995;50:89-94.
6. Masszi T, Gluckman E. Lack of correlation between the number of donor nucleated bone marrow cells or CFU-GM content and the rapidity of engraftment in allogeneic BMT. Acta Biomed Ateneo Parmanse 1993;64:221-6.
7. Miller CL, Lai B. Human and mouse hematopoietic colony forming cell assays. In: Helgason CD, Miller CL, eds. Basic cell culture protocols. 3rd ed. Totowa, NJ: Humana Press, 2005.
8. Eaves C, Lambie K. Atlas of human hematopoietic colonies. Vancouver, BC: StemCell Technologies, 1995.

Method 48-1. Hematopoietic Colony-Forming Cell Assays

Description

This procedure describes protocols for the detection and enumeration of multipotential progenitors and lineage-committed progenitors of the erythroid, granulocyte, and monocyte lineages in samples from various human hematopoietic tissues.

Time for Procedure

The time for the initial setup of the assay may vary based on the amount of processing required for the sample. If a sample of cord blood is provided following red cell depletion, the assay will likely take 30 to 45 minutes for trained personnel. If, however, an untreated marrow or peripheral blood sample is received, requiring the generation of a mononuclear cell suspension by density gradient centrifugation, the process will likely take 1.5 hours.

After the cells are plated in the methylcellulose, the cultures must be incubated for 7 to 16 days. The duration of the assay is in part related to the maturity stage of the progenitors. Mature progenitors (eg, colony-forming unit erythroid, or CFU-E) have limited proliferative potential and hence require a relatively short time to achieve maximal colony size (small), whereas the more immature progenitors (eg, burst-forming unit—erythroid, or BFU-E) require longer culture periods to allow their true proliferative potential to be expressed and their characteristically larger colonies to be formed. To ensure the accurate enumeration of both primitive and mature progenitors, the assay is typically read at days 14 to 16.

Summary of Procedure

1. Prepare colony-forming cell assay medium and tissue culture dishes.
2. Dilute the samples to be tested into the CFC assay medium.
3. Plate the samples.
4. Incubate the samples for 7-16 days.
5. Enumerate the colonies.

Equipment

1. Biological safety cabinet.
2. Light microscope and hemacytometer or automated cell counter.
3. Inverted microscope equipped with low- (2.5×) and higher- (4-5×, 10×) power objectives, 10 to 12.5× ocular eyepieces, and a blue filter (which enhances the red color of hemoglobinized erythroblasts for easier CFC identification).
4. Incubator (>95% humidity, water jacketed, 37 C, 5% CO_2) with an open pan of water placed in the incubator chamber to help maintain humidity.
5. Vortex.

Supplies and Reagents

1. Pipettor and sterile tips (20 µL, 200 µL, and 1000 µL).
2. 35-mm dishes, pretested for low cell adherence.
3. 150×25-mm tissue culture dishes or 245-mm square bioassay dishes.
4. 3- and 5-mL syringes with luer-lock fitting.
5. 16-gauge blunt-end needles.
6. 60-mm gridded scoring dish.
7. Methylcellulose-based CFC assay medium containing cytokines.
8. Iscove's modified Dulbecco's medium (IMDM) containing 2% fetal bovine serum (FBS).

Procedure

1. Prepare the CFC assay medium and tissue culture dishes.
   a. Thaw the appropriate numbers of tubes containing methylcellulose-based CFC assay medium. One tube (4 mL) is sufficient for triplicate cultures at a single cell concentration.

Note: If the medium has been purchased as a 100-mL bottle, thaw the contents of the bottle and shake vigorously to ensure it is mixed well and that all the nutrients and growth factors within it are dispersed evenly. Then let the medium stand for 10 minutes to allow the bubbles to dissipate. Accurately dispense the medium into replicate tubes (4 mL of medium into each), using a 5-cc syringe and a blunt-end needle. Keep out the number of tubes needed for the current assay, and freeze the rest at –20 C according to the manufacturer's instructions until required in the future.

   b. Place four sterile 35-mm culture dishes with lids inside a sterile 150 × 25-mm tissue culture dish with a lid. Three of these 35-mm dishes will be used for the assay, and one of the dishes will be used for water to ensure a local high humidity (remove the lid on the water dish for the duration of the assay). This set of dishes is sufficient for one triplicate assay. If plating multiple cell concentrations (see Note 1, below) or assays, the 35-mm dishes may be placed in 245-mm bioassay trays with two extra 35-mm dishes for water to ensure appropriate humidity.

   c. Label the edge of each 35-mm culture dish lid appropriately (eg, with experiment and assay number), using a permanent (water-resistant) fine-tip felt marker.

2. Dilute the samples to be tested in the CFC assay medium.

   a. Dilute the cells with IMDM containing 2% FBS to 10× the final concentration(s) required for plating.

   Note: When the correct plating cell concentration is difficult to anticipate, the use of two or more two- to threefold serially diluted cell concentrations is advised (see Note 1, below).

   b. Add 0.4 mL of diluted cells to a tube containing 4 mL methylcellulose medium.

   c. Vortex the tube vigorously for approximately 5 seconds and let it stand for at least 5 minutes to allow bubbles to dissipate.

3. Plate the samples.

   a. Prepare a 3-mL syringe with a 16-gauge blunt-end needle by drawing up approximately 1 mL of methylcellulose-based medium and dispensing it completely back into the tube (this helps remove air bubbles from the syringe; see Note 2, below).

   b. Draw the test sample (medium containing cells from Step 2b) up into the prepared syringe to the 2.6-mL mark. Use the opposite hand to remove the lid from the first 35-mm culture dish and dispense 1.1 mL into the center of the dish (plunger now at the 1.5-mL mark). Replace the lid. Similarly, dispense another 1.1 mL into the second 35-mm dish (plunger now at the 0.4-mL mark). Draw up more of the remaining test sample to the 1.5-mL mark and dispense 1.1 mL into the third dish.

   c. Tilt and rotate the dishes to spread the medium evenly over the surface of each dish. Allow the meniscus to attach to the dish wall evenly on all sides but avoid getting medium up the side wall.

   d. Repeat Steps 2 and 3 for each cell sample to be assayed. Use a new sterile disposable 3-mL syringe with a new 16-gauge blunt-end needle for each test sample tube plated (see Note 2, below).

   e. Place approximately 3 mL of sterile water in the empty, uncovered 35-mm dish(es) to maintain humidity.

4. Incubate the samples. Put the tray of cultures into the incubator (see Note 3, below) for 7 to 16 days, depending on the duration of the specific assay (Note 4).

5. Enumerate the colonies. After the appropriate incubation period, remove the trays of dishes from the incubator. Enumerate the colonies by placing, in turn, each of the 35-mm culture dishes onto a 60-mm gridded dish and evaluating the colonies using an inverted microscope. Adjust the focus under low power (2.5× objective) until the colonies are in focus (see Notes 5 and 6, below). If erythropoietin was absent from the culture medium, only the colony-forming units—granulocyte-macrophage (CFUs-

GM) will be present (except in some disease states). If erythropoietin was present in the culture medium, the following list of colonies may be present:

- CFU-E (not shown): This erythroid CFC generates a very small erythroid colony containing one to two clusters with a total number of 8 to 200 erythroblasts. Magnification of 125-150× is typically required to visualize these colonies.
- BFU-E (Fig 48-1-1): This more primitive CFC generates larger colonies containing more than 200 erythroblasts. Magnification of 25 to 50× is typically required to visualize these colonies.
- CFU-GM (Fig 48-1-2): This myeloid CFC is capable of producing colonies with 40 or more granulocyte-monocyte and/or macrophage cells. Magnification of 25 to 50× is typically required to visualize these colonies.
- Colony-forming unit—granulocyte-erythrocyte-macrophage-megakaryocyte (CFU-GEMM) (Fig 48-1-3): This primitive CFC is capable of producing colonies containing erythroid cells as well as 20 or more granulocytes, macrophages, and megakaryocytes. Magnification of 25 to 50× is typically required to visualize these colonies, though it is wise to confirm the presence of both erythroid and myeloid cell types at higher magnifications.

Anticipated Results

Considerable variability in CFC frequency can occur in samples derived from both normal donors and patients. Hence, the cells may sometimes need to be plated at multiple concentrations to ensure an accurate readout (see Note 1). For marrow, peripheral blood, and mobilized peripheral blood, 70-100 colonies per 35-mm culture dish will provide an excellent value from which to calculate the CFC content of a product or determine whether a specific treatment or procedure is deleterious to hematopoietic progenitors. Ideally, one would like the calculated standard deviation derived from the

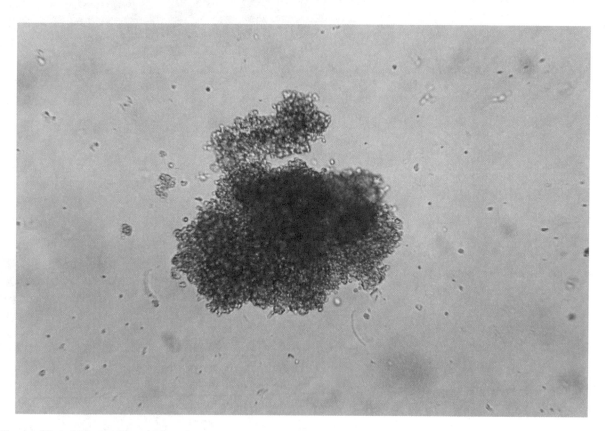

Figure 48-1-1. Burst-forming unit—erythroid (BFU-E).

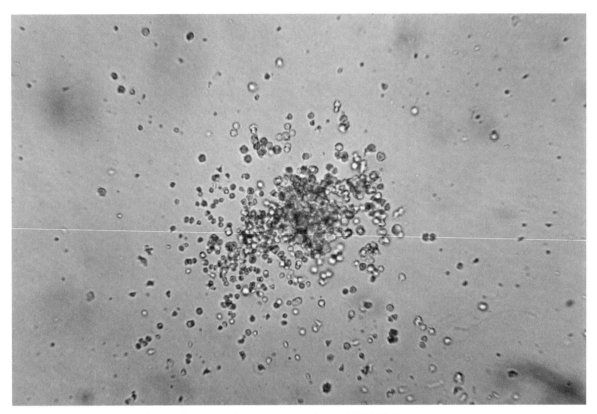

Figure 48-1-2. Colony-forming unit—granulocyte-macrophage (CFU-GM).

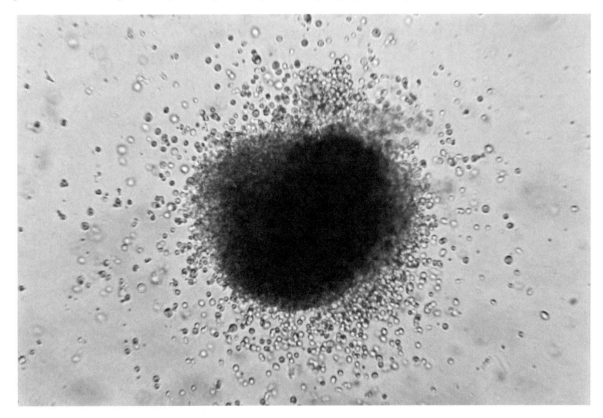

Figure 48-1-3. Colony-forming unit—granulocyte-erythrocyte-macrophage-megakaryocyte (CFU-GEMM).

number of colonies in the three replicate culture dishes to be less than 10% of the average colony number.

The colonies derived from cord blood progenitors are typically larger than colonies derived from other tissues. Therefore, if samples from cord blood are being tested, an average of 50 colonies per 35-mm dish is desirable. In addition, the red cell background (which is a feature of many cord blood assays) can make colony identification challenging, so increasing the space between colonies has an added benefit because it can facilitate more accurate counting. Again, the calculated standard deviation derived from the number of colonies in the three replicate culture dishes should be less than 10% of the average colony number. This method should provide a reliable value from which to calculate the CFC content per mL of cord blood or CFC content per product, as required.

Notes

1. The frequency of progenitors in tissue samples from normal donors and patients is variable. Therefore, one must try to plate an adequate cell number to get an appropriate number of colonies per 35-mm culture dish. Plating too few cells will result in a low colony number per dish, which in turn can result in an overestimation of CFCs per product. Plating too many cells results in a very high colony number per plate, making colony identification difficult and often resulting in an underestimation of CFCs per product. For these reasons, many laboratories elect to plate cells from patients at more than one concentration (threefold serial dilutions) to ensure appropriate colony numbers. Suggested plating cell concentrations for various tissues and cell populations have been described previously.[7]

2. Methylcellulose is a viscous solution and cannot be accurately dispensed using pipettes because the medium adheres to the inside of the pipette. Syringes fitted with blunt-end needles facilitate accurate dispensing of the medium and prevent injury caused by needle pricks. Accurate dispensing of medium containing cells ensures the numbers of colonies detected in each of the replicate dishes are similar and the resulting standard deviation is low.

3. Incubator conditions are extremely important for primary hematopoietic cells. The temperature (37 C) should be confirmed using a thermometer placed inside the incubator chamber, and CO_2 levels (5%) should be routinely monitored using a Fyrite (New Kensington, PA) CO_2 device. A water-jacketed incubator with an open pan of water placed in the incubator chamber to maintain humidity (>95%) is optimal. A suitable additive (ie, copper sulfate crystals) can be added to the water pan to inhibit microbial growth.

4. If the cultures will not be enumerated by day 16, they may be placed in an incubator at 33 C at that time to slow colony growth and temporarily maintain optimal morphology. Refill water dishes if necessary, and count as soon as possible (eg, within 3-4 days).

5. Microscopic enumeration of colonies is often perceived as difficult, but with some training, it becomes easier. The following suggestions may aid in the process:
   a. Scan the entire dish for relative placement of colonies to one another.
   b. Make note of overall appearance of the culture (presence or absence of red cell background) to help with the scoring and evaluation.
   c. Continually focus up and down to identify all colonies present in the three-dimensional culture and to distinguish individual colonies that are close together but present on different planes.
   d. Pay particular attention to the edges of dishes because colonies tend to grow along the medium meniscus and can be challenging to see.
   e. Start counting at one end of the dish and proceed to count all colonies in each column (up and down rather than side to side), which will minimize the sensation of motion sickness.

6. Colony descriptions provide information on typical colony morphologies.[8] However, a red cell background, which is often a feature of cord blood CFC assays, makes enumeration more challenging. In certain disease states, the colony morphology or colony size may be significantly different from colonies cultured

from samples derived from normal individuals.[2,8]

References/Resources

1. Eaves AC, Barnet MJ, Ponchio L, et al. Differences between normal and CML stem cells: Potential targets for clinical exploitation. Stem Cells 1998;16(Suppl 1):77-83(discussion 89).
2. Nissen-Drury C, Tichelli A, Meyer-Monard S. Human hematopoietic colonies in health and disease. Basel, Switzerland: S Kagler Medical and Scientific Publishers, 2005.
3. Bacigalupo A, Piaggio G, Podesta M, et al. Influence of marrow CFU-GM on engraftment and survival after allogeneic bone marrow transplantation. Bone Marrow Transplant 1995;15:221-6.
4. Cancelas JA, Querol S, Canals C, et al. Peripheral blood CD34+ cell immunomagnetic selection in breast cancer patients: Effect on hematopoietic progenitor content and hematologic recovery after high-dose chemotherapy and autotransplantation. Transfusion 1998;38:1063-70.
5. Torres A, Alonso MC, Gomez-Villagran JL, et al. No influence of number of donor CFU-GM on granulocyte recovery in bone marrow transplantation for acute leukemia. Blut 1995;50:89-94.
6. Masszi T, Gluckman E. Lack of correlation between the number of donor nucleated bone marrow cells or CFU-GM content and the rapidity of engraftment in allogeneic BMT. Acta Biomed Ateneo Parmanse 1993;64:221-6.
7. Miller CL, Lai B. Human and mouse hematopoietic colony forming cell assays. In: CD Helgason, CL Miller, eds. Basic cell culture protocols. 3rd ed. Totowa, NJ: Humana Press, 2005.
8. Eaves C, Lambie K. Atlas of human hematopoietic colonies. Vancouver, BC: StemCell Technologies, 1995.

In: Areman EM, Loper K, eds
Cellular Therapy: Principles, Methods, and Regulations
Bethesda, MD: AABB, 2009

♦♦♦   **49**   ♦♦♦

Bioluminescence Assays for Assessing Potency of Cellular Therapy Products

Karen M. Hall, MT(ASCP), and Ivan N. Rich, PhD

THE PROCESS OF CELL PROLIFERATION can be correlated with a number of markers, one of which is the intracellular adenosine triphosphate (i-ATP) concentration. In fact, i-ATP can be used as a biochemical marker for five cellular parameters: 1) proliferation/cytotoxicity, 2) cell number, 3) viability, 4) cellular/mitochondrial integrity, and 5) apoptosis because i-ATP is required for the initiation of programmed cell death. As a biochemical marker, the concentration of i-ATP can be calibrated against an external ATP standard. Furthermore, when the concentration of ATP is the limiting substrate, as in the case of i-ATP, the bioluminescence produced in a luciferin/luciferase reaction measured in a plate luminometer is directly proportional to the proliferation status of the cells. The two stem and progenitor cell—quality control (SPC-QC) platforms (see Table 49-1) and one potency assay platform described in this chapter have been designed and developed in reliance on this principle.

Calibration and Standardization of the Potency Assay

By measuring a biochemical marker of the proliferation process, namely, i-ATP concentration, and relying solely on an instrument-based readout, not only does the assay become nonsubjective, but it can also be calibrated and standardized. This, in turn, allows for assay validation and proficiency testing within and between laboratories.

Before measuring bioluminescence as a function of i-ATP concentration and therefore proliferation of the sample product, an ATP standard curve is performed using an external ATP source. There are several reasons why this step is of the utmost importance. First, it calibrates the plate luminometer. *Calibration* is defined here as the periodic activity to check and maintain the accuracy of measurements against a known standard. Second, it ensures that the reagents are working correctly. Third, it allows the instrument readout in non-

---

Karen M. Hall, MT(ASCP), Laboratory Manager/Project Manager, and Ivan N. Rich, PhD, Chairman and Chief Executive Officer, HemoGenix, Inc, Colorado Springs, Colorado

The authors have disclosed no conflicts of interest.

Table 49-1. SPC-QC Assay Platforms

Characteristics	HALO-96 MeC SPC-QC*	HALO-96 SEC SPC-QC*
Type of assay	Proliferation	Proliferation
Validated	Yes	Yes
Type of culture	Methylcellulose	Suspension expansion culture
Cell growth	Clonal	Expansion
Parameters measured	i-ATP	i-ATP
Assay readout type	Instrument based	Instrument based
Calibration	External ATP	External ATP
Readout	ATP concentration	ATP concentration
Subjectivity	Nonsubjective	Nonsubjective

*HemoGenix, Colorado Springs, Co.
SPC-QC = stem and progenitor cell—quality control; i-ATP = intracellular adenosine triphosphate.

standardized relative luminescence units (RLUs) to be converted to standardized ATP concentrations (microMolars, or µM), thereby standardizing the assay. Luminometers from different manufacturers exhibit different ranges of RLUs. By using an external ATP standard, results from different plate luminometers can be compared. Finally, by performing an ATP standard curve and providing results in ATP concentrations, not only can results from different instruments be compared, but results within and between laboratories of tests performed at different times can also be directly compared.

HALO-96 MeC SPC-QC

The HALO-96 MeC SPC-QC (HALO = hematopoietic/hemotoxicity assays via luminescence output; MeC = methylcellulose; HemoGenix, Colorado Springs, CO) was the first platform to be developed and is based on the traditional colony-forming cell (CFC) assay. It was designed specifically for 1) high-throughput hemotoxicity testing for biotechnology and pharmaceutical companies to test potential toxicity at any stage of drug development and 2) as a hematopoietic progenitor cell (HPC) potency assay for transplantation and umbilical cord blood (UCB) processing facilities.

HALO is a proliferation assay. Although the target cells are grown under clonal conditions in MeC, the 7-day incubation time for human peripheral blood (PB), UCB, and marrow cells does not allow the cells to differentiate. At 7 days, the cells stimulated with growth factor/cytokine cocktails (similar to those used in the CFC assay) are proliferating exponentially, but little if any differentiation occurs, and therefore colonies of mature cells cannot be enumerated. Indeed, the purpose of HALO was to design a CFC assay that did not require manually enumerating colonies, thereby eliminating the subjectivity of the assay.

If colonies are not counted because the cells have not been allowed to differentiate, however, how does one know that the stimulated cells are going to produce colonies of the proper cell types? The answer lies in the fact that HALO can be multiplexed with other assays using the same sample. If extra replicate wells are prepared, the cells from one set of replicates can be used to measure proliferation while the cells from the other set of replicates can be used for phenotypic analysis. In this case, the cells are removed from the wells of a 96-well plate by diluting the viscosity of the MeC medium following culture, processing the cells for various membrane-specific expression markers, and examining these markers by flow cytometry. Table 49-2 shows that if a colony-forming cell—granulocyte-erythrocyte-macrophage-megakaryocyte (CFU-GEMM) is allowed to grow under HALO conditions, the cell types that are expected to be produced from this stem cell population are indeed produced. Thus, some stem cell markers are present, as are markers corresponding to the erythroid cells (glycophorin-A+), macrophages (CD14+), neutrophils (CD15+), and megakaryocytes (CD41+/CD61+) that would be expected to be produced from this cell population. The same type

Table 49-2. Phenotypic Analysis of Cells Removed from HALO* Cultures†

Marker	CFC-GEMM	BFU-E	GM-CFC	M-CFC	Mk-CFC	T-CFC	B-CFC
CD34	0.05%	0.06%	0.08%	—	0.1%	—	—
CD117	2.55%	—	—	—	—	—	—
CD133	3.24%	—	—	—	—	—	—
Glycophorin	25%	54%	—	—	—	—	—
CD14	9.3%	3.9%	16.8%	—	9.7%	—	—
CD15	1.6%	1.1%	1.1%	17.8%	1.1%	—	—
CD41/61	9.2%	8.5%	—	—	48.1%	—	—
CD3	—	—	—	—	—	31.4%	—
CD3/CD4	—	—	—	—	—	17.9%	—
CD3/CD8	—	—	—	—	—	11.6%	—
CD3/CD56	—	—	—	—	—	7.0%	—
CD19	—	—	—	—	—	—	21.9%

*HemoGenix, Colorado Springs, CO.
†Percentages are of total cells gated through CD45.
CFC-GEMM = colony-forming cell—granulocyte-erythrocyte-macrophage-megakaryocyte; BFU-E = burst-forming unit—erythroid; GM-CFC = granulocyte-macrophage colony-forming cell; M-CFC = macrophage colony-forming cell; Mk-CFC = megakaryocyte colony-forming cell; T-CFC = T-lymphocyte colony-forming cell; B-CFC = B-lymphocyte colony-forming cell.

of analysis was performed for the other cultured cell populations as shown in Table 49-2.

HALO-96 SEC SPC-QC

In this MeC-free assay, all reagents are similar to those used in the HALO-96 MeC SPC-QC, except that MeC is replaced by a liquid reagent (suspension expansion culture, or SEC). This assay platform has several advantages compared to the MeC equivalent. First, the assay is easier and faster to perform because it is unnecessary to dispense viscous MeC, which can result in significant errors and high coefficients of variation. Second, because the cells are grown in suspension rather than under clonal conditions, cell-to-cell interactions take place. This has the advantage of reducing the lag time to initiation of proliferation. As a result, the assay takes only 5 days to complete, rather than the 7 days required for the MeC format. Third, culturing cells under suspension expansion conditions increases the sensitivity of the assay twofold over cultures grown in MeC.

Despite these changes in culture conditions and format, a direct correlation exists between the tra-ditional CFC assay, HALO-96 MeC, and HALO-96 SEC as a function of cell concentration. One example of this correlation is shown in Fig 49-1, which illustrates that the CFC assay performed at 14 days can be replaced by the HALO-96 MeC at 7 days. Moreover, HALO-96 MeC and HALO-96 SEC can be interchanged (Fig 49-2).

HALO-96 PQR

The HALO-96 PQR (Potency, Quality, Release) is a quality control assay that uses HALO-96 SEC technology, but it has been designed as a true stem cell potency assay for UCB and incorporates a UCB reference standard (RS). All potency assays require a dose response to be performed. For HALO-96 PQR, a cell dose response is performed for both the post-thaw sample segment and the RS that is provided with the kit. The slope of the linear regression of the cell dose response is compared to that of the RS slope. The potency ratio can then be estimated. In addition, HALO-96 PQR provides the ability to define the acceptance limits for release criteria of UCB before transplantation.

Relationship between the Colony-Forming Assay at 14 Days and HALO™-96 MeC at 7 Days for Human Bone Marrow CFC-GEMM

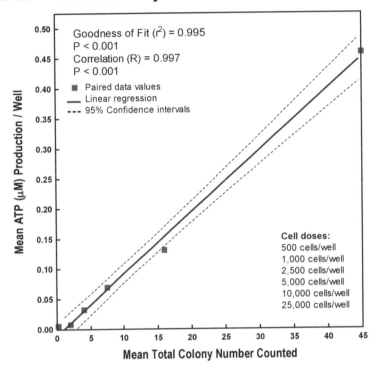

Figure 49-1. The individual sample points are a mean of four identical replicate cultures, using the 14-day colony-forming assay method, and eight identical replicate cultures of human marrow mononuclear cells from the same sample, stimulated to detect colony-forming cells—granulocyte-erythrocyte-macrophage-megakaryocyte (CFC-GEMM) using HALO-96 MeC technology (HemoGenix) and incubated for 7 days. The reagents and conditions to stimulate CFC-GEMM using both methodologies were exactly the same. MeC = methylcellulose; ATP = adenosine triphosphate.

Cell Populations

The three HPC potency assay platforms described in this chapter are available as kits with different media formulations that permit detection of the following hematopoietic cell populations in side-by-side cultures from the same sample.

- **High proliferative potential—stem and progenitor (HPP-SP) cell.** HPP-SP is a primitive stem cell population that is more mature than the long-term culture-initiating cell, but more primitive than the CFU-GEMM. The HPP-SP cell population is quiescent and either can be initially "primed" to induce the cells into cell cycle or can be "fully stimulated." The latter not only primes the cells but also expands the cells into

different lineages. Therefore, the HPP-SP can be used as an "expansion potency assay." When primed and fully stimulated, the HPP-SP should exhibit the highest proliferation status of all seven cell populations described here. The HPP-SP produces both hematopoietic and lymphopoietic cells and can be considered as occupying a stage of "stemness" that is approximately equivalent to the point at which divergence of these two systems occurs. Inclusion of the HPP-SP populations could provide valuable information on long-term engraftment and repopulation potential.

- **Colony-forming cell—granulocyte-erythrocyte-macrophage-megakaryocyte [CFC-GEMM (CFU-GEMM)].** This mutipotential stem cell has the

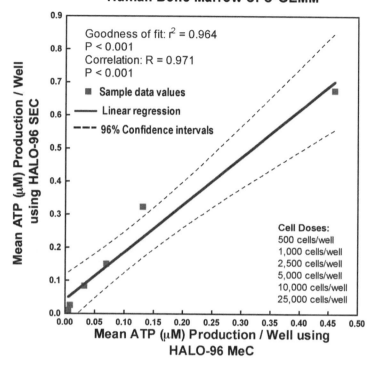

Figure 49-2. The individual sample points are means from eight identical replicate cultures of human marrow mononuclear cells stimulated to detect CFC-GEMM and incubated for 7 days using HALO-96 MeC and for 5 days using HALO-96 SEC technology. The graph depicts the correlation between i-ATP production of cells cultured in MeC and those cultured in suspension expansion conditions as a function of cell concentration. SEC = suspension expansion culture.

capability of producing cells of the granulocyte-macrophage, erythroid, and megakaryocytic lineages, but not cells of the lymphopoietic lineages. The CFC-GEMM population could be useful for short-term engraftment and reconstitution potential and should demonstrate a proliferation status lower than HPP-SP but higher than the three hematopoietic progenitor cell populations.

• **Burst-forming unit—erythroid (BFU-E).** This is a primitive erythropoietic progenitor cell population with high proliferative capacity.

• **Granulocyte-macrophage colony-forming cell [GM-CFC (CFU-GM)].** The GM-CFC is the population often detected using the conventional CFC/CFU assay.

• **Megakaryocyte colony-forming cell [Mk-CFC (CFU-Mk)].** The proliferation status of the Mk-

CFC is, like the BFU-E and GM-CFC, lower than the CFC-GEMM but greater than either of the lymphopoietic lineages.

• **T-lymphocyte colony-forming cell (T-CFC) and B-lymphocyte colony-forming cell (B-CFC).** Inclusion of the T- and B-lymphopoietic colony-forming cells could be useful for monitoring lymphopoiesis after transplantation.

The three hematopoietic lineages (BFU-E, GM-CFC, and CFU-Mk), when detected together, could provide information on engraftment status after transplantation. Figure 49-3 shows the mean proliferation status of each of these cell populations derived from normal human marrow. The combined use of all seven populations has previously been reported as a powerful in-vitro tool to predict hemotoxicity.[1]

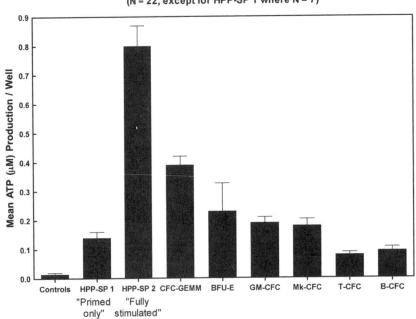

HALO 7-Population Response Profile Showing the Proliferation Status of Lympho-Hematopoietic Cells from Human Bone Marrow
(N = 22, except for HPP-SP 1 where N = 7)

Figure 49-3. The HALO-96 MeC SPC-QC potency assay was used to detect seven different stem and progenitor cell populations simultaneously from 22 human marrow samples. For 7 of the 22 samples analyzed, the primitive stem cell population HPP-SP (high proliferative potential—stem and progenitor; see text) was initially "primed" out of quiescence and into cell cycle over a 7-day incubation period. This primed population is referred to in the diagram as HPP-SP 1. All samples detected the "fully stimulated" HPP-SP population, referred to in the diagram as HPP-SP 2. The results indicate the expected difference in proliferation status of the different cell populations: HPP-SP > CFC-GEMM > BFU-E = CFU-GM = CFU-Mk > T-CFC >= B-CFC.

Bioluminescence technology has the following advantages over CFC assays used for quality control and stem cell potency of cellular therapy products:
- Nonsubjective, instrument-based readout with capability for compliance with good laboratory practice and current good manufacturing practice.
- Ability to calibrate and standardize the assay.
- Significantly shorter time to obtain results.
- High predictive value.
- Short (2-3 day) training period.
- Validation capability.
- Proficiency-testing capability.

Reference/Resource

1. Rich IN, Hall KM. Validation and development of a predictive paradigm for hemotoxicology using a multifunctional bioluminescence colony-forming proliferation assay. Tox Sci 2005;87:427-41.

Method 49-1. Measuring Proliferation Using Bioluminescence-Based ATP Assays

Description

Cell samples are prepared according to a user-defined or prevalidated protocol. After obtaining the mononuclear cell (MNC) count, the cells are adjusted to a specific cell concentration. All three assay platforms use premixed "master mixes" for each cell population to be detected, including the growth factor/cytokine cocktails that are predispensed into separate tubes for each sample. The cell suspension is added to the master mix, the tubes are vortexed, and 100 μL is dispensed into each of 6 replicate wells of the 96-well plate provided. The cultures are incubated for the requisite number of days at 37 C in a fully humidified atmosphere containing 5% CO_2 and, if possible, 5% O_2. The cultures are processed to release intracellular adenosine triphosphate (i-ATP) from the cells so that it can act as a substrate for a luciferin/luciferase reaction. After a 10-minute incubation at room temperature, bioluminescence is measured in a plate luminometer.

Time for Procedure

For all three platforms, the setup time is very similar and usually takes 15 to 45 minutes, depending on the number of samples being assayed. Cultures are then incubated for 5 to 7 days, depending on the platform.

Performance of the ATP standard curve usually takes approximately 15 to 20 minutes. Processing time for the samples will depend on the number of samples being assayed, but for a full 96-well plate, regardless of the cell populations being examined, the procedure can usually be completed in 15 to 20 minutes, including measurement.

Summary of Procedure

1. Prepare cells and adjust cell concentration.
2. Add the cells to the culture medium and plate in 96-well microtiter plates.
3. Culture the cells for the time required for the specific assay platform.
4. Construct an ATP standard curve and measure luminescence.
5. Measure luminescence for cultured samples.

Equipment and Supplies

1. Plate luminometer.
2. Single-channel pipettes, preferably electronic, for variable volumes between 1 μL and 1000 μL.
3. 8- or 12-channel pipette, preferably electronic, for fixed or variable volumes between 10 μL and 100 μL.
4. Repeater pipette with positive displacement.
5. Vortex mixer.
6. Tissue culture incubator, humidified at 37 C with 5% CO_2 (minimum requirement) and 5% O_2 (preferable).
7. Incubator, humidified at 23 C with 5% CO_2 (optional).
8. Hemacytometer or automated cell counter.
9. Flow cytometer for optional phenotypic analysis and viability assessment.
10. Inverted microscope (for 80 to 100× magnification) with a 96-well plate stage holder.

Supplies and Reagents

1. Sterile plastic tubes (5 mL).
2. Sterile pipette tips.
3. 1.5-mL plastic vials (five for each ATP standard curve).
4. Ficoll density gradient medium.
5. Iscove's Modified Dulbecco's Medium (IMDM).
6. Phosphate-buffered saline (PBS).
7. Syringe tips for repeater pipette (1.25 mL, 2.5 mL, 5 mL, or nearest volume depending on the repeater syringe used).

8. HALO-96 SEC, HALO-96 MeC, or HALO-96 PQR kits (HemoGenix, Colorado Springs, CO), as appropriate.

Procedure

1. Prepare the cells.
   a. All human bioluminescence quality control assay platforms can be used with peripheral blood (normal or mobilized), marrow, or umbilical cord blood (UCB); HALO-96 PQR is specific for UCB. Depletion of erythrocytes is essential because they can interfere with the luminescence reaction when present at high concentrations. In addition, if red cells are lysed, it is essential to wash the cells after lysis because the lysate contains free hemoglobin that can also interfere with the assay.
   b. UCB requires special attention. It is necessary to deplete the UCB of erythrocytes using hydroxyethylstarch (HES) or a density gradient separation per the manufacturer's protocol so that erythrocytes constitute less than 10% of the cell suspension. The small number of remaining enucleated and nucleated erythrocytes present should not interfere with the assay.
   c. Measure viability using trypan blue and a hemacytometer or by flow cytometry and use 7-amino-actinomycin D (7-AAD) or another vital stain. For this assay, a viability of 90% or greater is recommended for unfrozen cells as well as for cryopreserved and thawed cells.
   d. Determine the cell concentration using either a hemacytometer or electronic cell/particle counter.
   e. Adjust the cell concentration according to Table 49-1-1. Prepare 500 to 1000 µL (0.5-1 mL) of this working cell concentration. Note that the working cell concentration per mL is 100× the final cell concentration per well.
2. Set up the cell culture.
   Note: Figure 49-1-1 is a flow diagram for performing the ATP bioluminescence proliferation assay. Regardless of which assay is used, culture setup is the same.
   a. Tubes containing 900 µL of predispensed and premixed master mixes are supplied. The number of tubes depends on the number of samples and populations that can be evaluated using the assay kit. The contents of the tubes are supplied frozen. Remove the number of tubes equal to the number of samples to be analyzed, and thaw either in a waterbath at 37 C or at room temperature.

Table 49-1-1. Adjustment of Cell Concentration for Bioluminescence Assays

Cell Type	Cell Preparation	Cell State	Working Cell Concentration Required (100 × Final Cell Concentration)	Final Cell Concentration per Well
Marrow	Mononuclear cell	Fresh/frozen	7.5×10^4 to 7.5×10^5/mL	750-7500 cells/well
Peripheral blood	Mononuclear cell	Fresh/frozen	1 to 7.5×10^5/mL	1000-7500 cells/well
Umbilical cord blood	Mononuclear cell	Fresh/frozen	7.5×10^4 to 7.5×10^5/mL	750-7500 cells/well
Marrow	CD34+	Fresh/frozen	$1\text{-}5 \times 10^4$/mL	100-500 cells/well
Peripheral blood, mobilized	CD34+	Fresh/frozen	$1\text{-}5 \times 10^4$/mL	100-500 cells/well
Umbilical cord blood	CD34+	Fresh/frozen	2.5×10^3/mL to 5×10^4/mL	25-500 cells/well

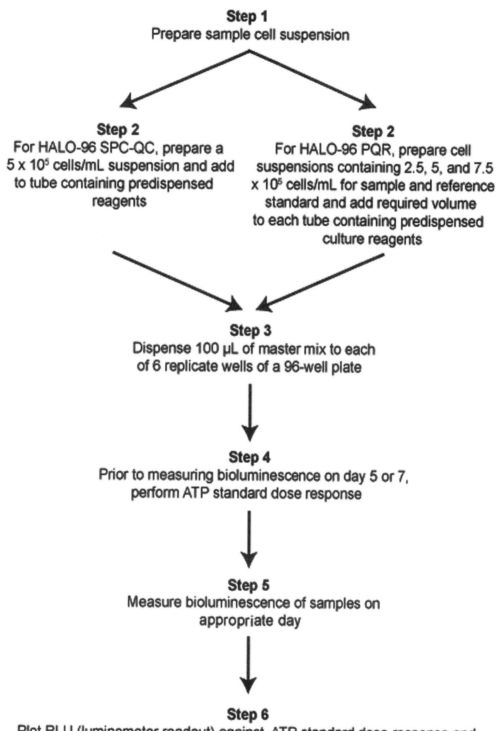

Figure 49-1-1. General flow diagram for using adenosine triphosphate (ATP)-based proliferation cell potency assays.
RLU = relative luminescence unit.

b. Using a calibrated (preferably electronic) pipette, add 100 µL (0.1 mL) of the sample working cell concentration to the completely thawed master mix. The total volume in the tube will now be 1000 µL (1 mL), but the working cell concentration will now be reduced 10-fold.

c. Mix the contents of the tube thoroughly by vortexing. If using MeC, allow the contents to settle for a few minutes.

d. Using a positive displacement repeater pipette, dispense 100 µL (0.1 mL) of the master mix containing the cell sample into the center of each of six replicate wells across the plate in rows. By dispensing only 100 µL (0.1 mL) of the master mix into each well, the sample working cell concentration has been decreased a further 10-fold, thus producing the final cell concentration required per well.

e. If all 96 wells have not been used, the empty wells can be covered with one of the sterile, adhesive foils supplied with the assay kit. If this is the case, remove the lid and attach the sterile adhesive foil over the empty wells to avoid any contamination so that the plate can be used at a later time. This step should be performed under aseptic conditions.

3. Culture cells.

a. Transfer the culture plate to a fully humidified incubator at 37 C containing an atmosphere of 5% CO_2. If possible, use an incubator gassed with nitrogen to reduce the atmospheric oxygen concentration (21%) to 5% O_2; this helps increase the plating efficiency by reducing oxygen toxicity.[2,3]

b. Incubation times are as follows:
   • 5 days for HALO-96 SEC SPC-QC and HALO-96 PQR.
   • 7 days for HALO-96 MeC SPC-QC.

4. Construct an ATP standard curve, and measure luminescence.

a. Before measuring the luminescence of the samples, an ATP standard curve is performed. This needs to be carried out once daily. Because the ATP standard curve is not performed under sterile conditions, a nonsterile, 96-well plate is used. When performing any part of this assay that involves ATP, always wear latex gloves.

b. Perform a serial dilution of ATP standard from the 10 µM stock solution: 1 µM, 0.5 µM, 0.1 µM, 0.05 µM, and 0.01 µM, using the medium provided as diluent. For each ATP concentration, a total of 4×100 µL is required.

c. Dispense 100 µL of the supplied medium alone into the first 4 wells of column 1.
   Note: This is to measure background luminescence.

d. Starting from the lowest ATP dilution, continue dispensing 100 µL into 4 replicate wells.

e. After dispensing all of the ATP concentrations of the standard curve, dispense 100 µL of the low and high controls provided into 4 replicate wells.

f. Using an eight-tip multichannel pipette, add 100 µL of ATP monitoring reagent mix to each column and mix the contents. Always change pipette tips after the contents of the wells are mixed.

g. For the ATP standard curve, no incubation time is needed.

h. Place the plate in the luminometer and, after 2 minutes for reaction development to occur, read the plate.

5. Measure luminescence for cultured samples.

a. Before processing the sample plate, transfer the plate to a humidified incubator set at 22 to 23 C, gassed with 5% CO_2 for 30 minutes to equilibrate, or simply allow the plate to reach room temperature.

b. Usually, only part of a plate is used because there are not enough samples to fill a 96-well plate.

c. Using an 8- or 12-tip multichannel pipette, add 100 µL of the ATP monitoring reagent mix to the first column. Mix the contents and discard the tips.

d. Repeat this procedure for each column, using new tips.

e. When the ATP monitoring reagent mix has been added to all wells, replace the plastic lid and incubate for 10 minutes at room temperature. During this time, cell lysis occurs and the luminescence signal is stabilized.

f. Transfer the plate to the luminometer and initiate luminescence measurement.

Anticipated Results

For the ATP standard curve, a linear regression with goodness of fit (r^2) of between 0.98 and 1 should be obtained. This usually represents percent coefficients of variation (%CV) of less than 5%. Increased CVs are an indication of pipetting error. For HALO-96 MeC, typical CVs usually range from 10% to 25%, but they can also exceed this range in both directions because of the imprecision in dispensing MeC. Even if self-calibrating electronic repeater pipettes are used, the error in dispensing MeC is much higher than if MeC is absent. For this reason, the %CVs obtained using HALO-96 SEC are usually between 5% and 15%.

To determine stem cell UCB potency using HALO-96 PQR, the slopes of the 3-point cell dose response linear regressions for the sample and reference standard have to be compared and the potency ratio calculated. At the time of writing, acceptance limits for colony-forming cells—granulocyte-erythrocyte-macrophage-megakaryocyte and high proliferative potential—stem and progenitor UCB stem cell populations were ATP values of 0.04 µM and 0.05 µM/5000 cells, respectively. Values lower than these indicate that the stem cells will not grow; therefore, the UCB must be rejected for further use.

Notes

1. The HALO technology used in this method was designed and developed for use as a cell potency assay in the quality control arena. The use of these assays as release tests for licensed cellular products should be discussed with the Food and Drug Administration and validated before implementation.

2. All procedures use human cells. Use universal precautions when handling any type of human cells. Steps 1 and 2 require sterile conditions, and all procedures should be performed in a biological safety cabinet.

3. Both calibrated pipettes and accurate dispensing are essential for these assays. For the traditional CFC assay, which requires 1 mL of reagents/35-mm petri dish, normal syringes and needles are used. These are inaccurate for the 96-well plate assays described here. Because small volumes are being dispensed, variations in dispensing caused by noncalibrated or manual-set pipettes can cause large discrepancies in the results. This in turn leads to loss of accuracy, precision, reliability, and reproducibility, all of which are essential to perform a potency assay correctly. Use a positive displacement repeater pipette (preferably electronic) for all dispensing operations involving MeC.

4. The majority of plate luminometers are controlled by computer software. Some plate luminometers are so-called stand-alone instruments and do not require a separate computer. Regardless of whether a computer is required or not, the software can usually be programmed so that sample RLU values can be automatically converted to standardized ATP concentrations from the external ATP standard dose response. In addition, most, if not all, statistical calculations can be performed, printed in tabular and graphical form, and stored.

References/Resources

1. Rich IN, Hall KM. Validation and development of a predictive paradigm for hemotoxicology using a multifunctional bioluminescence colony-forming proliferation assay. Tox Sci 2005;87:427-41.
2. Bradley TR, Hodgson GS, Rosendaal M. The effect of oxygen tension on haemopoietic and fibroblast cell proliferation in vitro. J Cell Physiol 1978;97:517-22.
3. Rich IN, Kubanek B. The effect of reduced oxygen tension on colony formation of erythropoietic cells in vitro. Brit J Haemat 1982;52:579-88.
4. Reems J, Hall KM, Gebru L, et al. Development of a novel assay to evaluate the functional potential of umbilical cord blood progenitors. Transfusion 2008;48:620-8.
5. Measurement of hematopoietic stem cell potency prior to transplantation. HemoGenix White Paper. (February 2009) Colorado Springs, CO: HemoGenix, 2009. [Available at http://www.hemogenix.com/downloads/files/DownloadsPage/WhitePaper2.pdf (accessed May 29, 2009).]

In: Areman EM, Loper K, eds
Cellular Therapy: Principles, Methods, and Regulations
Bethesda, MD: AABB, 2009

♦♦♦   50   ♦♦♦

Assessing the Function of Cellular Therapy Products by Measurement of Cytoplasmic Aldehyde Dehydrogenase

N. Rebecca Haley, MD

INTRACELLULAR ALDEHYDE DEHYDROGE-nase (ALDH) is an enzyme with activity in a number of functional areas of cell metabolism. It oxidizes aldehydes such as acetaldehyde, an intermediate in ethanol metabolism, and biogenic amines produced during catecholamine metabolism.[1-3] Of importance in immature cells undergoing maturation, ALDH converts vitamin A to retinoic acid, thus participating in the cell development/differentiation process.[4,5] High levels of the cytoplasmic enzyme are present in early hematopoietic cells, as was illustrated by Sahovic et al in purging experiments for autologous marrow transplantation in leukemia patients.[6] When the marrow was treated with 4-hydroperoxycyclophosphamide (4-HC), an activated form of cyclophosphamide, mature and leukemic cells did not survive, but the colony-forming hematopoietic cells remained.[6] This finding supported the clinical observation that patients undergoing autologous marrow transplantation for acute myelogenous leukemia with 4-HC

purged marrow had a better chance of recovering normal hematopoietic function without return of the leukemia.[7]

Background

Researchers developed a reagent reporting system to illustrate the presence of ALDH in cells. Storms et al found a boron-dipyrromethene (BODIPY)-labeled reagent that had the necessary characteristics for basic science and clinical investigation, BODIPY aminoacetaldehyde diethyl acetal.[8] It was a stable, dry fluorophore that, although not itself a substrate of ALDH, could be easily solubilized and turned into a single aldehyde liquid reagent. The liquid form was BODIPY aminoacetaldehyde (BAAA), a hydrophobic aldehyde that freely passed in and out of the cell membranes of the cells being analyzed as long as the cells had low levels of ALDH activity. Cells with high ALDH activity used BAAA

N. Rebecca Haley, MD, Associate Professor of Medicine, Division of Cellular Therapy, and Program Director, Cell Therapy Core, Duke Translational Medicine Institute, Durham, North Carolina

The author has disclosed no conflicts of interest.

as a substrate and turned the fluorescent aldehyde into an organic acid, BODIPY aminoacetate (BAA). Now the charged compound was no longer free to pass in and out of the cell wall in equilibrium but was trapped inside the cell, causing it to fluoresce. The cells identified using this reagent by flow cytometry were small, low side-scatter cells that appear on Giemsa stain and light microscopy as typical stem cells. Although the ALDH-bright cells fluoresced brightly after the reaction, if allowed to warm toward room temperature or higher, the cells' multiple drug resistance pump recognized the BAA as a substrate and effluxed the compound promptly with a clearance half-time of less than 20 minutes. Therefore, the reacted cells had to be kept cold until they were measured. An intact and functioning cell membrane was also necessary to retain the fluorescent, charged acetate compound, so dead or dying cells with damaged membranes did not fluoresce.[9]

Characteristics of Hematopoietic Cells with High ALDH

The ability to identify early repopulating hematopoietic cells was an interesting idea for several scientists to explore. Hess and colleagues[10] used human cord blood research units to experiment with the engrafting power of enriched ALDH-bright cells in nonobese diabetic/severe combined immune deficiency (NOD/SCID) mice, which were tolerant of the human cells and allowed them to grow to their innate capacity. For example, short-term repopulating cells were found for only 3 to 5 weeks, whereas the long-term repopulating cells remained in the mice until they were sacrificed. The researchers prepared lineage-negative cell preparations and then stained them with the BAAA reagent to allow high-speed fluorescence sorting to enrich the ALDH-bright cells for the repopulation experiments. They also counterstained the cells with CD34 in one set of experiments and with CD133 in an additional set of studies to determine which subpopulations were responsible for engraftment. The long-term repopulating cells were concentrated in the ALDH-bright, CD34+/CD38– populations. The CD34+, ALDH[lo] (also primarily CD38+) cells were responsible only for short-term engraftment. Researchers also found that the

ALDH-bright cells formed hematopoietic colonies at a rate of 1 in 4.4 cells plated. In additional experiments, they separated the ALDH-bright cells into CD133+ and CD133– cell populations. Although both phenotypes grew long-term culture-initiating cells efficiently, only the ALDH-bright, CD133+ cells engrafted the NOD/SCID mice long term.[11] The investigators concluded that the CD133+ cells must have a homing factor that facilitated their engraftment. In further studies, Hess et al found that after streptozotosin challenge, the NOD/SCID mice showed improvement in their diabetes after infusion of ALDH-bright human cord blood cells. Pathologic analysis of the kidney showed incorporation of the human stem cells into the endothelial lining of the capsule containing the cells of the islets of Langerhans. This repair of the supporting structure of the islets was sufficient to improve the blood sugar of the mice to near normal levels.

Another group, Christ et al, looked at ALDH-bright cells' repopulating ability using Lin– cord blood cells to see if the brightness of fluorescence of the cells identified a more primitive or highly active group of repopulating cells.[12] They found that the higher fluorescence did not indicate a higher concentration of long-term repopulating cells, but that both groups were equal.

Other types of stem cells also express high levels of ALDH. Mitchell et al found that human adipose-derived mesenchymal stem cells showed an enrichment of the ALDH-bright marker along with other accepted stem cell markers in the population with high colony-forming ability and considered this to be a marker of "stemness."[13] The ALDH-bright cell percentage gradually decreased with passages of colonies and differentiation into mature cell types such as fibroblasts, bone, cartilage, and fat cells. In another set of experiments, Cai et al used the BAAA reagent to find brightly fluorescing neuronal stem cells in developing rat embryos.[14] These discoveries led them to believe that ALDH brightness was likely a general marker of stemness not relegated solely to the hematopoietic system.[15]

Human experience reported to date confirms that the percentage of ALDH-bright cells in marrow transplant grafts has correlated with subsequent engraftment. Fallon et al studied the grafts of 21 patients undergoing autologous transplantation for cancer and found that the number of ALDH-bright cells infused with the graft was highly correlated with speed of neutrophil (p <0.015) and platelet (p <0.003) engraftment.[16] Lioznov et al studied the usefulness of ALDH-bright cell measurement under graft stress conditions in marrow and peripheral blood stem cell grafts. They found that in grafts that were delayed in shipment or in cases where transplantation was delayed, the ALDH-bright cell measurement predicted either prompt or delayed engraftment, or failure to achieve donor chimerism. Graft CD34+ cell content accurately predicted engraftment in the cases where transplantation was prompt and there was no stress on the graft, but it did not predict the difficulties encountered with the deteriorating grafts.[17] Clinical trials have been initiated to evaluate the therapeutic use of ALDH-bright enriched cell products in various clinical settings.

References/Resources

1. Russo JE, Hilton J. Characterization of cytosolic aldehyde dehydrogenase from cyclophosphamide resistant L1210 cells. Cancer Res 1998;48:2963.
2. Labrecque J, Bhat PJ, Lacroix A. Purification and partial characterization of a rat kidney aldehyde dehydrogenase that oxidizes retinal to retinoic acid. Biochem Cell Biol 1993;71:85-9.
3. Yoshida A, Hsu LC, Dave V. Retinal oxidation activity and biological role of human cytosolic aldehyde dehydrogenase. Enzyme 1992;46:239.
4. Kastan MB, Stone KD, et al. Direct demonstration of elevated aldehyde dehydrogenase in human hematopoietic progenitor cells. Blood 1990;75:1947-50.
5. Kohn FR, Sladek NE. Aldehyde dehydrogenase activity as the basis for the relative insensitivity of murine pluripotent hematopoietic stem cells to oxazaphosphorines. Biochem Pharmacol 1985;34:3465-71.
6. Sahovic EA, Colvin M, Hilton J, Ogawa M. Role for aldehyde dehydrogenase in survival of progenitors for murine blast cell colonies after treatment with 4-hydro-peroxycyclo-phosphamide in vitro. Cancer Res 1988;48:1223-6.
7. Colvin OM. Pharmacological purging of bone marrow. In: Thomas ED, Blume KG, Forman SJ, eds. Hematopoietic cell transplantation. 2nd ed. Malden, MA: Blackwell Sciences, 1999:217-24.
8. Storms RW, Trujillo AP, Springer JB, et al. Isolation of primitive human hematopoietic progenitors on the basis of aldehyde dehydrogenase activity. Proc Natl Acad Sci U S A 1999;96:9118-23.
9. Jones RJ, et al. Assessment of aldehyde dehydrogenase in viable cells. Blood 1995;85:2742-6.
10. Hess DA, Meryrose TE, Wirthlin L, et al. Functional characterization of highly purified human hematopoietic repopulating cells isolated based on aldehyde dehydrogenase activity. Blood 2004;104:1648-55.
11. Hess DA, Wirthlin L, Craft TP, et al. Selection based on high aldehyde dehydrogenase activity isolates long-term reconstituting human hematopoietic stem cells. Blood 2006;107:2162-9.
12. Christ O, Lucke K, Imren S, et al. Improved purification of hematopoietic stem cells based on their elevated aldehyde dehydrogenase activity. Haematologica 2007;92: 1165-72.
13. Mitchell J, McIntosh K, Zvonic S, et al. Immunophenotype of human adipose-derived cells: Temporal changes in stromal-associated and stem cell-associated markers. Stem Cell 2006;24:376-85.
14. Cai J, Cheng A, Luo Y, et al. Membrane properties of rat embryonic multipotent neural stem cells. J Neurochem 2004;88:212-26.
15. Cai J, Weiss ML, Rao M. In search of "stemness." Exp Hematol 2004;32:585-98.
16. Fallon P, Gentry T, Balber AE, et al. Mobilized peripheral blood SSCloALDHbr cells have the phenotypic and functional properties of primitive haematopoietic cells and their number correlates with engraftment following autologous transplantation. Br J Haematol 2003;122:99-108.
17. Lioznov MV, Freiberger P, Kröger N, et al. Aldehyde dehydrogenase activity as a marker for the quality of hematopoietic stem cell transplants. Bone Marrow Transplant 2005;35:909-14.
18. ALDEFLUOR product information circular. Durham, NC: Aldagen, Inc.

Method 50-1. Analyzing ALDH-Bright Cells by Flow Cytometry

Description

The test kits available for cytoplasmic aldehyde dehydrogenase (ALDH) testing are ALDEFLUOR (Aldagen, Durham, NC), a kit currently available for research use only, and ALDECOUNT (Aldagen), an in-vitro diagnostic.[18] The format of the kits differs to serve their intended purposes. Both use an aldehyde fluorophore that is changed from the hydrophobic, freely diffusing compound BODIPY aminoaldehyde (BAAA) to BODIPY aminoacetate (BAA), a polar compound that is trapped inside living cells with high levels of ALDH and intact membranes. The reagent is stored in the ALDECOUNT kit as a dried-down dialdehyde reagent, BAAA-DA. In the ALDEFLUOR kit, it is a bulk reagent. After activation it must be frozen at −20 C or below if not used promptly. The ALDE-COUNT kit contains 20 reagent tubes with dried-down reagent in each tube sufficient for one cell preparation measurement. Diethylaminobenzoate (DEAB) is used in the control tubes to stop the ALDH enzymatic action. Therefore, the control cell suspensions and the test cell suspensions are prepared at the same time and are the same except for the added DEAB in the controls. General directions are given below. Specific directions are contained in each kit.

Time for Procedure

Approximately 1 hour.

Summary of Procedure

1. Prepare the reagents.
2. Prepare the samples.
3. Perform the assay by incubating the cells with BAAA reagent.
4. Perform flow cytometric analysis.

Equipment

1. Centrifuge.
2. Automated cell counter.
3. Pipettors.
4. Flow cytometer.
5. Heat block or incubator at 37 C.

Supplies and Reagents

1. Test kit containing BODIPY-labeled reagent (BAAA-DA), DEAB, dimethyl sulfoxide (DMSO), HCl, and assay buffer.
2. Tubes for sample preparation and flow analysis (if not supplied with test kit).
3. Ammonium chloride lysis solution *without* fixative or detergent.

Procedure

1. Prepare the reagents.
   a. Allow all kit components to come to room temperature.
   b. Resuspend the dried BAAA-DA reagent by adding the supplied DMSO and wait 1 minute.
   c. Add HCl and mix well.
   d. Incubate for 15 to not more than 30 minutes at room temperature to convert BAAA-DA to the ALDH substrate BAAA.
   e. Add assay buffer per the manufacturer's instructions. If not used immediately, the ALDH substrate may be stored frozen in small aliquots for several months.
2. Prepare the samples.
   a. Fresh or frozen samples should be prepared according to standard procedures for that cell type.
   b. If the cell suspension contains red cells and the red-cell-to-white-cell ratio is >2:1, lyse the cells with an ammonium chloride buffer solution that *does not contain fixative or detergent.*
   c. Wash the cells after lysis by centrifuging 5 minutes at 250 × *g* and resuspend the cells in 1 mL of assay buffer.
   d. Perform a cell count and adjust the concentration to 1×10^6 cells/mL.

3. Perform the assay.
   a. Label a tube for "test" and "control" for each sample to be tested.
   b. Add DEAB to the "control" tube.
   c. Add ALDH substrate, then measured cell suspension, to the "test" tube.
   d. Immediately mix the "test" tube and transfer an aliquot to the "control" tube containing DEAB.
   e. Incubate at 37 C for 30 minutes. At the completion of incubation, place the cells on ice.
   f. If immunophenotyping is to be done, add antibodies at this point and incubate for 15 to 30 minutes at 2 to 8 C.
4. Perform flow cytometric analysis.
   a. Set up the selected flow cytometer per the manufacturer's instructions.
   b. In setup mode, place the DEAB "control" sample on the cytometer. Adjust the forward scatter (FSC) and side scatter (SSC) voltages to center the nucleated cell population within the FSC vs SSC plot. (See data plot in Fig 50-1-1.)
   c. On the FL1 vs SSC plot, adjust the photomultiplier tube voltage so that the right edge of the stained cells is placed at the second log decade on the dot plot. Note that all cells are fluorescent because of the intracellular pool of fluorescent substrate. (See data plot in Fig 50-1-2.)

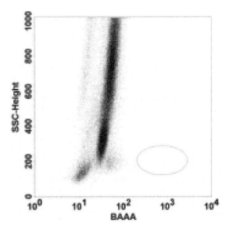

Figure 50-1-2. Data plot illustrating the right edge of the stained cells placed at the second log decade on the dot plot.

   d. Place the corresponding ALDH "test" sample on the cytometer. Create a region R2 to encompass the cell population that is side-scatter low (SSC^lo). (See data plot in Fig 50-1-3.)

Anticipated Results

Cells with high ALDH activity and intact membranes will be visible within R2 on analysis of the "test" samples (ie, ALDH^br SSC^lo cells). Manufacturer's instructions give specific directions for calculation of the percentage of ALDH^br SSC^lo cells in the sample.

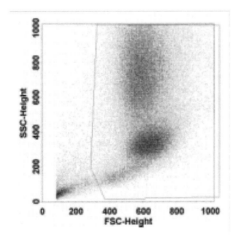

Figure 50-1-1. Data plot illustrating nucleated cell population centered within the FSC vs SSC plot.

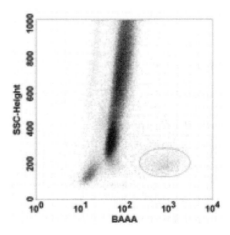

Figure 50-1-3. Data plot showing region (R2) encompassing the cell population that is side-scatter low (SSC^lo).

Notes

1. Cells to be analyzed should be kept at 4 C or, after thawing, should be washed to remove cryoprotectants and analyzed promptly. If samples are aging or poorly stored, the analysis will not give the desired information.

2. Using a red cell lysing agent with fixative or detergent will kill all the white cells, and no cells will appear to be ALDH^{br}SSc^{lo} because the reaction works with live cells only.

3. Gate-drawing around the cells of interest will be made impossible by failure to set up the photomultiplier tube settings to place the bulk of the cell population in the middle of the screen, with the right edge of the cell population at the second decade of fluorescence and to allow full view of the SSC^{lo} cells at the bottom of the plot.

In: Areman EM, Loper K, eds
Cellular Therapy: Principles, Methods, and Regulations
Bethesda, MD: AABB, 2009

◆◆◆ **51** ◆◆◆

Performance of Cytotoxicity Assays for Cellular Therapy Products

Ellen Areman, MS, SBB(ASCP)

APPLICATIONS OF CELL-BASED THERAPIES are continually expanding. Not long ago, the primary indication for their use was for marrow replacement in hematologic malignancies and for marrow rescue in patients receiving myeloablative cancer therapy. Cellular therapy (CT) products are now being developed to repair and regenerate a wide variety of tissues, as well as to target tumors and infected cells for destruction. The latter indications depend on the ability of the therapeutic product to lethally damage cancer cells and cells harboring infectious agents without harming normal cells and tissues. One way of evaluating these cytotoxic therapies is to perform in-vitro assays with cell types expected to be sensitive or resistant to the therapy. Although the results may not directly correlate with in-vivo effects, in-vitro methods of measuring the ability of cellular products to lethally damage target cells are important for the development of safe and effective cytotoxic celluar therapies.

Cytotoxicity assays have long been used in drug development to demonstrate whether certain compounds are toxic to living cells. For CT, the answer sought is whether the cellular product is toxic to the target cells or tissue and, if so, at what dose? It would be ideal if an exact correlation could be found between the in-vitro cytotoxicity assay and an in-vivo therapeutic effect, but this does not usually occur. However, a product demonstrating a high level of target-cell killing in vitro coupled with a lack of adverse effects in vivo would at least provide a rationale for further investigation of the product. If in-vivo surrogate measurements such as reduction in tumor size or number, normalization of relevant chemical or hematologic values, or improvement in certain physiological functions can be linked to in-vitro cytotoxicity, such an assay would be valuable for developing dose levels as well as for measuring potency for product release.

The basic concept of a cytotoxicity assay is quite simple:

- Target cells are placed in culture.
- The therapeutic (effector) cell product is added and incubated for approximately 2 to 48 hours.
- Dye or substrate is added and the mixture incubated for an appropriate period (this may also occur before the previous incubation).

Ellen Areman, MS, SBB(ASCP), Senior Consultant, Biologics Consulting Group, Inc, Alexandria, Virginia

The author has disclosed no conflicts of interest.

- The readout assay is performed.
- Data are analyzed.

Biologic parameters of the target cells, such as metabolic function, membrane integrity, DNA integrity or synthesis, or direct measurement of cell number, can be used to assess in-vitro cytotoxic effects of the CT effector cells. These biologic parameters can in turn be measured by a variety of readouts, including release of radioactive, fluorescent, or colorimetric material from target cells; release of materials detectable by antibodies or enzymatic assays from target cells; intracellular adenosine triphosphate levels measured by bioluminescence; cleavage of tetrazolium salts to form compounds that are measured colorimetrically; and detection of fragmented, labeled DNA released from the nucleus or cytoplasm by enzyme-linked immunosorbent assay. Care should be taken in selecting the appropriate assay based on the biologic properties of the target and effector cells. For example, increased metabolic activity of activated effector cells can mask decreased metabolic activity of the target cells.

Although every cytotoxicity assay used in CT development cannot be included in this chapter, the examples given in the methods that follow provide an idea of some of the options available for assessing cellular cytotoxicity.

Acknowledgments

Method 51-1 was submitted by Theresa L. Whiteside, PhD, Professor of Pathology, Immunology, and Otolaryngology, and Director, Immunologic Monitoring and Cellular Products Laboratory, University of Pittsburgh Cancer Institute, Hillman Cancer Center, Pittsburgh, Pennsylvania. Method 51-2 was submitted by Jeffrey S. Miller, MD, Professor, Department of Medicine, and Associate Director, Experimental Therapeutics Research Progams, and Sue Fautsch, MT(ASCP), CETI Administrative Coordinator, University of Minnesota Masonic Cancer Research Center, Minneapolis, Minnesota.

Method 51-1. Assessing Cytotoxic T- or Natural Killer Cell Function: ^{51}Chromium Release Assay

Description

The ^{51}chromium (^{51}Cr)-release assay is the classic method used to evaluate cytotoxic cell function. Effector [mononuclear, T-, or natural killer (NK)] cells are incubated with ^{51}Cr-labeled target cells at several effector-to-target cell (E:T) ratios. The amount of radioactivity released by lysed target cells is measured, and the percent specific lysis is calculated. This method describes NK-cell-mediated cytotoxicity but can be modified to evaluate other effector cells. For example, T-cell-mediated cytotoxicity can be measured using target cells expressing appropriate antigen-major-histocompatibility-complex (MHC) proteins. In addition, killing of additional targets such as patient leukemic cells may be evaluated.

Resting NK cells kill K562 cells without activation. Interleukin-2 (IL-2) or IL-15 enhances K562 killing and induces NK cells to kill targets that are not killed by resting NK cells (eg, Raji, Daudi, SKBR-3). The concentration of IL-2 and IL-15 and the duration of activation are important variables that determine how much target cell lysis will occur.

Time for Procedure

From 6 to 8 hours.

Summary of Procedure

1. Prepare the target cells.
2. Prepare the effector cells.
3. Combine the effector and target cells and incubate.
4. Collect the supernatants.
5. Count the amount of ^{51}Cr in the supernatants.
6. Calculate the percent specific lysis.

Equipment

1. Gamma scintillation counter.
2. CO_2 incubator: 37 C, 5% CO_2.
3. Centrifuge.
4. Hemacytometer.
5. Micropipettor and pipette tips.

Supplies and Reagents

1. Iscove's modified Dulbecco's medium (Invitrogen, Carlsbad, CA) + 10% fetal calf serum (IMDM-10%).
2. Target cells: K562 (or other targets) cells in IMDM-10%.
3. Effector cells: mononuclear or NK cells in IMDM-10%.
4. $Na_2{}^{51}CrO_4$ (^{51}Cr).
5. Triton X-100 (Dow Chemical, Midland, MI), 3% solution in phosphate-buffered saline.
6. 96-well microtiter plate.
7. Tubes: 50-mL conical screw cap and 5-mL snap cap.
8. Serologic pipettes.
9. Supernatant collection system.
10. Scintillation counting tubes.

Procedure

1. Prepare target cells:
   a. Transfer 10×10^6 cells from the active culture flask to a 50-mL conical tube.
   b. Centrifuge the tube and and remove the supernatant.
   c. Add 200 µCi ^{51}Cr to the cell pellet and mix.
   d. Incubate for 1 hour in a 5% CO_2 incubator at 37 C.
   e. Wash the cell suspension three times using IMDM-10%.
   f. Determine the number of viable cells, and adjust the cell concentration to 5×10^4/mL.
2. Prepare the effector cells:
   a. 1×10^6 effector cells are needed for the assay. Adjust effector cell suspension to 1×10^6/mL in IMDM-10% in a snap-cap tube. Fresh or cultured cells should be used

for this assay. When overnight storage is required, cells should be placed in serum-containing medium in the incubator. Cells taken out of the refrigerator or immediately thawed (after cryopreservation) have diminished NK cell cytotoxic function, some of which can be restored by placing cells in an incubator with IL-2 or IL-15 for 4 to 6 hours.

    b. Test the effector cells in at least three E:T ratios. The highest E:T ratio is typically 20:1 (with unseparated mononuclear cells), with each tested in triplicate.

    c. Perform serial threefold dilutions, thus testing E:T ratios as follows: 20:1, 6.6:1, 2.2:1, etc. E:T ratios can be modified for purified or activated cells to delete the highest E:T ratio if effector cells are limiting.

3. Combine the effector and target cells and incubate:

    a. Transfer 100 µL of each effector cell suspension to 3 wells of a 96-well round-bottom microtiter plate [test counts per minute (cpm)].

    b. Add 100 µL target cells to all wells containing effector cells plus 12 wells for total and spontaneous ^{51}Cr-release controls. Mix well.

    c. Add 100 µL IMDM-10% to 6 control wells (spontaneous-release cpm). Mix well.

    d. Add 100 µL Triton X-100, 3%, to 6 control wells (total-release cpm). Mix well.

    e. Cover the plate. Centrifuge for 5 minutes at $200 \times g$ at room temperature with no brake.

    f. Transfer the plate to the 5% CO_2 incubator (37 C) for 4 hours.

4. Collect the supernatants: using a micropipettor and tips or supernatant collection system, remove 100 µL supernatant from each well without disturbing the cell pellet, and transfer to scintillation counting tubes.

5. Count the amount of ^{51}Cr in the supernatants: using a gamma scintillation counter, measure the radioactivity in cpm from all supernatants.

6. Calculate the percent specific lysis:

    a. Calculate the mean cpm for all E:T ratios and the total and spontaneous wells.

    b. Calculate the percent specific lysis for each E:T ratio using the following formula:

$$\% \text{ specific lysis} = 100 \times \frac{(\text{mean test cpm} - \text{mean spontaneous cpm})}{(\text{mean total cpm} - \text{mean spontaneous cpm})}$$

Anticipated Results

The amount of ^{51}Cr release is proportional to the number of target cells killed. The percent specific lysis should generally be above 20%, with higher specific lysis for higher E:T ratios. The spontaneous divided by total cpm should be <15%.

Notes

1. Four-hour incubation times are standard. However, for lot release testing and other applications where time is limited and quantitative killing comparisons are not needed, shorter incubations (1, 2, 3 hours) can be used for easily killed targets such as K562. For example, after 2 hours, NK cells exhibit about half the specific lysis that occurs after 4 hours. Should this be used, standards in each laboratory must be established with shorter incubations times.

2. The most common cause for high spontaneous/total ratios is poor viability or unhealthy target cells. Some targets (adherent cells, for example) may have slightly higher spontaneous/total ratios and still yield interpretable results.

Safety

1. Refer to institutional guidelines for working with biological materials, bloodborne pathogens, and sources of ionizing radiation.

2. Work in an area designated for radioisotope use.

3. Use appropriate shielding and survey the work area frequently.

4. Wear protective clothing (lab coat and gloves) and dosimeters.

References/Resources

1. Whiteside TL. Measurement of NK-cell activity in humans. In: Detrick B, Hamilton RG, Folds JD, eds. Manual of molecular and clinical laboratory immunology. Washington, DC: ASM Press, 2006:296-300.

2. Cervantes F, McGlave PB, Verfaillie CM, Miller JS. Autologous activated natural killer cells suppress primitive chronic myeloid leukemia progenitors in long term culture. Blood 1996;87:2476-85.

Method 51-2. Assessing Cytotoxic T- or Natural Killer Cell Function: CD107A Degranulation Assay

Description

Lysosomal-associated membrane protein-1 (LAMP-1 or CD107a) is a marker of CD8+ cytolytic T- and natural killer (NK) cell degranulation and is strongly upregulated on the cell surface following stimulation with target cells. This method describes NK cell-mediated cytotoxicity, but it can be modified to evaluate other effector cells. For example, T-cell-mediated cytotoxicity can be measured using target cells expressing appropriate antigen-major-histocompatibility-complex (MHC) proteins. In addition, killing of additional targets such as patient leukemic cells may be evaluated.

CD107a can be used as a marker of NK cell activation and function, and it usually correlates well with other killing assays. One major advantage to this procedure is that it allows precise identification by flow cytometry of subsets of cells responsible for function.

Time for Procedure

From 8 to 10 hours.

Summary of Procedure

1. Effector cells are stimulated with target cells.
2. Cells are stained with CD107a and surface NK cell markers.
3. Flow-cytometric acquisition and analysis are performed.

Equipment

1. Flow cytometer.
2. CO_2 incubator: 37 C, 5% CO_2.
3. Centrifuge.
4. Refrigerator: 4 C.
5. Cell counter.
6. Micropipettor and pipette tips.

Supplies and Reagents

1. RPMI 1640 medium (Gibco, Grand Island, NY) + 10% fetal calf serum (RPMI-10%).
2. Target cells: K562 cells in RPMI-10% or 721 null cells in RPMI-10% as positive control cells, additional target cells of interest.
3. Effector cells: mononuclear cells (MNCs) or NK cells in RPMI-10%.
4. CD107a-fluorescein isothiocyanate (FITC) antibody.
5. CD3-peridinium chlorophyll protein (PerCP) antibody.
6. CD56-antigen-presenting cell (APC) antibody.
7. The phycoerythrin (PE) channel can be used for subsetting the populations using additional desired markers (eg, antibodies that recognize NK cell receptors)
8. Monensin
9. Tubes: 5-mL snap cap.
10. Serologic pipettes.

Procedure

1. Effector cells are stimulated with target cells at a 1:1 ratio.
   a. Adjust all cell suspensions to 2×10^6/mL with RPMI-10% in snap-cap tubes.
   b. Transfer 100 µL effector cells into each of three snap-cap tubes.
   c. Add 100 µL of the test target cells to one tube (test).
   d. Add 100 µL of K562 or 721.221 MHC Class-I-negative cells to one tube (positive control).
   e. Add 100 µL RPMI-10% to one tube (no effector cells, negative control).
2. Cells are stained with CD107a and surface NK cell markers.
   a. Add CD107a-FITC at a final concentration of 20 µL/mL to all tubes.

b. Incubate tubes for 1 hour in CO_2 incubator to initiate degranulation and CD107a surface expression.

c. Add monensin at a final concentration of 6 µg/mL to all tubes. Monensin blocks protein transport and internalization of CD107a and bound antibody.

d. Incubate tubes for 5 hours in the CO_2 incubator.

e. Stain all cells with CD3-PerCp and CD56-APC for 30 minutes at 4 C; wash and fix.

3. Flow-cytometric acquisition and analysis are performed.

a. For acquisition, gate on the MNCs. Acquire 50,000 MNC events.

b. For analysis, gate on the CD3–/CD56+ (NK) cells. Determine the percentage of NK cells that are CD107a+.

Anticipated Results

Positive control target cells (eg, K562 cells) typically result in 10% to 40% CD107a+ NK cells. Other targets will likely result in lower levels of CD107a expression.

Note

Although CD107a is upregulated after exposure to sensitive targets, nonspecific stimuli such as IL-2 and IL-15 will increase CD107a expression without targets. Specific CD107a expression is often reported as the CD107a expression in the test condition after subtracting the background CD107a expression in the effector cell tube without targets.

Reference/Resource

1. Alter G, Malenfant JM, Altfield M. CD107a as a functional marker for the identification of natural killer cell activity. J Immunol Meth 2004;94:15-22.

In: Areman EM, Loper K, eds
Cellular Therapy: Principles, Methods, and Regulations
Bethesda, MD: AABB, 2009

◆◆◆ **52** ◆◆◆

Assessing Cellular Therapy Products for Microbial Contamination

Hanh Khuu, MD

TESTING REQUIREMENTS FOR CELLULAR therapy (CT) products can be confusing and complex, as is the heterogeneous nature of the products themselves. AABB standards require that CT products be tested for microbial contamination in cultures that detect bacteria and fungi.[1] Although the Food and Drug Administration's (FDA's) good tissue practice regulations in the Code of Federal Regulations (Title 21 CFR, Part 1271[2]) do not explicitly require sterility testing, Section 1271.265(c) states "you must not make available for distribution an HCT/P that is...contaminated."[3] The implication is that testing for microorganisms should be done to ensure the product is not contaminated. The only explicit FDA requirement for testing of those CT products not considered biological drugs and regulated solely under Section 361 of the Public Health Service (PHS) Act (42 USC 264) ("361 products") is that testing must be performed by validated methods.

In contrast, for biological CT products regulated by Section 351(a) of the PHS Act [42 USC 262(a)] ("351 products"), sterility testing is required and must be performed by the method described in 21 CFR 610.12 (hereafter referred to as the CFR method) or methods demonstrated to be equivalent.[4] A similar method, described in the USP, is also directly applicable to the manufacture of drugs and biologics.[5] In summary, both the codified CFR method and the alternate USP methods rely on manual detection of turbidity in broth cultures and specify the type of medium, incubation conditions, and time frames for visual inspection of cultures throughout the 14-day incubation period. The CFR describes preparation of the broth, growth promotion tests with the broth, and organisms for which growth must be demonstrated. The USP compendium describes two test methods accepted by the FDA: direct inoculation and membrane filtration, as well as performance of bacteriostasis and fungistasis tests if samples were prepared with antibiotics. Method 52-1 provides a brief example of the procedure described in 21 CFR 610.12. For a complete description of the method, please see the reference at the end of Method 52-1. Although considered the standard by the FDA, this method is

---

Hanh Khuu, MD, Assistant Medical Director, Cell Processing Section, Department of Transfusion Medicine, National Institutes of Health, Bethesda, Maryland

The author has disclosed no conflicts of interest.

labor intensive and subjective, and little published data are available on its applicability to CT products.

In the approximately 30 years since the CFR method was codified, commercially available media and automated bacterial growth detection systems have been developed. Many of these systems are FDA 510(k)-cleared for performing human blood cultures and have also been used for testing other body fluids. At least one method, the BacT/ALERT Microbial Detection System (BTA; bioMerieux, Marcy L'Etoile, France), has received 510(k) clearance from the FDA for quality control testing of platelet products. These automated methods incorporate a computer-controlled incubation/detection system and a wide variety of media formulations, including some with proprietary substances for binding antibiotics, if present. The sensor-and-detection system is a noninvasive method that detects microbial growth via CO_2 production. As the microbes in the medium multiply, CO_2 is released and chemically alters the sensor in each culture medium bottle so that it may be detected through a color change or fluorescence production. The detection systems are more sensitive than visual inspection for turbidity, leading to more-rapid detection of positive results. Every bottle is monitored repeatedly by the detection unit, and the rate of color change is also measured. The computer systems use a proprietary algorithm to analyze the data and determine positivity. At the established positivity threshold, the instrument flags the bottle as positive. The bottle is then removed for further workup, which typically consists of performing a Gram's stain for preliminary morphologic description of the organism, followed by plating onto solid medium for identification and sensitivity testing, as needed.

In a survey performed by the International Society for Cellular Therapy[6] of 89 mostly North American, hospital-based cell-processing facilities, 76% used the automated methods available in the hospital's microbiology laboratory to perform sterility testing of their CT products. Modern automated culture methods were used by 83% of facilities for products that were minimally manipulated, by 84% for products manufactured within 12 hours of collection, and by 56% for products that were cultured or expanded. The most commonly used automated

methods were the BTA and the Bactec (Becton Dickinson, Franklin Lakes, NJ) systems; combined, they accounted for 90% of the automated culture systems used.

However, because sterility testing of CT products was not an approved application for these systems, each CT facility had to independently choose a method and validate it. In addition, if intended for use with "351 products," the user would have to show the method to be equivalent to the CFR method because of the lack of available data demonstrating equivalency between the methods when testing CT products. In 2004, the proof-of-principle concept that these automated culture methods can be used for sterility testing of CT products was demonstrated by Khuu et al.[7] Since that publication, several other groups have shown that automated culture methods perform as well or better than the compendial methods with shorter time to detection.[8,9]

The Gram's stain may be used clinically to detect infections; however, although the limit of detection is quite high at 10^5 colony-forming units per mL, this level is considerably lower than the concentration of microorganisms in the blood during bacteremia.[10] Gram's staining is useful for samples that contain a high level of microbial contaminants, such as wound exudates, or that may be concentrated before staining, such as synovial fluid and other body fluids. For CT products, the Gram's stain is most often used as a surrogate for a microbial growth-based assay to permit the immediate release of products for which culture results are not available at the time of infusion. However, because of the sensitivity of this assay, it is of limited value for detecting low-level microbial contamination of most CT products. Depending on the starting material, the initial bioburden may range from no organisms to a high level of contamination. For example, because of the collection process, most apheresis product starting materials are at very low risk for contamination. In contrast, pancreas tissue, with segments of bowel or spleen attached, may present with a significantly higher bioburden. For products that are infused or cryopreserved immediately after processing, even if contaminated during processing, insufficient time passes for the organisms to multiply adequately to reach a level detectable by Gram's stain.

Special Challenges Pertaining to Sterility Testing of CT Products

Heterogeneous Product Types

CT products represent a wide range of tissues and cells prepared using a variety of media and reagents, including antibiotics and other substances that potentially affect the growth and detection of organisms that may be present. The final product preparation may be a complex mixture of cells, dimethyl sulfoxide, DNAse, human serum albumin, acid (or anticoagulant)-citrate-dextrose, and heparin.

Sample Size

Each CT product often represents a batch of one, with the entire product required for administration in a single dose. Because sterility testing is only one of the assays required for product release, the sample volume required for testing may represent a substantial fraction of the entire product in terms of volume and cell content. The amount of material available for microbial testing might be substantially less than 1 mL. Removal of a volume of sample adequate to perform the necessary release testing could result in compromising the volume of product available to the patient. Although merely producing more product to "build in" the additional volume required would be ideal, this may be impossible based on a finite amount of available starting material.

Timing of Sampling

Ideally, sampling will occur from the final container after all reagents, including cryoprotectant solution, have been added. Testing of other "in-process" samples should be based on product type, processing performed, historical data, and deviation management practices. For example, a testing protocol may stipulate that sampling after thawing is performed only if a precryopreservation sample is positive or if a container breach is noted at thaw. A processing facility may decide to sample only starting material for marrow products if a collection container breach has been reported or if donor bacteremia is suspected by collection personnel.

Some CT products may need to be released for patient use before the completion of sterility testing because the products cannot be held for the amount of time required. This would occur with products that are to be infused immediately after processing or culture. For cultured products, sampling for sterility testing between 48 and 24 hours before product use is a widely accepted approach.

Inoculation of Cultures

Some CT facilities send product samples to the microbiology/testing laboratory for inoculation into culture medium bottles. Others choose to inoculate the culture medium bottles in the CT facility and transport inoculated bottles to the testing laboratory for incubation and workup of positive cultures. The advantage of the latter method is that once the culture bottles are inoculated, they are not entered unless flagged as positive. Inoculation in the CT facility is typically in a more controlled environment with less risk of contamination of culture medium during inoculation.

Length of Culture Period

Although the CFR method requires 14 days of incubation, some disagreement exists about how long samples tested in automated blood culture systems should be incubated. When these devices are used for testing patient blood cultures, clinical microbiology laboratories often incubate culture bottles for as few as 5 days. Results of studies performed at the National Institutes of Health using several different CT product formulations[7,8] indicated that most organisms were detected within 3 days.

For 361 products, many of these issues can often be factored into validation plans. For 351 products, microbial testing issues should be considered in the product development plan and clearly addressed in the investigational new drug application and biologic license application. Validation of any microbial testing method should demonstrate the system's ability to detect a wide range of organisms, including aerobes, anaerobes, yeasts, and fungi.

Interpretation of Results

A true-positive culture is one from which organism(s) have been isolated. A true-positive culture may be the result of actual product contamination or contamination of the test sample during handling. However, ruling out true product contamination and attributing the positive test result to improper sample handling is nearly impossible. Therefore, positive cultures that are suspected of resulting from handling errors would be interpreted as "indeterminate" culture results. A false positive is defined as a culture result where the instrument has flagged the bottle as positive but no organism was isolated. (See Table 52-1.)

The interpretation of a culture result often influences the treatment of the product recipient. Consultation with the treating physician is critical whether the positive test result is received before or after the product has been administered. The identity of the organism is only one factor in the interpretation of the culture result. Other factors to be considered include from which bottle the organism was isolated (if both aerobic and anaerobic), time to detection, product starting material, extent of ex-vivo manipulation, and results from other samples from the same parent product. Investigation of all positive culture results includes review of batch process records and all factors mentioned above. The most commonly cultured organisms are skin contaminants, such as coagulase-negative *Staphylococcus* spp.

Use of a culture-positive product, whether as a result of true product contamination or handling contamination, must be carefully considered in light of regulatory implications. As previously stated, use of a contaminated product is prohibited in 21 CFR 1271. Although a number of publications have described the lack of serious adverse reactions after administration of contaminated products,[11-13] the benefits and risks to the patient must be thoroughly evaluated and documented before deciding whether to perform the infusion. Because most CT products are unique and irreplaceable, alternative products may not be available. For example, if the patient has already undergone myeloablative preparative conditioning, rejecting a culture-positive product from apheresis or marrow might subject the recipient to a greater risk than infusing it.

Future Directions

Molecular methods or DNA-based technologies, such as polymerase chain reaction and microarrays, are being developed for the detection of microorganisms in the patient-care setting. Most of these methods are specific for detecting particular organisms or differentiating among species of related organisms. A few methods are being developed for pan-detection of all members of large classes of microorganisms, comparable to culture-based methods. Although these methods may eventually be able to identify microbial contaminants within hours instead of days, this potential has not yet been met.

Table 52-1. Interpretation of Microbial Testing Results

Result	Culture Report	Interpretation	Possible Cause
True-positive culture	Organism(s) isolated; repeat sample also tests positive	Confirmed product contamination	1. Product container breached 2. Contaminated during processing 3. Problematic collection
True-positive culture	Organism(s) isolated; repeat sample tests negative	Indeterminate culture	1, 2, 3, or 4. Sample contaminated at time of culture inoculation
True-positive culture	Organism(s) isolated; no repeat sample available	Product contamination	1, 2, 3, or 4
False-positive culture	No organism isolated	No contamination	High white celll count causes detectable CO_2 production

The FDA has recently published a draft guidance for industry addressing considerations for validation of growth-based rapid microbiologic methods for sterility testing of CT products that are subject to licensure.[14] This guidance includes discussion of the automated culture methods previously described but excludes molecular methods that do not rely on the ability to detect viable microorganisms multiplying in liquid media. The document provides valuable information on validation parameters such as limit of detection, specificity, ruggedness and robustness, appropriate microbial challenge organisms, necessary controls, and method comparison studies. Pending implementation of the final guidance document, validation data will be expected before using growth-based rapid microbial methods in place of compendial methods.

References/Resources

1. Padley D, ed. Standards for cellular therapy product services. 3rd ed. Bethesda, MD: AABB, 2008.
2. Code of federal regulations. Human cells, tissues, and cellular and tissue-based products. Title 21, CFR Part 1271: Subpart A (general provisions). Washington, DC: US Government Printing Office, 2009 (revised annually).
3. Code of federal regulations. Human cells, tissues, and cellular and tissue-based products. Title 21, CFR Part 1271: Subpart D (current good tissue practice). Washington, DC: US Government Printing Office, 2009 (revised annually).
4. Code of federal regulations. General biological products standards. Title 21, CFR Part 610.12 (sterility). Washington, DC: US Government Printing Office, 2009 (revised annually).
5. Microbiology and Sterility Assurance Expert Committee. General chapter <71>. Sterility tests. In: USP 32-NF27. Rockville, MD: United States Pharmacopeial Convention, 2008.
6. Davis-Sproul J. ISCT sterility testing survey. ISCT Telegraft Newsletter 2002;9:1-3.
7. Khuu HM, Stock F, McGann M, et al. Comparison of automated culture systems with a CFR/USP-compliant method for sterility testing of cell-therapy products. Cytotherapy 2004;6:183-95.
8. Khuu HM, Patel N, Carter CS, et al. Sterility testing of cellular therapy products: Parallel comparison of automated methods with a CFR-compliant method. Transfusion 2006;46:2071-82.
9. Keilpinski G, Prinzi S, Duguid J, et al. Roadmap to approval: Use of an automated sterility test method as a lot release test for Carticel, autologous cultured chondrocytes. Cytotherapy 2005;7:531-41.
10. Tilton RC. The laboratory approach to the detection of bacteremia. Annu Rev Microbiol 1982;36:467-93.
11. Padley DJ, Dietz AB, Gastineau DA. Sterility testing of hematopoietic progenitor cell products: A single-institution series of culture-positive rates and successful infusion of culture-positive products. Transfusion 2007;47:636-43.
12. Klein MA, Kadidlo D, McCullough J, et al. Microbial contamination of hematopoietic stem cell products: Incidence and clinical sequelae. Biol Blood Marrow Transplant 2006;12:1142-9.
13. Patah PA, Parmar S, McMannis J, et al. Microbial contamination of hematopoietic progenitor cell products: Clinical outcome. Bone Marrow Transplant 2007;40:365-8.
14. Food and Drug Administration. Draft guidance for industry: Validation of growth-based rapid microbiological methods for sterility testing of cellular and gene therapy products. (February 2008) Rockville, MD: Center for Biologics Evaluation and Research, 2008.

Method 52-1. Cellular Therapy Product Sterility Testing (As Described in 21 CFR 610.12)

Description

Sterility testing of licensed cellular therapy products is required and should be performed as described in the Code of Federal Regulations (CFR), Title 21, Part 610.12. The method uses tryptic soy broth (TSB) incubated at 20 to 25 C and fluid thioglycollate broth incubated at 30 to 35 C, assessed at three time points during 14 days. No growth at the end of 14 days is the desired outcome.

Time for Procedure

1. Day of inoculation: 1 hour.
2. Duration of culture incubation: 14 days.

Summary of Procedure

1. Inoculate a sample of the CT product into the culture medium.
2. Incubate, assess for turbidity or microbial growth, and subculture as needed.

Equipment

1. Incubator: 20 to 25 C.
2. Incubator: 30 to 35 C.
3. Sterile syringes and needles.

Supplies and Reagents

1. Soybean-casein digest medium (also known as TSB).
2. Fluid thioglycollate medium.

Procedure

1. Inoculate a sample of the CT product into the culture medium:

    a. If culture bottles have a plastic or metallic cover over the septum, remove the septum cover.

    b. Disinfect the septum.

    c. Using the sterile needle and syringe, draw up the sample and inoculate half into the TSB bottle and half into the thioglycollate bottle.

2. Incubate, assess for turbidity or microbial growth, and subculture as needed.

    a. Incubate the TSB bottle at 20 to 25 C. Incubate the thioglycollate bottle at 30 to 35 C. Incubation duration is 14 days.

    b. Assess each bottle for turbidity or microbial growth on day 3 or 4; day 5, 7, or 8; and at the end of the incubation period, day 14.

    c. If turbidity or growth is observed, perform a Gram's stain and subculture onto solid media for identification of the organism.

    d. If no growth is observed after 14 days of incubation, the product passes the test and is reported as "no growth."

Anticipated Results

No growth (after 14 days of incubation).

Note

Each lot of medium must be tested for growth promotion using specified microbial species as defined in the CFR.

Reference/Resource

1. Code of federal regulations. General biological products standards. Title 21, CFR Part 610.12 (sterility). Washington, DC: US Government Printing Office, 2009 (revised annually).

Method 52-2. Cellular Therapy Product Sterility Testing Using an Automated Microbial Detection System (Alternate Method)

Description

Sterility testing of licensed cellular therapy (CT) products is required and should be performed as described in the Code of Federal Regulations (21 CFR 610.12). Federal regulations permit use of alternative methods if validated with the test material and shown to be equivalent to the standard method (21 CFR 610.9). Multiple automated systems are in use; this method describes one of them. The BacT/ALERT Microbial Detection System (bioMerieux, Marcy L'Etoile, France) uses a colorimetric sensor and reflected light to monitor the presence and production of carbon dioxide (CO_2). If microorganisms are present, CO_2 will be produced as the organisms metabolize substrates in the culture medium. When CO_2 is produced, the color of the sensor in the bottom of the bottle changes to yellow, activating the alert.

Time for Procedure

1. Day of inoculation: 15 minutes.
2. Duration of culture incubation: 7 to 14 days.

Summary of Procedure

1. Inoculate a sample of the CT product into the culture medium.
2. Incubate, monitoring continuously for microbial growth, and subculture as needed.

Equipment

1. BacT/ALERT Microbial Detection System.
2. Sterile syringes and needles.
3. Disposable gloves.
4. Appropriate biohazardous waste containers.

Supplies and Reagents

1. BacT/ALERT aerobic culture medium.
2. BacT/ALERT anaerobic culture medium.

Procedure

1. Inoculate a sample of the CT product into the culture media:
   a. Collect samples aseptically and maintain under sterile conditions before testing.
   b. Visually inspect culture bottles before testing.
   c. Discard any bottles showing evidence of leakage, exhibiting turbidity, or with yellow sensors.
   d. Label bottle appropriately and disinfect septum.
      Note: Bottles must be at room temperature.
   e. Inoculate the liquid sample directly into the culture bottle using a needle and syringe. Alternatively, the septum may be aseptically removed and a pipette used to transfer the sample.
2. Incubate, monitoring continuously for microbial growth, and subculture as needed.
   a. Load inoculated culture bodies promptly into the BacT/ALERT instrument.
   b. Bottles should remain in the instrument from 7 to 14 days, depending on institutional protocol, or until designated positive.
3. Positive bottles should be Gram's stained and subcultured.

Anticipated Results

No growth at the end of the incubation period.

Notes

1. Because samples for testing may contain interfering substances that could result in false-negative results, each sample type and volume should be validated with the BacT/ALERT culture bottles to ensure the sample type is free from bacteriostatic or fungistatic activity.

2. Follow the operator's manual procedures for loading and unloading the instrument.

3. See the media package insert for limitations of the test and specific performance characteristics.

4. The manufacturer has shown the ability of BacT/ALERT media to detect a wide range of microorganisms, including aerobes, anaerobes, yeast, and fungi. However, individual CT manufacturers should validate the system with their specific product type(s) to demonstrate appropriate performance.

References/Resources

1. BacT/ALERT iAST and iNST culture bottle package insert. Marcy L'Etoile, France: bioMerieux.

2. Keilpinski G, Prinzi S, Duguid J, et al. Roadmap to approval: Use of an automated sterility test method as a lot release test for Carticel, autologous cultured chondrocytes. Cytotherapy 2005;7:531-41.

3. Khuu HM, Patel N, Carter CS, et al. Sterility testing of cellular therapy products: Parallel comparison of automated methods with a CFR-compliant method. Transfusion 2006;46:2071-82.

In: Areman EM, Loper K, eds
Cellular Therapy: Principles, Methods, and Regulations
Bethesda, MD: AABB, 2009

◆◆◆　53　◆◆◆

Detection of Mycoplasma Contamination

Peter Bugert, PhD

MYCOPLASMA CONTAMINATION IS AMONG the most frequently occurring problems associated with cell cultures. It poses a recurrent threat to cell cultures and biological materials. Contamination by members of the class Mollicutes (including *Mycoplasma, Ureaplasma,* and *Acholeplasma* species) can render experimental results unreliable and biological products defective.[1,2] Quality control as well as safety concepts were developed to ensure the purity and safety of biopharmaceuticals and cellular therapeutics. In spite of the European Pharmocopoeia and the Food and Drug Administration requirements for frequent testing for mycoplasmas, confusion still exists about how to translate these requirements into practical application.[3,4] Many methods have been described that deal with the detection of contaminant mollicutes.[5,6] This chapter summarizes different approaches to mycoplasma detection and provides protocols for microbiologic culture-based and polymerase chain reaction (PCR)-based mycoplasma detection. The testing of cellular therapeutics for mycoplasma contamination represents an important contribution to the quality and safety of these products. Validated PCR-based techniques may also be valuable for release testing of applicable cellular therapy (CT) products before distribution to patients.

Common Characteristics of *Mycoplasma* Species

Common characteristics of *Mycoplasma* species are the complete lack of a bacterial cell wall, resistance to penicillin, osmotic fragility, colony shape, and the ability to pass through 200-nm-pore-diameter membrane filters.[7] Mollicute contamination is not always easy to detect because the medium does not demonstrate turbidity caused by bacterial growth, and cytopathic effects are also rare. Therefore, the risk of overlooking a contamination is very high, and 15% to 80% of cell cultures have been reported to be contaminated with mollicutes.[8] Of 20 Mollicute species known to cause cell culture contamination, 5 (*Mycoplasma arginini, M. fermentas, M.*

Peter Bugert, PhD, Associate Professor and Head, Molecular Biology Department, Heidelberg University Institute of Transfusion Medicine and Immunology, Mannheim, Germany

The author has disclosed no conflicts of interest.

hyorhinis, M. orale, and *Acholeplasma laidlawii*) account for about 95% of episodes, whereas *M. pneumoniae, M. hominis, M. genitalium, Ureaplasma parvum,* and *U. urealyticum* are most frequently found in clinical specimens.[9,10]

Methods for Mycoplasma Detection

The microbiologic approach of incubating cell culture supernatants in specific media and subsequently plating on agar plates represents the "gold standard" of mycoplasma detection and remains the reference method in good manufacturing practice protocols and in pharmacopoeias. Viable mycoplasma cells can be determined as colony-forming units (CFUs) or color-changing units (CCUs). However, the quality of CFU data may be inaccurate because of the subjective interpretation of the results[11] and because not all *Mycoplasma* species grow in all media, especially solid media.[12] CCU determination gives higher estimates of cell numbers and correlates better with the DNA content.[11] Both CFU and CCU techniques are time consuming, however, requiring an incubation period of 21 days. As a consequence, nonculture methods have been developed for the detection and identification of mollicutes in clinical specimens and cell culture. They include immunologic techniques,[13,14] DNA staining techniques,[15,16] nucleic acid hybridization,[17,18] and PCR assays.[19-24] The author and others developed PCR assays with primers targeting the mollicute 16S ribosomal RNA (rRNA) gene to detect the *Mycoplasma* species that were the most common cause of cell culture contaminations.[19,20,24] That PCR assay was validated with CCUs determined from *M. orale* and *M. pneumoniae* strains as references.

Validation of New Methods for Mycoplasma Detection

Determination of CCUs represents the gold standard in detection and quantification of biologically active mycoplasma. The author established a validation concept according to the guidelines of the European Pharmacopoeia, Section 2.6.7, and validated a PCR system with reference species *M. orale* and *M. pneumoniae.*[24] The validation for PCR-based mycoplasma detection is in agreement with the European Pharmacopoeia and provides data from direct correlation of microbiologic data with PCR results. In general, validation of a new method for mycoplasma detection should consider all steps of the procedure, including mode of sampling, sample preparation, analysis of samples, and evaluation of results. The determination of CCUs achieved by serial dilutions of liquid mycoplasma cultures should be used as the reference method for validation. The validation experiments should be performed in at least three independent runs by different staff members.

The data obtained in validation experiments represent the basis for calculation of the detection probability of the new method by a probit (predicted proportion positive) analysis as a model of nonlinear regression. The probit analysis determines a continuous 95% confidence interval of the probability of achieving a positive result at any given input mycoplasma concentration (CCU/mL). The different test concentrations of CCUs (1 to 10^6 CCU/mL) constitute the experimental input data. For example, the validation of the author's PCR-based mycoplasma detection revealed a detection probability of 95% for a mean concentration (range) of 1222 (935-1844) CCU/mL for *M. pneumoniae* and 2547 (1584-10,352) CCU/mL for *M. orale.*[24]

Future Directions of PCR-Based Mycoplasma Detection

PCR-based mycoplasma detection assays represent an attractive diagnostic tool that is superior to microbiologic testing with regard to speed, convenience, and throughput of samples. After the detection probability of a PCR method has been determined by validation experiments, the method can be implemented by routine laboratories with standard PCR equipment. However, the sensitivity of standard PCR approaches with detection of amplification products by agarose gel electrophoresis may not be sufficient. PCR methods that target 16S and 23S rRNA genes of mycoplasma, as previously described,[19,20,22-24] reported a higher sensitivity compared to PCR methods with other targets, such as the P1 adhesin gene.[21,25,26] Further improvement of sensitivity may be achieved by the use of real-time PCR with SYBR Green (Molecular Probes, Eugene, OR)[27] or fluorescently labeled probes.[28,29]

Different repetitive sequences (repMp1 to 5) have been identified all over the *M. pneumoniae* genome.[30] The repetitive sequences differ in size, number of copies, and sequence. Investigation of the repetitive sequences may increase the sensitivity of a PCR approach by amplifying a multicopy target. Compared to a monocopy gene locus (P1 adhesin), a real-time PCR system based on amplification of a part of the repetitive element repMp1 of *M. pneumoniae* showed an increased sensitivity by a factor of 22.[29]

Mycoplasma detection assays based on multicopy target amplification and real-time PCR may represent the most reliable, sensitive, and rapid tools for testing CT products. Among other test results, a negative mycoplasma result is an important parameter that contributes to the quality and safety of the CT product.

Acknowledgments

Method 53-1 was submitted by Elsbeth Pirkl, Technician, Center for Molecular Biology, University of Heidelberg, Heidelberg, Germany. Method 53-2 was submitted by Karen Bieback, PhD, Head, Stem Cell Research Laboratory, Institute of Transfusion Medicine and Immunology, Heidelberg University, Mannheim, Germany, and Hermann Eichler, MD, Professor of Medicine and Director, Institute of Clinical Hemostaseology and Transfusion Medicine, Saarland University, University Hospital, Homburg/Saar, Germany. The author wishes to thank K. Bieback and H. Eichler for critical review of the manuscript.

References/Resources

1. Hay RJ, Macy M, Chen TR. Mycoplasma infection of cultured cells. Nature 1989;339:487-8.
2. Drexler HG, Uphoff CC. Contamination of cell culture, mycoplasma. In: Spier E, ed. Encyclopedia of cell technology. New York: Wiley-Interscience, 2000:609-27.
3. European pharmacopoeia. Section 2.6.7 (*Mycoplasma*). 5th ed. Strasbourg, France: Council of Europe, 2004.
4. Code of federal regulations. Test for *Mycoplasma*. Title 21, CFR Part 610.30. Washington, DC: US Government Printing Office, 2009 (updated annually).

5. Tully JG, Razin S, eds. Molecular and diagnostic procedures in mycoplasmology. Vol 2. Diagnostic procedures. San Diego, CA: Academic Press, 1996.
6. Waites KB, Talkington DF, Bebear CM. Mycoplasmas. In: Truant AL, ed. Manual of commercial methods in clinical microbiology. Washington, DC: American Society for Microbiology, 2002:201-24.
7. Razin S, Herrmann R, eds. Molecular biology and pathogenicity of mycoplasmas. New York: Kluwer Academic and Plenum, 2002.
8. Langdon SP. Cell culture contamination: An overview. Methods Mol Med 2004;88:309-17.
9. Tully JG. Current status of the mollicute flora of humans. Clin Infect Dis 1993;17(Suppl 1):S2-9.
10. Waites KB, Talkington DF. *Mycoplasma pneumoniae* and its role as human pathogen. Clin Microbiol Rev 2004;17:697-728.
11. Stemke GW, Robertson JA. Comparison of two methods for enumeration of mycoplasmas. J Clin Microbiol 1982;16:959-61.
12. Robertson AJ, Stemke GW. Measurement of mollicute growth by ATP-dependent luminometry. In: Tully JG, Razin S, eds. Molecular and diagnostic procedures in mycoplasmology. Vol 2. San Diego, CA: Academic Press, 1996:65-72.
13. Blazek R, Schmitt K, Krafft U, et al. Fast and simple procedure for the detection of cell culture mycoplasmas using a single monoclonal antibody. J Immunol Methods 1990;131:203-12.
14. Radka SF, Hester DM, Polak-Vogelzang AA, et al. Detection of mycoplasma contamination in lymphoblastoid cell lines by monoclonal antibodies. Hum Immunol 1984;9:111-6.
15. McGarrity GJ, Kotani H, Carson D. Comparative studies to determine the efficiency of 6 methylpurine deoxyriboside to detect cell culture mycoplasmas. In Vitro Cell Dev Biol 1986;22:301-4.
16. Payment P, Corbeil M, Chagnon A. Detection of *Mycoplasma hominis* and *Mycoplasma orale* in cell cultures by immunofluorescence. Can J Microbiol 1978;24:689-92.
17. Mattsson JG, Johansson KE. Oligonucleotide probes complementary to 16S rRNA for rapid detection of mycoplasma contamination in cell cultures. FEMS Microbiol Lett 1993;107:139-44.
18. McGarrity GJ, Kotani H. Detection of cell culture mycoplasmas by a genetic probe. Exp Cell Res 1986;163:273-8.
19. van Kuppeveld FJ, van der Logt JT, Angulo AF, et al. Genus-species-specific identification of mycoplasmas by 16S rRNA amplification. Appl Environ Microbiol 1992;58:2606-15.
20. van Kuppeveld FJ, Johansson KE, Galama JM, et al. Detection of mycoplasma contamination in cell cultures by a mycoplasma group-specific PCR. Appl Environ Microbiol 1994;60:149-52.
21. Kong F, Gordon S, Gilbert GL. Rapid-cycle PCR for detection and typing of *Mycoplasma pneumoniae* in clinical specimens. J Clin Microbiol 2000;38:4256-9.

22. Kong F, James G, Gordon S, et al. Species-specific PCR for identification of common contaminant mollicutes in cell culture. Appl Environ Microbiol 2001;67:3195-200.

23. Ossewaarde JM, de Vries A, Bestebroer T, et al. Application of a mycoplasma group-specific PCR for monitoring decontamination of mycoplasma-infected *Chlamydia* sp. strains. Appl Environ Microbiol 1996;62:328-31.

24. Bruchmüller I, Pirkl E, Herrmann R, et al. Introduction of a validation concept for a PCR-based mycoplasma detection assay. Cytotherapy 2006;8:62-9.

25. Jensen JS, Sondergard-Andersen J, Uldum SA, Lind K. Detection of *Mycoplasma pneumoniae* in simulated clinical samples by polymerase chain reaction. APMIS 1989;97:1046-8.

26. de Barbeyrac BC, Bernet-Poggi C, Febrer F, et al. Detection of *Mycoplasma genitalium* in clinical samples by polymerase chain reaction. Clin Infect Dis 1993;17 (Suppl 1):S83-9.

27. Ishikawa Y, Kozakai T, Morita H, et al. Rapid detection of mycoplasma contamination in cell cultures using SYBR Green-based real-time polymerase chain reaction. In Vitro Cell Dev Biol Anim 2006;42:63-9.

28. Pitcher D, Chalker VJ, Sheppard C, et al. Real-time detection of *Mycoplasma pneumoniae* in respiratory samples with an internal processing control. J Med Microbiol 2006;55:149-55.

29. Dumke R, Schurwanz N, Lenz M, et al. Sensitive detection of *Mycoplasma pneumoniae* in human respiratory tract samples by optimized real-time PCR approach. J Clin Microbiol 2007;45:2726-30.

30. Himmelreich R, Hilbert H, Plagens H, et al. Complete sequence analysis of the genome of the bacterium *Mycoplasma pneumoniae*. Nucleic Acids Res 1996;24:4420-49.

Method 53-1. Determining Color-Changing Units for Microbiologic Culture-Based Mycoplasma Detection

Description

The color-changing test is done in modified Hay-flick medium containing phenol red.[1] Bacterial metabolism leads to a decrease of pH (from pH 7.6 to pH 6.2) that subsequently causes a color change from red to orange and then to yellow. The yellow-colored medium remains stable for weeks, but, depending on the species, mycoplasma does not survive under these lower pH conditions. The assay requires long incubation times (up to 21 days) at 37 C with periodic inspection of the tubes.

Time for Procedure

1. Preparation of media stocks: 2 days.
2. Preparation of dilution series: 2 hours.
3. Duration of culture incubation: up to 21 days. Samples with a high mycoplasma content may lead to a color change of the first dilution tubes within a few days.

Summary of Procedure

1. Prepare the modified Hayflick liquid medium.
2. Prepare sample dilutions and inoculate into Hayflick medium.
3. Incubate the microbiologic cultures, inspecting regularly for color change.
4. Determine the number of color-changing units (CCUs).

Equipment

1. Incubator at 37 C.
2. Vortex mixer.

Supplies and Reagents

1. Modified Hayflick medium[2]
   a. Pleuropneumonia-like organism (PPLO) broth without crystal violet (CV).
   b. Phenol red.
   c. HEPES buffer.
   d. Glucose.
   e. Horse serum.
   f. Penicillin G.
   g. 2 M NaOH.
2. Sterile, disposable culture tubes with screw caps or sterile glass tubes with silicone stoppers.
3. Sterile, graduated pipettes.
4. Sterile filters (200-nm pore size), for 250-mL or 500-mL volume.

Procedure

1. Prepare modified Hayflick liquid medium.
   a. Solution I (dissolved in sterile water with pH adjusted to 7.6):
      • PPLO broth without CV.
      • Phenol red solution.
      • HEPES.
   b. Solution II:
      • Horse serum (heat inactivated).
      • Glucose solution.
      • Penicillin G.
   c. Aseptically mix equal volumes of solutions I and II in a biological safety cabinet. The complete medium can be stored at 4 C for about 1 month.
2. Prepare sample dilutions (eg, cell culture supernatant of a cellular therapy product), and inoculate into the Hayflick medium.
   a. For each sample solution to be tested, prepare three replicate series of 10 tubes, each with 1.8 mL modified Hayflick medium.
   b. Prepare eight serial dilutions (1:10) by pipetting 0.2 mL of sample solution into the first tube and continuously pipetting 0.2-mL volumes through the dilution series. Use a new pipette for each dilution.
   c. Inoculate 2 additional tubes with medium only as negative controls to test the sterility of the medium.

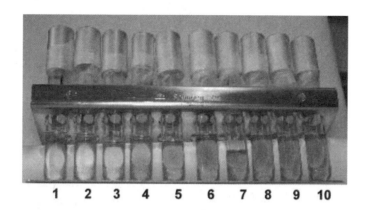

Figure 53-1-1. Representative result of culture-based mycoplasma detection. A 1:10 dilution series of *Myco-plasma pneumoniae* was incubated in modified Hayflick liquid medium at 37 C for 21 days. A color shift from red to orange/yellow was seen in tubes 1 through 5. Tube 5 (10^{-5} dilution) was defined to have 1 color-changing unit (CCU)/mL, with the undiluted sample solution (tube 1) containing 100,000 CCU/mL. Tubes 6 through 10 represent negative results; that is, no color change (tubes 9 and 10 were negative controls).

3. Incubate the microbiologic cultures.
   a. Seal the airtight tubes and incubate at 37 C for up to 3 weeks or until a color change from red to orange/yellow is observed.
   b. Inspect the color of the cultures once every day over a period of up to 21 days.
4. Determine number of CCUs.
   a. Growth of mycoplasma is indicated by a change in color of the medium from red to orange/yellow (see Fig 53-1-1). Red color indicates a negative result, that is, no mycoplasma contamination. A color shift to orange or yellow indicates mycoplasma contamination.
   b. The highest dilution that shows a color change is defined as 1 CCU.[3] The estimated number of CCUs for a sample is the reciprocal of the highest dilution in which a color change was observed.

Anticipated Results

If cellular therapy products are free from myco-plasma contamination, no color change should occur (over that seen in negative control tubes) after 21 days of incubation.

Notes

1. The CCU value of a mycoplasma sample should be determined in at least three independent dilution series and reported as a mean value.
2. Incubation of medium over a period of 21 days causes a slight color change.
3. The use of at least one reference mycoplasma strain as a positive control is recommended to prove the quality of culture media.

References/Resources

1. Purcell RH, Taylor-Robinson D, Wong D, Chanock RM. Color test for the measurement of antibody to T-strain mycoplasmas. J Bacteriol 1966;92:6-12.
2. Hayflick L. Tissue culture and mycoplasma. Tex Rep Biol Med 1965;23(Suppl 1):285-303.
3. Rodwell AW, Whitcomb RF. Methods for direct and indirect measurement of mycoplasma growth. In: Razin S, Tully JG, eds. Methods in mycoplasmology. Vol 1. San Diego, CA: Academic Press, 1983:185-96.

Method 53-2. Detecting Mycoplasma by Conventional PCR

Description

The polymerase chain reaction (PCR) assay uses conventional detection of amplification product after size separation by agarose gel electrophoresis and ethidium bromide staining. The primers were designed from reference *Mycoplasma* DNA sequences of the gene coding for the 16S ribosomal DNA (rDNA). Specific amplification of a 278-bp DNA fragment occurs in samples containing *Mycoplasma* DNA. Simultaneous amplification of a 119-bp DNA fragment from a synthetic oligonucleotide template containing primer binding sites allows control of the efficacy of the PCR assay.

Time for Procedure

Approximately 4 hours.

Summary of Procedure

1. Isolate the total DNA from the cell culture supernatant of the cellular therapy (CT) product.
2. Perform PCR.
3. Analyze PCR products by agarose gel electrophoresis.

Equipment

1. Bench-top centrifuge for 1.5-mL reaction tubes.
2. Thermal block incubator or waterbath at 56 C.
3. PCR cycler with 96-well block for 0.2-mL PCR tubes.
4. Agarose gel electrophoresis unit.
5. UV-documentation device equipped with digital camera.

Supplies and Reagents

1. DNA extraction kit (eg, QIAamp DNA Blood Mini Kit, Qiagen, Hilden, Germany).
2. Primers (100-µM solutions):
   a. Forward: 5'-GAGCAAAYAGGATTAGATAC-3'.

   b. Reverse: 5'-ACCATGCACCAYCTGT-CAYTC-3'.
3. Internal control oligonucleotide (1 pg/µl).
   Note: binding sites of primers are underlined:
   5'-TGGG<u>GAGCAAACAGGATTAGATAC</u>CC TGGTAGTCCACGCCGTAAACGATATGCTC GCAAGAGTAACCTTCGCAAAGCTATAGAG ATATAGTGGAGGTTAACG<u>GAGTGACAGAT GGTGCATGG</u>TTGTCG-3'
4. PCR buffer (10× concentrate): 100 mM Tris/HCl pH 8.3, 500 mM KCl, 15 mM $MgCl_2$, 0.1% bovine serum albumin.
5. Deoxynucleotide triphosphate (dNTP) mix (10× concentrate): 2 mM each of deoxyadenosine triphosphate (dATP), deoxycitidine triphosphate (dCTP), deoxyguanosine triphosphate (dGTP), deoxythymidine triphosphate (dTTP).
6. Taq DNA polymerase (5 units/µL).
7. PCR-grade water.
8. Tris-acetic acid-EDTA (TAE) gel electrophoresis buffer (50× concentrate): 2 M Tris/acetic acid pH 8, 50 mM EDTA.
9. Sample buffer for gel electrophoresis (10× concentrate): 50% glycerol, 10× TAE, 1 mg/mL bromphenol blue, 1 mg/mL xylene cyanol.
10. Standard agarose.
11. Ethidium bromide stock solution (10 mg/mL).

Procedure

1. Isolate the total DNA from the cell culture supernatant of the CT product.
   a. Take a 1-mL sample from the cell culture supernatant, then centrifuge, carefully remove 800 µL from the top of the supernatant, and resuspend the remaining sample.
   b. Extract DNA from the 200-µL sample with the use of a commercial kit (eg, QIAamp DNA Blood Mini Kit) according to the manufacturer's protocol for isolation of genomic DNA from bacterial cultures.

c. Elute DNA using 50 μL PCR-grade water with a prolonged incubation time of 5 minutes to increase the DNA yield.

2. Perform PCR.

a. Set up PCRs following institutional procedures. Sample reactions will include a 5-μL DNA sample, 0.5 μM of each primer, 0.1 pg internal control oligo, 1× PCR buffer, 200 μM dNTP, and 1 unit of Taq DNA polymerase.

b. Set the PCR cycling protocol as follows: 2 minutes initial denaturation at 95 C, followed by 30 cycles with 30 seconds denaturing at 94 C, 60 seconds annealing at 55 C, and 60 seconds extension at 72 C.

3. Analyze PCR products by agarose gel electrophoresis.

a. After cycling, add 2 μL 10 × sample buffer to each reaction tube.

b. Analyze 10 μL of each reaction in 2% agarose gels containing 0.5 ng/mL ethidium bromide in a gel electrophoresis chamber.

c. Visualize the gels under ultraviolet (UV) light and document using a UV documentation system (see Fig 53-2-1).

Anticipated Results

If CT products are free from mycoplasma contamination, the control 119-bp fragment should be visible, but no 278-bp PCR fragment should be visible. If a CT product is contaminated with mycoplasma at a level higher than the detection limit of the PCR system, both PCR fragments or only the 278-bp fragment should be visible. The detection probability of the PCR system for *M. pneumoniae* is 1222 CCU/mL [95% confidence interval (CI); 935-1844 CCU/mL] and for *M. orale,* 2547 CCU/mL (95% CI; 1584-10,352 CCU/mL).[1]

Notes

1. A negative control tube with water in place of a DNA sample should always be included.

2. It is recommended to use reference mycoplasma DNA samples as positive controls to prove the functionality of the PCR system.

Reference/Resource

1. Bruchmüller I, Pirkl E, Herrmann R, et al. Introduction of a validation concept for a PCR-based mycoplasma detection assay. Cytotherapy 2006;8:62-9.

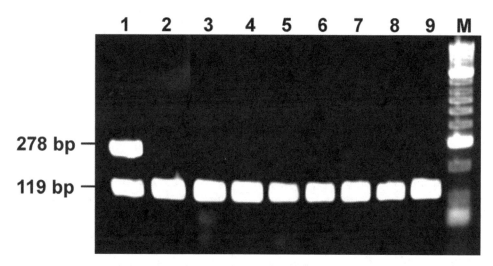

Figure 53-2-1. Representative result of PCR-based mycoplasma detection. DNA was extracted from 1 mL of different cell culture supernatants (lanes 3-9). The positive control (lane 1) contained DNA isolated from *Mycoplasma pneumoniae*. The negative control (lane 2) contained sterile water instead of a DNA sample. The internal control fragment (119 bp) generated from the synthetic oligonucleotide template added to the reaction mix could be observed in each lane. The test amplicon (278 bp) generated from the 16S rDNA of mycoplasma was found only in the positive control. Thus, each cell culture supernatant revealed a negative result. M = DNA size marker.

In: Areman EM, Loper K, eds
Cellular Therapy: Principles, Methods, and Regulations
Bethesda, MD: AABB, 2009

♦♦♦   54   ♦♦♦

Endotoxin Testing of Cellular Therapy Products

Diane Kadidlo, MT(ASCP)SBB

ENDOTOXIN IS A COMPLEX LIPOPOLYSAC-charide found in the outer membrane of the cell wall of most gram-negative bacteria. Well known to be toxic to humans, endotoxin can induce pyrogenic responses ranging from fever, chills, and hypotension to disseminated intravascular coagulation, tumor necrosis, shock, and death. Endotoxin is released from the cells when the bacteria are actively growing or disintegrating, with the greatest amount released during cell death (autolysis, external lysis, and phagocytic digestion).[1]

Endotoxin contamination is of significant concern to manufacturers of cellular and tissue-based products. Gram-negative bacteria and endotoxin can be introduced into the cellular therapy (CT) product through an infected donor. They can also be introduced into the product during the manufacturing process through the use of contaminated media, water used for washing glassware, and human and animal sera. Poor laboratory sanitation and inadequate environmental controls can increase the risk of product contamination. Food and Drug Administration (FDA) regulations require that biologics be free from extraneous material.[2] Pyrogenicity testing and testing for residual contamination from reagents, proteins, peptides, sera, cytokines, antibodies, and cellular phenotypes are typically required for somatic cell and tissue products that have undergone more-than-minimal manipulation and in which immediate administration of the product is necessary following processing.[3]

The rabbit pyrogenicity test developed in the 1940s was the first FDA-approved method for the detection of endotoxin.[4] Since that time, an alternative and more sensitive method for the detection and quantification of endotoxin has been developed. The limulus amebocye lysate (LAL) assay is based upon the findings of Frederick Bang, in which he determined that gram-negative bacteria cause intravascular coagulation in the horseshoe crab, *Limulus polyphemus*.[5] Levin and Bang later proved that this coagulation was caused by an enzymatic reaction between the horseshoe crab amebocytes and endotoxin.[6] Today several LAL assay kits are commercially available involving turbidemetric,

Diane Kadidlo, MT(ASCP)SBB, Director, Molecular and Cellular Therapeutics, University of Minnesota, and Technical Supervisor, Cell Therapy Clinical Laboratory, University of Minnesota Medical Center Fairview, St Paul, Minnesota

The author has disclosed no conflicts of interest.

gel-clot, and kinetic-chromogenic methods for the detection and quantification of endotoxin.

The endotoxin assay is relatively straightforward and can be performed in most CT facilities. The principles behind the endotoxin assay are similar regardless of the method selected (ie, gel clot, turbidemetric, or kinetic chromogenic). The typical endotoxin assay involves combining the test sample with a reagent containing LAL. If endotoxin is present in the test sample, an activation of a proenzyme in the limulus amebocyte reagent will occur, resulting in opacity and formation of a gelatinous clot. The time required for a reaction (turbidity, color change, or clot) is inversely proportional to the amount of endotoxin present in the sample. Therefore, the more endotoxin present in the test sample, the faster a color change or clot will occur. On the basis of the reaction time, the amount of endotoxin in the sample is then calculated against a standard curve of known concentrations of endotoxin controls. For the gel-clot method, the clotting is visibly observed by the operator, and the concentration of endotoxin is determined by multiplying the lowest dilution of sample in which clotting is observed by the lysate sensitivity. The turbidemetric and kinetic-chromogenic methods require the aid of a spectrophotometer to assess turbidity and color change. In the kinetic-chromogenic method, the enzymatic activation caused by lysate reagent and endotoxin sample catalyzes the splitting of a colorless substrate Ac-Ile-Glu-Ala-Arg-pNa by cleaving the p-nitroaniline. P-nitroaniline is a yellow color and is measured photometrically at 385 to 410 nm.[7] The turbidemetric method measures the increase in turbidity/optical density that precedes the formation of the gel clot.[8] For the turbidemetric and the kinetic-chromogeneic methods, the concentration of endotoxin is determined by the intensity of the turbidity or color change. The concentration of endotoxin in the sample is expressed as the number of endotoxin units (EU) per milliliter or per kilogram of patient body weight.

The potential for adverse effects from endotoxin correlates with the amount of endotoxin in the product administered. For that reason, for licensed CT products and for those being studied under investigational new drug exemptions, the FDA has established an upper limit of 5 EU/kg of body weight/dose for intravenous drugs, biological products, and medical devices. Intrathecal product administration permits a much lower limit of 0.2 EU/kg/dose.[3,9] The procedure in Method 54-1 is an example of a kinetic-chromogenic LAL assay, in this case using the Kinetic-QCL kit (Lonza, Walkersville, MD).

References/Resources

1. Todar K. Online textbook of bacteriology. Madison, WI: University of Wisconsin—Madison, Department of Bacteriology, 2006. [Available at http://www.textbookofbacteriology.net (accessed April 16, 2009).]
2. Code of federal regulations. General biological products standards. Title 21, CFR Part 610.13. Washington, DC: US Government Printing Office, 2009 (updated annually).
3. Food and Drug Administration. Guidance for FDA reviewers and sponsors: Content and review of chemistry, manufacturing, and control (CMC) information for human somatic cell therapy investigational new drug applications (INDs). (April 2008) Rockville, MD: Center for Biologics Evaluation and Research, 2008. [Available at http://www.fda.gov/cber/gdlns/cmcsomcell.htm (accessed April 16, 2009).]
4. Ryan J. Endotoxins and cell culture. Technical bulletin. Lowell, MA: Corning Incorporated Life Sciences, 2008.
5. Bang FB. A bacterial disease of Limulus polyphemus. Bull Johns Hopkins Hosp 1956;98:325.
6. Levin J, Bang FB. Clottable protein in Limulus: Its localization and kinetics of its coagulation by endotoxin. Thromb Diath Haemorrh 1968;19:186.
7. Limulus Amebocyte Lysate (LAL) Kinetic QCL. Assay package insert. Walkersville, MD: Lonza, 2007.
8. Pyrogent-5000 user manual. Catalog Nos: N383, N384, N588, N688. Walkersville, MD: Lonza.
9. Food and Drug Administration. Guideline on validation of the limulus amebocyte lysate test as an end-product endotoxin test for human and animal parenteral drugs, biological products and medical devices. (December 1987) Rockville, MD: Center for Drug Evaluation and Research, 1987.

Method 54-1. Kinetic-Chromogenic LAL Assay

Description

In the kinetic-chromogenic limulus amebocyte lysate (LAL) assay, the test sample is mixed with the LAL/substrate reagent, placed in the plate reader, and automatically monitored over time for the appearance of a yellow color. The concentration of endotoxin in a sample is calculated from a standard curve. It is critical that all materials coming in contact with the sample be pyrogen free. Positive product controls (PPCs) must be included in the assay to verify the absence of product inhibition or enhancement. PPCs consist of the specimen to be tested spiked with a known amount of positive control.

Time for Procedure

Procedure takes 90 to 120 minutes.

Summary of Procedure

1. Set up the instrument and prepare supplies for the assay.
2. Dilute standards.
3. Prepare samples.
4. Prepare PPCs.
5. Add samples to the microtiter plate and preincubate.
6. Reconstitute the lysate and add to wells.
7. Incubate the microtiter plate.
8. Review the results and determine the endotoxin concentration of samples.

Equipment

1. Incubating plate reader.
2. Appropriate software.
3. Multichannel pipettor.
4. Adjustable-volume pipettor.
5. Vortex mixer.
6. Drybath.

Reagents and Supplies

1. 13 × 100-mm glass test tubes, pyrogen free.
2. Pipette tips: 200 μL, pyrogen free.
3. Pipette tips: 1000 μL, pyrogen free.
4. 96-well microplates: flat bottom, pyrogen free.
5. Reagent reservoirs: pyrogen free.
6. Kinetic-QCL test kit (Lonza, Walkersville, MD): includes LAL reagent, control standard endotoxin (CSE), and other reagents.
7. Pyrosperse (Lonza).
8. 50-mM Tris buffer.
9. LAL reagent water (LRW).

Procedure

1. Set up the instrument and prepare supplies for the assay.
   a. Turn on the plate reader and allow it to warm up to 37 ±1 C.
   b. From the test kit, prepare CSE if reconstituted standard is not available. The endotoxin concentration of the reconstituted CSE will be 50 EU/mL.
   c. Vortex the reconstituted standard for at least 5 minutes on high speed.
   d. Prepare a template for the assay plate using the appropriate software program. This typically involves entering information and microtiter plate locations for standards, products, PPCs, and negative controls.
   e. Label a 96-well microplate according to the template. Label wells A1 and A2 as "BL" (blank). Wells B1, B2, C1, C2, D1, D2, and so on will contain dilutions of the standard. Label wells to correspond with dilutions indicated on the template.
2. Dilute the CSE for the standard curve. For standard dilutions of 0.05 EU/mL, 0.5 EU/mL, and 5.0 EU/mL, dilutions may be made as follows:
   a. Add 900 μL LRW to each dilution tube.
   b. Remove the CSE from the vortex mixer after the 5-minute vortex period has been completed. Add 100 μL of the CSE stock

solution to the tube labeled "5.0." Vortex the tube for at least 1 minute.

c. Add 100 μL of sample from the 5.0 tube to the 0.5 tube. Vortex the tube for at least 1 minute.

d. Add 100 μL of sample from the 0.5 tube to the 0.05 tube. Vortex the tube for at least 1 minute.

3. Prepare the samples.

a. Perform pretreatment of the samples if necessary to eliminate interfering substances (see "Notes").

b. Add an appropriate volume of LRW and sample to each dilution tube. Vortex tubes for at least 1 minute after adding sample. Each sample dilution should be run in duplicate.

4. Prepare PPCs.

a. Vortex the CSE standard solution that is 10-fold more concentrated than the selected PPC value for 1 minute.

b. Add 10 μL of the CSE solution to each PPC well. When mixed with the 100-μL sample volume, a 1:10 dilution is made, resulting in the expected PPC value. For example, if a PPC value of 0.5 EU/mL is selected, vortex the 5.0-EU/mL standard and add 10 μL to the appropriate wells. Spike all PPC wells *before* adding any products or standards into the wells.

5. Add the samples to the microtiter plate and preincubate.

a. Add the samples to the 96-well microplate: Vortex each standard and sample dilution for at least 30 seconds before use. Pipette 100 μL of blank, standard, sample, or negative control into the appropriate wells on the microplate. Refer to the template map. Cover the microplate.

b. For preincubation, verify that the temperature of the plate reader is 3 C, and insert the covered microwell plate into the plate reader.

6. Reconstitute the lysate and add to the wells.

a. Reconstitute the lysate reagent during the preincubation period. Each well on the microplate will require 100 μL of reconstituted lysate reagent. Transfer the lysate reagent to a reagent reservoir. If more than

one vial is added to the reservoir, mix by gently rocking the reservoir.

b. After the microplate has incubated 10 minutes, add 100 μL lysate reagent to each of the wells containing blanks, standards, samples, and PPCs.

c. Do not change pipette tips between samples. Avoid causing bubbles. Do *not* replace the microplate cover.

7. Incubate the microtiter plate. Close the cover of the reader and initiate the assay procedure. The progress of color development will be monitored by the optics system in the reader and testing software as the plate is incubated. The assay will end after the lowest concentration standard reaches its predefined threshold. The threshold is defined as the onset optical density plus the required change (Delta) in the optical density.

8. Review results and determine endotoxin concentration of samples.

a. Acceptance criteria: For an assay to be valid, all criteria for the standard curve, PPCs, negative control, and the test sample must have been met (see "Anticipated Results" for details).

b. Results for samples are expressed as reaction time in seconds. The amount of endotoxin expressed as EUs is determined by taking the average reaction time of the duplicate samples and comparing it to the standard endotoxin curve. The concentration of endotoxin in the test sample is determined by selecting the lowest sample dilution in which the coefficients of variation (CVs) for sample and PPC and the percent PPC recovery are valid. The concentration of endotoxin is calculated by multiplying the endotoxin result by the dilution. To calculate the amount of endotoxin in the product per kilogram of patient weight, multiply the endotoxin concentration by the product volume and divide the result by the patient weight.

Anticipated Results

1. Standard curve: All three parameters (correlation coefficient, slope, and Y intercept) must

be within established specifications or the assay is invalid and must be repeated.

2. Diluted standards: All dilutions must be within 10% of expected result for the standard curve results to be acceptable. If any standard is out of specification, the assay is invalid and must be repeated.

3. Product test results: Each sample dilution tested is evaluated along with the results of the corresponding PPC for that dilution.

   a. If a sample does not react, then the result will be reported as "<the lowest standard." If the sample does react, then the CV for the two replicates must be <10%. If the sample dilution has a CV >10%, the results from that dilution are unacceptable. If the samples did not react during the test period, a percent CV cannot be calculated and the result is still valid.

   b. The results for each PPC dilution are reported as percent CV and PPC recovered. The PPC recovered must be 50% to 200% of the expected spike concentration. This result confirms that the sample contains no interfering substance. The CV between the PPC replicates must be <10%. The PPC must meet both criteria for the dilution to be acceptable.

4. Negative control: For the results of the negative control to be valid, the CVs (for the control sample and PPC) must be <10% and percent PPC recovery between 50% and 200%.

Notes

1. The Food and Drug Administration *Guideline on Validation of the Limulus Amebocyte Lysate Test as an End-Product Endotoxin Test for Human and Animal Parenteral Drugs, Biological Products and Medical Devices* specifies that all test operators must perform an initial qualification before being considered authorized to run the assay.[1] This initial qualification must also be performed with each new lot of test reagents, and the guideline requires that a

PPC be run with each dilution of a test sample and that the PPC recovered be within 50% to 200% of the known spike concentration.

2. Generally, five standards are available for the test: 0.005, 0.05, 0.5, 5.0, and 50. Most laboratories routinely use the 0.05-, 0.5-, and 5.0-EU/mL standards.

3. For most cellular therapy assays, a PPC concentration of 0.5 EU/mL is used. It is important to note that the PPC concentration must fall within the standard curve with a standard on both the high and low side. If not, the software will not allow the assay to proceed.

4. Eliminating inhibition or enhancement:

   a. If the PPC recovery status for all dilutions is not acceptable, the sample may contain a substance that is interfering with the test. Serum albumin, EDTA, and high or low pH are common conditions that interfere with LAL assays. Several techniques may help eliminate interference with the assay, including the following:

      • Heat inactivation (100 C for at least 10 minutes) to eliminate interference from albumin.

      • Addition of a dispersing agent to the sample to eliminate interference from EDTA.

      • Addition of a buffer to eliminate interference from pH.

   b. These techniques can be used individually or in combination to achieve an acceptable PPC recovery, but every effort should be made to limit sample pretreatment as much as possible. Do not use pretreatment techniques on the standard dilutions.

References/Resources

1. Food and Drug Administration. Guideline on validation of the limulus amebocyte lysate test as an end-product endotoxin test for human and animal parenteral drugs, biological products and medical devices. (December 1987) Rockville, MD: Center for Drug Evaluation and Research, 1987.

2. Limulus Amebocyte Lysate (LAL) Kinetic QCL. Assay package insert. Walkersville, MD: Lonza, 2007.

In: Areman EM, Loper K, eds
Cellular Therapy: Principles, Methods, and Regulations
Bethesda, MD: AABB, 2009

◆◆◆   55   ◆◆◆

The Use of Blood Grouping for Identity Testing of Cellular Therapy Products

Ellen Areman, MS, SBB(ASCP)

CELLULAR THERAPY (CT) PRODUCTS COL-lected from hematopoietic progenitor cell (HPC) donors contain the same red cell antigens and serum/plasma antibodies found in the blood circulating in the donor. Because humans have only a few major blood groups (A, B, AB, O), one cannot always depend on this characteristic alone for confirming the identity of a CT product. However, because ABO typing is often performed on HPC donors and products as part of the product characterization process, the results can be combined with those of other tests such as flow cytometry and HLA typing to differentiate one HPC product from others produced in the same facility.

In most situations, a peripheral blood sample from the donor, rather than from the CT product itself, is used for testing. One way of confirming identity before processing is to perform an ABO test on a sample from the product as well as from the donor. In the case of umbilical cord blood products, although a sample from the donor mother is tested for infectious disease markers, the red cells from the cord blood itself must be typed for ABO because they will not necessarily be the

same as those of the mother. HPC products or donors are sometimes tested for D (Rh) antigen, but unless a reason exists to anticipate transplant problems from a red cell incompatibility, phenotyping for other red cell markers is usually not performed.

Samples for grouping and typing should be removed before the unit undergoes processing, because any manipulation may remove or reduce the intact red cells, serum, or plasma required for accurate and reliable testing. As long as the CT product contains adequate mature red cells and plasma for the assay, test kits and reagents labeled for testing human blood and blood products can be expected to produce a reliable test result. However, before implementing a testing procedure using materials or reagents not labeled for use with a CT product or its donor, the laboratory should first validate the test system.

ABO typing may also be used as one test for confirming the identity of a final CT product before release. However, this confirmatory testing can be used only for products with an adequate volume of intact red cells to perform the assay. It may not be

---

Ellen Areman, MS, SBB(ASCP), Senior Consultant, Biologics Consulting Group, Inc, Alexandria, Virginia

The author has disclosed no conflicts of interest.

appropriate for thawed or red-cell-depleted CT products.

The procedure depends on agglutination or hemolysis of donor or product red cells when combined with commercial antibody reagents (anti-A, anti-B, anti-A,B) and donor plasma or serum combined with commercial red cells (A, B, O). The pattern of agglutination or hemolysis indicates the ABO group of the sample. Various technologies are available for performing the assay in test tubes, on slides, in multiwell plates, or on automated systems. Manufacturers' instructions should be followed for the various blood grouping systems.

Discussion of the ABO blood groups and descriptions of some common procedures can be found in the AABB *Technical Manual.*[1]

Reference/Resource

1. Roback JD, Combs MR, Grossman BJ, Hillyer CD, eds. Technical manual. 16th ed. Bethesda, MD: AABB, 2008.

In: Areman EM, Loper K, eds
Cellular Therapy: Principles, Methods, and Regulations
Bethesda, MD: AABB, 2009

◆ ◆ ◆   56   ◆ ◆ ◆

HLA Typing for Cellular Product Characterization and Identity Testing

Terry O. Harville, MD, PhD

THE ABBREVIATION *HLA* STANDS FOR *human leukocyte antigen* and is based on the discovery of a group of proteins expressed on human white blood cells (leukocytes).[1] The discovery of the HLA family of proteins had its roots in early attempts to transplant skin tumors, and subsequently skin, from one unrelated, inbred strain of a "fancy breeders' mouse" to another.[2] With inbred members of the same strain, the tissue would be accepted, but in unrelated mice, transplanted tissue was found to become necrotic within a few weeks of transplantation, and subsequent attempts at transplantation from the same donor to the same recipient would result in necrosis within a few days. Through breeding studies, the ability to accept or reject tissue or skin grafts (*histocompatibility)* was recognized as inherited in a Mendelian fashion. Unfortunately, early transplantation attempts between unrelated human beings yielded the same unacceptable results as with transplantation of skin or tissue between unrelated mice. Thus, the major histocompatibility complex (MHC) of immune response genes was recognized. With further use of highly inbred strains of fancy breeders' mice, where the characteristics could be followed in the offspring, George Snell performed specific antigen-recognition experiments and determined specific MHC gene components in mice.[3]

Karl Landsteiner's pioneering work illustrated that antibodies can cause agglutination of red cells as well as hemolytic reactions.[4] With regard to tissue rejection, it was demonstrated that white cells infiltrated rejected tissue, indicating that a cellular reaction was involved.[5] These findings prompted studies mixing serum from one individual with lymphocytes from another to determine the type of reaction that would occur. In such studies, it was found that sera from young men rarely resulted in agglutination of lymphocytes from other individuals. In contrast, a mother of several children was not uncommonly found to have serum that would agglutinate the lymphocytes from her children's father. Such serum might fail to agglutinate cells from nonfamily members, but frequently it would

Terry O. Harville, MD, PhD, Medical Director, Special Immunology Laboratory, Medical Director, Histocompatibility Laboratory, Medical Director, Immunogenetics and Transplantation Laboratory, Departments of Pathology and Laboratory Services and Pediatrics, University of Arkansas for Medical Sciences, Little Rock, Arkansas

The author has disclosed no conflicts of interest.

result in agglutination of cells from the father's siblings, parents, or even extended family members. This finding led to the recognition that sera of previously pregnant women might be used as reagents for identifying specific polymorphic components expressed on human cells and to the discovery of the HLA protein components.[6] It was subsequently determined that HLA antigens act as protein receptacles for the presentation of self-antigens and foreign antigens in immune system recognition. This antigen presentation allows activation of immunity in the case of potential pathogens, or lack of activation and toleration in the case of self-antigens.

HLA Terminology

The first serum identified in the study of HLA was initially called "serum Hu1." The serum was shared with other researchers who were able reproduce the results. Researchers identified other sera that appeared to recognize unique subsets of related individual cells, but not others, and not on the same cells recognized by serum Hu1, and so forth. After a number of apparently unique sera were found, a first international workshop was organized by Bernard Amos and convened in 1964 to discuss and compare the findings. By the third workshop in 1967, the consensus was to change the name of Hu1 to A1, thus establishing the HLA nomenclature. Each new serum would be assigned a new "workshop" designation (eg, Aw3), until it was clearly identified as a unique serum, when it would lose the "w" designation. For example, Aw3 would become A3. Through the massive efforts of many individuals, a panel of HLA sera was identified and cataloged, thereby providing a manner for developing standardized typing procedures.[7]

HLA is the human subset of the MHC proteins, which are present in one form or another on the cell surfaces of essentially all animals and even of some more primitive creatures. MHC/HLA genes in contiguous grouping on one chromosome are termed a *haplotype*. Each individual normally possesses two haplotypes, one associated with each chromosome, and each representing the alleles of the HLA genes on their respective chromosomes. The antigen-presenting components of the HLA locus are divided into two major groupings, Class I and Class II. The major antigen-presenting compo-

nents of Class I are the *A, B,* and *C* gene loci, and the major antigen-presenting components of Class II are the *DR, DQ,* and *DP* gene loci. Within the overall HLA locus is a Class III locus with genes for proteins that do not present antigens but are involved with immune function (Fig 56-1). Class I MHC is composed of a protein chain (with $\alpha 1$, $\alpha 2$, and $\alpha 3$ domains) that associates in a noncovalent fashion with $\beta 2$ microglobulin on the surface of cells [Fig 56-2(A)]. Class II MHC is composed of α and β subunit chains, each with two domains ($\alpha 1$ and $\alpha 2$, and $\beta 1$ and $\beta 2$, respectively), which are expressed together on the cell surface, providing a three-dimensional conformation very similar to that of the Class I MHC [Fig 56-2(B)]. Class I HLA presents *endogenous* antigens to CD8 T lymphocytes and is found expressed on most cells within the body, except most notably for red cells. Class II HLA is found expressed on specific subsets of white cells, which are defined as "professional" antigen-presenting cells (APCs), and presents *exogenous* antigens to CD4 T lymphocytes. B lymphocytes and monocytes are two of the more common cells in the blood that act as APCs and express Class II HLA. Polymorphisms exist within the HLA genes, most of which result in specific amino acid substitutions.

Serologic, "Low-Resolution" HLA Typing

After sufficient sera were identified for standardization, in 1964 Paul Terasaki developed a technique for HLA typing, which has been termed CDC (complement-dependent cytotoxicity) HLA typing.[8] Each of the individual wells of a microtiter tray is coated with an individual typing serum. Lymphocytes from the person to be typed are isolated, and a small number are placed into each well. Rabbit serum complement proteins are added to each well, and the reaction is incubated for about half an hour. Cells remaining intact exclude a dye in the reaction mixture, considered a negative reaction. For cells with the HLA type to which the serum contains antibodies, the corresponding antibodies bind to the cell-surface HLA proteins. With the addition and fixation of complement, holes develop in the cell membrane, making these cells unable to exclude the dye, and thus producing a

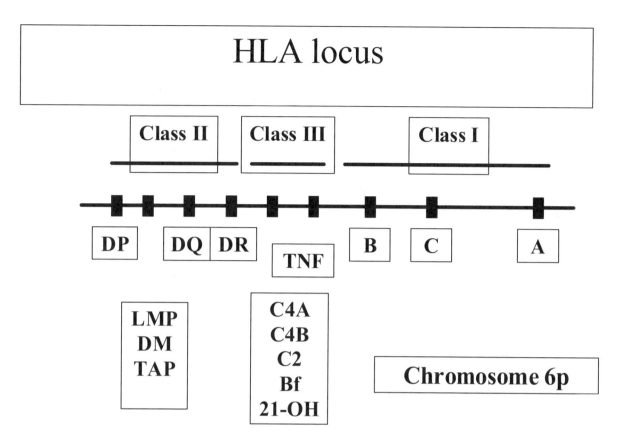

Figure 56-1. HLA gene locus on chromosome 6p. The HLA gene locus contains three major regions, two of which have genes to encode antigen-presenting proteins: Class I (*A, B,* and *C*) and Class II (*DR, DQ,* and *DP*). The third region, Class III, is for nonantigen-presenting proteins, which for the most part are involved with immune system function. Genes for proteins involved with the formation and assembly of HLA proteins are found in the Class II region (*LMP, DM,* and *TAP*).

positive reaction. Reactions are scored as in Table 56-1. Wells recorded as 6 or 8 are considered to be "true" reactions for routine typing purposes.

This well-established approach to HLA typing has been in common use for nearly 45 years. An experienced technologist can produce a result within an hour after lymphocytes have been isolated, making this a valuable technique for use in organ transplantation or cell and tissue identity testing, where time may be a critical factor.

Before the development of HLA typing, only transplantation of an "identical-twin" donor kidney could be performed successfully.[9] With the advent of the HLA-typing approach, related, nontwin, apparently HLA-identical donors could be identified, resulting in successful kidney transplantation for a larger population.

As with solid organs, an identical twin could also donate marrow to a twin sibling without complications. With the inception of the HLA-typing technique, related, nonidentical twin siblings could be identified as apparent HLA-identical matches. Although many of these transplants were successful, these HLA-matched donor marrow transplants sometimes resulted in complications such as failure to engraft, graft rejection, or graft-vs-host disease (GVHD).

Attempts to use HLA-matched unrelated donors by this low-resolution HLA-typing approach resulted in unacceptable rates of GVHD, indicating that higher-resolution typing results might be needed for better patient outcomes. Indeed, in the author's experience using umbilical cord blood as a source of unrelated donor stem cells, HLA typing

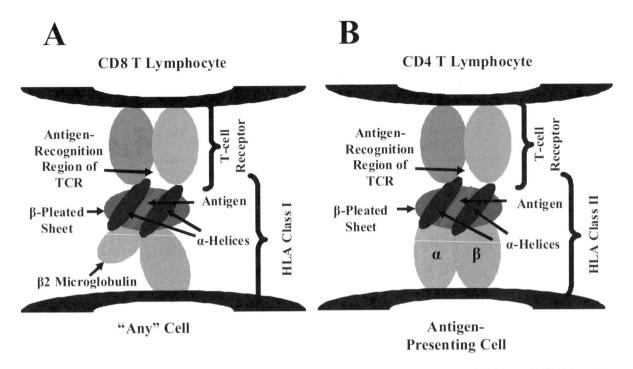

Figure 56-2. Part A represents Class I HLA-presenting antigen to T-cell receptor (TCR) on CD8 T lymphocyte. Antigen (red) is presented between two α-helices on a β-pleated sheet (in the three-dimensional conformation of HLA) to a TCR. Part B represents Class II HLA-presenting antigen to TCR on CD4 T lymphocyte. Antigen (red) is presented between two α-helices, one contributed by the α chain and one contributed by the β chain, on a β-pleated sheet also composed of part α chain and part β chain. Cognate interaction occurs between the TCR and HLA α-helices, allowing for initial attraction of HLA and TCR, and this allows subsequent antigen recognition (or not) by the TCR antigen-binding region. Most of the polymorphisms are found around the α-helices.

by serology indicated that at least 75% of units were 5 out of 6 (5/6) or 6 out of 6 (6/6) HLA-A, B, and DR matches. When they were subsequently typed by molecular techniques, only 30% of the units were found to be 5/6, 50% were 4/6, and 13% were 3/6 A, B, and DR matches. Therefore, it was apparent that polymorphisms of HLA were present that could not be distinguished by serologic typing techniques and that higher-resolution HLA typing was required to allow successful matched-unrelated-donor transplantation, especially with adult marrow or apheresis stem cell donors.[10]

HLA Typing by DNA Analysis Techniques

As the complexity of the polymorphisms of HLA have become better understood, relevant HLA components in hematopoietic progenitor cell transplantation have been found to include the *A, B, C, DRB1, DRB3, DRB4, DRB5,* and *DQB* gene loci, and possibly also *DQA, DPA,* and *DPB.* There are ~600 *A* genes currently identified, ~1000 *B* genes, >300 *C* genes, ~600 *DRB1* genes, >30 *DQA* genes, ~90 *DQB* genes, >20 *DPA* genes, ~130 *DPB*

Table 56-1. Reaction Scoring for CDC HLA Typing

Score	1	2	4	6	8
Percentage of cells reactive	≤10	11 to 20	21 to 50	51 to 80	>80

genes, and >70 *DRB3, DRB4,* and *DRB5* genes,[11] making many thousands of combinations possible. Typically, the common and well-documented alleles are used for potential patient-donor selection.[11]

Traditional molecular biologic techniques, such as Southern blotting, have limited use for determining an individual's HLA type. With the advent of the polymerase chain reaction (PCR) for amplifying small amounts of DNA, analyzing specific gene segments became easier. Most of the diversity of HLA Class I is located in exons 2 and 3, which make up the 1 and 2 domains, respectively, with each contributing to the two α-helices and β-pleated sheet structure in the three-dimensional structure. Class II DRB has most of its diversity in the 1 domain, encoded by its exon 2. Therefore, primer sets could be designed to amplify the diversity regions found in exons 2 and 3 of the various HLA genes. Specific identification based on the detected differences could be used as a basis for higher-resolution typing. With this concept in mind, three major approaches have been developed: 1) single-strand oligonucleotide (SSO) specificity-probe binding, 2) sequence-specific primer (SSP) PCR priming, and 3) sequence-based technology (SBT).

Medium-to-High-Resolution HLA Typing by SSO

The basic premise for the SSO approach is that the entire or most relevant portions of exons 2 and 3 can be amplified using primers for each major gene locus (*A, B, C, DR, and DQ*). Oligonucleotide probes with specific sequences unique to each individual HLA type can then be hybridized to the PCR product, with subsequent detection, allowing the HLA type to be identified. One platform, Luminex (Luminex Corp, Austin, TX), can be used to perform this analysis in a convenient manner. The Luminex device is a small bench-top fluorescence cytometer specifically designed to analyze 100 beads simultaneously, each with a slightly different inherent color. Each bead can have a probe attached, and the extent of binding to the probe can be quantified by the extent of fluorescence associated with the PCR product binding to the specific probe. The pattern of probe binding, as determined by which beads display the Streptavidin-fluores-cent-tag-associated fluorescence, can then be used to determine which HLA type is present.

Overall, this procedure is relatively quick, amenable to batching large numbers of samples while minimizing direct technologist time required for performing each of the steps of the assay. It gives much better HLA-type resolution than serologic testing.

High-Resolution HLA Typing by SSP PCR Technique

SSP PCR takes advantage of the fact that the 3′ terminal base of a primer must hybridize to the target DNA for Taq polymerase to initiate the DNA polymerization reaction. Therefore, single nucleotide differences between HLA alleles can be used to distinguish between the alleles (Figs 56-3 and 56-4). If the 3′ terminal base of the primer can bind, then a PCR product can be produced; if it cannot bind, then no product results (Fig 56-5). The DNA concentration is determined by absorption spectrometry at A260. At least 25×10^6 cells are typically required to extract sufficient DNA, a possible problem when attempting to HLA-type a leukopenic patient. Primer sets come prealiquoted into the wells of a 96-well tray (UniTray, Invitrogen, Carlsbad, CA). An 8-μL volume of "master mix," with added genomic DNA, is added to each well to facilitate the amplification reaction.

After the amplification reaction on the thermocycler, an aliquot is removed from each well and analyzed by agarose gel electrophoresis. Typically, a photograph of the gel is obtained and positive wells are identified. Because more than 400 amplification reactions are set up for each DNA typing, problems may arise. The pattern of SSP amplification products is analyzed to determine the likely alleles that are present. Two common and well-documented alleles are expected to be distinguished. When this is not the case, the specimen should be reanalyzed, preferably with an alternative technique.

From the point that a blood specimen is available, obtaining the complete HLA typing results by SSP may take 6 to 8 hours. SSP requires more hands-on labor for the technologist than the SSO technique, but typically a higher-resolution result is obtained. Because of the number of gels that need

```
      10    20    30    40    50    60
    1 GAT GAG GAG TTC TAC GTG GAC CTG GAG AGG AAG GAG ACT GCC TGG CGG TGG CCT GAG TTC AGC
    a CTA CTC C                   GAG TTC AGC

    2 --- --- C-- --- --- --- --- --- --- --- --- --- --- --- --- --- --- --- --- --- ---
    3 --- --- C-- --- --- --- --- --- -A- --- --- --- --- --- --- --- --- --- --- --- ---
    4 --- --- C-- --- --- --- --- --- --- G-- --- --- --- --- --- --- --- --- --- --- ---
    b CTA CTC G                   GAG TTC AGC

    5 --C --- --- --- --T --- --- --- --- --- --- --- -T- --- AA- -T- --- CT- --- CA-
    6 --C --- --- --- --T --- --- --- --- --- --- --- -T- --- -A- -T- --- CT- --- C--
    c CTA CTC C                   CTG TTC AGC

    7 --C --- C-- --- --- --- -G- --- --- --- --- --- -T- --- T-T -T- --- TT C-- --A
    8 --- --- C-- --- --- --- -G- --- --- --- --- --- -T- --- T-T -T- --- TT C-- --A
    9 --C --- C-- --- --- --- -G- --- --- --- --- --- -T- --- T-T -T- --- TT C-- --A
    d CTA CTC G                   TT TTC AGC
```

Figure 56-3. HLA DNA sequences demonstrating single-nucleotide substitutions in closely related alleles, which can be used to produce sequence-specific primer (SSP) pairs. The prototypical sequence is listed as number 1. Related alleles are listed as 2 through 9. Single-nucleotide changes that can act for SSP are noted in the vertical boxes. Primer sets exploiting these single-nucleotide differences are labeled a, b, c, and d and indicated in the horizontal boxes.

to be electrophoresed, the SSP technique is not good for batching a large number of specimens.

HLA Typing by Sequence-Based Technology

Sequencing the HLA genes could be expected to be the ideal way of obtaining an accurate HLA type. Although this is basically true, some issues should be considered. Perhaps the foremost issue is the cost of the 16-channel sequencer, which may exceed US$175,000. The sequencer is a high-resolution capillary electrophoresis unit capable of detecting four different fluorescence signals in each capillary unit, which allows simultaneous detection

of the four DNA bases of a DNA sequence for each capillary tube. Up to a thousand bases may be resolved, so that the entire exon 2 or exon 3 can be sequenced for analysis. Primers for each gene locus are used in separate amplification reactions to amplify the entire exon of each locus. Two aliquots of each are transferred to two new reaction wells for chain-terminating sequencing-amplification reactions of each DNA strand.

Dideoxynucleotides, which are conjugated with a different fluorescent dye for each base, are used to allow detection of all four bases in the same capillary electrophoresis tube. Both strands of each initial amplified product are sequenced. Therefore, for high-resolution HLA typing, initial A, B, C, DR,

Primer Set	HLA DNA Sequence								
	1	2	3	4	5	6	7	8	9
a	X								
b		X	X	X					
c					X	X			
d							X	X	X

Figure 56-4. Patterns of detection of the primer sets denoted in Fig 56-3 with the specific HLA DNA sequences in Fig 56-3. Primer set *a* can uniquely identify sequence 1. In this example, primer set *b* can amplify sequences 2, 3, and 4 but cannot distinguish between them. Likewise for *c* and 5 and 6, and *d* and 7, 8, and 9, respectively.

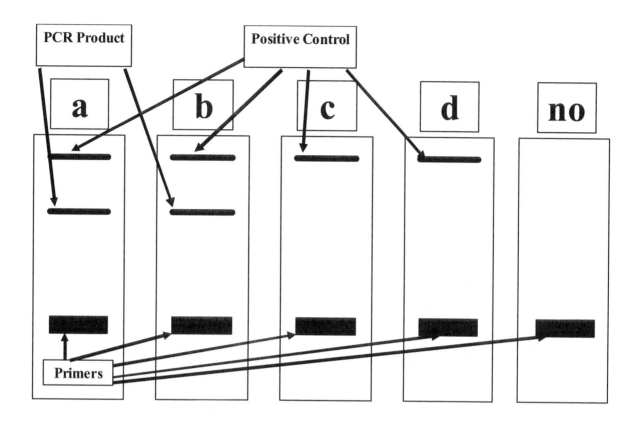

Figure 56-5. Representation of an electropherogram with the polymerase chain reaction (PCR) primer sets from Figs 56-3 and 56-4. Lanes *a, b, c,* and *d* denote the primer set used. The lane labeled *no* is the no-DNA-added control well for detecting contamination in the reaction. Each reaction is designed to have a separate internal positive control to verify that amplifiable DNA is present in the sample. In this example, the amplification reaction has resulted in the detection of product in lanes *a* and *b*. Based on Figs 56-3 and 56-4, primer sets *a* and *b* are expected to identify DNA sequences 1, and 2, and 3, respectively.

and DQ exon 2 amplification reactions are required, and typically additional reactions are required for A, B, and C, so that, minimally, eight individual amplification reactions are performed. For the sequencing reaction, each sample is split in two, which allows sequencing of both DNA strands, so that the final number of specimens to be analyzed by the sequencer is 16. A 16-channel sequencer contains 16 capillary electrophoresis units, each with a four-channel fluorescence detector, which allows one blood sample to be analyzed for all the HLA genes simultaneously. Sequence analysis software permits relatively easy interpretation of the results.

Depending on various factors, obtaining the HLA-typing results may take 4 to 8 hours. Because both alleles are being amplified in the same reac-

tion, and being sequenced simultaneously, ambiguities may arise. Various methods may be used to resolve these ambiguities, including use of additional specific primer sets for amplifying and sequencing subsegments of an exon or nontranslated DNA regions of the genes. Alternatively, a different technique can be used for clarification of an ambiguous result.

Comparisons of DNA Typing Techniques

The SSO, SSP, and SBT techniques can all provide high-resolution results 50% to 75%, 70% to 75%, and 75% to 80% of the time (as reported by the manufacturers), respectively (see Table 56-2). SBT

Table 56-2. Comparison of DNA Typing Techniques

Characteristic	SSO	SSP	SBT
Frequency of achieving high-resolution typing results	50%-75%	70%-75%	75%-80%, but >90% with additional primer sets and sequencing reactions
Procedure time	4 hrs	6-8 hrs	4-8 hrs
Technologist hands-on time	Low	High	Moderate
Batching	Easy	Amplification reactions, but numerous electro-phoreseis runs per sample	Amplification and sequencing reactions, single gel run per sample
Sample needed	Blood or buccal swab	5 mL blood; more if neutropenic	Blood or buccal swab
DNA needed	<1 µg	25 µg	<1 µg
Detection method	Fluorescence plate reader (eg, Luminex*)	Agarose gel electrophoresis	Sequencing gel (capillary electrophoresis)
Capital outlay	High	Low	High

*Luminex Corp, Austin, TX.
SSO = single-strand oligonucleotide; SSP = sequence-specific primer; SBT = sequence-based technology.

may provide unambiguous results more than 90% of the time through the use of additional primer sets and sequencing reactions. Although supply costs for each method are similar, differences arise when considering the amount of technologist time and dedicated equipment required. Manufacturers are sometimes willing to bundle the devices in reagent lease programs, which can make SSO and SBT techniques more accessible to a smaller laboratory. SSP requires more technologist time and effort to complete the assay and is also the least amenable to batching specimens, whereas the SSO technique readily allows batching a significant number of specimens. The SBT technique is limited by the time required to determine each complete HLA type (16 individual sequence reactions in a 16-channel analyzer) for each sample run through the sequencer, perhaps four to six samples in an 8-hour period. The amount of initial genomic DNA needed may be considerably different for the different techniques, with SSO and SBT requiring <1 µg of genomic DNA each, and SSP, approximately 25 µg. SSO and SBT can readily use genomic DNA isolated from buccal cell swabs, whereas SSP requires at least 5 mL of blood to obtain approximately 25 × 10^6 white cells, with much more blood required from a patient with significant leukopenia.

Overall, a significant number of HLA types for which the high-resolution typing cannot be performed exist for each molecular HLA typing technique, and these vary among the techniques. Therefore, using two or more techniques in combination (including serologic typing) may be best to obtain the most reliable HLA-typing results.

HLA Typing as an Identity Test

HLA typing and matching allow cellular therapy products from both related and unrelated donors to be successfully administered to patients with a variety of serious conditions. The high-resolution molecular techniques available today can provide greater confidence that the donor and recipient are more closely matched than could the earlier serologic methods, resulting in less risk of graft rejection or severe GVHD. In addition to donor selection, HLA typing can play an important role in confirming the identity or source of the cellular therapy product, for example, from cells that are shipped for infusion or when considering autologous therapy of stored material. The uniqueness of each HLA phenotype at the molecular level makes this an ideal characteristic for determining whether a discrepancy exists. If a sample were taken from the stored product or from the prospective donor at the time of actual donation and reassessed for HLA type, even by low-resolution technique, the results would indicate any inconsistency before infusion of the material into the patient. The chance of multiple HLA antigens from two different, unrelated individuals being identical at the molecular level is extremely remote, considering the polymorphic nature of the HLA system. Therefore, whenever possible, a confirmation of the HLA type of the donor should be performed before the donated product is cleared for patient administration.

References/Resources

1. Marsh SGE, Parham P, Barber L. The HLA factsbook. San Diego, CA: Academic Press, 2000.
2. Little CC, Tyzzer EE. Further studies on the inheritance of susceptibility to a transplantable tumor in Japanese waltzing mice. J Med Res 1916;33:393.
3. Snell GD, Smith P, Gabrielson F. Analysis of the histocompatibility-2 locus in the mouse. J Natl Cancer Inst 1953;14:457-80.
4. Landsteiner K. The specificity of serologic reactions. Boston: Harvard University Press, 1945.
5. Medawar PB. The behavior and fate of skin autografts and skin homografts in rabbits. J Anat 1944;78:176-99.
6. Dausset J. Iso-leuco-anticorps. Acta Haematol 1959;20:156.
7. Terasaki PI, ed. History of HLA: Ten recollections. Los Angeles: University of California Los Angeles Tissue Typing Laboratory, 1990.
8. Terasaki PI, Mandell M, Vandewater J, Edgington TS. Human blood lymphocyte cytotoxicity reactions with allogenic antisera. Ann N Y Acad Sci 1964;120:322-34.
9. Murray G, Holden R. Transplantation of kidneys, experimentally and in human cases. Am J Surg 1954;87:508-15.
10. Charron D. HLA: Genetic diversity of HLA: Functional and medical implications. Paris, France: EDK, 1997.
11. Cano P, Klitz W, Mack SJ, et al. Common and well-documented HLA alleles. Hum Immunol 2007;68:392-417.

Appendix 56-1. Selected Internet Resources on the HLA System and HLA Typing

Organization	URL
American Society of Histocompatibility and Immunogenetics (ASHI)	http://www.ashi-hla.org
National Marrow Donor Program (NMDP)	http://www.marrow.org
United Network for Organ Sharing (UNOS)	http://www.unos.org
Complete Human MHC Sequence, Wellcome Trust Sanger Institute	http://www.sanger.ac.uk/HGP/Chr6/MHC.shtml
HistoCheck (Institute for Transfusion Medicine, Hanover Medical School, Hanover, Germany)	http://www.histocheck.org
IMGT/HLA Database	http://www.ebi.ac.uk/imgt/hla
Abbott Molecular (Abbott Laboratories)	http://international.abbottmolecular.com/Transplantation_1600.aspx
Applied Biosystems	http://www.appliedbiosystems.com/?abhomepage=na
Biotest	http://www.biotestusa.com
Genome Diagnostics BV	http://www.gendx.com/index.php?option=com_content&task=view&id=48&Itemid=69
GTI Diagnostics	http://www.gtidiagnostics.com/products/transplantation/
Innogenetics	http://www.innogenetics.com/transplantation.html
Invitrogen	http://www.invitrogen.com/
Luminex	http://www.luminexcorp.com/
One Lambda	http://www.onelambda.com/
Promega Corporation	http://www.promega.com/Default.asp
Qiagen	http://www1.qiagen.com/Search/Search.aspx?SearchTerm=HLA
Tepnel Life Sciences	http://www.tepnel.com/

Method 56-1. Serologic HLA Typing by Complement-Dependent Cytotoxicity

Description

HLA Class I (CD8+) lymphocytes are isolated from a diluted buffy coat prepared from whole blood maintained in acid (or anticoagulant)-citrate-dextrose (ACD) solution using Dynabeads HLA Cell Prep (Invitrogen Dynal, Oslo, Norway). The rosetted cells are removed from the cell suspension with the aid of a rare-earth magnet, stained with carboxyfluorescein diacetic acid (CFDA), suspended in enriched cell culture medium, and incubated on commercially prepared antisera trays. Rabbit complement is added, causing cell lysis where an antigen-antibody complex occurred and subsequent leakage of CFDA out of the cell. Ethidium bromide (EB) is added and taken up by the lysed cells. The reactions are read on an inverted fluorescent microscope and recorded, and a phenotype is assigned.

Time for Procedure

Approximately 1 hour.

Summary of Procedure

1. Prepare the buffy coat.
2. Isolate and stain HLA Class I lymphocytes.
3. Perform complement-dependent lysis and analyze.

Equipment

1. Multifuge centrifuge or equivalent.
2. Vacuum apparatus.
3. Rotator.
4. Magnetic separation device.
5. 100-μL MLA pipette (VistaLab Technologies, Mt Kisco, NY).
6. 1-μL single-channel cell-dispensing pipette.
7. Illuminated light box.
8. 5-μL multichannel pipette for complement.
9. 2-μL multichannel pipette for EB.
10. 21-C incubator.

Supplies and Reagents

1. 10-mL polypropylene screw-cap tubes.
2. Phosphate-buffered saline (PBS): pH 7.2 to 7.6, plain and with 6% sodium citrate.
3. Dynabeads HLA Cell Prep I.
4. CFDA working solution.
5. RPMI with 5% fetal calf serum.
6. EB working solution.
7. Commercially prepared HLA-ABC typing trays.
8. Commercially prepared HLA-ABC rabbit complement.

Procedure

1. Prepare the buffy coat.
   a. Centrifuge the blood sample and remove the upper 80% of plasma with the vacuum apparatus. Transfer the remaining 20% of plasma, buffy coat, and upper layer of red cells to a 10-mL polypropylene screw-cap tube. Total volume should be 1 to 2 mL.
   b. Add 5 mL of PBS with 6% sodium citrate to the tube, cap tube, and mix well by gentle inversion. Cool in an ice bath for 8 to 10 minutes.
2. Isolate and stain HLA Class I lymphocytes.
   a. Resuspend the Dynabeads HLA Cell Prep I product by gently swirling. Add 100 μL of well-mixed cell suspension to the cooled buffy coat/PBS mixture. Cap tube and place on the rotator for 5 minutes at 2 to 8 C.
   b. Remove the tube from the rotator, remove the cap, and position the tube on the magnet for 3 minutes. Do not bump or disturb the specimen.
   c. Without moving the tube from the magnet, remove the supernatant with the vacuum. Pull the tube from the magnet immediately after removing the supernatant.

d. Wash the isolated cells with PBS and resuspend in 200 µL of freshly prepared CFDA working solution. Replace the cap. Incubate the tube vertically for 15 minutes at 37 C.

e. Remove the tube from the incubator, wash the cells twice with cold PBS/sodium citrate solution, and resuspend cells in 200 µL of RPMI with 5% heat-inactivated fetal-calf serum.

f. Isolated, CFDA-labeled cells must be kept in the dark at 2 to 8 C and plated within 4 hours.

3. Perform complement-dependent lysis and analyze.

a. With the light box turned on, dispense 1 µL of well-mixed cell suspension into each well of the appropriate ABC trays with a single-channel cell-dispensing pipette.

b. Incubate the cells and sera in the 21 C incubator for 30 minutes, and dispense 5 µL of cold complement into each well.

c. Pipette 2 µL of EB working solution into each well, and incubate trays for 30 minutes in the incubator at 21 C.

d. Read trays under fluorescence using the 10× objective.

e. Score and record reactions in each well on the worksheet by using the American Society for Histocompatibility and Immunogenetics (ASHI) standards method of estimating the percentage of cell death. Record results according to the scale in Table 56-1-1.

Anticipated Results

1. A negative reaction (1 or 2) will contain mostly viable cells, which will retain CFDA, exclude EB, and fluoresce bright green.

2. Positive reactions (4, 6, or 8) will contain mostly nonviable cells, which will leak CFDA, absorb EB, and fluoresce reddish orange. The Dynal beads will be visible and appear black or rusty in color.

Notes

1. The discussion of a specific manufacturer's reagents, kits, or equipment is not meant to be an endorsement of the manufacturer or the manufacturer's products. Several manufacturers may have products that perform comparably. The protocols supplied should be used as guides, which can be modified as needed, depending on the specific reagents, kits, and equipment used.

2. One filled 7- or 10-mL ACD tube of blood is kept at room temperature and tested within 72 hours of collection. A sample that is clotted, refrigerated, or frozen is not acceptable.

3. Patients/donors must have a minimum lymphocyte count of 1×10^6/mL.

4. Quality control:

a. Each antisera tray contains a positive control. The purpose of this control is to verify that all reagents and procedures required to produce a complement-dependent lymphocytotoxic reaction are present. EB staining affinity is verified each day of use through the positive control staining characteristics.

Table 56-1-1. ASHI Scale for Recording Reactions in HLA Typing

Score	Interpretation	% Dead Cells
1	Negative	0-10
2	Doubtful negative	11-20
4	Weak positive	21-50
6	Positive	51-80
8	Strong positive	81-100
0	Unreadable	—

b. The negative control on an antisera tray is used to demonstrate viability of the lymphocytes in the absence of HLA antibodies and to determine the degree of background contamination. CFDA staining affinity is verified each day of use through the negative control staining characteristics.

Troubleshooting

1. Fluorescent intensity is too low or too high: Increase or decrease the concentration of CFDA (green) or EB (red).
2. Low viability of cells on typing trays: May be caused by abnormal cell damage. If tray is unreadable because of excessive cytolysis, submission of a new sample will be necessary, or HLA Class I SSP-PCR molecular typing may be performed.
3. Weak reactivity:
   a. Ensure that antiserum is present in all wells when thawing trays and that complement is added and thoroughly mixed with cells.
   b. Increase the incubation time.
   c. Ensure that cell suspension is at the proper concentration. Antigen excess caused by an excessive number of cells can cause false-negative or weak reactions.
   d. The complement lot may have weak lability.
   e. There may be a specific antigen problem.
   f. Typing trays may be approaching expiration.

g. Cytotoxicity negative, absorption positive (CYNAP) phenomenon may be present. CYNAP occurs when anti-HLA antibody is absorbed by the lymphocytes, but the cells are not lysed, resulting in false-negative reactions. SSP-PCR molecular typing is recommended in suspected CYNAP cases in which a homozygous result is obtained at the HLA-A, -B, and/or -Cw locus to verify that a second antigen was not missed.
4. Antisera, on trays, that turn bright yellow when thawed have been exposed to CO_2 and must be discarded.
5. The pretest viability of the cell suspension is critical for accurate scoring. Any damage to the cell membrane will allow vital dye to "leak" into the cell and cause false-positive reactions. Proper positive and negative controls can aid the technologist in assessing the extent of this damage.

References/Resources

1. Dynabeads HLA Cell Prep I package insert. Oslo, Norway: Invitrogen Dynal, 2008.
2. Sections I.A5.1 - I.A5.7. In: Phelan DL, Micleelson EM, Noreen HS, et al, eds. ASHI laboratory manual. 3rd ed. Lenexa, KS: American Society of Histocompatibility and Immunogenetics, 1993.
3. Sections I.A.5 and I.C.1. In: Land GA, Strothman RM, eds. ASHI laboratory manual. 4th ed. Lenexa, KS: American Society of Histocompatibility and Immunogenetics, 2001.
4. Hurley CK. DNA-based typing of HLA for transplantation. In: Leffell MS, Donnenberg AD, Rose NR, eds. Handbook of human immunology. Boca Raton, FL: CRC Press, 1997.

Method 56-2. Performing Medium-to-High-Resolution HLA DNA Typing by SSO Luminex Technique

Description

DNA is purified from human leukocytes by any acceptable method. The DNA sample to be used for a polymerase chain reaction (PCR) assay should be resuspended in sterile water or in 10 mM Tris-HCl (pH 8.0-9.0), at an optimal concentration of 20 ng/L with the A260/A280 ratio of 1.65 to 1.80. LAB-Type (One Lambda, Canoga Park, CA) applies Luminex (Luminex Corp, Austin, TX) technology to the reverse single-strand oligonucleotide (SSO) DNA typing method. Target DNA is PCR-amplified using a group-specific primer. The PCR product is biotinylated, which allows it to be detected using R-phycoerythrin-conjugated streptavidin (SAPE). The PCR product is denatured and allowed to rehybridize to complementary DNA probes conjugated to fluorescently coded microspheres. For this procedure, a flow analyzer, the LABScan 100 (Luminex), identifies the fluorescence intensity of PE (phycoerythrin) on each microsphere. The assignment of the HLA typing is based on the reaction pattern compared to patterns associated with published HLA gene sequences.

Time for Procedure

1. DNA isolation: 30-60 minutes.
2. Amplification setup: 15-30 minutes.
3. Thermocycler amplification: ~110 minutes.
4. Preparing and allowing SSO bead hybridization: ~30 minutes.
5. Completing analysis and report generation: ~30 minutes (depends on the number of specimens being analyzed).
6. Total: ~4 hours.

Summary of Procedure

1. Amplify DNA.
2. Hybridize amplified DNA to SSO beads.
3. Label and analyze.

Equipment

1. LABScan 100 flow analyzer.
2. Luminex XY Platform (optional accessory for automated 96-sample reading on the LABScan 100 flow analyzer).
3. Centrifuge:
   a. Rotor for 1.5-mL microfuge tube (14,000 to 18,000 *g*).
   b. Swing bucket rotor for 96-well microplate (1000 to 1300 *g*).
4. Vortex mixer with adjustable speed.
5. Thermocycler equipped with a heated lid and with adjustable ramp speed (equivalent to 9600 ramp speed).
6. Pipettors and pipette tips.

Supplies and Reagents

1. 96-well, thin-walled PCR tray, or tubes, and holder that can withstand 1000 to 1300 *g* in a centrifuge.
   Caution: PCR plate must have tight contact with the heating block.
2. Tray seals.
3. 1.5-mL microfuge tubes.
4. 96-well, 250-μL V-bottom, white polystyrene microplate with a nontreated surface.
5. Microspheres with DNA probes specific for HLA alleles covalently attached.
6. Hybridization reaction buffers to facilitate the binding of target DNA to the probe.
7. R-phycoerythrin-conjugated streptavidin (SAPE) solution.
8. SAPE buffer for diluting stock SAPE solution.
9. HLA loci-specific primer mixes.
10. D-mix (contains deoxynucleotide triphosphates and other ingredients necessary for PCR).
11. Denaturation buffer.
12. Neutralization buffer.
13. Hybridization buffer.

14. Wash buffer.
15. Deionized water.
16. 70% ethanol.
17. 20% chlorine bleach.
18. Sheath fluid.
19. Recombinant Taq polymerase.

Procedure

A. *Amplify DNA*

1. Adjust the concentration of genomic DNA to 20 ng/µL using sterile water.
2. Pipette 2 µL of DNA (at 20 ng/µL) into the bottom of a tube (for a final volume of 20 µL per PCR reaction).
3. Mix the appropriate volume of D-mix and primers. Vortex for 15 seconds.
4. Add Taq polymerase immediately before use. Thoroughly vortex.
5. Aliquot 18 µL of amplification mixture into each well containing DNA.
   Caution: To prevent cross contamination, avoid touching the prealiquoted DNA at the bottom.
6. Seal with a PCR seal, making sure it is pressed tightly against the rim of each well.
7. Place the PCR tray containing the PCR cocktail into the freezer at –20 C until ready for amplification.
8. Place the tray in the thermocycler and start the run.
9. At the completion of thermocycling, the DNA is ready for denaturation and hybridization. The amplified DNA tray can be stored at 4 C for 5 days or at –80 C to –20 C for up to 1 month.

B. *Hybridize Amplified DNA to SSO Beads*

1. Denaturation/neutralization:
   a. Transfer 5 µL of each amplified DNA sample into a well of a clean 96-well plate.
   b. Add 2.5 µL denaturation buffer. Mix thoroughly and incubate at room temperature for 10 minutes.
   c. Add 5 µL neutralization buffer with pipette, and mix thoroughly. Note the color change to clear or pale yellow.
   d. Place the PCR plate with neutralized PCR product in an ice bath.
2. Hybridization:
   a. Combine appropriate volumes of bead mixture and hybridization buffer to prepare a hybridization mixture, and add to each well.
   b. Cover the tray with a tray seal and vortex thoroughly at low speed.
   c. Place the PCR tray in the thermocycler at 60 C. Close and tighten the lid. Incubate for 15 minutes.
   d. Remove PCR tray from the thermocycler, place in the tray holder, and remove the tray seal.
   e. Quickly add 100 µL wash buffer to each well. Cover the tray with a clean tray seal. Centrifuge the tray for 5 minutes at 1000 to 1300 *g*. Flick tray upside down into sink to remove wash buffer. Repeat twice.

C. *Label and Analyze*

1. Labeling:
   a. Add 50 µL of 1× SAPE solution to each well. Cover the tray with a tray seal and vortex thoroughly at low speed. Remove the tray from the base and place the tray in the 60-C thermocycler. Close and tighten lid. Incubate for 5 minutes.
   b. Wash tray and transfer to V-bottom microplate.
   c. Keep tray in the dark and at 4 C until placed in the LABScan 100 for reading.
   d. For best results, read samples as soon as possible. Prolonged storage of samples (more than 4 hours) may result in loss of signal.
   e. Store samples overnight at 4 C in the dark with a tray seal if they cannot be read immediately. Be sure to thoroughly mix the samples immediately before reading.
2. Data acquisition and analysis:
   a. Run the samples according to the LABScan 100 manufacturer's instructions.

b. Analyze the data using the appropriate software.

Quality Control

1. Before each assay, two calibrators and two controls are run. These must fall within the expected range before proceeding with testing.

2. Each bead set contains control beads. For the assay to be valid, the positive and negative control beads must adhere to the manufacturer's cutoff values.

Notes

1. A list of resolution limitations is provided for each lot of the LABType SSO Typing Test to aid in interpretation of the reaction pattern and assignment of HLA typing.

2. Samples should not be resuspended in solutions containing chelating agents, such as EDTA, above 0.5 mM in concentration.

3. When compared to SSP, SSO has more ambiguities because the probes used in SSO can interrogate sample DNA at only one region per test, and SSP can interrogate sample DNA at two regions per test.

4. DNA samples may be used immediately after isolation or stored at 6 C or below for extended periods of time (up to 1 year) with minimal adverse effects on results.

Limitations of the Procedure

1. The LABType SSO system combines an HLA locus-specific DNA amplification process and DNA-DNA hybridization process. The procedure, as well as the equipment calibration described in this product, must be strictly followed.

2. DNA amplification is a dynamic process that requires highly controlled conditions to obtain PCR products that are specific to a target segment of HLA gene(s). The procedure provided for the DNA amplification process must be strictly followed. In particular, because sample DNA quantity and quality can significantly affect the amplification reaction, a standardized DNA extraction procedure and spectrophotometric measurement of DNA quantity and quality are strongly recommended.

3. The DNA-DNA hybridization-based assay is a very temperature-sensitive process. Strict adherence to the temperatures and incubation times described in this procedure is critical for obtaining optimal results.

4. LABType SSO microspheres are light sensitive and must be protected from light as much as possible. Avoid freezing and thawing to ensure maximum shelf life.

5. Because of the complexity of the HLA allelic definitions, a certified HLA technician or specialist should review and interpret the data and assign the HLA typing.

References/Resources

1. LABType SSO Typing Tests product insert. Canoga Park, CA: One Lambda.
2. Luminex 200 System user manual. Austin, TX: Luminex.
3. Luminex IS software manual for version 2.3. Austin, TX: Luminex.

Method 56-3. High-Resolution HLA Typing by SSP-PCR

Description

High resolution typing of *HLA-A, -B, -Cw, -DR,* and *-DQ* gene products is obtained through testing of amplified genomic DNA using SSP-PCR Uni-Trays (Invitrogen Dynal, Oslo, Norway). This method is based on sequence-specific primer (SSP) amplification of all Class I and Class II alleles with a known sequence as described by the World Health Organization Nomenclature Committee for Factors of the HLA System. The procedure involves mixing a commercially prepared polymerase chain reaction (PCR) buffer with a human genomic DNA sample and Taq polymerase, dispensing the mixture into the UniTray, then thermocycling for amplification of specific DNA products. After thermocycling is complete, the amplified PCR products are loaded into a 2% agarose gel for electrophoresis. After electrophoresis, the gel is photographed and interpreted using the Dynal UniTray computer software and worksheet.

Time for Procedure

Approximately 6 to 8 hours from the time a blood specimen is received.

Summary of Procedure

1. Amplify DNA.
2. Analyze PCR products by agarose gel electrophoresis.

Equipment

1. Adjustable pipettes and tips.
2. Repeater pipette and 50-µL-capacity tips.
3. Eight-channel pipette and tips.
4. Aluminum heat-equalizing block.
5. Thermocycler.

Supplies and Reagents

1. 0.75× Tris-borate-EDTA (TBE) buffer
2. Dynal DNA molecular weight markers.
3. Dynal DNA grade agarose.
4. Ethidium bromide (10 mg/mL).
5. Dynal UniTray PCR tray(s) containing 5 µL/well of primer solution overlaid with paraffin oil.
6. Prealiquoted PCR buffer containing deoxynucleotide triphosphates and gel loading buffer.
7. PCR sealing film.
8. Taq polymerase: 5 units/µL.
9. DNA-grade water.

Procedure

1. Amplify DNA.
   a. Perform DNA isolation according to institutional procedure. DNA at a concentration of 50-125 µg/mL is preferred; however, DNA at a lower concentration may be used, provided that electrophoretic bands are discernible and a phenotype assignment is possible.
   b. Turn on the thermocycler, and input the appropriate information according to the laboratory standard operating procedure (SOP) and manufacturer's directions. When the thermocycler sample block has reached 96 C, the instrument is ready for use.
   c. Remove the tray(s), PCR buffer aliquot(s), and Taq from the −20 C freezer.
   d. Add appropriate amounts of Taq and water to an aliquot of PCR buffer. Vortex briefly.
   e. Remove 8 µL from the preceding mixture and add to the last well containing primer mixes on the tray. This well is the contamination (negative) control and contains no genomic DNA.
   f. Add an appropriate volume of vortexed DNA sample to the remaining buffer mixture, and vortex again briefly.
   g. Using a repeater pipette, dispense 8 µL of the master mix into each of the remaining wells. Note that after sample addition, the

primer mixture, below the paraffin oil, will turn from yellow to pink.

h. Firmly press the PCR sealing film onto the tray to attain complete adherence, and place the tray(s) in a freezer at –20 C. If more trays are to be set up, prepared trays may be stored in a freezer at –20 C for up to 72 hours before proceeding to postamplification steps.

i. Place the tray in the thermocycler and start the run. It will take approximately 1 hour and 50 minutes for the thermocycler to complete the program.

2. Analyze PCR products.

a. Analyze the PCR products by agarose gel electrophoresis according to the appropriate procedure.

b. Photograph the gel according to laboratory SOP.

Interpretation of Results

Analyzing the results of PCR amplification involves many factors. The following criteria can be used to interpret and verify results:

1. Compare the photodocumentation of PCR results with the standards in the example shown in Fig 56-3-1.

a. Lane 1 and Lane 8 are molecular size markers.

b. Lane 2 demonstrates a reaction grade of 8. This reaction exhibits a strong positive specificity band and a strong to weak internal control band.

c. Lane 3 demonstrates a reaction grade of 6. This reaction exhibits a specificity band where the signal strength is approximately 20% less than that of an 8 and a strong to weak internal control band.

d. Lane 4 demonstrates a reaction grade of 4. This reaction exhibits a specificity band where the signal strength is approximately 50% less than that of an 8 and a strong to weak internal control.

e. Lane 5 demonstrates a reaction grade of 2. This reaction exhibits a specificity band where the signal strength is approximately 80% less than an 8 and a strong to weak internal control band.

f. Lane 6 demonstrates a reaction grade of 1. This reaction exhibits no specificity band and a strong to moderate internal control band.

g. Lane 7 demonstrates a reaction grade of 0. This reaction exhibits no specificity band or internal control band present. This represents a reaction failure. (This lane may also be the no-DNA-added control, which must be negative for the assay to be valid.)

2. Enter the positive reactions into the computer software. Based on the pattern of specificity bands for the various primer mixes, alleles or groups of alleles can be determined. To assign an allele, all of the primer mixes that amplify that allele should have a specific PCR product.

Notes

1. Acid (or anticoagulant)-citrate-dextrose is the preferred anticoagulant for isolating DNA, but EDTA may also be used. Do *not* use heparinized blood for DNA isolation because heparin may inhibit DNA amplification.

2. False-negative reactions can be caused by inefficient amplification, poor DNA quality, uneven placement of the plate in the block, temperature variations across the wells of the thermocycler, loss of electrophoretically sepa-

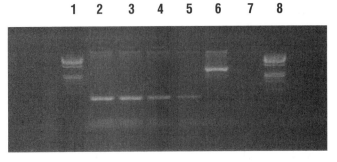

Figure 56-3-1. Standards for interpreting PCR results.

rated PCR product caused by uneven agarose gel, or inadequate thermocycler calibration.

3. A complete HLA Class I and Class II typing using the Dynal UniTray is primarily used for typing unrelated donors and recipients. Other instances where this method would be used include, but are not limited to, the following:

a. Verification of a homozygous serologic result obtained at a locus or loci.

b. Verification of a suspected serologically typed antigen of low frequency, of which appropriate antisera are limited or unavailable.

c. Supplementation of an incomplete serologic type caused by insufficient lymphocyte count, poor cell quality, or poor serologic reactions.

d. Verification of a previously obtained serologic type.

Quality Control

1. The negative control well contains pairs of contamination primers that detect amplicons produced by specific amplifications as well as genomic DNA. If the negative buffer/Taq mixture was added as directed, any band in this lane is evidence of contamination, and the results of the test are invalid. The exception to this outcome would be a primer dimer band of <80 base pairs, which occurs rarely.

2. Every lane of the gel should show a control band, except for the negative control well. If a well does not exhibit a control band or a specificity band, the test reaction failed.

3. Invitrogen Dynal prepares allele updates approximately every 3 months. The allele updates add new alleles and their reaction patterns to the current lot(s) of primer kits. The updates are downloaded from the Invitrogen Dynal Web site and added to the UniMatch software program. Updated interpretation tables are also available on the Web site and are printed with each allele update.

Reference/Resource

1. SSP UniTray instructions. Oslo, Norway: Invitrogen Dynal.

A P P E N D I C E S

◆

Appendix 1. Global Cellular Therapy Regulatory Bodies and Organizations

International Regulatory Resources

- International Conference on Harmonisation of Technical Requirements for Registration of Pharmaceuticals for Human Use (ICH) http://www.ich.org
- Specific Guidelines on Stem Cells, Cell Therapy and Xenotransplantation in the World http://www.biosafety.be/GT/Regulatory/Guidelines_CTXeno.html

European Union

- European Medicines Agency http://www.emea.europa.eu/
- European Commission: Advanced Therapies http://ec.europa.eu/enterprise/pharmaceuticals/advtherapies/index.htm
- Joint Accreditation Committee EBMT-ISCT Europe (JACIE) http://www.jacie.org/

Australia

- Australia—Therapeutic Goods Administration, Blood and Tissues http://www.tga.gov.au/bt/index.htm

Canada

- Health Canada Biologics and Genetic Therapies Directorate http://www.hc-sc.gc.ca/ahc-asc/branch-dirgen/hpfb-dgpsa/bgtd-dpbtg/index_e.html
- Canadian Standards Association: Cells, Tissues, and Organs for Transplantation and Assisted Reproduction: General Requirements http://www.csa-intl.org/onlinestore/GetCatalogDrillDown.asp?Parent=3244

China

- State Food and Drug Administration of China http://eng.sfda.gov.cn/eng/

India

- Ministry of Health and Family Welfare (India) http://mohfw.nic.in/
- Indian Council of Medical Research Proposed Guidelines for Stem Cell Research and Therapy (2006) http://www.icmr.nic.in/stem_cell/stem_cell_guidelines.pdf

Japan

- Ministry of Health, Labour, and Welfare http://www.mhlw.go.jp/english/
- National Institute of Health Sciences Division of Cellular and Gene Therapy Products http://www.nihs.go.jp/cgtp/cgtp/home.html

Korea

- Korea Food and Drug Administration http://www.kfda.go.kr/
- Korea Food and Drug Administration Biologics Evaluation Department http://www.kfda.go.kr/open_content/english/index.html

New Zealand

- Ministry of Health http://www.moh.govt.nz
- Bioethics Council Focus on Stem Cells http://www.bioethics.org.nz/about-bioethics/issues-in-focus/stem-cells/

Singapore

- Health Sciences Authority http://www.hsa.gov.sg
- Singapore Position on Stem Cells and Human Tissue Research http://www.bioethics-singapore.org/old/resources/articles.html

Taiwan

- Bureau of Food and Drug Analysis
  http://www.nlfd.gov.tw/english/index.aspx

USP

- <1046> Cell and Tissue-Based Products
  http://www.usp.org
- <1043> Ancillary Materials for Cell, Gene, and
  Tissue-Engineered Therapy Products
  http://www.usp.org

Appendix 2. Glossary

Note: Definitions of words and phrases not credited with a reference number were taken from the Merriam-Webster OnLine Dictionary.[1]

351 products: HCT/Ps that do not meet the FDA's criteria that are set forth in 21 CFR 1271 for regulation solely under Section 361 of the PHS Act. These products are regulated as drugs, devices, or biological products.

361 products: HCT/Ps that are regulated solely under Section 361 of the PHS Act (for preventing the introduction, transmission, and spread of communicable disease) and 21 CFR 1271. To be regulated solely under Section 361 of the PHS Act and 21 CFR 1271, an HCT/P must meet all four criteria:
- Be minimally manipulated.
- Be intended for homologous use only.
- Not be combined with a device or drug, except for sterilizing, preserving, or storage agents that do not raise clinical safety concerns.
- Not have a systemic effect or depend on the metabolic activity of living cells for its primary function, unless the HCT/P is for a) autologous use, b) allogeneic use in a first-degree or second-degree blood relative, or c) reproductive use.

7-aminoactinomycin D (7-AAD): A fluorescent chemical compound with a strong affinity for DNA. It is used as a fluorescent marker for DNA in fluorescence microscopy and flow cytometry. It intercalates in double-stranded DNA, with a high affinity for guanosine-and-cytidine-rich regions.

Adverse reaction: A noxious or unintended response to any cellular therapy product for which there is a reasonable possibility that the response may have been caused by the product.

Adoptive immunotherapy: The use of a cellular therapy to produce an immune reaction against malignant or virally infected cells.

Agreement: A contract, order, or understanding between two or more parties, such as between a facility and one of its customers.

Agreement review: Systematic activities carried out by a supplier before finalizing an agreement to ensure that requirements are adequately defined, free from ambiguity, documented, and achievable.

Aldehyde dehydrogenase (ALDH): An enzyme with activity in a number of functional areas of cell metabolism and expressed at high levels in human hematopoietic progenitor cells.

Allogeneic donor: An individual from whom cellular therapy products are procured for transplantation to another. This individual may or may not be genetically related to the recipient.

Allograft: A graft or transplant from an allogeneic donor.

Allotolerance: The capacity of the body to endure or become less responsive to a cellular therapy product from an allogeneic donor.

Amplification: Massive replication of genetic material and especially of a gene or DNA sequence (as in a polymerase chain reaction).

Analyte: A substance or chemical constituent that is assayed.

Anaphylaxis: An acute and severe systemic type I hypersensitivity allergic reaction.

Ancillary materials: Materials that are used in the manufacture of cellular therapy products but do not remain in or are not intended to be part of the final product.

Apheresis: Removal of a blood component, either cellular or noncellular in composition, from circulation.

Apoptosis: Programmed cell death.

Aseptic methods: Methods designed to minimize the risk of microbial contamination to a product, reagent, specimen, or person in a laboratory or clinical care setting.

Aseptic processing facility: A building or a segregated segment of a building that contains rooms in which air supply, materials, and equipment are regulated to control microbial and particle contamination.

Aseptic technique: Practices that are designed to reduce and prevent the risk of contamination of products, reagents, or specimens during processing and handling of cellular materials.

Assessment: A systematic and independent examination to determine whether quality activities comply with planned activities and whether these activities are implemented effectively and are suitable to achieve objectives.

Autograft: A cellular therapy product that originates from the same (autologous) individual who will receive it.

Autologous use: The implantation, transplantation, infusion, or transfer of a human cellular or tissue-based product back into the individual from whom the cells or tissue that compose the product were removed.

Basal medium: An unsupplemented medium that promotes the growth of many types of microorganisms or cells that do not require special nutrient supplements.

Biologic mother: The female who is the source of the fertilized ovum.

Bioluminescence: Production and emission of light by a living organism.

Birth mother: The female who carries the fetus to term.

Bolus: A single, relatively large quantity of a substance, such as a dose of a drug.

Boolean: A complete mathematical system for logical operations, which is named after George Boole, who first defined an algebraic system of logic in the mid-19th century. Boolean logic has many applications in electronics, computer hardware, and software and is the basis of digital electronics.

Buffy coat: The portion of an HPC product that contains the nucleated cells after the bulk of the plasma and mature red cells have been removed by sedimentation or centrifugation.

Burst-forming unit-erythroid (BFU-E): A primitive erythropoietic progenitor cell that in vitro forms daughter cells arranged in the form of a burst. It may contain more than 2 clusters.

Cadaveric donor: A deceased individual from whom cellular therapy products are procured.

Calibration: Periodic activity to check and maintain the accuracy of measurements against a known standard.

Cannula: A small tube for insertion into a body cavity or into a duct or vessel.

Cannulate: To insert a cannula.

CAPA (corrective and preventive action): A systematic approach that includes actions that are needed to correct, prevent the recurrence of, and eliminate the cause of a potentially nonconforming product and other quality problems.[2]

CD (cluster of differentiation): A nomenclature system for a group of cell surface markers.
- CD3: Cell surface marker for mature lymphocytes; a component of the T-cell receptor complex.
- CD4: Glycoprotein that is expressed on the surface of helper and regulatory T lymphocytes.
- CD8: Transmembrane glycoprotein that is predominantly expressed on cytotoxic T cells but is also found on natural killer (NK) cells.
- CD14: Membrane-associated glycoprotein that is found on the surface of monocytes and macrophages.
- CD34: Transmembrane glycoprotein that is constitutively expressed on endothelial cells and on HPCs.
- CD45: Tyrosine phosphatase, also known as the leukocyte common antigen (LCA). CD45 is present on all human cells of hematopoietic origin, except erythroid cells, platelets, and their precursor cells.

Cell bank: A homogeneous population of cells that are frozen at the same population-doubling level.
- Master cell bank (MCB): A culture of cells from the primary or accession cell bank. The cells are processed and frozen at the same time to ensure uniformity and stability and are used to prepare the working cell banks or clinical product.
- Working cell bank (WCB): A population of cells generated by culturing or expanding one or more vials of a master cell bank and used to produce the manufactured product (clinical lot).

Cellular therapy product: A somatic cell- or tissue-based product intended for administration to an allogeneic, syngeneic, or autologous recipient.

Cell washer: A machine that removes extraneous material from a cell suspension or cellular therapy preparation.

CMS certified: Having met the requirements of the Clinical Laboratory Improvement Amendments of 1988 through inspection by the Centers for Medicare and Medicaid Services (CMS), a deemed organization, or an exempt state agency.

Chemokine (chemotactic cytokine): One of a group of cytokines produced by various cells (eg, at sites of inflammation) that stimulate chemotaxis in white blood cells.

Chemotaxis: The orientation or movement of an organism or cell in relation to stimulating agents.

Chimerism: The presence of cells or tissues of different genetic composition than those of the host. Chimerism may occur as a result of an allogeneic HPC transplant.

Chromogenic: Pigment or color-producing.

CLIA [Clinical Laboratory Improvement Amendments (1988)]: Passed by the US Congress in 1988 to establish quality standards to ensure the accuracy, reliability, and timeliness of patient test results regardless of where the test is performed.

Clonogenic: See "colony-forming cell."

CMC (chemistry, manufacturing, and controls): Information included in an investigational new drug (IND) application that describes the composition, manufacture, and control of the cellular therapy product.

CMS (Centers for Medicare and Medicaid Services): US federal agency that administers Medicare and Medicaid.

Collection: See "recovery."

Colony-forming cell (CFC) or colony-forming unit (CFU): A cell that has the potential to proliferate and give rise to a colony of cells.

- Colony-forming unit—erythroid (CFU-E/CFC-E): A more differentiated erythroid precursor than BFU-E that forms only erythroid elements in culture.

- Colony-forming unit—granulocyte, erythroid, megakaryocyte, macrophage (CFU-GEMM/CFC-GEMM): Hematopoietic precursor cells that in vitro form colonies containing cells of the four lineages indicated.

- Colony-forming unit—granulocyte-macrophage (CFU-GM, GM-CFC, CFU-Mix): A precursor cell that in vitro forms cells of both granulocytic and macrophage morphology, which are capable of producing colonies that have 40 or more granulocyte-monocyte or -macrophage cells.

Colony-stimulating factors: See "growth factors."

Compendial methods: Analytical methods that are described in the USP National Formulary (USP-NF).[3] The FDA considers these to be established methods, not requiring validation if unmodified, but requiring verification under actual conditions of use.[4]

Competence or competency: The ability of an individual to perform a specific task according to procedures.

Compliance: See "conformance."

Complement: A multicomponent enzyme system that is involved in the lysis of cells.

Confluent culture: A cell culture in which all the cells are in contact and the entire surface of the culture vessel is covered.

Conformance: The fulfillment of requirements.

Consenter: An individual whose consent is obtained for cord blood collection activities. Examples of consenters are the birth mother, biologic mother, surrogate mother, and legal custodians.

Controlled environment: A manufacturing space in which air quality, proper garb, aseptic technique, and personnel movement are specified and monitored. Permissible levels of particulates in the air depend on the classification requirements of the space.

Controlled-rate freezing: A procedure that uses a device to control the temperature of a product during the freezing process.

Cord blood: The portion of the blood of a fetus or neonate that remains in the placenta or umbilical cord after delivery of the neonate and clamping of the umbilical cord.

Cord blood donor: The infant who is the source of collected cord blood.

Cord blood service: The facility that is involved in any of the following activities: collection, processing, and storage of cord blood products.

Cord blood unit: HPCs that are collected from a single cord blood, processed, and cryopreserved for subsequent use as a clinical transplantation product.

Corrective action: Action that is taken to eliminate the causes of an existing discrepancy or other undesirable situation to prevent its recurrence.[2]

Counterflow centrifugation (elutriation): A centrifuge separation method by which cells are separated owing to centrifugal forces, as well as to size and density, in a physiologic environment.

Critical equipment: A piece of equipment that can affect the quality of the facility's products or services.

Critical material: A reagent or supply item that can affect the quality of a facility's products or services and is used in the preparation of the cellular therapy product or service.

Critical tasks: Elements (such as materials, equipment, or tasks) that directly affect the quality of the product or service.

Cross-contamination: Transmission of infectious or contaminating agents among reagents, products, or supplies.

Cryopreservation: The process of low-temperature freezing and storage of cellular products, which preserves cells so that, after thawing, they retain a significant measure of their prefreeze viability and function.

Cryoprotectant: A solution or additive that, when combined with living cells, provides protection from damage otherwise induced by the freezing or thawing process.

Cytocentrifuge: A device that uses low-speed centrifugal force to separate and deposit a mono-layer of cells on a slide while maintaining cellular integrity.

Cytokine: A soluble substance that mediates signals among different cell populations or within the same cell population (eg, interleukin-l, interleukin-2).

Defined medium: Medium for which all of the ingredients are known.

Depletion: Ex-vivo removal of one or more cell populations from a cellular therapy preparation.

Design controls: The systems and procedures incorporated into the design and development process that ensure a new or changed cellular therapy product or service can be used safely and effectively while meeting the needs of the customer.

Design output: Documents, records, and evidence in any format that can be used to verify that design goals have been met.

Design qualification (DQ): The act of identifying and qualifiying the critical parameters and conditions of the product.

Design validation: All efforts to ensure that the design will meet customer needs for the intended use of the product, given the expected variations in components, materials, manufacturing processes, personnel, and environmental conditions.

Design verification: The confirmation and provision of objective evidence that functional and operational requirements have been fulfilled. Verification is the process of checking at each stage whether the design output is safe and effective and conforms to defined user needs and intended uses.

Deviation: A departure from the appropriate policies, processes, or procedures. Deviations can be planned or unplanned. Not all deviations result in an unacceptable product or result.

Differential: A technical term used to describe a white cell count by providing the relative proportion of cells of different morphology in the total cell number.

Differentiation: The process by which a less-specialized cell divides and creates more-specialized daughter cells.

Dimethyl sulfoxide (DMSO): A cryoprotectant; a chemical that is used together with other agents to protect cells from injury that otherwise would be sustained during the cryopreservation or thawing processes.

DNAse: An enzyme that digests DNA.

Disposition: The final status or control of a cellular therapy product in a given facility. For records, disposition occurs at the end of their retention period.

Distribution: The act of transferring a cellular therapy product that meets applicable product release criteria from 1) a location of processing or manufacture or 2) an intermediate separate holding location for storage to either 1) the location of medical administration or 2) another intermediate separate holding location for temporary storage before infusion.

Document: Written or electronically generated information. Examples of documents include quality manuals, policies, processes, procedures, labels, and forms.

Donor: A living or deceased person who is the source of a cellular therapy product.

Donor eligibility: Suitability to donate a cellular therapy product after evaluation for risk factors and clinical evidence of relevant communicable disease agents or diseases for the purpose of preventing the introduction, transmission, and spread of communicable disease.

Elutriation: See "counterflow centrifugation."

Engraftment: In-vivo proliferation and differentiation of infused autologous or allogeneic HPCs, which is typically assessed by the recovery of circulating blood cell counts.
- Neutrophil engraftment: An absolute neutrophil count of ≥500 cells/μL on three consecutive days. The first of the three days is designated as the day of neutrophil engraftment.[5]
- Platelet engraftment: A transfusion-independent platelet count of ≥20,000 platelets/μL on the first of three consecutive days.[5]

Enrichment: The removal of contaminating cell populations to increase the concentration of the cell type of interest in a cell suspension or culture system.

Environmental monitoring: Policies, processes, and procedures for monitoring any of the following: temperature, humidity, particulates, and microbial contamination in a specific area.

Establish: To define, document, and implement.

Eutectic: Relating to a solution's freezing (or melting) point.

Exception: An action or condition that is not part of normal operations.

Excipient: An inert substance that is used as a diluent or vehicle in a drug or biologic substance.

Expiration date: The date beyond which there are no data to ensure that the product will perform safely or effectively and beyond which the manufacturer states that the product should not be used.

Ex-utero cord blood collection: Collection of cord blood after the placenta is expelled from the uterus.

Ex-vivo: Outside of a living body; denoting the removal of cells or tissues for manipulation, after which they are returned to the living body.

Ficoll-hypaque: A material that is used in density gradient media for separating cell populations that have different densities.

Final cellular therapy product: A cellular therapy product that is ready for issue or final distribution.

Firmware: A computer program that is embedded in a hardware device (as read-only memory).

Flow cytometry (cytofluorometry): A technique that uses the principles of light scattering, light excitation, and emission of fluorochrome molecules to generate specific multiparameter data from cells.

Forcing function: In interaction design, a behavior-shaping constraint; a means of preventing undesirable user input usually made by mistake.

Function: The special, normal, or proper physiologic activity of a cellular therapy product that can be qualitatively or quantitatively evaluated.

Glycophorin-A: A 131 amino acid protein that spans the membrane once and presents its amino-terminal end at the extracellular surface of the human red cell.

GCP (good clinical practice): A standard for the design, conduct, performance, monitoring, auditing, recording, analysis, and reporting of clinical trials that ensures that the data and reported results are credible and accurate and that the rights, integrity, and confidentiality of trial subjects are protected.

GLP (good laboratory practice): Scientifically sound practices for conducting nonclinical laboratory studies supporting research for marketing applications for products regulated by the FDA.[6]

GMP (good manufacturing practice): A set of scientifically sound methods, practices, or principles that are implemented and documented during product development and production to ensure the consistent manufacture of safe, pure, and potent products. cGMP refers to the most current good manufacturing practice.

GTP (good tissue practice): Requirements that govern the methods used in, and the facilities and controls used for, the manufacture of HCT/Ps. The requirements are intended to prevent the introduction, transmission, or spread of communicable diseases by HCT/Ps.

Graft: An implant or infusion of living cells or tissue.

Graft-vs-Host Disease: A common complication of allogeneic HPC transplantation in which functional immune cells in the transplanted HPC graft recognize the recipient as "foreign" and mount an immunologic attack.

Growth factors: Recombinant cytokines that promote the proliferation or differentiation of specific cell types or lineages.

Harvest: In the setting of marrow transplantation, usually describes the collection of marrow cells or peripheral blood stem cells to be used for transplantation. Also see "recovery."

Hemacytometer: A counting chamber that is used in the laboratory to determine the number of leukocytes or red cells in a blood sample.

Hematopoietic: Pertaining to the production of blood.

Hematopoietic progenitor cells (HPCs): Primitive pluripotent hematopoietic cells that are capable of self-renewal or differentiation as well as maturation into any of the hematopoietic lineages.

HPC and cellular product service: A facility that is involved in a) qualifying donors, b) performing one or more of the manufacturing steps for HPC products (including collection, processing, and storage), or 3) distributing these products.

Hemotoxicity: The destruction of red cells, the disruption of blood clotting, or organ degeneration and generalized tissue damage.

HEPA filter: A high-efficiency particulate air filter with a minimum 0.3-μm particle-retaining efficiency of 99.97%.

HEPES: A zwitterionic organic chemical buffering agent used in cell culture.

Histocompatibility: A state of immunologic similarity (or identity) that permits successful allogeneic transplantation. The best-known histocompatibility antigens are those of the major histocompatibility complex, termed "HLA" in humans.

Homologous use: The use of a cellular or tissue-based product for a normal function that is analogous to that of the cells or tissues being replaced or supplemented.

Human cells, tissues, and cellular and tissue-based products (HCT/Ps): Products that contain human cells or tissues or any cell or tissue-based component of such a product that is intended for implantation, transplantation, infusion, or transfer into a recipient.[7]

Hydroxyethyl starch: A chemical used for mobilization and separation of leukocytes as well as in some cryopreservation techniques.

Hypocalcemia: A condition characterized by low-serum calcium levels in the blood.

Hypotension: Abnormally low blood pressure.

Immunophenotype: The type of a cell as determined by immunologic methods, usually by the use of monoclonal antibodies that recognize cell surface antigens.

Impedance: That which restrains the flow an electric current, making it more difficult for the current to move through a circuit.

Incoming materials: Materials at the time of receipt into a facility.

Incompatibility, major: ABO incompatibility in which the recipient of a graft has antibodies against donor red cell antigens.

Incompatibility, minor: ABO or other red cell antigen incompatibility in which the donor of a graft (or transfusion) has antibodies against recipient red cells.

Indication for use: "A general description of the disease or condition the device will diagnose, treat, prevent, cure, or mitigate, including a description of the patient population for which the device is intended."[8]

In-utero cord blood collection: The collection of blood from the umbilical cord while the placenta is still in the uterus.

In vitro: Observable in an artificial environment.

In vivo: Within the living body.

Inner shipping container: A box, container, or bag that holds a labeled product during shipping inside an outer shipping container.

Inspect: To measure, examine, or test one or more characteristics of a product or service and compare the results with specific requirements.

Installation qualification (IQ): The act of ensuring that systems are installed in accordance with approved design, specifications, and regulatory codes and that the manufacturer's installation recommendations have been taken into consideration.

Intended use: "The objective intent of the persons legally responsible for the labeling of devices. The intent is determined by such persons' expressions or may be shown by the circumstances surrounding the distribution of the article."[9]

Intermediary facility: Any facility other than the original procurement (collection) service and transplant program that manipulates or performs any activity that relates to a cellular therapy product.

Intrathecal: Introduced into or occurring in the space under the arachnoid membrane, which covers the brain and spinal cord.

Investigator: An individual under whose immediate direction a clinical study is performed.

Issue: To release a final cellular therapy product for clinical use.

Issuing facility: The facility that issues the cellular therapy product for clinical use.

Kinetic: Pertaining to or producing motion.

Labeling: Information that is required or selected to accompany a product, which may include identification of the product, the product content, a description of processes performed, storage requirements, the expiration date, cautionary statements, and indications for use.

Laboratory director: A qualified individual who holds a relevant doctoral degree and who is responsible for all technical aspects of the cellular therapy product service.

Laminar flow: An airflow that is moving in a single direction and in parallel layers at a constant velocity from the beginning to the end of a straight-line vector.

Legal custodian: The person legally responsible for the donor until the donor reaches the age of majority.

Leukostasis: Increased blood viscosity and tendency to clot.

Life-cycle requirements: The stages and time span of a computer software program from initial planning of the program to retirement.

Linearity: The ability of a method to elicit results that are directly proportional to the quantity of the article contained in the sample being analyzed within a given range.

Limiting dilution analysis (LDA): A laboratory assay in which the examination of progressively lower concentrations of cells allows frequency of certain precursor cells (for example, cytotoxic T cells) to be determined.

Line clearance (product changeover): The activities involved in changing a work area and the associated equipment from the preparation of one product batch to another.

Lineage negative (Lin-) cells: Cells that lack all hematopoietic lineage cell markers.

Listmode: A correlated flow cytometry data file in which each event is listed sequentially, parameter by parameter. Listmode files may be edited or gated to include or exclude events.

Luciferin or luciferase reaction: An enzymatic reaction in which the enzyme luciferase, in the presence of ATP, catalyzes oxidation of the photoprotein luciferin, producing light.

Luminometer: A sensitive photometer that is used for measuring very low levels of light (such as produced in a luminescent process).

Maintain: To keep in the current state; to preserve or retain; to keep in a state of validity.

Manufacture: All the steps in the preparation and testing of a cellular therapy product, from donor evaluation and procurement to the final release of the product for administration.

Materials: Goods or supplies that are used to prepare the cellular therapy product or service.

Meconium: Dark green mucilaginous material in the intestine of the full-term fetus. This is the first type of feces passed by the newborn infant.

Medical director: A qualified licensed physician who has overall responsibility and authority for all medical aspects of the cellular therapy product service.

Methylcellulose: An organic chemical that is used to grow hematopoietic cells in vitro.

Microbial contamination: The presence of infectious organisms that render a cellular therapy product or preparation impure or harmful.

Minimal manipulation: The processing of cells and nonstructural tissues in a manner that does not alter the relevant biological characteristics of the cells or tissues.[7]

Mobilization (stem/progenitor cell): The recruitment of HPCs from the marrow into the blood.

Mole: The amount of a substance that contains as many atoms, molecules, ions, or other elementary units as the number of atoms in 0.012 kg of carbon 12.

Mollicutes: A group of bacteria that is distinguished by the absence of a cell wall. A few mollicutes cause diseases in humans (eg, certain species of mycoplasma, ureaplasma, and erysipelothrix).

Monoclonal antibody (MAb): A single type of antibody that is directed against a specific epitope (antigen or antigenic determinant) and is produced by a single clone of B cells or a single hybridoma cell line.

Mononuclear cells: Usually refers to blood and marrow cells other than granulocytes and erythrocytes.

Myeloablative therapy: Treatment of a patient with an agent (eg, chemotherapy or gamma irradiation) that causes marrow aplasia that is reversible only with administration and engraftment of HPCs.

Myeloproliferative disorders: Conditions that are characterized by the clonal proliferation of one or more hematopoietic cell lineages, predominantly in the marrow.

Necrosis: Traumatic cell death that results from acute cellular injury.

Nonconforming: A product or service that does not satisfy one or more specified requirements.

Nonconformity (nonconformance): A deficiency in a characteristic, product specification, process parameter, record, or procedure that renders the quality of a product unacceptable, indeterminate, or not in accordance with specified requirements.[2]

Nucleated cells: Any cells in a cellular therapy product other than mature red cells.

Operational qualification (OQ): ". . . The process of demonstrating that an instrument will function according to its operational specification in the selected environment."[10]

Organization: An institution, a part thereof, or an entity bridging several institutions that has its own functions and executive management.

Output: The product or service that results from the performance of a process or procedure.

Pancreatic islet cells: A cellular therapy product that consists of partially purified pancreatic islets of Langerhans. Insulin-producing beta cells within such islets make up the functional component of the product. This product is obtained from a living or cadaveric donor pancreas by one or more isolation and purification steps.

Patient-specific product: A product collected or prepared exclusively for a particular autologous or allogeneic recipient.

Peripheral blood stem cell (PBSC): A hematopoietic cell with multilineage potential obtained from peripheral blood rather than from marrow, usually from a mobilized allogeneic or autologous donor. PBSCs are commonly referred to as HPC-A (HPCs from apheresis).

Pluripotent: Capable of producing daughter cells of different lineages.

Policy: A documented general principle that guides present and future decisions.

Polymerase chain reaction (PCR): A procedure that amplifies a particular DNA sequence in multiple cycles of denaturation, renaturation, and DNA synthesis.

Potency: The therapeutic activity of a product as indicated by appropriate laboratory tests or adequately developed or controlled clinical data.

Precision: A measure of the degree of repeatability of a method under normal operation.

Preventive action: Action taken to eliminate the cause of a potential discrepancy or other undesirable situation to prevent such an occurrence.[2]

Preventive maintenance (PM): An orderly program of activities (eg, cleaning, adjustments, and checks) to prevent equipment failure.

Primagravida: A woman who is pregnant for the first time or has been pregnant one time.

Procedure: A description of how an activity is to be performed, ie, a standard operating procedure.

Process: A set of related tasks and activities that accomplish a goal, ie, which transforms input into output products and services.

Process control: Efforts to standardize and control processes to produce a predictable output.

Process qualification (PQ): Determination and documentation that processes operate consistently and reliably as required at the normal operating limits of critical parameters, especially when likely challenges are encountered.

Process simulation (media fill): The use of a microbiological growth medium in place of a product, and then the exposing of the medium to product contact surfaces of equipment, container closure systems, critical environments, and process manipulations to closely simulate the exposure that the product itself will undergo. The sealed containers filled with the medium are then incubated to detect microbial contamination.

Procurement: See "recovery."

Product: A tangible result of a process or procedure.

Proficiency testing: The structured evaluation of laboratory methods that assesses the suitability of the test system. Proficiency testing is performed to ensure the adequacy of analytical methods, procedures, and equipment and the competency of personnel.

Progenitor cell: An early descendant of a stem cell that can differentiate into one or more cell types but cannot renew itself.

Proliferation: The production of new cells from a given precursor.

Prophylaxis: Protective or preventive treatment.

Pulse oximetry: A noninvasive method for monitoring blood oxygenation.

Purge: To remove one or several undesirable cell populations from a cell suspension.

Purity: Freedom from microbial, chemical, and physical contamination.

Pyrogen: A substance that induces a febrile reaction.

Qualification (equipment): Verification that specified attributes required to accomplish the desired task have been met.

Quality: The characteristics of a product or service that affect its ability to meet requirements, including those defined during an agreement review. A measure of a product's or service's ability to satisfy the customer's stated or implied needs.[2]

Quality assurance: Confidence that the policies, processes, and procedures that influence the quality of the product and service are working as expected, both individually and collectively.

Quality control: The steps taken during the generation of a product or service to ensure that it meets requirements and is reproducible.[2]

Quality management: Accountability for the successful implementation of the quality system.[2]

Quality manual: A document that describes the facility's quality policies, objectives, practices, resources, and activities.

Quality system: The organizational structure, responsibilities, policies, processes, procedures, and resources established by executive management to achieve the quality policy.

Quality Unit: A group within an organization that is responsible for promoting quality in general practice.[2]

Quarantine: The storage of a cellular therapy product in a physically separate and clearly identified area, or the identification of a product through the use of procedures such as automated designation to prevent its improper release.

Raw materials: Supplies that indirectly or directly enter into the production of finished products.

Reagent: A substance that is used to perform an analytical or manufacturing procedure; also a substance that is used (eg, in detecting or measuring a component or preparing a product) because of its biological or chemical activity.

Record: Information that has been captured in writing or electronically that provides objective evidence of activities that have been performed or results that have been achieved, such as test records or audit results. Records do not exist until the activity has been performed.

Recovery: The act of obtaining a cellular therapy product from a donor by facility-approved methods, including apheresis, marrow harvest, cord blood procurement, and organ or tissue harvest.

Registry: An organization that maintains a database of cellular therapy donors or products and coordinates the acquisition of cellular therapy products for transplantation.

Regulation: Law that is promulgated by federal, state, or local authorities.

Related donor: An allogeneic donor who is a blood relative of the recipient.

Release: Removal of a product from quarantine or in-process status for distribution.

Release criteria: Predetermined specifications and limits for the safety, purity, potency, and identity of a biological product. Licensed biologics cannot be distributed unless they meet all release criteria.

Release testing: The testing of one or more characteristics of a cellular product that compares the results with specified requirements to establish whether the product meets the requirements for release.

Repeatability: A measure of precision in which results are achieved by a method when operating in the same assay run, or during a short interval under the same conditions.

Reproducibility: The ability to duplicate measurements over long periods by different laboratories

Risk: The combination of the probability of occurrence of harm and the severity of that harm.[2]

Risk assessment: A systematic process for organizing information to support a risk decision that is made within a risk management process. The process consists of the identification of hazards and the analysis and evaluation of the risks associated with exposure to those hazards.[2]

Risk management: The systematic application of quality management policies, procedures, and practices to the tasks of assessing, controlling, communicating, and reviewing risk.[2]

Sedimentation: The gradual settling of cells by gravity.

Sensitivity: The proportion of reference-test-positive (diseased) subjects who test positive according to the screening test.

Sepsis: A systemic inflammatory response owing to an infectious agent and accompanied by characteristic clinical and laboratory findings.

Service: Work or activities performed to fulfill the needs of a customer.

Shall: A term used to indicate a regulatory or accreditation requirement.

Shipping facility: A facility that is responsible for delivering a product in its custody to another location.

Somatic cell: Any cell within the developing or developed organism with the exception of germline (egg and sperm) cells.

Source material: Cells, tissue, or organs procured from a donor that have not been manipulated or processed.

Specified requirements: The expectations for products or services. Specified requirements may be defined by customers, regulatory agencies (such as the FDA), practice standards, or accrediting organizations.

Specificity: The proportion of reference-test-negative (healthy) subjects who test negative according to the screening test.

Sponsor: An individual, company, institution, or organization that takes responsibility for and initiates a clinical study.

Stability: The ability of a sample or product to maintain its quality characteristics and resist change or deterioration.

Standards: A set of specified requirements upon which a facility may base its criteria for the products, components, or services it provides.

Standard curve: A method of plotting assay data that is used to determine the concentration of a substance.

Statistical techniques: Established mathematical methods for collecting, analyzing, and presenting data.

Stem cell: The cell that is thought to be capable of producing all necessary components in a given tissue.

Sterility: Freedom from living microorganisms.

Streptavidin: A protein isolated from Streptomycetes avidinii that has a high affinity for biotin. It is used to detect biotin markers.

Streptozotocin: An agent that is used to induce a form of diabetes in experimental animals.

Summary of records: A condensed version of the required testing and screening records that contains the identity of the testing laboratory, the listing and interpretation of all required infectious disease tests, a listing of the documents reviewed as part of the relevant medical records, and the name of the person or establishment who is determining the suitability of the product for transplantation.

Supernatant: The fluid component of a culture system produced in part by the cells in suspension; also, the clear liquid from a cell suspension, the cellular portion of which is deposited at the bottom of a vessel by centrifugation, sedimentation, or precipitation.

Supplier: An organization or individual that provides a product or service.

Surrogate mother: The female who carries the fertilized ovum of another woman.

Syngeneic: Referring to genetically identical individuals (ie, identical twins); also called monozygotic.

Taq polymerase: A heat-stable DNA polymerase that is normally used in the polymerase chain reaction.

Test script: Test script in software testing is a set of instructions that will be performed to test that the system functions as expected. It is often written in programming language.

Thrombocytopenia: A persistent decrease in the number of blood platelets.

Tissue: Any aggregation of morphologically similar cells and associated intercellular matter that is intended for transfusion, transplantation, or other therapy.

Tissue culture: The propagation of cells and tissues in an artificial laboratory environment.

Total nucleated cells (TNCs): The total number of nucleated cells in a volume of a cellular therapy product.

Tolerance: The lack of an immune response to an antigen. See also "allotolerance."

Traceability: The degree to which the history of a process, product, or service can be followed by the review of documents.

Tracking: Following all steps of a process or procedure from beginning to end.

Transfer: The act of relocating a final cellular therapy product or its intermediate in-process precursors.

Transportation: The act of transferring a cellular therapy product (at any stage in manufacturing) within a facility or between facilities.

Trend: A movement of measurement data in a specific direction over time.

Tritiated thymidine: A DNA precursor to which tritium, a radioactive isotope of hydrogen (H3), is attached that is used to label proliferating cells in vitro.

Trypan blue: A dye that is absorbed by nonviable cells and excluded by viable cells.

Unidirectional flow: An airflow moving in a single direction, in a robust and uniform manner, and at a sufficient speed to reproducibly sweep particles away from the critical processing or testing area.

Validation: The confirmation by examination and provision of objective evidence that particular requirements can consistently be fulfilled. Validation of a process, or process validation, means establishing by objective evidence that a process consistently produces a result or product that meets its predetermined specifications.[5]

- Prospective validation: Validation that is conducted before the distribution of either a new product or a product made under a revised manufacturing process, where the revisions may affect the product's characteristics.
- Retrospective validation: Validation of a process for a product that is already in distribution on the basis of accumulated production, testing, and control data.

Validation protocol: A written plan that states how validation will be conducted, including test parameters, product characteristics, production equipment, and decisions about what constitutes acceptable test results.

Verification: The confirmation by examination and provision of objective evidence that specified requirements have been fulfilled.

Viability: Demonstrated capability of living; the ability (indicated either in vivo or in vitro) to perform physiologic functions.

Workflow: The planned physical movement of people, materials, or data that are associated with a process, or the planned temporal sequence of activities associated with a process.

Worst case: A set of conditions encompassing the upper and lower processing limits and circumstances, including those conditions within standard operating procedures, that pose the greatest chance of process or product failure when compared to ideal conditions.

Xenogeneic: Referring to a donor and recipient of a tissue or other graft who are of different species.

References/Resources

1. Merriam-Webster Online Dictionary (includes medical dictionary). Springfield, MA: Merriam-Webster, 2009. [Available at http://www.merriam-webster.com (accessed April 21, 2009).]
2. Food and Drug Administration. Glossary. In: Guidance for industry: Quality systems approach to pharmaceutical CGMP regulations. (September 2006) Rockville, MD: CDER, CBER, CVM, and ORA, 2006. [Available at http://www.fda.gov/cber/gdlns/qualsystem.htm#glos (accessed April 21, 2009).]
3. USP 31-NF 26. Rockville, MD: The United States Pharmacopeial Convention, 2008.
4. Code of federal regulations. Title 21, CFR Part 211.194(a)(2). Washington, DC: US Government Printing Office, 2009 (revised annually).
5. Food and Drug Administration. Definitions. In: Draft guidance for industry: Minimally manipulated, unrelated, allogeneic placental/umbilical cord blood intended for hematopoietic reconstitution in patients with hematological malignancies. (December 2006) Rockville, MD: CBER Office of Communication, Training, and Manufacturers Assistance, 2006. [Available at http://www.fda.gov/cber/gdlns/cordbld.htm#ix (accessed April 21, 2009).]
6. Code of federal regulations. Title 21, CFR Part 58. Washington, DC: US Government Printing Office, 2009 (revised annually).
7. Food and Drug Administration. Request for proposed standards for unrelated allogeneic peripheral and placental/umbilical cord blood hematopoietic stem/progenitor cell products; request for comments. Docket No. 97N-0497. (January 20, 1998) Fed Regist 1998;63:2985-8.
8. Code of federal regulations. Title 21, CFR Part 814.20(b)(3)(i). Washington, DC: US Government Printing Office, 2009 (revised annually).
9. Code of federal regulations. Title 21, CFR Part 801.4. Washington, DC: US Government Printing Office, 2009 (revised annually).
10. Bedson P, Sargent M. The development and application of guidance on equipment qualification of analytical instruments. Accreditation and Quality Assurance 1996; 1:265-74.

Index